Biology and Biomechanics of the Traumatized Synovial Joint: The Knee as a Model

American Academy of
Orthopaedic Surgeons
Symposium

Biology and Biomechanics of the Traumatized Synovial Joint: The Knee as a Model

Edited by
Gerald A.M. Finerman, MD
Professor and Acting Chief
Division of Orthopaedic Surgery
Dorothy and Leonard Straus Scholar
University of California at Los Angeles
Los Angeles, California

Frank R. Noyes, MD
Clinical Professor
Department of Orthopaedic Surgery
University of Cincinnati
Cincinnati, Ohio

with 202 illustrations

Workshop
Scottsdale, Arizona
November 1991

Supported by the
American Academy of Orthopaedic Surgeons

and the
National Institute of Arthritis and
Musculoskeletal and Skin Diseases

and the
American Orthopaedic Society
for Sports Medicine

American Academy of Orthopaedic Surgeons
6300 North River Road
Rosemont, IL 60018

Biology and Biomechanics of the Traumatized Synovial Joint: The Knee as a Model

Library of Congress Cataloging-in-Publication Data

Biology and biomechanics of the traumatized synovial joint: the knee as a model / edited by Gerald A.M. Finerman, Frank R. Noyes.
    "Workshop, Scottsdale, Arizona, November 1991, supported by the American Academy of Orthopaedic Surgeons, and the National Institute of Arthritis and Musculoskeletal and Skin Disease, and the American Orthopaedic Society for Sports Medicine."
    Includes bibliographical references and index.
    ISBN 0-89203-070-4 : $75.00
    1. Knee—Wounds and injuries—Treatment—Congresses.   2. Knee—Mechanical properties—Congresses.   I. Finerman, Gerald.   II. Noyes, Frank R.   III. American Academy of Orthopaedic Surgeons.   IV. National Institute of Arthritis and Musculoskeletal and Skin Diseases (U.S.)   V. American Orthopaedic Society for Sports Medicine.
    [DNLM: 1. Biomechanics—congresses.   2. Knee Injuries—rehabilitation—congresses.   3. Models, Biological—congresses.   4. Synovial Membrane—Physiopathology—congresses.   WE 870 B615 1991]
RD561.B56   1992
617.5′82044—dc20
DNLM/DLC   92-48242
for Library of Congress   CIP

Contributors

Allen F. Anderson, MD†
Director
The Lipscomb Clinic Foundation for
   Education and Research and
Lipscomb Sports Medicine Fellowship
St. Thomas Hospital
Nashville, Tennessee

Steven P. Arnoczky, DVM*†
Wade O. Brinker Endowed Professor of
   Surgery
Director, Laboratory for Comparative
   Orthopaedic Research
College of Veterinary Medicine
Michigan State University
East Lansing, Michigan

Gerard A. Ateshian, PhD†
Assistant Professor of Mechanical
   Engineering
Associate in Orthopaedic Research
Columbia University
New York, New York

Richard J. Beaver, MD, FRACS†
Clinical Fellow
Mount Sinai Hospital
Toronto, Ontario, Canada

Charles Beck, MD*†
Co-Director Orthopedic Biomechanics
   Institute
Co-Director Orthopedic Specialty Clinic
   Sports Medicine Fellowship
The Orthopedic Specialty Hospital
Salt Lake City, Utah

Thomas M. Best, MD, PhD†
Department of Biomedical Engineering
   and Orthopaedic Surgery
Duke University Medical Center
Durham, North Carolina

Bruce D. Beynnon, PhD†
Research Assistant Professor
Department of Orthopaedics
University of Vermont College of
   Medicine
Burlington, Vermont

Mark Bolander, MD*
Senior Associate Consultant and
   Associate Professor of Orthopaedic
   Surgery
Mayo Medical School
Rochester, Minnesota

Joseph A. Buckwalter, MD*†
Professor of Orthopaedic Surgery
University of Iowa
Iowa City, Iowa

Arnold I. Caplan, PhD
Director, Skeletal Research Center
Professor of Biology
Case Western Reserve University
Cleveland, Ohio

Dale M. Daniel, MD*†
Staff Surgeon
Kaiser Permanente Medical Group
San Diego, California

Kenneth E. DeHaven, MD*†
Professor of Orthopaedic Surgery
Department of Orthopaedics
University of Rochester Medical Center
Rochester, New York

Christopher H. Evans, PhD*†
Ferguson Laboratory for Orthopaedic
   Research
Department of Orthopaedic Surgery
University of Pittsburgh School of
   Medicine
Pittsburgh, Pennsylvania

Contributors

Gerald A.M. Finerman, MD*
Professor and Acting Chief
Division of Orthopaedic Surgery
Dorothy and Leonard Straus Scholar
University of California at Los Angeles
Los Angeles, California

Braden C. Fleming, MS†
McClure Musculoskeletal Research
  Center
Department of Orthopaedics &
  Rehabilitation
University of Vermont College of
  Medicine
Burlington, Vermont

Freddie H. Fu, MD*†
Blue Cross of Western Pennsylvania
  Professor of Orthopaedic Surgery
Vice Chairman/Clinical
Department of Orthopaedic Surgery
University of Pittsburgh
Pittsburgh, Pennsylvania

Marc T. Galloway, MD*†
Assistant Professor of Orthopaedic
  Surgery
Section Sports Medicine
Yale University School of Medicine
New Haven, Connecticut

William Garrett, Jr, MD, PhD*†
Associate Professor of Orthopaedic
  Surgery and Cell Biology
Duke University
Durham, North Carolina

Jan Gillquist, MD, PhD*†
Professor of Sports Medicine
University Hospital
Linkoping, Sweden

Victor M. Goldberg, MD*†
Professor and Chairman, Department of
  Orthopaedics
Case Western Reserve University
Cleveland, Ohio

Stephen L. Gordon, PhD*
Musculoskeletal Diseases Program
  Director
National Institute of Arthritis and
  Musculoskeletal and Skin Diseases
National Institutes of Health
Besthesda, Maryland

Tatsuhiko Goto, MD†
Orthopaedic Surgeon
Department of Orthopaedic Surgery
National Defense Medical College
Tokorozawa, Japan

J. David Grauer, MD*†
Assistant Clinical Professor of
  Orthopaedic Surgery
University of Colorado School of
  Medicine
Louisville, Colorado

Peter Grigg, PhD*†
Professor of Physiology
University of Massachusetts Medical
  School
Worcester, Massachusetts

Edward S. Grood, PhD*†
Director, Noyes-Giannestras
  Biomechanics Laboratories
Department of Aerospace Engineering
  and Engineering Mechanics
University of Cincinnati
Cincinnati, Ohio

Allan E. Gross, MD, FRCS (C)*†
A. J. Latner Professor and Chairman
Division of Orthopaedic Surgery
University of Toronto
Toronto, Ontario, Canada

Stephen E. Haynesworth, PhD†
Assistant Professor
Departments of Biology and Orthopaedics
Case Western Reserve University
Cleveland, Ohio

James G. Howe, MD†
McClure Musculoskeletal Research
  Center
Department of Orthopaedics &
  Rehabilitation
University of Vermont College of
  Medicine
Burlington, Vermont

Rik Huiskes, PhD*†
Professor of Musculoskeletal
  Biomechanics
Institute of Orthopaedics
University of Nijmegen
Nijmegen, The Netherlands

Robert J. Johnson, MD*†
Professor of Orthopaedic Surgery
Department of Orthopaedics &
  Rehabilitation
University of Vermont College of
  Medicine
Burlington, Vermont

David J. Kuester, MD†
Orthopaedic Associates of Manitowoc
Manitowoc, Wisconsin

William D. Lew, MS†
Research Fellow
University of Minnesota
Minneapolis, Minnesota

Jack L. Lewis, PhD*†
Professor of Orthopaedic Surgery and
  Mechanical Engineering
University of Minnesota
Minneapolis, Minnesota

Mohammed N. Mahomed, MD†
Intern
Toronto East General Hospital
Toronto, Ontario, Canada

Charles J. Malemud, PhD†
Professor of Medicine and Anatomy
Department of Medicine
Division of Rheumatic Diseases
Case Western Reserve University
Cleveland, Ohio

Joseph Mansour, PhD†
Department of Bioengineering and
  Aerospace
Case Western Reserve University
Cleveland, Ohio

Keith L. Markolf, PhD*†
Adjunct Professor
Department of Orthopaedic Surgery
University of California at Los Angeles
Los Angeles, California

Patrick J. McMahon, MD†
Orthopaedic Resident
Musculoskeletal Research Laboratories
Department of Orthopaedic Surgery
University of Pittsburgh
Pittsburgh, Pennsylvania

Roland W. Moskowitz, MD†
Professor, Department of Medicine
Division of Rheumatic Diseases
Case Western Reserve University
Cleveland, Ohio

Van C. Mow, PhD*†
Professor of Mechanical Engineering and
  Orthopaedic Bioengineering
Director, Orthopaedic Research
  Laboratory
Columbia University
New York, New York

James T. Ninomiya, MD, MS†
McClure Musculoskeletal Research
  Center
Department of Orthopaedics &
  Rehabilitation
University of Vermont College of
  Medicine
Burlington, Vermont

Frank R. Noyes, MD*†
Director, Cincinnati Sports Medicine
  Orthopaedic Center
Cincinnati, Ohio

Karen J. Ohland, MS†
Coordinator
Musculoskeletal Research Laboratories
Department of Orthopaedic Surgery
University of Pittsburgh
Pittsburgh, Pennsylvania

Lonnie E. Paulos, MD*†
The Orthopedic Specialty Hospital
Salt Lake City, Utah

Steven J. Pineda, MD†
Skeletal Research Center
Department of Biology and Orthopaedics
Case Western Reserve University
Cleveland, Ohio

John Pinkowski, MD*†
Assistant Clinical Instructor
Northeastern Ohio University College of
  Medicine
Akron, Ohio

Malcolm H. Pope, DMSc, PhD*†
McClure Professor of Musculoskeletal
  Research
Director of Orthopaedic Research
Department of Orthopaedics &
  Rehabilitation
University of Vermont College of
  Medicine
Burlington, Vermont

Christopher Rangger, MD†
University of Innsbruck
Department of Traumatology
Innsbruck, Austria

Anthony Ratcliffe, PhD†
Associate Professor, Orthopaedic
  Biochemistry
Head, Biochemistry Section, Orthopaedic
  Research Laboratory
Columbia University
New York, New York

Per A.F.H. Renström, MD, PhD*†
Professor
Department of Orthopaedics &
  Rehabilitation
University of Vermont College of
  Medicine
Burlington, Vermont

William G. Rodkey, DVM*†
Director, Research and Education
Steadman Sports Medicine Foundation
Vail, Colorado

Peter A. Simkin, MD*†
Professor of Medicine
Adjunct Professor of Orthopaedics
University of Washington
Seattle, Washington

J. Richard Steadman, MD†
Orthopaedic Surgeon
Steadman Hawkins Clinic
Vail, Colorado

Kevin R. Stone, MD†
Orthopaedic Surgeon
California Pacific Medical Center
San Francisco, California

Mary Lou Stone, RPT, BS†
Clinical Specialist II (Physical Therapy)
Kaiser Permanente Medical Group
San Diego, California

William O. Thompson, MD†
Orthopaedic Surgery Research Resident
Department of Orthopaedic Surgery
University of Pittsburgh
Pittsburgh, Pennsylvania

Shigeyuki Wakitani, MD†
Assistant Professor
Department of Orthopaedic Surgery
Osaka University Medical School
Osaka, Japan

Savio L-Y. Woo, PhD†*
Professor and Vice Chairman for
  Research
Musculoskeletal Research Laboratories
Department of Orthopaedic Surgery
University of Pittsburgh
Pittsburgh, Pennsylvania

---

* Workshop Participant
† Contributor to this volume

Contents

Contents

Preface

Injuries to the musculoskeletal system have a frequent and serious impact on the health and quality of life of those who are affected. In the population from 25 to 74 years of age, 46% of the population experienced knee pain, which was reported to be second in frequency of all musculoskeletal conditions, surpassed only by back or neck pain.[1] In this age range, almost one-third of all reported joint pain occurred in the knee. Knee joint related disorders, when combined represent the most frequent musculoskeletal disorder requiring surgery, with the next most frequent disorder being disk excision. In an assessment of the 30 most frequent operations performed (according to ICD codes), arthroscopy of the knee was the third most frequent, total knee replacement was fifth on the list, meniscectomy was seventh, repair of the knee ligaments was 14th and 15th, and excisions of other lesions of the knee was 27th.[1]

With the growing national interest in physical fitness and athletics, the diagnosis and treatment of sports-related injuries has become a major health concern. The majority of sports injuries occur to the lower extremity, with a large proportion of these involving the knee. As much as 77% of all confirmed knee ligament tears involve injury to the anterior cruciate ligament. These data vividly paint the high frequency of knee-related disorders, which span a wide variety of causative factors, including trauma, inflammatory causes, and poorly understood degenerative causes, and which span all age groups in both males and females. It is thus entirely appropriate that disorders of the knee joint was selected as the focus for this collaborative workshop effort among physicians, scientists, and scholars of the many scientific disciplines represented.

The workshop on the *Biology and Biomechanics of the Traumatized Synovial Joint: The Knee as a Model* is part of the continuing cooperative series between the American Academy of Orthopaedic Surgeons and the National Institute of Arthritis and Musculoskeletal and Skin Diseases of the National Institutes of Health, and has also been cosponsored by the American Orthopaedic Society for Sports Medicine. These workshops have gathered leading basic and clinical scientists from multidisciplinary backgrounds for important intellectual exchanges and development of state-of-the-art books in various areas of orthopaedics. The recommendations for future research serve to guide investigators towards projects that may resolve important scientific issues.

The workshop was held in Tucson, Arizona, November 16-19, 1991. The individual presentations were outstanding and stimulated spirited and intense discussions. The participants enjoyed the opportunity to present, defend, and debate investigative findings and research strategies. New ideas were generated, and the participants truly learned from each other given the diversity and multidisciplinary backgrounds of those who attended. Special thanks must be given to the efforts of each of the group leaders who had the responsibility of organizing their sections and leading and formulating the Overview and Future Research Directions sections.

Disorders of the knee joint, such as loss of a meniscus or chronic ligament deficiency, may frequently show the highest incidence of injury in the second and third decade of life. Yet the ramifications of these injuries, arthrosis of the knee joint, the attendant symptomatic state, and its occupational effects, are frequently manifest 10 to 20 years later. Because the options for successful treatment of advanced arthrosis are few and a salvage clinical situation is often present, clinicians have established a major effort to diagnose and treat knee joint related traumatic conditions, particularly of ligaments and menisci, at an early stage. Significant clinical and research advances have allowed arthroscopically-assisted anterior cruciate ligament reconstructions and meniscus repairs to be undertaken with relatively high success rates, as measured by patient outcome scales. Aggressive postoperative rehabilitation programs with early return of joint function have prevented or lessened disuse-related disorders and postoperative arthrofibrosis. This more aggressive approach to these common knee injuries has proven to be clinically effective. These early advances have now opened the door to address in a much more complete manner a host of other more complex knee disorders concerning which insufficient basic science information is currently available.

The clinician is faced with performing, in certain instances, surgical procedures that, although more successful than in the past, still carry a 20% to 30% failure rate. The reasons for this were debated at the workshop. What accounts for late stretching out of anterior cruciate and posterior cruciate reconstructions? What are the actual forces on cruciate ligament grafts and how should they be implanted in terms of initial tension and placement to optimize results? What are the biologic mechanisms that control ligament graft remodeling? How can these biologic mechanisms be controlled to enhance healing? When is it too late to perform an anterior cruciate reconstruction in a knee with arthrosis present? Will the ligament reconstruction decrease the rate of arthrosis? What are the articular cartilage biologic mechanisms for injury and repair and how does joint instability affect these mechanisms? Do ligament reconstructions need to "fine tune" joint kinematics to be successful or are the "check rein" effects of the ligament reconstruction in preventing gross displacement all that is required? How does the clinician truly replace the delicate function of the posterior cruciate ligament and posterolateral ligament structures? How do neuromuscular control mechanisms enhance joint stability and lessen injury?

The workshop participants discussed the biology and response of all the various components of the knee joint to improve understanding of how one tissue component reacts to and affects the other components. Thus, the first section in this book deals with the biology, function, and response of the knee synovium. The next section deals with the properties, function, responses, and repair of knee cartilage. Section three presents the biomechanics, repair and replacement of knee menisci. In Section four, the biology, healing, and repair

mechanisms of knee ligament disorders are addressed. In Section five, knee instability problems are discussed, specifically addressing ligament function, force measurements in ligaments, in-vivo ligament strain, placement of ligament grafts, and knee modeling studies. In Section six, clinical investigations of specific ligament-deficient states are discussed, including studies on objective measurements of knee instability and evaluation methods to assess clinical results.

The specific objectives of the workshop were to (1) disseminate new information concerning the restoration of function following injury to synovial joints, with the knee as a model; (2) stimulate communication among scientists and clinicians concerning the problems of synovial joint function following injury, with particular attention to knee-related disorders; and (3) identify new research directions that will improve the care of patients with synovial joint injuries.

This book follows a format in which a succinct overview of each section is first provided. This allows the reader to focus on the primary aspects of each section and the relationship of each paper or research study to the other studies. Finally, important recommendations and suggestions for future research are provided at the end of each section. These recommendations are important to researchers who wish to focus on the most important problems at hand; to the young researcher who may wish to select one particular problem for long-term, in-depth studies; and to appropriate grant and review boards for the funding of the more important unresolved clinical and basic science problems that require investigation.

The participants agree that cell biology must be integrated with biomechanics to understand normal homeostatic mechanisms and the response to injury and subsequent repair. For example, after anterior cruciate ligament reconstruction, the true in-vivo state of the stress or strain of the graft and the change with time and remodeling require intense investigation. It is becoming apparent that repair of ligament tissues and remodeling of autografts are highly dependent on the forces and deformations that tissue undergoes; however, the biologic signals, factors, and mechanisms coordinating the repair process are only in the initial investigative stage. New in-vivo measurement sensors implanted in knee ligaments may, for the first time, provide surgeons who implant ligament grafts with precise knowledge of the forces and elongations the graft undergoes. Rehabilitation programs could then be designed to maximize muscle and lower-limb function without unduly loading the reconstructed ligament and producing graft stretching with diminished function or complete failure.

The advances in cartilage repair, including growth factors, interrelationships of cells and extracellular matrix, and control factors for homeostasis and response to injury represent important advances. Less is known of ligament and meniscus cell biology; response to mechanical stimuli; and control mechanisms for homeostasis, remodeling, or turnover.

The participants agree that ligament reconstruction, such as for the anterior cruciate ligament, still requires much clinical and investigative study. Current surgical procedures do not truly restore knee joint kinematics and, thus, abnormal cartilage loadings can still be inferred. Even with apparently successful ligament reconstructions, a certain percentage of knees show an occurrence of synovial effusions, low-grade chronic inflammation of synovial tissues, and development of articular cartilage deterioration over time. What mechanisms explain these changes and what treatment is indicated? Are such knees in an early state of arthrosis in which all activities must be avoided, thereby lessening the chronic inflammatory state, or are there more specific biomechanical and biologic mechanisms that can be understood and controlled to achieve more predictable clinical outcomes? Ligament surgery replaces static restraints, yet the function at the knee joint represents a delicate balance between static and dynamic forces. Muscular mechanisms undoubtedly play a major role in preventing injury by limiting and controlling joint displacements. All participants agreed that insufficient data exist to measure, diagnose, and treat neuromuscular abnormalities in control of knee joint stability. This is a new and exciting area for research that has highly important clinical application.

The development and wide application of tools for objectively measuring knee joint rotations and translations, joint kinematics, and neuromuscular control is needed for defining the success of surgical procedures. Standardization and objective measurement are needed for clinical evaluation of symptoms, physical examination for stability, and assessment of lower limb function, so that results can be compared between studies and clinical conclusions reached on effectiveness of surgical procedures. Clinical rating systems require strict application of epidemiologic principles in defining and controlling populations and eliminating bias in data collection and analysis. Short-form clinical analysis of only a few clinical variables as related to symptoms, signs, or function may provide the treating physician with sufficient information, but often provide insufficient data to base treatment decisions on rigorous scientific analysis, particularly in more complex knee conditions involving injury to cartilage, ligaments, and menisci. Examples of the application of more strict clinical evaluation methodologies are presented, which require careful consideration by clinicians conducting or contemplating clinical trials.

To be able to publish the workshop manuscripts and recommendations in a timely manner requires a special effort. The participants at this workshop represented experienced and seasoned investigators from both basic science and clinical backgrounds. We learned from each other and it is our hope that this text will provide a similar review of the current state of knowledge, as well as stimulate successful new research methodologies and investigations.

FRANK R. NOYES, MD
GERALD A. M. FINERMAN, MD

Reference

1. Praemer A, Furner S, Rice DP: *Musculoskeletal Conditions in the United States.* Park Ridge, IL, American Academy of Orthopaedic Surgeons, 1992.

Acknowledgments

This publication and the workshop on which it is based would not have taken place without the intellectual and financial support provided by the American Academy of Orthopaedic Surgeons, The National Institute of Arthritis and Musculoskeletal and Skin Diseases of the National Institutes of Health, and the American Orthopaedic Society for Sports Medicine.

We would like to thank the participants from these organizations who contributed unselfishly to the completion of this project. We especially want to thank Stephen L. Gordon, PhD, the Director of the Musculoskeletal Diseases Program at NIH, for his commitment to and encouragement of the project. Nancy Peacock Heath, PhD, director of the Academy's Division of State and Specialty Societies and former director of the Center on Research, and Marilyn L. Fox, PhD, director, publications, helped to initiate and organize the workshop.

Joan Abern, associate senior medical editor, managed the publications project and with the assistance of Lisa Moore, editor, edited the manuscripts; Loraine Edwalds and Monica Trocker handled book production; and Geraldine Dubberke and EmLee Lambos did the word processing. Karen Schneider, the workshop coordinator deserves special recognition for organizing and planning the workshop.

Lastly, we want to thank the physicians and scientists who generously contributed their expertise and time. Their enthusiasm for their work, willingness to accept additional assignments, and openness to share not only their work but also their ideas and theories at the workshop and here in print made the symposium a scientific success.

FRANK R. NOYES, MD
GERALD A. M. FINERMAN, MD

Section One
Synovium

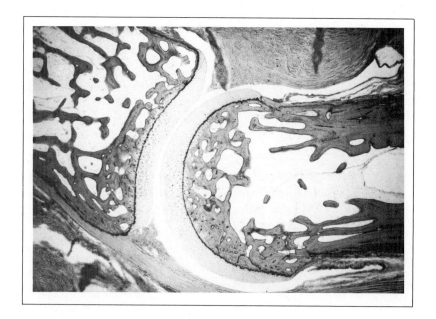

Overview

Although normal synovial tissue is an exceptionally thin and seemingly inconsequential lining, it plays important roles in the lubrication of both synovium and cartilage, the nutrition of cartilage, and the stabilization of the joint. The tissue elaborates synovial fluid that forms a film between intra-articular structures and fills the normally small joint space. The microvascular physiology of synovial fluid formation and transsynovial exchange of solutes varies significantly and symmetrically among the normal joints of each individual. Normal synovial functions are served less well when the tissue becomes inflamed with arthritis. In synovitis, there is increased microvascular leakage of water and of protein with resultant effusions. Ischemia may be a complicating factor in some rheumatoid effusions with resultant impairment in the delivery and clearance both of normal metabolites and of therapeutic agents.

Synovium plays no known biomechanical role and has been poorly investigated in the context of mechanical injury. In view of the paucity of literature on this subject, much of the material on mechanical injury is conjectural.

Synovium has the potential to respond both directly to mechanical trauma and indirectly to injury elsewhere in the joint. Direct mechanical trauma can take the form of increased intra-articular pressure and twisting or tearing during inappropriate joint kinematics. By analogy with other types of cells, the metabolism of synoviocytes may be sensitive to mechanical stress. Excessive stresses may lead to metabolic alterations with pathophysiologic consequences. Extremely high intra-articular pressures, sometimes sufficient to rupture the capsule, occur in inflamed joints with large effusions. The high intra-articular pressures generated when such joints are flexed can impair perfusion of the synovium, leading to reperfusion injury when the joint is relaxed.

Trauma to the synovium also increases vascular permeability, leading to clear effusions. When damage is severe enough to violate the synovial blood vessels, bloody effusions result. Direct mechanical disruption of the synoviocytes within the synovium will liberate into the joint lysosomal enzymes, cytokines, and, perhaps, other intra-articular mediators of articular pathology.

Damage to the other structures within the joint releases wear particles and, perhaps, soluble breakdown products. Such materials activate synoviocytes, resulting in the excessive production of proteinases, prostaglandins, cytokines, and other biochemical mediators. Clearly, the biochemical homeostasis of the joints can be greatly disrupted following damage to the synovium.

Arthrofibrosis

Increased interest has been focused on the loss of motion after knee ligament surgery. It is recognized that loss of full extension not only will have a deleterious effect on gait and muscle function, but also will increase the risk for overuse injuries. Knee ligament surgery is difficult and requires experience. The use of meticulous surgical techniques with the aid of arthroscopy should be emphasized. The selection of a strong graft along with proper placement and fixation are required to avoid graft impingement and to allow early motion, which is of greatest importance in the avoidance of arthrofibrosis. Early motion and aggressive physical therapy are being accepted as important factors in obtaining a successful outcome.

Arthrofibrosis may still be a complication in spite of proper surgical technique and rehabilitation, but the etiology of this arthrofibrosis is still unknown. It may result from increased numbers of collagen synthesizing cells, increased synthesis of matrix by existing cells, or diminished degradation of collagen molecules. However, a net imbalance of collagen synthesis and degradation leads to the accumulation of excess collagen.

Reversal or modulation of the fibrotic process might be possible by inhibiting the actions or synthesis of the many chemotactic and growth stimulating compounds that are released in response to injury. The roles that these factors play in normal and excess cartilage formation has yet to be elucidated.

If arthrofibrosis is present, arthroscopy should be considered as one of the initial treatment modalities, with lysis of adhesions. Manipulation should be carried out with great care to avoid creating further damage and injury. Finally, open surgery including posterior capsular releases or even removal of grafts might be required to restore motion.

Chapter 1

Biology and Function of Synovium

Peter A. Simkin, MD

Introduction

The synovium is a tissue lining all intra-articular structures except the contact surfaces of articular cartilage and menisci.[1,2] It is characterized by a well-organized, highly fibrillar, interstitial matrix that is approximately 25 microns deep and contains loosely interdigitating synovial cells; however, the biochemistry of the synovial matrix is not well defined. The principal collagens are types I and III, but "minor" types, especially VI, are represented as well. These fibrous elements provide an elastic framework for the tissue as it expands and contracts in response to the intermittent tensile stresses of joint motion. The proteoglycans of synovium are also thought to be confined within this collagenous mesh. The components of the proteoglycan gel and the nature of their intermolecular bonds remain unknown. Physiologic evidence suggests, however, that this matrix is important as a diffusion barrier between plasma and synovial fluid and as a critical factor maintaining the subatmospheric pressures found within most synovial joints.

The synovium is composed of cells that are often said to be up to three layers deep, but their arrangement is not laminar and they do not share the tight junctions characteristic of epithelial tissues. Traditionally, synovial cells have been classified by morphologic criteria into macrophage-like A cells, which are relatively rich in lysosomal structure, and fibroblast-like B cells, which have abundant endoplasmic reticulum. The presumed respective roles of phagocytosis and of matrix synthesis became clouded first by recognition of intermediate Type C cells, then by the discovery that hyaluronate release appears more a function of A than of B cells, and finally by the recognition of "stellate" synovial cells that also did not fit the traditional classification. More recent analyses of genetic markers suggest that most synovial cells share a common origin in the bone marrow and may also share the potential for most synovial functions. In addition, scattered mast cells are normally present, and the various leukocytes are rarely found.

There is no basement membrane to mark the point of demarcation between the synovial lining and deeper, subsynovial tissues. These may be fibrous, fatty, or areolar depending on their location and function within the articulation. The absence of a basement membrane is the principal feature distinguishing the synovium from the epithelial tissues lining other hollow organs, indicating that synovial fluid is directly continuous with the interstitial fluid of the lining matrix and of deeper intracapsular tissues. This continuity means that findings in synovial aspirates can be considered representative of interstitial events, a property relevant to the microvascular work to be discussed later. The tissue is served by a rich meshwork of fenestrated microvessels and by a complementary system of lymphatics.

Microvascular fenestrations, analogous to those found in glomeruli, are characteristic of microvascular beds that effectively retain plasma proteins but permit a rapid, bidirectional exchange of smaller solutes between plasma and interstitial fluids. Both sets of draining vessels, venous and lymphatic, contain one-way valves. Capsular and subsynovial tissues also include a generous number of small nerve fibers. This innervation plays a central role in proprioception, which is vital to effective musculoskeletal function. These nerves have recently generated more interest as a source of substance P and other neuropeptides that appear to participate in at least some forms of joint inflammation, that is, arthritis.

The normal anatomic features of synovial tissue are obscured by the cellular infiltration and hyperplasia characteristic of long-term inflammatory disease. Thus, the synovial tissues defined by the histologist and evaluated by the physiologist may be quite different from those palpated by the rheumatologist or removed by the orthopaedist during synovectomy. These distinctions must be kept in mind as clinicians and scientists exchange perspectives in a common effort to better understand the workings of joints.

Synovial Fluid

Synovial fluid occupies the cavity within the synovium and over the opposing cartilaginous surfaces (Fig. 1); this space is small. When peripheral joints, such as those of the fingers, are opened, the presence of fluid is recognizable not by a pool of readily available fluid but by the fact that the exposed surfaces are moist. Because the synovial fluid is inaccessible, full characterization of synovial aspirates has been limited to those from the knee.

Synovial fluid is largely composed of the same constituents as plasma. The concentrations of small molecules are essentially the same in both fluids, an observation that for some time has led interested clinicians to characterize synovial fluid as an ultrafiltrate or dialysate of plasma. Synovial fluid proteins are also those of plasma; however, their concentrations are lower and are inversely related to their radii. For instance, a relatively small protein such as albumin is

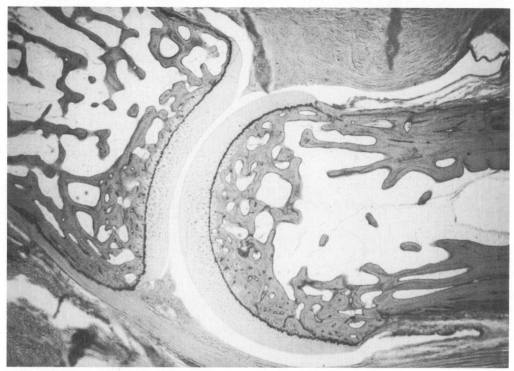

Fig. 1   *A normal interphalangeal joint. The synovial lining overlies all intra-articular surfaces except for the contact surfaces of articular cartilage. Synovial recesses above and below the joint facilitate the expansion and contraction required by the normal range of articular motion. The small articular cavity normally occupied by synovial fluid is somewhat exaggerated by fixation of this specimen. (Reprinted from the Clinical Slide Collection on the Rheumatic Diseases, copyright 1991. Used by permission of the American College of Rheumatology.)*

normally present at a concentration much closer to that of plasma than is the much larger α_2 macroglobulin. The mechanism for this differentiation is not entirely clear but appears most consistent with restricted diffusion overlying a very small element of unrestricted filtration. When the protein content rises, as it does in pathologic effusions, the principal change is an increase in this nonselective filtration or plasma leak.

Certain synovial fluid proteins may also be synthesized locally. In normal fluid, the only established example is that of lubricin, an important factor in joint lubrication. In chronically inflamed synovial tissues, additional proteins may be released. The best example of this is that of immunoglobulins in rheumatoid fluids. The antigenic targets of these antibodies remain an interesting focus of ongoing efforts to understand the pathogenesis of this disease.

Hyaluronan, or hyaluronic acid, is the constituent that provides synovial fluid with its characteristic viscosity. The word "synovium'' is derived from Latin, meaning ''like egg'' in reference to the consistency of the normal fluid, which resembles that of the white of an egg. This prominent viscosity originates from the interaction of the long glycosaminoglycan polymers of hyaluronan. When inflammation is severe, these polymers shorten, with a corresponding decrement in the viscosity of pathologic effusions.

Joint Motion

Fundamentally, synovial joints serve as the bearings in the intricate machine that is the human body. In response to the changing articular geometry of motion, large areas of synovium are normally subjected to repeated expansion and contraction. The histologic implications of motion have not yet been evaluated. It seems likely, however, that synovium stretched by the normal range of motion in humans will reveal changes analogous to those observed when rabbit joints are distended and fixed under increased internal pressure. In this case, the cells move apart from each other and become more stellate in appearance, while the vessels move closer to the synovial surface.[3] These changes should substantially reduce the interstitial diffusion barrier between plasma and synovial fluid.

The expansile capabilities of synovium impose a severe challenge to the lubricating capabilities of synovial fluid. As the tissue adapts to flexion, extension, and additional ranges of motion, it does so in direct apposition to large areas of articular cartilage. Despite this intimate contact, synovial tissue is almost never entrapped and traumatized as the joint goes through its working cycles. This highly effective lubrication of synovium on cartilage may well involve hyaluronan.[4] The system is as impressive as the separate and better-known lubrication of cartilage on cartilage. The latter appears to be predominantly a boundary-layer system involving a specialized glycoprotein, lubricin, and perhaps lipid factors as well.[5] For both synovium on cartilage and cartilage on cartilage, effective lubrication is provided not by a large pool of interposed lubricant, but by a thin film of fluid between the opposing surfaces. Thus, the volume of synovial fluid is small in normal joints.

Joint Stability and Intra-articular Pressure

The thinness of the film between opposing surfaces suggests that synovial fluid plays another mechanical role in addition to lubrication. Boundary layer lubricants are known to be effective adhesives as well.[6] In a seeming paradox, such systems do not resist shearing forces but are highly resistant to distraction. The adhesive properties of synovial fluid probably play a role in maintaining close apposition of both synovium on cartilage and cartilage on cartilage. In the latter role, the normal synovial fluid film may contribute significantly to both normal tracking and joint stability as the opposing cartilages make contact. These properties are readily demonstrated at the base of an extended index finger. Relaxed tendons and collateral ligaments permit deviation in any direction, but distraction is resisted by the synovial fluid bond. It is the rupture of this bond that provides the best explanation for the familiar sound when people "crack" their knuckles. The bond is also lost in the presence of a significant synovial effusion. When effusions are chronic, the lack of normal adhesion can be expected to cause sloppy joint action with increased stress on adjacent ligaments and resultant articular instability.

In normal articulations, the volume of free synovial fluid appears to be minimized by a continuous suction exerted through the interstitial matrix of the investing synovial lining. This force also lowers the intra-articular pressure to the subatmospheric values routinely observed in normal knees.[7] The mechanism driving this suction remains unclear; it probably reflects an osmotic effect exerted by the structured gel of the synovial matrix. It seems likely that the osmotic differential is in turn sustained by regular articular motion that pumps the valved draining vessels of both the venous and the lymphatic vascular systems. In effect, the synovial matrix acts like a sponge that is regularly wrung out by the moving joint. These systems prove inadequate or fail in inflamed tissues where articular clearance cannot stay ahead of microvascular leakage, and the results are synovial edema, joint stiffness, and pathologic effusions.

When effusions are present, the intra-articular pressure is no longer subatmospheric. Resting values of 20 mm Hg or more are especially common in patients with rheumatoid arthritis. As these joints are used, pressures rise dramatically. Clearly, such load-induced pressure pulses may impair synovial blood flow by tamponade of the microvascular bed. It is not yet clear, however, whether this intermittent interruption of flow causes any overall impairment of solute exchange between plasma and interstitial fluids.

Another complication of increased pressure with more clearly established clinical consequences is synovial rupture or herniation. Although rise in pressure and synovial rupture may occur in any joint, they are recognized most often in patients with chronic knee effusions. In these patients, acute rupture of the synovium leads to drainage of effusion fluid into soft-tissue planes in the calf where it causes an inflammatory response that is often misinterpreted as thrombophlebitis. When the same synovial lining bulges but does not break, the result is a Baker's cyst, which may be chronically symptomatic.

Pathophysiology of Effusions

Presumably, a small volume of synovial fluid, well mixed by continued joint movement, provides an optimal vehicle for the transport of oxygen, glucose, and other micronutrients from the blood in synovial microvessels to the chondrocytes of avascular articular cartilage. Conversely, the same path carries carbon dioxide, lactate, and other metabolic wastes from the tissues back to the bloodstream. In normal joints, this system maintains healthy chondrocytes at remarkably great distances from their nurturing microvasculature.

In rheumatoid arthritis, however, the system often fails. The protein content of synovial fluid rises toward that of plasma, and the small molecules give evidence of local ischemia manifested by low glucose, low PO_2, low pH, high lactate, and high PCO_2 levels.[8,9] Thus, an altered microvasculature appears to be more permeable to proteins, but less effective in transporting smaller molecules. That, in fact, is exactly the case.

Plasma proteins continuously escape through the microvascular endothelium and diffuse toward the joint space, where they are removed by lymphatic clearance. The synovial fluid concentration of total protein (or of any individual plasma protein) reflects both sides of this balance. Concentrations may rise in response to either increased vascular permeability or decreased lymphatic clearance, or a combination of the two. In rheumatoid knee effusions, the protein content is higher than in osteoarthritis, but not significantly so. Quantitative kinetic evaluation demonstrates that the rheumatoid microvasculature is twice as permeable to protein as is that of osteo-arthritis (Fig. 2).[10] This striking difference in vascular permeability is largely obscured by a corresponding increase in lymphatic drainage from the rheumatoid knee, an important point for clinicians and scientists interested in evaluating synovial events by measuring the concentrations of individual proteins in synovial fluid. The synovial arrival of any protein will be underestimated by concentration when lymphatic clearance is high, and, conversely, may be overestimated if clearance is low. Thus, local production and/or release of any protein can only be evaluated when concentrations are measured in concert with kinetics.

The best available evidence indicates that rheumatoid synovial ischemia is real. For instance, those knee effusions having low glucose or low pH levels also have a plasma flow that is significantly lower than that of rheumatoid effusions not showing such changes. Furthermore, and of particular relevance to clinicians, the ischemic knees are also colder than their better perfused counterparts (Fig. 3).[11] This finding implies that temperature may not be a valid index of the severity of inflammation in joints involved in chronic rheumatoid arthritis.

Most rheumatologists have seen too many rheumatoid patients who had progressive destruction of their wrists despite the fact that these joints were not warm to the touch. From what is known about rheumatoid knees, it seems reasonable to suspect that cool wrists with boggy swelling are significantly ischemic. At the University of Washington, Andrew Holman, Peter Dewire, John Bassett, and I are pursuing the hypothesis that rheumatoid ischemia may be exacerbated by therapy with nonsteroidal anti-inflammatory drugs (NSAIDs). We suspect that many rheumatoid joints resemble mar-

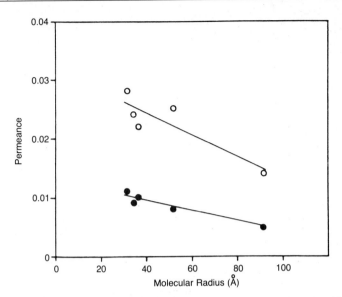

Fig. 2 *Microvascular permeability to five marker proteins in rheumatoid (open circles) and osteoarthritic (closed circles) knees. Synovial permeance (the decimal fraction of perfusing protein that escapes into the joint space during each microvascular passage) is more than twice as great in the rheumatoid joints over a wide range of molecular sizes. (Reproduced with permission from Wallis WJ, Simkin PA, Nelp WB: Protein traffic in human synovial effusions.* Arthritis Rheum *1987:30:57-63.)*

ginal kidneys in that their baseline perfusion has become prostaglandin-dependent. When such patients are treated with NSAIDs, inhibition of cyclo-oxygenase removes the prostaglandin prop, and the hitherto sufficient circulation no longer keeps pace with demand. When this happens to the kidney, ensuing renal insufficiency makes recognition of the problem all too easy.[12] In the joint, however, the resultant fall in temperature that may be accompanied by a decrease in swelling and pain will be interpreted as a significant therapeutic achievement. Recent Swedish radiographic studies have established that the most ischemic knee joints suffer the greatest destruction.[13] If such changes are potentiated by NSAIDs, we may have to reevaluate the role of these drugs, which are the cornerstone of current therapy.

Intrasynovial Pharmacokinetics

A working knowledge of synovial physiology is useful in interpreting the pharmacokinetics of antirheumatic drugs. For most of the agents used by rheumatologists and orthopaedists, data are available on drug concentrations in synovial fluid as well as in plasma or serum.[14] With rare exceptions, this information was de-

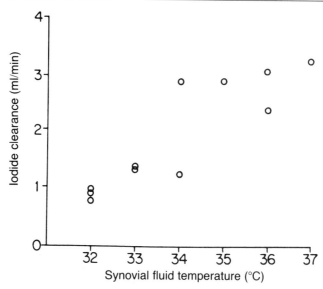

Fig. 3 *Iodide clearance, a measure of effective synovial blood flow, correlates highly with synovial fluid temperature in rheumatoid knee effusions. Together with comparable relationships between perfusions and synovial fluid lactate, pH, and glucose, this finding strongly indicates that local ischemia causes metabolic compromise in this disease. (Reproduced with permission from Wallis WJ, Simkin PA, Nelp WB: Low synovial clearance of iodide provides evidence of hypoperfusion in chronic rheumatoid synovitis. Arthritis Rheum 1985;28:1096-1104.)*

rived from serial studies of knee effusions in people with rheumatoid disease. Such studies are valuable because of the insights they provide on drug availability in distended interstitial spaces. However, the rheumatoid knee is not representative of other connective tissues. Its relatively limited blood supply and large fluid volume imply that the intra-articular concentration will lag well behind changing plasma levels. This will be true during the absorptive phase when plasma levels rise rapidly with gastrointestinal uptake, and during the later clearance phase when tissue (and synovial fluid) levels normally exceed those in plasma. Such patterns can be expected, and have been observed, with virtually all antirheumatic agents. Because rational subjects are unlikely to consent to serial retrieval of fluid samples from their normal joints, pharmacokinetic information from joints without effusions cannot be expected. When such studies have been carried out in large animals, however, the synovial fluid levels have closely followed those in plasma. By inference, NSAID levels in uninflamed osteoarthritic joints, for example, are more likely to resemble those of normal plasma than those found in swollen rheumatoid knees.

Physiologic Differences Among Normal Joints

In considering the structure and function of synovium, it is important to remember that all synovial joints need not be the same. In

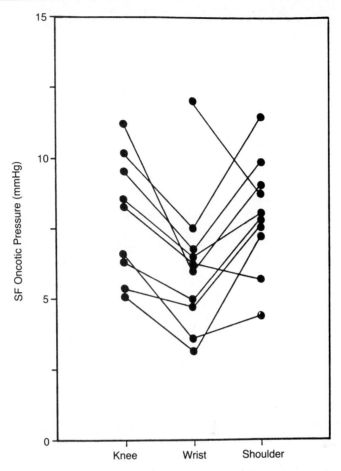

Fig. 4   *The oncotic pressure in canine "wrists" is consistently lower than that in "knee" (stifle) and shoulder joints. Comparable wrist/knee differences in hydrostatic pressure and in microvascular permeability confirm a highly significant, interarticular difference in microvascular physiology. Such physiologic differences may be important determinants of resistance or susceptibility of individual joints to specific rheumatic disease. (Reproduced with permission from Simkin PA, Benedict RS: Hydrostatic and oncotic determinants of microvascular fluid balance in normal canine joints.* Arthritis Rheum *1990;33:80-86.)*

fact, existing evidence reveals highly significant interarticular differences between the wrists and knees of normal dogs;[15] the protein concentration and the corresponding oncotic pressure of synovial fluid aspirates are consistently higher in the knees (stifle joints) than in the wrists (Fig.4). Further, the hydrostatic pressures in the wrists are higher than those in the knees. When analyzed in the classic Sterling formulation of microvascular function, these differences are additive rather than offsetting. Together, they indicate a relatively high-pressure microvascular bed in the wrist as opposed to a remarkably low-pressure microvascular bed in the knee. The same two joints were compared in isotopic studies of microvascular function.[16] The results of these studies showed that the high-pressure microvascular bed of the wrist was significantly more permeable to water and protein than the low-pressure vessels of the knee. Thus, the synovial physiology of these joints differs markedly with solute exchange in the wrist being more filtration-dependent than the diffusion-based system of the knee. Other animals have not been studied in comparable detail, but significant interarticular differences in protein concentration have been found in every species that has been studied. This includes humans, who have higher protein concentrations in shoulders and hips than in elbows, wrists, knees, or ankles.

The reason for contrasting physiology of large joints in the same individual lies in the patterns of involvement that characterize specific rheumatic diseases. Every clinician recognizes that each pathologic entity tends to affect some joints and to spare others. Rheumatoid arthritis, for instance, regularly attacks metacarpophalangeal joints and spares the distal interphalangeals, while interphalangeal osteoarthritis reverses this pattern. These patterns do not happen by chance and cannot result from systemic factors that should involve all joints in the same way. The possibility that physiologic differences make some joints relatively susceptible and others resistant to each pathogenetic mechanism is being pursued. However, corresponding interarticular differences in innervation, mechanics, or the biochemistry of constituent tissues may be equally or more important than the features chosen for study in this chapter. Ultimately, no form of arthritis will be understood until the logic of its patterns has been deciphered.

Conclusions

Although swollen joints are the cardinal feature of arthritis, the cause of swelling is unknown. A wealth of information has developed over the years about the involved cells and their potential responses to a host of demonstrated mediators. In the final analysis, some (or all) of these factors interact with each other and with synovial microvessels to produce swelling, redness, and sometimes heat. A further focus on synovial physiology and on the vascular response to disease and to therapy seems likely to produce progress, in practice as well as in theory.

Acknowledgments

This work was supported in part by NIH Grant No. AM32811. This chapter was adapted with permission from Simkin PA: Physiology of normal and abnormal synovium. *Semin Arthritis Rheum* 1991;21:179-183.

References

1. Ghadially FN: Fine structure of joints, in Sokoloff L (ed): *The Joints and Synovial Fluid.* New York, Academic Press, 1978, vol I, pp 105-176.

2. Henderson B, Edwards JCW: *The Synovial Lining: In Health and Disease*. London, Chapman & Hall, 1987.

3. Levick JR, McDonald JN: Synovial capillary distribution in relation to altered pressure and permeability in knees of anaesthetized rabbits. *J Physiol (Lond)* 1989;419:477-492.

4. Swann DA, Radin EL, Nazimiec M, et al: Role of hyaluronic acid in joint lubrication. *Ann Rheum Dis* 1974;33:318-326.

5. Swann DA, Silver FH, Slayter HS, et al: The molecular structure and lubricating activity of lubridin isolated from bovine and human synovial fluids. *Biochem J* 1985;225:195-201.

6. Salomon G: The adhesion of liquids to solids, in Houwink S, Salomon G (eds): *Adhesion and Adhesives*. Amsterdam, Elsevier Publishing Company, 1965, vol 1, pp 29-52.

7. Levick JR: Joint pressure-volume studies: Their importance, design and interpretation. *J Rheumatol* 1983;10:353-357.

8. Levick JR: Hypoxia and acidosis in chronic inflammatory arthritis: Relation to vascular supply and dynamic effusion pressure. *J Rheumatol* 1990;17:579-582.

9. Stevens CR, Williams RB, Farrell AJ, et al: Hypoxia and inflammatory synovitis: Observations and speculation. *Ann Rheum Dis* 1991;50:124-132.

10. Wallis WJ, Simkin PA, Nelp WB: Protein traffic in human synovial effusions. *Arthritis Rheum* 1987;30:57-63.

11. Wallis WJ, Simkin PA, Nelp WB: Low synovial clearance of iodide provides evidence of hypoperfusion in chronic rheumatoid synovitis. *Arthritis Rheum* 1985;28:1096-1104.

12. Clive DM, Stoff JS: Renal syndromes associated with nonsteroidal antiinflammatory drugs. *N Engl J Med* 1984;310:563-572.

13. Geborek P, Saxne T, Pettersson H, et al: Synovial fluid acidosis correlates with radiological joint destruction in rheumatoid arthritis knee joints. *J Rheumatol* 1989;16:468-472.

14. Netter P, Bannwarth B, Royer-Morrot MJ: Recent findings on the pharmacokinetics of nonsteroidal anti-inflammatory drugs in synovial fluid. *Clin Pharmacokinet* 1989;17:145-162.

15. Simkin PA, Benedict RS: Hydrostatic and oncotic determinants of microvascular fluid balance in normal canine joints. *Arthritis Rheum* 1990;33:80-86.

16. Simkin PA, Benedict RS: Iodide and albumin kinetics in normal canine wrists and knees. *Arthritis Rheum* 1990;33:73-79.

Chapter 2

Response of Synovium to Mechanical Injury

C. H. Evans, PhD

Introduction

Normal synovium is a thin membrane, only two to three cell layers thick, covering the internal surfaces of all diarthrodial joints. It overlies the fibrous, fatty, or areolar subsynovial tissue that exists between it and the surrounding joint capsule.

Synovium can be viewed as a tissue whose function is to regulate the intra-articular biochemical environment. It does this in two main ways (Fig. 1). The first is a passive process involving the trans-synovial diffusion of substances between the synovial fluid and capillaries within the synovium; the second is an active process involving the secretion and uptake of substances by the synoviocytes that line the joint space.

The rates at which molecules diffuse between the blood vessels and the synovial fluid are determined by a number of factors, including the permeabilities of both the vascular endothelium and the synovial interstitium. Diffusion of proteins into the joint occurs as a function of their molecular sizes, with smaller proteins entering the joint more readily. The rate of efflux from the joint, in contrast, is the same for all proteins and occurs via the lymph.[1-4] Because these topics are dealt with extensively in Chapter 1, they will not be discussed here.

Superimposed upon this trafficking of chemicals between the blood, synovial fluid, and lymph are the active contributions made by the synoviocytes. Because the synovial membrane has such a large surface area, the cells that line it have the potential to modify considerably the chemistry of the synovial fluid. The most obvious example is their secretion of hyaluronate, which is almost absent from serum but present in synovial fluid at a concentration of approximately 3 mg/ml. Of relevance is the ability of activated synoviocytes to secrete various cytokines, proteolytic enzymes, and eicosanoids, among other mediators, into the joint space. In addition,

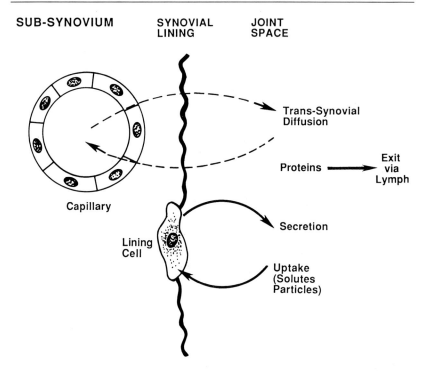

SUB-SYNOVIUM   **SYNOVIAL**   **JOINT**
                       LINING   **SPACE**

Trans-Synovial
Diffusion

Exit
Proteins ➡ via
Lymph

Capillary

Secretion

Lining
Cell

Uptake
(Solutes
Particles)

Fig. 1 *Major routes by which synovium regulates the intra-articular biochemical environment.*

synoviocytes modify the intra-articular biochemical environment subtractively via selective metabolic uptake from synovial fluid.

Synovium is mechanically weak and has no known biomechanical role. Thus, although the joint's vulnerability to mechanical injury is widely appreciated, attention has been focused on damage to those weightbearing tissues that suffer the most macroscopically obvious disruption, namely cartilage, ligaments, and tendons. Nevertheless, there is reason to suspect that synovial injury also occurs, with consequences important to the physiology and pathophysiology of the joint. Some of these injuries will affect diffusion across the synovium, while others primarily will affect synoviocyte metabolism. Both will alter the biochemistry of the intra-articular milieu, leading to possible joint dysfunction.

This chapter discusses the responses of synovium to indirect and direct mechanical injury. Obtaining information for this chapter was difficult because, as confirmed by a recent MEDLINE search of the literature since 1966, there are few publications on this subject. As a result, much of this chapter is of hypothetical nature. However, I hope that the following hypotheses and speculations will provoke greater experimental analysis of the normal physiology of the synovium and its dysfunction following injury and disease.

Injuries That Alter Transsynovial Diffusion

Three parameters contribute fundamentally to determining the rates of transsynovial diffusion between the synovial capillaries and synovial fluid: the permeability of the vessel wall, the distance between the capillary and the joint space, and the chemical composition of the extracellular matrix through which the diffusing molecules must pass. Mechanical injuries have the capacity, directly or indirectly, to alter each of these.

Altered permeability of the capillary wall following trauma is most obvious in the bloody effusions that occur when the integrity of the vessel has been violated. Because such effusions are highly inflammatory,[5] it is not surprising that synovitis is a common consequence of injury to the joint.[6,7]

Clear effusions reflect more subtle changes in capillary permeability. Although these could result from limited mechanical damage, they are more likely to reflect the secretion of vasoactive mediators, such as leukotrienes, histamine, bradykinin, and certain cytokines, which are potent inducers of microvascular leakage. Rheumatoid synovial fluid contains substances that increase the permeability of vascular endothelial cells in vitro; a 92 kd gelatinase has been implicated in this process.[8] It is also possible that the higher protein content of inflammatory synovial fluids contributes to these effusions by lowering the oncotic gradient between plasma and synovial fluid.[4]

The cellular origins of vasoactive mediators and the ways in which trauma stimulates their production are unknown. It could reflect a direct effect of altered mechanical forces on the cells that produce vasoactive mediators. An indirect mechanism is also possible, with attention having been drawn to the involvement of microcrystals released from bone or deep cartilage, fat from the bone marrow or subsynovial tissues,[9] and cartilaginous wear particles.

Quantitative and qualitative alterations in the synthesis and degradation of the synovial extracellular matrix will affect both the permeability of the matrix to diffusion and the distance between the capillaries and the joint space. The matrix presents considerable resistance to fluid flow, and it confines the synovial fluid within the joint cavity.[10] Its macromolecular composition includes hyaluronic acid, proteoglycan, fibronectin, laminin, and collagen types I, III, IV, V, and VI.[11,12] Scarring of synovium following injury could alter the chemical composition of the matrix and also its thickness. The factors that promote deposition of the synovial extracellular matrix are unknown but, as with vasodilation, they could be produced as part of a direct cellular response to mechanical forces or an indirect response to injury elsewhere in the joint. Of particular relevance is the observation that certain cytokines, such as interleukin-1 (IL-1), strongly increase the synthesis of type I collagen and other matrix macromolecules by synovial fibroblasts.[13] As discussed later in this chapter, IL-1 and other cytokines can be released from mechanically damaged synoviocytes.

Table 1 Cellular responses to mechanical stress
Cell Type

Response	Reference	
Endothelial	Cell division	14
Endothelial	Prostacyclin synthesis	15
Endothelial	Morphology changes	16
Endothelial	Cytoskeletal changes	16
Endothelial	Collagen synthesis	17
Endothelial	Contracting factor synthesis	18
Endothelial	Adenylate cyclase activity	19
Smooth muscle	Collagen synthesis	20
Osteoblast	Cell division	21
Osteoblast	Mineralization	*
Fibroblast	Alignment to force	**
Chondrocytes	Proteoglycan synthesis	22-24

*M. J. Buckley, A. J. Banes, R.D. Jordan, et al, unpublished data, 1992.
**A.J. Banes, R. Henderson, D. Donion, unpublished data, 1992.

Injuries That Alter Synoviocyte Metabolism

Mechanical Disruption

As the tissue that lines the internal surface of all diarthrodial joints, synovium is presumably subjected to considerable and varying mechanical forces during movement. It would be unusual if cells within the synovium were not metabolically responsive to these forces. Thus, mechanical stimulation is probably an important regulator of synovial metabolism, although this matter has received no experimental attention.

In vitro experiments with osteoblasts, endothelial cells, smooth muscle cells, fibroblasts, chondrocytes, and other types of cells recovered from mechanically active environments clearly demonstrate the metabolic responsiveness of cells to loading (Table 1). There are no published data concerning the responses of synoviocytes to such forces, despite the likelihood that the synovium is exposed to stretching, torque, and perhaps other types of mechanical distortion in vivo. Several of the metabolic responses mounted by cells when subjected to force (Table 1) would be of importance to the physiology of both the synovium and the joint.

Because there are few data on the mechanics of synovium during normal use of the joint, it is not surprising that little information is available on the circumstances under which mechanical forces become excessive. Such circumstances might occur when the joint goes through abnormal motions during, for example, certain types of sporting injury, or in the presence of effusions where the synovium is greatly distended. The intra-articular pressure of the normal knee at rest is below atmospheric pressure.[25] When an effusion is present, the intra-articular pressure increases. For example, injection of 20 ml of physiologic saline into the normal human knee produces 25 mm Hg positive pressure on quadriceps contraction.[26] Effusions are greatest in highly inflamed joints. Because the synovium and capsule of such joints are less compliant, considerable intra-articular pressures result. Quadriceps contraction of such joints can generate pressures over 500 mm Hg, leading to rupture of the joint capsule.[26] The formation of Baker's cysts may be linked to chronically high intra-articular pressures.

Cell Lysis

Recent laboratory research suggests a further consequence of mechanical insult to the synovium, namely the release of cytokines and other mediators from intracellular reservoirs. Synoviocytes produce a variety of cytokines, including IL-1, fibroblast growth factor, transforming growth factor-β, β_2-microglobulin, amyloid A, and other unidentified factors.[27,28] These mediators are capable of producing the synovial changes previously noted. Collectively, they are also able to increase the synthesis of neutral metalloproteinases and prostaglandin E_2 by chondrocytes and synoviocytes via paracrine and autocrine pathways.[29,30] The responses of chondrocytes and synoviocytes to these factors lead to breakdown of the articular cartilage.[31] Synovial cytokines are also inflammatory. In studying the synthesis and secretion of these cytokines in vitro, we have observed that the lapine synovial fibroblasts store them intracellularly. Mechanical disruption of the cells leads to release of the cytokines in a biologically active form. If such reservoirs exist in vivo, direct mechanical damage to the synovium could release these factors into the joint, where they have the potential to trigger inflammation, synovial hypertrophy, and cartilage breakdown. Of particular relevance is the ability of synovial cytokines to promote their own synthesis in an autocrine fashion.[29] In this way the effects of limited cellular damage could be magnified and prolonged (Fig. 2).

Ischemia and Reperfusion Injury

The high intra-articular pressures previously described are sometimes sufficient to impair the flow of blood through the synovial capillaries. This has two consequences.

During ischemic episodes the PO_2 of the synovial fluid falls, thereby engendering anaerobic metabolism. Lactate production thus increases, producing a fall in pH. There is evidence that the integrity of the joint is at particularly high risk under acidotic conditions of low oxygen tension.

Recent evidence suggests that synovium may also be susceptible to reperfusion injury.[32] According to this hypothesis, flexion of a joint with a sufficiently large effusion raises the intra-articular pressure to levels that impair blood flow through the synovial capillaries. During the resulting period of ischemia, adenosine triphosphate (ATP) is broken down to hypoxanthine and the enzyme xanthine reductase is converted to xanthine oxidase. Subsequent relaxation of the joint permits synovial reperfusion, during which

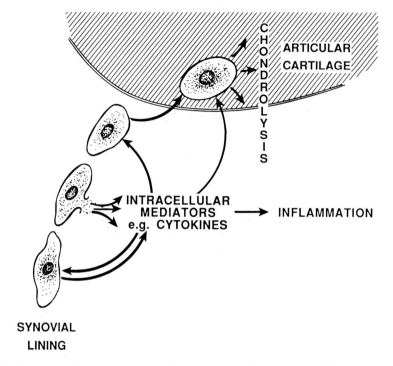

Fig. 2   *A possible mechanism for the production of arthropathy following mechanical damage to synoviocytes.*

xanthine oxidase converts hypoxanthine to uric acid, with the production of oxygen-derived free radicals that damage both cellular and matrix macromolecules. Similar series of events are postulated to occur during the reperfusion of ischemic heart and brain.

Experimental findings support this hypothesis. As discussed earlier, flexion or contraction of muscles around joints with effusions can generate very high intra-articular pressures. Under certain conditions, these pressures can exceed systolic blood pressure. Doppler flow measurements confirm that high intra-articular pressures impair periarticular blood flow, leading to decreased PO_2 values. Electron spin resonance spectroscopic data are consistent with the notion that hypoxic synovia produce the superoxide radical (O_2^-) in vitro through the action of xanthine oxidase.[33]

Synovial Responses to Mechanical Injury Elsewhere in the Joint

In addition to responding to the types of direct injury discussed so far, synovium has the capacity to mount an indirect response to the mechanical disruption of other intra-articular tissues. When mechanically degraded, these tissues release wear particles and possibly soluble breakdown products into the joint. These materials are captured by the synovium, where they provoke a cellular reaction. Best studied in this regard are the wear particles produced by abrasion of the articular cartilage.[34,35]

Addition of cartilaginous wear particles to cultures of synoviocytes increases the cellular production of prostaglandin E_2, cytokines, and the neutral metalloproteinases collagenase, gelatinase, and stromelysin.[36] Between them, these products have the potential to cause synovial inflammation and cartilage breakdown. Studies in which cartilaginous particles have been injected intra-articularly into rabbits' knees confirm that these pathologies are indeed provoked by the particles.[37] Examination of human synovial fluid and synovium has demonstrated that cartilaginous wear particles occur in vivo,[34,35] where they can contribute to the pathophysiology of certain arthritides. Lavage of joints during arthroscopy flushes wear particles from the joint, which may account for the reported symptomatic relief resulting from joint irrigation. Further studies have shown that soluble products of cartilage erosion, such as proteoglycan fragments, may also provoke synovial responses.[38]

The reactions of synoviocytes to wear particles may also be involved in the pathophysiology of two additional clinical problems. One is the poor performance of prosthetic anterior cruciate ligament replacements. There is evidence that these prostheses shed wear particles which, following their capture by the synovium, provoke the persistent synovitis and effusions that result from insertion of these devices.[39]

A second area of possible involvement is in the aseptic loosening of prosthetic joint replacements. Loosened prostheses are often coated with a pseudosynovium that forms at the interface between the bone and the inserted device. Such pseudosynovia often secrete considerable amounts of neutral metalloproteinases, prostaglandin E_2, and various cytokines that have the capacity to resorb bone. Particles of metal, polyethylene and, in cemented prostheses, bone cement are likely to be responsible for activating cells within this membrane.[40]

Summary and Conclusions

Although the synovium is not generally discussed in the context of mechanical injury to the joint, this tissue is likely to suffer considerable damage during certain types of joint trauma. Mechanical insults probably range from subtle changes in intra-articular pressure to macroscopically evident tearing of the tissue during injury. Furthermore, synovium is probably responsive to the mechanical injury of other structures within the joint.

The main physiologic role of synovium is biochemical rather than biomechanical. Thus, damage to this tissue is unlikely to have a major, direct effect on joint biomechanics, although its indirect consequences can be large. Synovial damage is likely to alter the joint's biochemistry in important ways. In particular, disturbances in the metabolism of the synoviocytes in direct or indirect response to the various types of injury described here could lead to the production of cytokines, proteinases, eicosanoids, free radicals, and other mediators of joint pathology. Coupled with altered transsynovial trafficking of materials between the circulation and the joint, such alterations would greatly change the intra-articular biochemical environment.

Thus, there are a variety of theoretical ways in which synovium could sustain injury and disrupt the physiologic homeostasis of the joint. Although the literature is sparse, there are suggestions that the joint may be more susceptible to synovial injury than generally believed. For example, Frost and Ghosh[41] have reported that a single intra-articular injection of saline into the knee of a rabbit provokes disaggregation of cartilage proteoglycans. In addition, the "sham operated" rabbit knees studied by Lukoschek and associates[42] sustained a synovitis with accompanying cartilaginous changes. In both of these examples, the changes spontaneously resolved, suggesting that joints have the capacity to reverse at least some of the sequelae of synovial insult. These mechanisms may be impaired in certain individuals, leading to chronic synovial and articular changes that are difficult to treat clinically.

This is clearly an underinvestigated area of orthopaedic research.

References

1. Simkin P, Pizzorno JE: Transsynovial exchange of small molecules in normal human subjects. *J Appl Physiol* 1974;36:581-587.
2. Levick JR: Permeability of rheumatoid and normal human synovium to specific plasma proteins. *Arthritis Rheum* 1981;24:1550-1560.
3. Sallis JG, Perry BJ: Absorption from the synovial cavity in rabbits and cats: The influence of different environments and drugs. *S Afr J Med Sci* 1967;32:83-95.
4. Wallis WJ, Simkin PA, Nelp WB: Protein traffic in human synovial effusions. *Arthritis Rheum* 1987;30:57-63.
5. Bignold LP, Lykke AW: Increased vascular permeability evoked by mechanical trauma and haemarthrosis in synovium of the rat. *Pathology* 1975;7:263-271.
6. Roy S, Ghadially FN, Crane WAJ: Synovial membrane in traumatic effusion. Ultrastructure and autoradiography with tritiated leucine. *Ann Rheum Dis* 1966;25:259-271.
7. Soren A, Rosenbauer KA, Klein W: Morphological examinations of so-called posttraumatic synovitis. *Beitr Pathol* 1973;150:11-30.
8. Koolwijk P, van Laar JM, Miltenburg AMR, et al: The presence of active 92-kDa type IV collagenase and factor(s) in synovial fluids of arthritis patients that induce vascular leakage, abstract. *Arthritis Rheum* 1991;34(suppl):S143.
9. Weinberger A, Schumacher HR: Experimental joint trauma: Synovial response to blunt trauma and inflammatory reaction to intraarticular injection of fat. *J Rheumatol* 1981;8:380-389.
10. Levick JR: Synovial fluid exchange: A case of flow through fibrous materials. *News Physiol Soc* 1989;4:198-202.

11. Ashhurst DE, Bland YS, Levick JR: An immunohistochemical study of the collagens of rabbit synovial interstitium. *J Rheumatol* 1991;18:1669-1672.

12. Pollock LE, Lalor O, Revell PA: Type IV collagen and laminin in the synovial intimal layer: An immunohistochemical study. *Rheumatol Int* 1990:9:277-280.

13. Goldring MB, Krane SM: Modulation by recombinant interleukin 1 of synthesis of types I and III collagens and associated procollagen mRNA levels in cultured human cells. *J Biol Chem* 1987;262:16724-16729.

14. Sumpio BE, Banes AJ, Levin LG, et al: Mechanical stress stimulates aortic endothelial cells to proliferate. *J Vasc Surg* 1987;6:252-256.

15. Sumpio BE, Banes AJ: Prostacyclin synthetic activity in cultured aortic endothelial cells undergoing cyclic mechanical deformation. *Surgery* 1988;104:383-389.

16. Sumpio BE, Banes AJ, Buckley MJ, et al: Alterations in aortic endothelial cell morphology and cytoskeletal protein synthesis during cyclic tensional deformation. *J Vasc Surg* 1988;7:130-138.

17. Sumpio BE, Banes AJ, Link GW, et al: Modulation of endothelial cell phenotype by cyclic stretch: Inhibition of collagen production. *J Surg Res* 1990;48:415-420.

18. Sumpio BE, Widmann MD: Enhanced production of endothelium-derived contracting factor by endothelial cells subjected to pulsatile stretch. *Surgery* 1990;108:277-282.

19. Letsou GV, Rosales O, Maitz S, et al: Stimulation of adenylate cyclase activity in cultured endothelial cells subjected to cyclic stretch. *J Cardiovasc Surg* 1990;31:634-639.

20. Sumpio BE, Banes AJ, Link WG, et al: Enhanced collagen production by smooth muscle cells during repetitive mechanical stretching. *Arch Surg* 1988;123:1233-1236.

21. Buckley MJ, Banes AJ, Levin LG, et al: Osteoblasts increase their rate of division and align in response to cyclic, mechanical tension in vitro. *J Bone Miner* 1988;4:225-236.

22. Hall AC, Urban JPG, Gehl KA: The effects of hydrostatic pressure on matrix synthesis in articular cartilage. *J Orthop Res* 1991;9:1-10.

23. Vasan N: Effects of physical stress on the synthesis and degradation of cartilage matrix. *Connect Tissue Res* 1983;12:49-58.

24. Sah RL, Kim YJ, Doong JY, et al: Biosynthetic response of cartilage explants to dynamic compression. *J Orthop Res* 1989;7:619-636.

25. Levick JR: An investigation into the validity of subatmospheric pressure recordings from synovial fluid and their dependence on joint angle. *J Physiol* 1979;289:55-67.

26. Jayson MIV, Dixon A StJ: Intra-articular pressure in rheumatoid arthritis of the knee III. Pressure changes during joint use. *Ann Rheum Dis* 1970;29:401-408.

27. Bandara G, Lin CW, Georgescu HI, et al: The synovial activation of chondrocytes: Evidence for complex cytokine interactions involving a possible novel factor. *Biochim Biophys Acta* 1992;1134:309-318.

28. Brinckerhoff CE, Mitchell TI, Karmilowicz MJ, et al: Autocrine induction of collagenase by serum amyloid A-like and B$_2$-microglobulin-like proteins. *Science* 1989;243:655-657.

29. Baratz ME, Georgescu HI, Evans CH: Studies on the autocrine activation of a synovial cell line. *J Orthop Res* 1991;9:651-657.

30. Sung K, Mendelow D, Georgescu HI, et al: Characterisation of chondrocyte activation in response to cytokines synthesised by a synovial cell line. *Biochim Biophys Acta* 1988;971:148-156.

31. Dingle JT, Saklatvala J, Hembry R, et al: A cartilage catabolic factor from synovium. *Biochem J* 1979;184:177-180.
32. Levick JR: Hypoxia and acidosis in chronic inflammatory arthritis; relation to vascular supply and dynamic effusion pressure. *J Rheumatol* 1990;17:579-582.
33. Allen RE, Blake DR, Nazhat NB, et al: Superoxide radical generation by inflamed human synovium after hypoxia. *Lancet* 1989;2:282-283.
34. Evans CH, Mears DC, McKnight JL: A preliminary ferrographic survey of the wear particles in human synovial fluid. *Arthritis Rheum* 1981;24:912-918.
35. Evans CH, Mears DC, Stanitski CL: Ferrographic analysis of wear in human joints: Evaluation by comparison with arthroscopic examination of symptomatic knee joints. *J Bone Joint Surg* 1982;64B:572-578.
36. Evans CH, Mears DC, Cosgrove JL: Release of neutral proteinases from mononuclear phagocytes and synovial cells in response to cartilaginous wear particles in vitro. *Biochim Biophys Acta* 1981;677:287-294.
37. Evans CH, Mazzocchi RA, Nelson DD, et al: Experimental arthritis induced by intraarticular injection of allogenic cartilaginous particles into rabbit knees. *Arthritis Rheum* 1984;27:200-207.
38. Boniface RJ, Cain PR, Evans CH: Articular responses to purified cartilage proteoglycans. *Arthritis Rheum* 1988;31:258-266.
39. Olson EJ, Kang JD, Fu FH, et al: The biochemical and histological effects of artificial ligament wear particles: In vitro and in vivo studies. *Am J Sports Med* 1988;16:558-570.
40. Galante JO, Lemons J, Spector M, et al: The biologic effects of implant materials. *J Orthop Res* 1991;9:760-775.
41. Frost L, Ghosh P: Microinjury to the synovial membrane may cause disaggregation of proteoglycans in rabbit knee joint articular cartilage. *J Orthop Res* 1984;2:207-220.
42. Lukoschek M, Schaffler MB, Burr DB, et al: Synovial membrane and cartilage changes in experimental osteoarthrosis. *J Orthop Res* 1988;6:475-492.

Chapter 3

Mechanism of Postoperative and Posttraumatic Arthrofibrosis

Per A. Renström, MD, PhD
James T. Ninomiya, MD, MS

Knee ligament injuries are very common; however, their treatment is still open to discussion. Reconstructive surgery is generally accepted as the treatment of choice for anterior cruciate ligament (ACL) injuries in young, active patients. Surgical techniques for treatment of these injuries have developed rapidly over the last 20 years, culminating in the introduction of arthroscopically assisted techniques. These techniques are technically demanding, but are routinely used because the outcome is now predictable, although there is still a risk of complications. Limitation of knee motion, which is the single most common and difficult of these complications,[1-6] can be caused by arthrofibrosis of the knee.

The main problem associated with knee arthrofibrosis is a flexion contracture or an inability to fully extend the knee. The normal knee extends to at least 0 degrees or into a few degrees of hyperextension; a patient has a flexion contracture when there is a 5-cm heel-side difference measured in the prone position. Loss of full extension can be a disaster for the knee and the lower extremity because it makes normal gait impossible. A flexion contracture from more than 5 to 20 degrees will cause a limp, and a contracture of more than 20 degrees will cause a leg-length discrepancy leading to serious secondary problems.

Loss of full extension generates increased load on the knee. Weightbearing on a flexed knee significantly increases the load on the posterior distal femoral condyles and the posterior half of the tibial plateau; moreover, the quadriceps force needed to stabilize the flexed knee during weightbearing increases with increasing knee flexion.[7] Inability to fully contract the quadriceps muscles results in reduced muscle strength and atrophy, especially of the vastus medialis, and greatly increases the risks for both intra-articular and interarticular overuse problems.

Limited knee flexion can be experienced as a problem in sports such as gymnastics, wrestling, skiing, and track and field events, but is, in general, better tolerated than limited knee extension. Inability to flex the knee more than 125 degrees will result in decreased running speed.

Harner and associates[8] found an 11.1% incidence of lost knee motion after ACL surgery. Risk factors included acute surgery carried out within one month after trauma and performance of additional extra-articular surgery. Age, meniscal repair, and tourniquet time were not related to loss of motion.[8] However, DeHaven[9] considers increased acute knee ligament surgery on patients over age 25 to be a risk factor.

Although arthrofibrosis can occur after any type of knee surgery, the literature has focused on complications after ACL surgery. Routine arthroscopic meniscectomy, patellofemoral surgery, knee replacement surgery, or high tibial osteotomies can also result in a major loss of motion. Other possible causes of arthrofibrosis include trauma such as fractures around the knee, long-term immobilization, poor rehabilitation, reflex sympathetic dystrophy, infection, and sepsis.

According to Paulos and associates,[10] 5% to 10% of patients going through intra-articular ACL surgery may develop primary arthrofibrosis or fibrotic healing response. Another 10% may develop arthrofibrosis secondary to nonisometric positioning or long-term casting, allowing the fat pad to become fibrotic.

Pathology of Arthrofibrosis

In his 1917 discussion of the morbid anatomy of knee stiffness, Payr[11] concluded that the suprapatellar tissues were involved first, and resulted in quadriceps sclerosis and patellofemoral adhesions. The final stage was a fixed patella with patellar, femoral, and tibial articular cartilage destruction secondary to invasion by fibrosclerotic pannus.

In 1963, Nicoll[12] described loss of knee motion caused by fibrosis of the vastus intermedius, intracapsular adhesions between the patella and femur, fibrosis of the vastus lateralis with adhesions to the condyles, and shortening of the rectus femoris.

O'Connor[13] attributed loss of knee motion to an extracapsular band extending from the proximal pole of the patella to the anterior femur. This band has also been described by Sprague and associates,[5] who categorized 24 patients with restricted knee motion into three groups: (1) those with discrete bands or a single sheet of adhesions; (2) those with complete obliteration of the suprapatellar pouch and gutters with massive adhesions; and (3) those with multiple bands of adhesions or obliteration of the suprapatellar pouch with an additional extracapsular band about 1 cm wide, which was considered important in restricting motion.

Flexion contracture can be caused by the posterior capsule adhering to itself and to the posterior femoral condyle.[14] Hamstring muscle and cruciate ligament contractures play only a minor role.

Jackson and Schaefer[15] have described a nodule of peripheral fibrous tissue located anterolateral to the tibial tunnel placement of the ACL graft. These nodules, called cyclops, may cause impingement, resulting in a postoperative loss of full extension and a notable clunking sound that can be heard with terminal extension. The authors believe that cartilaginous tissue lifted from the tibia during the drilling of the tibial tunnel may then form a nidus for a fibroproliferative process, resulting in cyclops formation.[15]

Arthrofibrosis may be present in intra-articular or extra-articular tissues. Richmond and Al Assal[16] have identified three areas that may contribute to loss of mobility: (1) intra-articular adhesions; (2) extracapsular bands of O'Connor; and (3) patellar entrapment syndrome, which they define as a subcategory of arthrofibrosis. The patellar entrapment syndromes have also been called developmental patella infera syndrome and infrapatellar contracture syndrome.

The intra-articular arthrofibrosis usually involves the medial and lateral peripatellar recesses, the anterior structures, and the suprapatellar pouch; a cyclops lesion can be present. This intra-articular involvement usually limits flexion and causes only mild limitations of extension.

Developmental patella infera syndrome was first described in 1982 by Caton and associates.[17] Surgery or trauma produced secondary low patella position that resulted in a disabling condition in half of 128 cases. The origin was iatrogenic, mechanical, natural, or inflammatory.

Wojtys and associates[18] reported on 11 patients who had patella infera syndrome following trauma of surgery with symptoms such as: (1) transient patella infera resulting from peripatellar and fat pad soft-tissue contractures and quadriceps weakness; (2) joint stiffness resulting from associated arthrofibrosis; (3) permanent shortening of the patellar ligament when the condition was not effectively treated; and (4) eventual onset of patellofemoral arthrosis. Noyes and associates'[19] pathomechanics for developmental patella infera, patellar tendon shortening, and arthrosis are presented in Figure 1.[19]

According to Noyes and associates,[20,21] ACL surgery seems to be the most frequent factor initiating patella infera syndrome. Limited knee motion, joint stiffness, and significant quadriceps muscle weakness were found in the postoperative period. The two most significant contributing factors were soft-tissue contracture of peripatellar tissues and quadriceps weakness. Case reports showed that adaptive shortening of the patellar ligament may occur shortly after surgery.

Paulos and associates[10] have described an entrapment of the patella in association with loss of extension and flexion caused primarily by an exaggerated pathologic fibrous hyperplasia of the anterior soft tissue of the knee, which they call infrapatellar contracture syndrome (Fig. 2). This syndrome can also be secondary to the prolonged immobility and lack of extension associated with intra-articular surgery. Failure to improve with rehabilitation is an important clue to its presence.

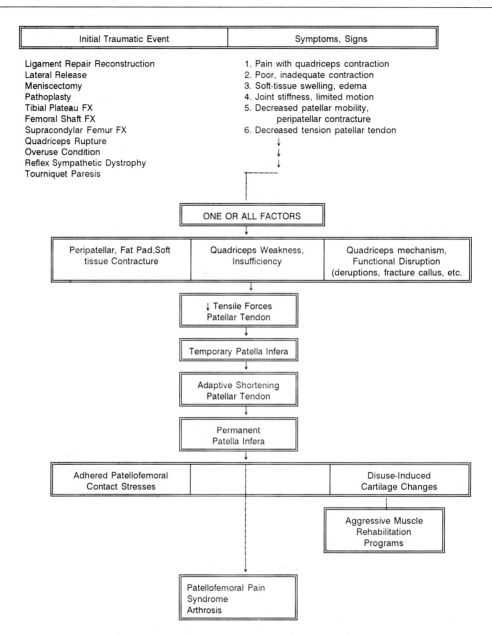

Initial Traumatic Event	Symptoms, Signs

Ligament Repair Reconstruction
Lateral Release
Meniscectomy
Pathoplasty
Tibial Plateau FX
Femoral Shaft FX
Supracondylar Femur FX
Quadriceps Rupture
Overuse Condition
Reflex Sympathetic Dystrophy
Tourniquet Paresis

1. Pain with quadriceps contraction
2. Poor, inadequate contraction
3. Soft-tissue swelling, edema
4. Joint stiffness, limited motion
5. Decreased patellar mobility,
    peripatellar contracture
6. Decreased tension patellar tendon

ONE OR ALL FACTORS

Peripatellar, Fat Pad, Soft tissue Contracture	Quadriceps Weakness, Insufficiency	Quadriceps mechanism, Functional Disruption (deruptions, fracture callus, etc.

↓ Tensile Forces
Patellar Tendon

Temporary Patella Infera

Adaptive Shortening
Patellar Tendon

Permanent
Patella Infera

Adhered Patellofemoral Contact Stresses		Disuse-Induced Cartilage Changes

Aggressive Muscle
Rehabilitation
Programs

Patellofemoral Pain
Syndrome
Arthrosis

Fig. 1 *Pathomechanics for developmental patella infera, patellar tendon shortening, and arthrosis. (Reproduced with permission from Noyes FR, Wojtys EM, Marshall MT: The early diagnosis and treatment of developmental patella infera syndrome. Clin Orthop 1991;265:241-252.)*

Infrapatellar contracture syndrome has three stages. Stage 1, called the prodromal stage, includes induration of the synovial fat pad and retinacular tissues. Motion is painful, patellar mobility is restricted, and quadriceps lag is present. Stage 2, called the active stage, involves continued peripatellar swelling with severely re-

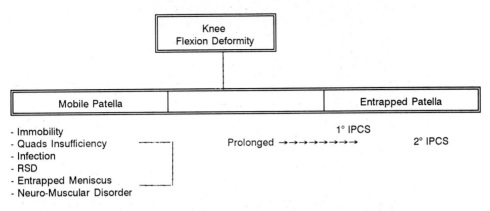

Fig. 2 *Etiology of infrapatellar contracture syndrome. RSD = reflex sympathetic dystrophy; IPCS = infrapatellar contracture syndrome. (Reproduced with permission from Paulos LE, Rosenberg TD, Drawbert J, et al: Infrapatellar contracture syndrome. An unrecognized cause of knee stiffness with patella entrapment and patella infera. Am J Sports Med 1987;15:331-341.)*

stricted patellar motion. It is at Stage 3, called the burned-out stage, that the development of patellar infera is the key finding.

Paulos and associates[10] reported that patella infera occurred in 16% of their cases; these were the majority of their Stage 3 patients. They found that a very specific set of conditions must occur simultaneously for patella infera to develop. First, there must be a constricting scarification caused by a peritendinous inflammatory reaction in the tissues surrounding the patellar tendon. Second, the patella must become entrapped in the lower femoral sulcus, secondary to patellofemoral adhesions in the medial/lateral and superpatellar areas as well as to infrapatellar contracture.

Prolonged patellar entrapment also resulted in destructive changes in the articular surface of the tibia, femur, and patella. These changes were caused by a pressure alteration that appeared whenever the fibrosclerotic fat pad impinged against a medial or lateral femoral condyle, or appeared as an infiltrating inflammatory pannus extending from the medial and lateral gutters over the noncontact surfaces of the joint. This pannus was extremely adherent, and the cartilage below was discolored, softened, and fibrillated. Cadaver studies have shown that fibrosclerosis in the fat pad results in a firm tissue block to normal knee extension.[10] Because the fat pad extends into the intracondylar notch throughout the ligamentum mucosum, and is firmly attached to the anterior aspect of the medial and lateral menisci, tibial impingement becomes prominent and locks extension.

Paulos and associates'[10] belief that developmental patella infera is a consequence of patellar entrapment in infrapatellar contracture syndrome is supported by the fact that patients with quadriceps hypertonia are extremely common, yet developmental patella infera is very rare. Noyes and associates[19] believe that infrapatellar contracture syndrome actually represents patella infera syndrome, and that the former term is incorrect because contractures involve all the tissues about the knee. Why some patients get arthrofibrosis as a postoperative or posttraumatic complication is still unknown.

Cause of Arthrofibrosis

Immobilization of joints with inflamed soft tissue can produce joint stiffness. The mechanism for this is still under debate. Peacock[22] concluded that joint stiffness was secondary to changes affecting the joint capsular tissues, and that new collagen synthesis caused shortening of capsular and collateral tissues. Akeson and associates[23,24] found no change in total collagen content, and they concluded, "The mechanism which changed the physical characteristics of periarticular connective tissue seemed to be the cross-linking of existing fibers, or deposition of a small amount of new collagen, disposed randomly in the connective tissue weave without regard to the usual constraints imposed by physical forces." Loss of motion results in decreased water content and causes glycosaminoglycans; increased collagen fiber cross-linking causes changes in the fat pad and retinacular tissues.[10]

Limitation of knee motion in combination with trauma, such as acute intra-articular surgery, may cause an excessive fibrotic response in the repair process. Although little is known about the cause of this arthrofibrosis, some information is available about the mechanism of fibrogenesis in the lung, liver, and skin. Fibrosis is recognized as the end stage of a variety of systemic or organ-specific diseases such as pulmonary fibrosis, hepatic cirrhosis, and scleroderma.[25] Infectious diseases such as filariasis and schistosomiasis, along with iatrogenic causes such as bleomycin and irradiation therapies are also associated with fibrosis.[26-30] Hypertrophic scar formation in the skin can result in keloid formation, which can present as much difficulty as the original injury.[31] The phenomenon occurring within these fibrotic structures is probably quite similar to the proliferation of myofibroblast-like cells characterizing injury and repair in other tissues, such as the synovium and capsular structures of the knee.

The Synovium

The involvement of the synovium is not fully clear. This layer of cells, which lines articular joints, forms an interface between the joint space and the articular cartilage. Histologically, the synovium is generally from one to three cells in depth, with the cells loosely arranged in sheets. Morphologically, there appear to be two principal types of synovial cells, which have been designated type A and type B cells. The type A cell is characterized by prominent Golgi apparatus, many intracellular vacuoles, and scant endoplasmic reticulum. In contrast, the type B cell has scant Golgi apparatus and abundant rough endoplasmic reticulum. It is not clear whether these two types of cells represent different states of maturation or differentiation of a single cell lineage or, in fact, are distinct in their origins.[32-34]

The two main functions of these cells are to remove debris from within the joint space and to produce synovial fluid hyaluronic acid. The synovial cells are able to phagocytose small particles, including ferritin, colloidal gold, and other substances such as red blood cells and their fragments. However, type A cells are believed to be more active in the uptake and processing of particulate material than type B cells.[35]

Another important function attributed to synovial cells is the presentation of antigens for activation of the immune response. In addition, macrophage-like cells in the synovial layer are capable of releasing a variety of cytokines, which could influence the ingrowth and proliferation of fibroblasts and chondroblasts.[36-38] This is important in the pathogenesis of arthrofibrosis.

Merry and associates[39] have suggested a mechanism of chronic synovitis in rheumatoid arthritis that may also be applicable to the synovitis seen after knee surgery. They suggest that the chronic synovitis in rheumatoid arthritis is an example of a hypoxic-reperfusion injury.[39,40] This mechanism, which has been demonstrated in heart disease and in the gut, is characterized by a period of temporary ischemia followed by reperfusion of the tissue, which results in the production of reactive oxygen species that are then responsible for tissue damage and subsequent inflammation.[41]

Pressure of synovial fluid in both resting and exercising volunteers and animals was shown to be slightly below atmospheric pressure at rest, and increased to as high as 800 mm Hg during quadriceps setting.[42-45] Additionally, there was a mean rise in synovial fluid pressure of over 160 mm Hg during exercise in a group of patients with rheumatoid arthritis, accompanied by a fall in synovial fluid oxygen pressure from a mean resting level of 61 mm Hg to 41 mm Hg. The hydrostatic pressure in normal synovial cavities is about 30 mm Hg, and it can be increased to 60 mm Hg in inflamed tissues. Therefore, after injury and the resulting hemarthrosis or effusion, there is a potential for temporary occlusion of the synovial capillary bed, producing a temporary hypoxic environment.[46,47]

The mechanism of this effect is believed to involve the formation of reactive oxygen species such as superoxide anion, hydrogen peroxide, and the hydroxyl radical. These highly chemically reactive species have been shown to form products of joint damage such as lipid peroxidation products as well as alterations in the structure of the immunoglobulin TgF. Results of other in vitro studies have shown that these reactive oxygen species can also denature proteoglycans, leading to cartilage damage and causing denaturation of glycosaminoglycans such as hyaluronic acid.[48-51] Thus, hemarthrosis could result in an increase in intracapsular pressure, which might produce a transient ischemia of the synovium, resulting in a generalized joint reaction that would include the activation and pro-liferation of fibroblasts and the formation of arthrofibrosis.

Wound Healing

Wound healing and the response to injury involve a complex se-ries of events characterized by interactions between cellular and biochemical elements. Historically, this series has been divided chronologically into three basic phases that actually represent a continuum of events.[52] The first phase is characterized by an inflam-matory response, followed by the formation of granulation tissues, and then a remodeling phase with matrix formation.

The initial events in the inflammatory phase of acute traumatic wound repair are characterized by bleeding, resulting in activation of the blood coagulation cascade and associated platelet aggregation and activation.[53,54] A blood clot is formed for hemostasis, numerous factors for chemotaxis and growth stimulation are released, and there is a rapid influx of both monocytes and leukocytes. These cell types are attracted by a variety of chemotactic factors, many of which are contained and released by platelets, such as fibronectin and fibrinogen, along with growth factors such as platelet-derived growth factor and transforming growth factors.[55-58]

The second phase of wound healing, which occurs after approxi-mately 48 hours, includes the formation of granulation tissue. This tissue consists of an amorphous mixture of fibroblasts, macro-phages, neovessels, and collagenous extracellular matrix. Among the major cell types of granulation tissue are myofibroblasts, which play an important role in wound contraction.[59]

The third phase of wound healing is remodeling, which is charac-terized by an alteration in the extracellular matrix. This alteration in composition can affect the phenotypic expression of a variety of cell types, thereby influencing the final distribution of cells in a healing wound.

One of the most extensively studied models for fibrosis is the human disease scleroderma. Although neither its cause nor its pathogenesis is known, the disease demonstrates cellular and bio-chemical interactions that ultimately result in extensive fibrosis.[60-63] Hallmarks of the disease include alterations in endothelial cells lin-ing the microcirculation, along with intimal fibrosis of arteries, re-sulting in partial obstruction. Another major characteristic of sclero-derma is the presence of autoantibodies that are similar to those in other autoimmune processes such as systemic lupus erythematosus. Although attempts have been made to isolate and identify a specific immunologic cause of scleroderma, it still remains unclear whether autoantibodies result from or cause the disease.[64]

Clearly, one of the most important characteristics of scleroderma is fibrosis and the resulting tissue damage. Studies of fibroblasts in vitro have shown that these cells produce more collagen in persons with scleroderma than in those without the disease.[65,66] Claman[25]

Outline 1 Fibroblast activities in wound repair

Wound Contraction
    Phenotypic alteration
        Retraction of Golgi and endoplasmic reticulum
        Formation of large actin bundles
    Migration into wound defect
    Deposition of fibronectin and types III/I collagen
    Formation of fibronexus
    Contraction

Formation and Remodeling of Matrix
    Fibronectin
    Hyaluronic acid
    Collagen, types III/I
    Proteoglycans
    Proteases and other enzymes

(Adapted with permission from Clark RAF: Cutaneous tissue repair: Basic biologic considerations: I. *J Am Acad Dermatol* 1985;13:701-725.)

has suggested that mast cells may play an important role in the fibrosis of scleroderma. He based his model on the observations of other workers that mast cells have been prominent in a number of conditions characterized by fibrosis, such as keloids, hypertrophic scars, and neurofibrosis. Additionally, an increase in these cells has been noted in the pulmonary fibrosis seen with bleomycin therapy or radiation therapy, along with the increase in macrophages, lymphocytes, and neutrophils.

Claman[60] postulated that heparin, which was released from mast cells bound to endothelial cells, caused the release of endothelial cell-derived growth factors[60,67] and that the heparin also served as a potent angiogenic stimulus for neovascularization. The resulting presence of these growth factors, along with heparin-binding growth factors such as fibroblast growth factors, could then play a role in the stimulation of mesenchymal cells, including fibroblasts, which would ultimately result in fibrosis.

Although fibroblasts have traditionally been believed to have somewhat uniform morphology, they apparently are able to perform a variety of functions, in addition to their established role in the synthesis of extracellular matrix (Outline 1).[68-70] Stromal cells, which are predominant in mesenchymal tissue, are able to produce the various types of collagen molecules, along with proteoglycans such as hyaluronic acid, chondroitin sulfates, heparan sulfates, and dermatan sulfates.[71,72] They are even capable of synthesizing growth factors.[73]

Ultrastructural studies have also revealed several different forms of fibroblasts.[74] One of the most interesting forms of fibroblasts is the myofibroblast, with morphologic characteristics combining those of fibroblasts and smooth muscle cells.[75] Myofibroblasts are seen in the granulation phase of wound healing and clearly play a key role in wound contraction. They contain the contractile elements of actin and myosin, and they respond to a variety of pharmacologic agents in a fashion similar to the smooth muscle reactions to serotonin, angiotensin, epinephrine, and vasopressin.[76]

One of the major advances in the cellular differentiation of fibroblasts has been the use of cytoskeletal markers.[77] Four main phenotypes of fibroblasts have been identified: (1) those expressing vimentin; (2) those co-expressing vimentin and desmin; (3) those expressing vimentin and smooth-muscle actin; and (4) those expressing vimentin, actin, and smooth-muscle actin. During wound healing, a transition of cell types has been demonstrated, which leads toward the formation of actin-containing cells with the characteristics of smooth muscle cells. These cells are believed to act as myofibroblasts in wound contraction in granulation tissue. As a corollary, when the wound is closed, these myofibroblasts disappear. However, the myofibroblasts persist in hypertrophic scars, as well as in lesions such as scleroderma, nodule fasciitis, and tenosynovitis. In Dupuytren's disease, myofibroblast-like cells proliferate within nodules at the disease site.

However, despite the ultrastructural information regarding the alteration of phenotypic expression during wound healing, the exact origin of myofibroblasts has yet to be determined. It is not clear whether the proliferation of myofibroblasts in wound healing results from clonal expansion of a subpopulation of cells, or whether these cells arise from pluripotent mesenchymal cells under the influence of growth factors. The stimuli and possible signal mechanisms responsible for the proliferation and reorganization of these factors are not well known. Several underlying mechanisms including roles for extracellular matrix, mechanical stress, growth factors, and mediators will be discussed.

The extracellular matrix is altered considerably in the disease stage. There are increased amounts and probably altered forms of fibronectin,[78] collagen,[79] elastin,[80] and glycosaminoglycans[80] in granulation tissue and fibrotic lengths. This could be a key stimulus, modulating both proliferation and differentiation of myofibroblast-like cells in the fibrotic lung.[81] Mechanical stress is an important factor regulating cell and tissue growth;[82] passive tension or stretch can affect tissue metabolism and induce collagen deposition in several organs.[83] Stretching can provoke the development of myofibroblast-like cells in skin tissue, although stretching by itself resulted in no evidence of inflammation and wounding alone did not stimulate proliferation of these cells. However, a combination of stretching and wounding provoked such a response.[84] Myofibroblast cells may thus develop from a modulation of existing fibroblasts brought about by mechanical tension within the material.

Biochemically, several factors play an important role in the etiology of fibrosis. One of the most exciting areas of research has been the study of transforming growth factor-β (TGF-β), which has multiple effects on virtually every cell type. Originally isolated from platelets, the mature form of TGF-β consists of two identical chains of 112 amino acids and is highly conserved in different species. Five additional types of TGF-β have been identified and cloned as well.[85,86]

Initial studies revealed that TGF-β could enhance the growth of fibroblasts in tissue culture. More recent evidence indicates that TGF-β can stimulate cell proliferation in some tissues, as shown with fibroblasts, while in other tissues, such as lymphocytes and epithelial cells, it can be a potent inhibitor.[87] In fact most eucaryotic cells seem to have TGF-β receptors.

The role of TGF-β in the inflammatory response has been widely investigated.[31] This protein, which is concentrated in the platelet alpha granule, is released at the time of injury. Upon its release, TGF-β has very potent positive chemotactic properties for macrophages, cells that play an important role in inflammation and fibrosis. In addition, it stimulates growth factor synthesis, as well as fibroblast growth and differentiation. Thus, TGF-β may play a pivotal role in the regulation of the many steps in wound healing and the development of fibrosis.[88]

Platelet-derived growth factor (PDGF), another potent mitogen for all mesenchymal cells, was first identified in platelets.[89] In organ culture, it has been shown to stimulate cell replication and collagenous and noncollagenous protein synthesis. The presence of PDGF in early as well as chronic stages of wound healing may contribute to normal, abnormal, and excessive tissue repair. There is probably a connection between PDGF and TGF-β.[90,91]

Proteins associated with adhesive properties, such as fibronectin, may also play an important role in the deposition and formation of granulation tissue. Several studies have indicated that a fibronectin matrix is initially formed, which can then act as a scaffold or template upon which collagen can be deposited. Results of in vitro studies have shown that in the absence of ascorbate, a dense fibronectin network will form but no collagen will be deposited.[92-95]

While the accumulation of collagen in fibrosis may result from excessive formation, another equally important cause might be altered or diminished matrix degradation. During the dynamic process of wound healing, the remodeling process also requires the presence of a variety of degradative enzymes such as collagenase and hyaluronidase. PDGF, tumor necrosis factor, and interleukin-1 have all been shown to increase the production of collagenase and other degradative proteins. In contrast, TGF-β has been shown to inhibit the degradation of newly synthesized matrix by inhibiting protein synthesis.[96]

Other cytokines such as interleukin-1 seem to play an important role in the activation of protease-secreting cells such as chondrocytes or synovial cells. Interleukin-1 can also decrease the production of a tissue inhibitor of metalloproteinases, especially collagenase. Thus, a deficiency of cytokines such as interleukin-1 could result in a decrease in the turnover of granulation tissue in wound healing, resulting in a net accumulation of collagen, and ultimately, fibrosis.[97-100]

Clearly, wound healing and fibrosis are complex combinations of multiple cellular and biochemical interactions. Simplistically, fibrosis might result from an individual's hereditary predisposition to form exuberant granulation tissues and scars, such as keloids. An acquired or autoimmune alteration also might lead to excessive collagen formation or deficient collagen degradation with continued collagen synthesis, resulting in arthrofibrosis. Finally, local effects such as persistent, profound bleeding at the time of initial insult or at surgery might result in overstimulation of the healing cascade, ultimately leading to excessive collagen formation. The potential role of growth factors and the molecular biology of healing offer a number of exciting possibilities in the understanding of both wound healing and fibrosis.

Prevention of Arthrofibrosis

Prevention of arthrofibrosis is, in many cases, probably possible. Surgical technique, meticulous surgical management, and aggressive rehabilitation are of major importance.

Timing of Surgery

Timing of the surgery is critical. Arthrofibrosis occurs more in the acutely reconstructed anterior cruciate ligament (ACL) than in the reconstructed chronic ACL-deficient knee.[101] In a retrospective study of 169 acute ACL reconstructions, a population of young athletes whose ligaments were reconstructed within the first week of injury were compared with patients who had ACL reconstructions at least 21 days or more after the trauma. Shelbourne and associates[6] found that the patients with ligaments reconstructed within the first week of injury had a statistically increased incidence of arthrofibrosis that was characterized by limited extension and increased formation of scar tissue. The evidence suggests that delaying reconstructive surgery until three weeks after the time of the trauma will result in earlier return of strength and, more importantly, in a significantly decreased incidence of arthrofibrosis and lack of full extension.

At the time of acute injury, there is blood surrounding the ACL stump. Initially, there is a clot matrix that is replaced by neovascularization after a few days.[102] This is accompanied by an ingrowth of fibroblasts that migrate into the wound. By the middle of the second week, inflammation and vascularity regress while, simultaneously, fibroblasts proliferate and secrete collagen into the extracellular space. If the surgery is carried out after this regression, the risk of arthrofibrosis seems to decrease.

A delay in reconstruction also is beneficial for the patient in other ways. Preoperative physical therapy, which emphasizes the same important principles as postoperative physical therapy, can be carried out to restore good range of motion. Also, the patient is more prepared psychologically for surgical treatment after waiting a couple of weeks.

Surgical Techniques

Meticulous surgical techniques involve the use of arthroscopy, proper graft placement and tension, and adequate notchplasty. The use of the arthroscope in the reconstruction of cruciate ligament injuries has improved the surgeon's view of the surgical site, allowing increased evaluation of the graft placement. There is less arthrofibrosis with arthroscopically-assisted techniques.[15] Restricted final motion has been shown to be correlated with open surgery and surgery performed within seven days.[103] Graft placement is considered essential in successful ACL surgery. Even a somewhat (above 1 cm) anteriorly placed graft on the femur results in problems with flexion and lengthening of the ligament. Successful surgical reconstruction of the ACL may depend on an appropriate initial tension of the graft at the time of fixation,[104] because there is a complex link between reconstructed ACL tension and tibiofemoral joint kinematics.

Graft impingement caused by graft hypertrophy or notch osteophytes can result in motion problems. ACL surgery techniques currently used include primary repair; augmented repair; and primary, allograft, and artificial graft reconstruction with prosthetic devices or a composite reconstruction with a ligament augmentation device. The most common technique is the bone-patellar tendon-bone autograft, which has excellent results in strength, stability, and long-term effectiveness. There is a theoretical advantage in using a semitendinosus and gracilis autograft, an allograft, or a prosthetic ligament. Autografts seem to result in loss of motion twice as often as allografts.[8] According to Cannon and Vittori,[105] notchplasty should be carried out high enough superiorly to allow for accommodation of the ACL graft during full extension, and there should be approximately 2 mm between the graft and the top of the notch with the knee in full extension.

Adequate graft fixation techniques are essential to allow early motion. Bone-to-bone healing is preferable, and interference screw technique will secure good fixation. The double-staple technique is also a valid clinical choice for graft fixation.[106] Surgery of the cruciate ligaments has become technically very demanding; it is considered difficult and highly specialized and should be performed by experienced surgeons.

Aggressive Rehabilitation

Aggressive rehabilitation emphasizes early motion because motion improves the mechanical and structural properties of the ligaments of the knee.[107] The early phase includes control of pain and swelling to prevent inhibition of the muscles. Shelbourne and associates[108] have used an aggressive accelerated rehabilitation program that emphasizes full passive extension, muscle control, management of swelling, early motion, and exercise. This program has been demonstrated to improve knee function more rapidly than more conventional protocols.

Joint stiffness after ligament reconstruction has been attributed to surgeons' failure to ensure early motion of the joint. The concept of early motion after knee ligament surgery was recognized by Eriksson and Häggmark,[107] but it was not until the end of the 1980s that this practice was considered safe by most orthopaedic surgeons. Today, early motion is considered necessary and, therefore, it is routine.

Continuous passive motion significantly stimulates the healing of articular tissues, including cartilage, tendons, and ligaments. The use of continuous passive motion after conventional knee ligament surgery is probably beneficial, but it has not been shown to be of significant long-term benefit.

Treatment of Arthrofibrosis

Recognition

Recognition of arthrofibrosis is extremely important. Patients at risk have exaggerated inflammatory soft-tissue response with excessive pain, warmth about the knee, some swelling, and limitation of knee motion. These patients should be treated immediately to control pain and swelling that, if untreated, will lead to muscle inhibition and other secondary reactions.

Physical Therapy

Physical therapy is very important, and the therapy program should be closely supervised. Joint effusion should be aspirated. Patella mobilization should be a routine aspect of the rehabilitation program, with medial lateral and proximal distal patella mobilization performed four to six times daily.[19] Quadriceps and hamstring exercises should be done, and sometimes electrical stimulation is valuable.

Manipulation

The degree of joint manipulation is also important. A joint with arthrofibrosis is often a joint with adhesions to the articular cartilage, and vigorous manipulation can result in major damage by either avulsing articular cartilage or leaving fibrous tissue covering the hyaline cartilage.[109,110] Therefore, arthroscopy always should be done before manipulation to evaluate the intra-articular damage and to treat the arthrofibrosis.

Surgery

Surgery is sometimes necessary. Indications for surgery include extension limitation of more than 10 degrees, flexion limitation of less than 125 degrees, failure with physical therapy, and functional impairment.

Open intra-articular surgical procedures have been used in improving flexion.[12,111-113] However, during the last decade, use of arthroscopic surgical techniques has increased, with good results including marked improvement of mobility.[5,13,114-116] Intra-articular surgery can include arthroscopy, percutaneous lysis, manipulation, and excision of scar tissue.[9] With this type of surgery, DeHaven improved flexion contraction from 17 degrees preoperatively to 2 degrees postoperatively with follow-up results of 5 degrees.[9] Parisien[117] and Del Pizzo and associates[118] used capsular releases in addition to lysis of adhesions and manipulation to increase motion. Arthrofibrosis surgery has been carried out successfully by Jackson and associates[15] whose patients' range of motion was 16 to 103 degrees before surgery and improved to 6 to 130 degrees after surgery.

The extra-articular surgery includes resection of the dense fibrosis around the patellar tendon in combination with manipulation into extension, continuous passive motion, and physical therapy. Paulos and associates[10] defined infrapatellar contracture syndrome as a subcategory of arthrofibrosis, with the patient having a loss of both extension and flexion, and recommended open treatment of these patients.

Richmond and Al Assal[16] developed an arthroscopic technique that includes systematic resection of adhesions, followed by freeing the vastus intermedius and any bands from the anterior femur. They follow resection of the scarred and contractive fat pad by lateral retinacular release if the passive patella glide is abnormal, and they reserve medial retinacular release for those whose patella glide remains limited at the lateral release. Improperly positioned ACL grafts should be resected if all else has failed to gain adequate motion at surgery. The use of continuous passive motion was the key in maintaining motion gains and minimizing mobility and hospitalization. By using this technique, they obtained a 50-degree increase in total range of motion in the routine arthrofibrosis patient and a 45-degree increase in patients with infrapatellar contracture syndrome.[16]

If full extension is not achieved after resection of the fat pad and anterior adhesions, an additional posterior approach can be attempted. Wilson[114] described posterior capsulotomy in certain flexion contractures of the knee; his technique has been modified by Bhan and associates.[116] Posterior release, in these arthrofibrotic cases, can be carried out through a posterior medial incision with release of posterior synovium adhesions and the posterior capsule. Manipulation is often needed to achieve full extension. In seven patients, we achieved full extension by means of a posterior release of the medial and lateral capsule from the bone. After surgery, the patients are immobilized in a cast locked in full extension for seven days.

The results of arthrofibrosis surgery vary. The functional outcome is not always good. In 35 cases reported by DeHaven,[9] results were excellent in 15%, good in 38%, fair in 32%, and poor in 15%. Most had significant gains in extension and flexion, but the degree of functional capacity was often disappointing. Degenerative changes and patella infera are not uncommon.

Discussion

The limitation of knee motion can be secondary to faulty surgical technique and poor rehabilitation, but in many cases there is an excessive fibrotic response in the repair process causing arthrofibrosis. Wahl and associates[119] theorized that fibrosis in soft-tissue injury may result from increased numbers (proliferation and recruitment) of collagen-synthesizing cells, increased matrix synthesis by existing cells, and/or deficient collagen degradation with continued collagen synthesis. An imbalance between synthesis and degradation leads to collagen accumulation. Important information is, however, still needed on the role of known biomechanical and cellular mechanisms as they apply to the fibrotic knee. It is necessary to determine which cells secrete and synthesize a large area of products affecting fibroblasts, and inflammatory and immune cells. Little is known about the biologic interactions between cell mediators and enzymes. Details may vary from organ to organ, but the basic patterns in producing fibrosis seem to be similar.

Although the incidence of knee arthrofibrosis seems to decrease with improved surgical technique, early motion, and increased awareness of the disorder, arthrofibrosis continues to be a problem. Clinicians must concentrate on early recognition of this problem, and basic scientists need to address some of the basic questions regarding its etiology.

References

1. Fullerton LR Jr, Andrews JR: Mechanical block to extension following augmentation of the anterior cruciate ligament: A case report. *Am J Sports Med* 1984;12:166-168.

2. Graf B, Uhr F: Complications of intra-articular anterior cruciate reconstruction. *Clin Sports Med* 1988;7:835-848.

3. Hughston JC: Complications of anterior cruciate ligament surgery. *Orthop Clin North Am* 1985;16:237-240.

4. Noyes FR, Mangine RE, Barber S: Early knee motion after open and arthroscopic anterior cruciate ligament reconstruction. *Am J Sports Med* 1987;15:149-160.

5. Sprague NF, O'Connor RL, Fox JM: Arthroscopic treatment of postoperative knee fibroarthrosis. *Clin Orthop* 1982;166:165-172.

6. Shelbourne KD, Wilckens JH, Mollabashy A, et al: Arthrofibrosis in acute anterior cruciate ligament reconstruction: The effect of timing of reconstruction and rehabilitation. *Am J Sports Med* 1991;19:332-336.

7. Perry J, Antonelli D, Ford W: Analysis of knee-joint forces during flexed-knee stance. *J Bone Joint Surg* 1975;57A:961-967.

8. Harner CD, Paul JJ, Fu FH, et al: Loss of knee motion following arthroscopic anterior cruciate ligament reconstruction. Presented at the 58th Annual Meeting of the American Academy of Orthopaedic Surgeons, Anaheim, CA, March 7-12, 1991.

9. DeHaven K: Arthrofibrosis of the knee. Proceedings of Sports Medicine Course, *Current Concepts of Sports Medicine*, University of Vermont, Burlington, VT, October 2-4, 1991.

10. Paulos LE, Rosenberg TD, Drawbert J, et al: Infrapatellar contracture syndrome. An unrecognized cause of knee stiffness with patella entrapment and patella infera. *Am J Sports Med* 1987;15:331-341.

11. Payr E: Zur operativen Behandlung der Kniegelenksteife nach langdauernder Ruhigstellung. *Zentralbl Chir* 1917;44:809-816.

12. Nicoll EA: Quadricepsplasty. *J Bone Joint Surg* 1963;45B:483-490.

13. O'Connor RL: *Arthroscopy*. Philadelphia, JB Lippincott, 1977, pp 14-22.

14. Insall J (ed): *Surgery of the Knee*. New York, Churchill Livingstone, 1984, pp 516-517, pp 639-643.

15. Jackson DW, Schaefer RK: Cyclops syndrome: Loss of extension following intra-articular anterior cruciate ligament reconstruction. *Arthroscopy* 1990;6:171-178.

16. Richmond JC, Al Assal M: Arthroscopic management of arthrofibrosis of the knee, including infrapatellar contraction syndrome. *Arthroscopy* 1991;7:144-147.

17. Caton J, Deschamps G, Chambat P, et al: Les rotules basses. A propos de 128 observations, English abstract. *Rev Chir Orthop* 1982;68: 317-325.

18. Wojtys EM, Noyes FR, Gikas P: Patella baja syndrome. Presented at the 53rd Annual Meeting of the American Academy of Orthopaedic Surgeons, New Orleans, LA, February 20-25, 1986.

19. Noyes FR, Wojtys EM, Marshall MT: The early diagnosis and treatment of developmental patella infera syndrome. *Clin Orthop* 1991;265:241-252.

20. Noyes FR, Mangine RE, Barber S: Early knee motion after open and arthroscopic anterior cruciate ligament reconstruction. *Am J Sports Med* 1987;15:149-160.

21. Noyes FR, Torvik PJ, Hyde WB, et al: Biomechanics of ligament failure: II. An analysis of immobilization, exercise, and reconditioning effects in primates. *J Bone Joint Surg* 1974;56A:1406-1418.

22. Peacock EE: Some biochemical and biophysical aspects of joint stiffness: Role of collagen synthesis as opposed to altered molecular bonding. *Ann Surg* 1986;64:1-12.

23. Akeson WH, Woo SL-Y, Amiel D, et al: The connective tissue response to immobility: Biochemical changes in periarticular connective tissue of the immobilized rabbit knee. *Clin Orthop* 1973;93:356-362.

24. Akeson WH, Woo SL-Y, Amiel D, et al: Biomechanical and biochemical changes in the periarticular connective tissue during contracture development in the immobilized rabbit knee. *Connect Tissue Res* 1974;2:315-323.

25. Claman HN: Mast cells and fibrosis: The relevance to scleroderma. *Rheum Dis Clin North Am* 1990;16:141-151.

26. Sylven B: Ester sulphuric acids of high molecular weight and mast cells in mesenchymal tumors. *Acta Radiol* 1945;59(suppl):1-99.

27. Goto T, Befus D, Low R, et al: Mast cell heterogeneity and hyperplasia of bleomycin-induced pulmonary fibrosis of rats. *Am Rev Resp Dis* 1984;130:797-802.

28. Kischer CW, Bailey JF: The mast cell in hypertrophic scars. *Tex Rep Biol Med* 1972;30:327-338.
29. Kawanami O, Ferrans VJ, Fulmer JD, et al: Ultrastructure of pulmonary mast cells in patients with fibrotic lung disorders. *Lab Invest* 1979;40:717-734.
30. Agius RM, Godfrey RC, Holgate ST: Mast cell and histamine content of human bronchoalveolar lavage fluid. *Thorax* 1985;40:760-767.
31. Smith CJ, Smith JC, Finn MC: The possible role of mast cells (allergy) in the production of keloid and hypertrophic scarring. *J Burn Care Rehab* 1987;8:126.
32. Henderson B: The synovial lining cell and synovitis. *Scand J Rheumatol Suppl* 1988;76:33-38.
33. Barland P, Novikoff AB, Hamerman D: Electron microscopy of the human synovial membrane. *J Cell Biol* 1962;14:207-220.
34. Castor CW: The microscopic structure of normal human synovial tissue. *Arthritis Rheum* 1960;3:140-151.
35. Castor CW: The rate of hyaluronic acid production by human synovial cells studied in tissue culture. *Arthritis Rheum* 1959;2:259-265.
36. Henderson B, Pettipher ER: The synovial lining cell: Biology and pathobiology. *Semin Arthritis Rheum* 1985;15:1-32.
37. Henderson B, Edwards JCW: *The Synovial Lining: In Health and Disease*. London, Chapman & Hall, 1987.
38. Henderson B, Revell PA, Edwards JC: Synovial lining cell hyperplasia in rheumatoid arthritis: Dogma and fact. *Ann Rheum Dis* 1988;47:348-349.
39. Merry P, Kidd BL, Mapp PI, et al: Mechanisms of persistent synovitis. *Scand J Rheumatol Suppl* 1988;76:85-93.
40. Woodruff T, Blake DR, Freeman J, et al: Is chronic synovitis an example of reperfusion injury? *Ann Rheum Dis* 1986;45:608-611.
41. McCord JM: Oxygen-derived free radicals in postischemic tissue injury. *N Engl J Med* 1985;312:159-163.
42. Jayson MIV, Dixon A StJ: Intra-articular pressure in rheumatoid arthritis of the knee: I. Pressure changes during passive joint distension. *Ann Rheum Dis* 1970;29:261-265.
43. Levick JR: An investigation into the validity of subatmospheric pressure recordings from synovial fluid and their dependence on joint angle. *J Physiol* 1979;289:55-67.
44. Jayson MIV, Dixon A StJ: Intra-articular pressure in rheumatoid arthritis of the knee: III. Pressure changes during joint use. *Ann Rheum Dis* 1970;29:401-408.
45. Jayson MIV, Dixon A StJ: Intra-articular pressure in rheumatoid arthritis of the knee: II. Effect of intra-articular pressure on blood circulation to the synovium. *Ann Rheum Dis* 1970;29:266-268.
46. Unsworth J, Outhwaite J, Blake DR, et al: Dynamic studies of the relationship between intra-articular pressure, synovial fluid oxygen tension, and lipid peroxidation in the inflamed knee: An example of reperfusion injury. *Ann Clin Biochem* 1988;25(suppl):8-11.
47. Lund-Olesen K: Oxygen tension in synovial fluids. *Arthritis Rheum* 1970;13:769-776.
48. Granger DN, Sennett M, McElearney P, et al: Effect of local arterial hypotension on cat intestinal capillary permeability. *Gastroenterology* 1980;79:474-480.
49. Granger DN, Rutili G, McCord JM: Superoxide radicals in feline intestinal ischemia. *Gastroenterology* 1981;81:22-29.

50. Granger DN, Höllwarth ME, Parks DA: Ischemia-reperfusion injury: Role of oxygen-derived free radicals. *Acta Physiol Scand Suppl* 1986;548:47-63.
51. Greenwald RA, Moy WW: Effect of oxygen-derived free radicals on hyaluronic acid. *Arthritis Rheum* 1980;23:455-463.
52. Clark RAF: Cutaneous tissue repair: Basic biologic considerations: I. *J Am Acad Dermatol* 1985;13:701-725.
53. Assoian RK, Sporn MB: Type beta transforming growth factor in human platelets: Release during platelet degranulation and action on vascular smooth muscle cells. *J Cell Biol* 1986;102:1217-1223.
54. Ginsberg M: Role of platelets in inflammation and rheumatic disease. *Adv Inflam Res* 1981;2:53-71.
55. Wahl SM, Hunt DA, Wakefield LM, et al: Transforming growth factor beta induces monocyte chemotaxis and growth factor production. *Proc Natl Acad Sci USA* 1987;84:5788-5792.
56. Norris DA, Clark RA, Swigart LM, et al: Fibronectin fragment(s) are chemotactic for human peripheral blood monocytes. *J Immunol* 1982;129:1612-1618.
57. Postlethwaite AE, Keski-Oja J, Moses HL, et al: Stimulation of the chemotactic migration of human fibroblasts by transforming growth factor beta. *J Exp Med* 1987;165:251-256.
58. Sporn MB, Roberts AB: Transforming growth factor-beta: Multiple actions and potential clinical applications. *JAMA* 1989;262:938-941.
59. Sappino AP, Schürch W, Gabbiani G: Differentiation repertoire of fibroblastic cells: Expression of cytoskeletal proteins as marker of phenotypic modulations. *Lab Invest* 1990;63:144-161.
60. Claman HN: On scleroderma: Mast cells, endothelial cells, and fibroblasts. *JAMA* 1989;262:1206-1209.
61. Campbell PM, LeRoy EC: Pathogenesis of systemic sclerosis: A vascular hypothesis. *Semin Arthritis Rheum* 1975;4:351-368.
62. Fleischmajer R: The pathophysiology of scleroderma. *Int J Dermatol* 1977;16:310-318.
63. Sternberg EM: Pathogenesis of scleroderma: The interrelationship of the immune and vascular hypotheses. *Surv Immunol Res* 1985;4:69-80.
64. Krieg T, Meurer M: Systemic scleroderma: Clinical and pathophysiologic aspects. *J Am Acad Dermatol* 1988;18:457-481.
65. Buckingham RB, Prince RK, Rodnan GP, et al: Increased collagen accumulation in dermal fibroblast cultures from patients with progressive systemic sclerosis (scleroderma). *J Lab Clin Med* 1978;92:5-21.
66. LeRoy EC: Connective tissue synthesis by scleroderma skin fibroblasts in cell culture. *J Exp Med* 1972;135:1351-1362.
67. Fernex M: *The Mast-Cell System. Its Relationship to Atherosclerosis, Fibrosis and Eosinophils.* Baltimore, Williams & Wilkins, 1968.
68. Bernfield M: Extracellular matrix: Editorial overview. *Current Opinion Cell Biol* 1989;1:953.
69. Bornstein P, Sage H: Structurally distinct collagen types. *Ann Rev Biochem* 1980;49:957-1003.
70. Gabbiani G, Rungger-Brändle E: The fibroblast, in Glynn LE, Houck JC, Weissman G (eds): *Handbook of Inflammation: Tissue Repair and Regeneration.* Amsterdam, Elsevier North-Holland Biomedical Press, 1981, vol 3, pp 1-50.
71. Iozzo RV: Proteoglycans: Structure, function, and role in neoplasia. *Lab Invest* 1985;53:373-396.
72. Werb Z, Burleigh MC: A specific collagenase from rabbit fibroblasts in monolayer culture. *Biochem J* 1974;137:373-385.

73. Sporn MB, Roberts AB: Peptide growth factors and inflammation, tissue repair, and cancer. *J Clin Invest* 1986;78:329-332.

74. Gabbiani G, Ryan GB, Majne G: Presence of modified fibroblasts in granulation tissue and their possible role in wound contraction. *Experientia* 1971;27:549-550.

75. Gabbiani G, Hirschel BJ, Ryan GB, et al: Granulation tissue as a contractile organ: A study of structure and function. *J Exp Med* 1972;135:719-734.

76. Skalli O, Gabbiani G: The biology of the myofibroblast relationship to wound contraction and fibrocontractive diseases, in Clark RAF, Henson PM (eds): *The Molecular and Cellular Biology of Wound Repair.* New York, Plenum Press, 1988, pp 373-402.

77. Skalli O, Schürch W, Seemayer T, et al: Myofibroblasts from diverse pathologic settings are heterogeneous in their content of actin isoforms and intermediate filament proteins. *Lab Invest* 1989;60:275-285.

78. Dubaybo BA, Thet LA: Changes in lung tissue and lavage fibronectin after paraquat injury in rats. *Res Commun Chem Pathol Pharmacol* 1986;51:211-220.

79. Clark JG, Overton JE, Marino BA, et al: Collagen biosynthesis in bleomycin-induced pulmonary fibrosis in hamsters. *J Lab Clin Med* 1980;96:943-953.

80. Goldstein RH, Fine A: Fibrotic reactions in the lung: The activation of the lung fibroblast. *Exp Lung Res* 1986;11:245-261.

81. Adler KB, Low RB, Leslie KO, et al: Contractile cells in normal and fibrotic lung. *Lab Invest* 1989;60:473-485.

82. Rodbard S: Negative feedback mechanisms in the architecture and function of the connective and cardiovascular tissues. *Perspect Biol Med* 1970;13:507-527.

83. Gabbiani G, Majne G: Dupuytren's contracture: Fibroblast contraction? An ultrastructural study. *Am J Pathol* 1972;66:131-146.

84. Squier CA: The effect of stretching on formation of myofibroblasts in mouse skin. *Cell Tissue Res* 1981;220:325-335.

85. Roberts AB, Flanders KC, Kondaiah P, et al: Transforming growth factor beta: Biochemistry and roles in embryogenesis, tissue repair and remodeling, and carcinogenesis. *Recent Prog Horm Res* 1988;44:157-197.

86. Sporn MB, Roberts AB, Wakefield LM, et al: Some recent advances in the chemistry and biology of transforming growth factor-beta. *J Cell Biol* 1987;105:1039-1045.

87. Roberts AB, Sporn MB, Assoian RK, et al: Transforming growth factor type beta: Rapid induction of fibrosis and angiogenesis in vivo and stimulation of collagen formation in vitro. *Proc Natl Acad Sci USA* 1986;83:4167-4171.

88. Centrella M, McCarthy TL, Canalis E: Skeletal tissue and transforming growth factor beta. *FASEB J* 1988;2:3066-3973.

89. Ross R, Raines EW, Bowen-Pope DF: The biology of platelet-derived growth factor. *Cell* 1986;46:155-169.

90. Owen AJ III, Geyer RP, Antoniades HN: Human platelet-derived growth factor stimulates amino acid transport and protein synthesis by human diploid fibroblasts in plasma-free media. *Proc Natl Acad Sci USA* 1982;79:3203-3207.

91. Rubbia L, Sappino PA, Hansson HK, et al: Action of different cytokines on actin-isoforms expression fibroblasts in vitro, abstract. *Experientia* 1989;45:A49.

92. Clark RA: Potential roles of fibronectin in cutaneous wound repair. *Arch Dermatol* 1988;124:201-206.

93. Hynes RO, Yamada KM: Fibronectins: Multifunctional modular glycoproteins. *J Cell Biol* 1982;95:369-377.

94. Hølund B, Clemmensen I, Junker P, et al: Fibronectin in experimental granulation tissue. *Acta Pathol Microbiol Immunol Scand [A]* 1982;90:159-165.

95. Viljanto J, Penttinen R, Raekallio J: Fibronectin in early phases of wound healing in children. *Acta Chir Scand* 1981;147:7-13.

96. Bevilacqua MP, Schleef RR, Gimbrone MA Jr, et al: Regulation of the fibrinolytic system of cultured human vascular endothelium by interleukin 1. *J Clin Invest* 1986;78:587-591.

97. Tryggvason K, Höyhtyä M, Salo T: Proteolytic degradation of extracellular matrix in tumor invasion. *Biochem Biophys Acta* 1987;907:191-217.

98. Canalis E, McCarthy T, Centrella M: Growth factors and the regulation of bone remodeling. *J Clin Invest* 1988;81:277-281.

99. Masure S, Opdenakker G: Cytokine-mediated proteolysis in tissue remodeling. *Experientia* 1989;45:542-549.

100. McGuire-Goldring MK, Murphy G, Gowen M, et al: Effects of retinol and dexamethasone on cytokine-mediated control of metalloproteinases and their inhibitors by human articular chondrocytes and synovial cells in culture. *Biochem Biophys Acta* 1983;763:129-139.

101. Mohtadi NGH, Webster-Bogaert S, Fowler PJ: Limitation of motion following anterior cruciate ligament reconstruction: A case control study. *Am J Sports Med* 1991;19:620-625.

102. Leslie KO, Mitchell J, Low R: Lung myofibroblasts. *Cell Motil Cytoskeleton* 1992;22:92-98.

103. Ott JW, Graf BK, Keene JS, et al: Risk factors for restricted motion after anterior cruciate ligament reconstruction: A retrospective study of 373 patients. Presented at the 58th Annual Meeting of the American Academy of Orthopaedic Surgeons, Anaheim, CA, March 7-12, 1991.

104. Beynnon BD, Huston DR, Pope MH, et al: The effect of ACL reconstruction tension on the knee and cruciate ligaments. Presented at the 38th Annual Meeting of the Orthopaedic Research Society, Washington, DC, February 17-20, 1992.

105. Cannon WD Jr, Vittori JM: The role of arthroscopic debridement after anterior cruciate ligament reconstruction. *Arthroscopy* 1991;7:344-349.

106. Pyne J, Gottlieb D, Beynnon B, et al: Semitendinosus and gracilis tendon graft fixation in ACL reconstructions. Presented at the 58th Annual Meeting of the American Academy of Orthopaedic Surgeons, Anaheim, CA, March 7-12, 1991.

107. Häggmark T, Eriksson E: Cylinder or mobile cast brace after knee ligament surgery. *Am J Sports Med* 1979;7:48-56.

108. Shelbourne KD, Nitz P: Accelerated rehabilitation after anterior cruciate ligament reconstruction. *Am J Sports Med* 1990;18:292-299.

109. Evans EB, Eggers GWN, Butler JK: Experimental immobilization and remobilization of rat knee joints. *J Bone Joint Surg* 1960;42A:737-758.

110. Enneking WF, Horowitz M: The intra-articular effects of immobilization on the human knee. *J Bone Joint Surg* 1072;54A:973-985.

111. Thompson TC: Quadricepsplasty to improve knee function. *J Bone Joint Surg* 1944;26A:366-379.

112. Hesketh KT: Experiences with the Thompson quadricepsplasty. *J Bone Joint Surg* 1963;45B:491-495.

113. Daoud H, O'Farrell T, Cruess RL: Quadricepsplasty: The Judet technique and results of six cases. *J Bone Joint Surg* 1982;64B:194-197.

114. Wilson PD: Posterior capsuloplasty in certain flexion contractures of the knee. *J Bone Joint Surg* 1929;11A:40-58.

115. Sprague NF III: Motion-limiting arthrofibrosis of the knee: The role of arthroscopic management. *Clin Sports Med* 1987;6:537-549.

116. Bhan S, Rath S: Modified posterior soft tissue release for management of severe knee flexion contracture. *Orthopedics* 1989;12:703-708.

117. Parisien JS: The role of arthroscopy in the treatment of postoperative fibroarthrosis of the knee joint. *Clin Orthop* 1988;229:185-192.

118. Del Pizzo W, Fox JM, Friedman MJ: Operative arthroscopy for the treatment of arthrofibrosis of the knee. *Contemp Orthop* 1985;10:67-72.

119. Wahl S, Renström P: Fibrosis in soft-tissue injuries, in Leadbetter WB, Buckwalter JA, Gordon SL (eds): *Sports-Induced Inflammation: Clinical and Basic Science Concepts*. Park Ridge, IL, American Academy of Orthopaedic Surgeons, 1990, pp 637-647.

Future Directions

Identify and characterize interarticular differences in the structure and function of synovial joints.

Each rheumatic disease tends to spare some joints and to involve others, usually in a symmetric pattern. The explanations for these differences in susceptibility presumably lie in local differences in the structure and/or function of normal joints. Reasonable starting points in the search for such factors include the studies of normal microvascular physiology, synovial innervation, and matrix biochemistry of articular tissues. Consistent interarticular differences that correlate with patterns of disease may ultimately provide insights into the pathophysiology of those diseases.

Determine the causes and the consequences of local ischemia in rheumatoid joints.

Intrasynovial indices of ischemia, such as low pH, high lactate, etc. correlate strongly with radiographic evidence of destruction in rheumatoid knees. It is not known, however, whether this relationship is causal or incidental. Appropriate areas for study include the possibility that increased intra-articular pressure, at least transiently, promotes ischemia, the hypothesis that prostaglandin-dependent blood flow may be compromised by nonsteroidal anti-inflammatory drug (NSAID) therapy, and the effects of local hypoxia and acidosis on articular tissues.

Establish the mechanism underlying pathologic crystallization in joints.

Crystallization of sodium urate, calcium pyrophosphate, and hydroxyapatite preferentially occurs in joints, and may induce severe arthritis. The biochemical bases of these pathologic precipitations are not well-established. A better understanding of these processes should lead to more effective therapy and ultimately to prevention.

Evaluate the role of normal synovial fluid in the preservation of joint stability.

Tendons, ligaments, and joint configuration are not entirely responsible for preventing distraction of metacarpophalangeal joints. A simple experiment is needed to demonstrate adhesive properties of the synovial fluid film between opposing cartilages. Study of this property in normal, trouble-free joints may confirm an important mechanism and explain the instability accompanying chronic effusions.

Determine the effect of mechanical forces on synovial cells.

Changes in the mechanical stresses experienced by cells within the normal and diseased synovium are thought to influence cellular function. However, this influence has never been investigated. In vitro and in vivo studies are needed to define the metabolic responses of synoviocytes to their mechanical environment. Similar studies of osteoblasts, chondrocytes, and smooth muscle cells have proved fruitful.

49

Delineate the pathophysiology of the mechanism of effusion.

Effusion represents an imbalance between entry and clearance of water or proteins through synovial tissue. Investigation is needed to identify the specifics of this imbalance. Delineation of the mechanisms by which cartilage wear particles, synovial tissue, mechanical stress, and inflammation contribute to effusion will assist in the understanding and treatment of the phenomenon. In addition, the effects of chronic effusion on synovium and cartilage metabolism must be determined.

Identify the risk factors of posttraumatic arthrofibrosis.

Arthrofibrosis with limited joint function occurs after trauma and surgical intervention. It is necessary to delineate the expression of the disorder and the risk factors associated with its occurrence. The study of factors such as timing of surgery, joint condition, joint motion, injury patterns, genetic factors, and surgical and rehabilitative techniques would assist in early identification of patients at risk.

Delineate the response of synovium to trauma.

Trauma frequently results in a synovial response, with the production of cytokines (PDGF, TGFb, FGF, IL-1) and prostaglandins. The study of the effects of cytokines on the biology and biochemistry of synovial matrix, cartilage, and bone following trauma would facilitate treatment. The mechanisms that assist in modifying and limiting IL-1 mediated inflammation must be investigated. Identifying the effects of NSAIDs and cytokine agonists and antagonists on healing processes and inflammation could lead to more effective treatment.

Define the pathophysiology of posttraumatic arthrofibrosis (PTA).

The etiology of PTA is not well understood. In addition to synovial changes, there are changes in fat pad, capsule, and other joint structures. The techniques of molecular biology should be used to identify the tissues and cells involved, the alterations in matrix production, and the specific growth factors and inflammatory mechanisms.

Determine the consequences of persistent joint effusion and possible synovial ischemia.

Persistent effusion causes significant changes in joint lubrication function and hydrostatic patterns in the cells of the synovial lining. This pressure and, perhaps, agents used to relieve synovitis, may lead to alterations of blood flow to the synovium. Synovial fluid is the primary source of cell metabolites. Appropriate studies should examine the effects of large effusions and hemarthrosis on joint surfaces and on ligament and meniscal healing.

Section Two
Cartilage

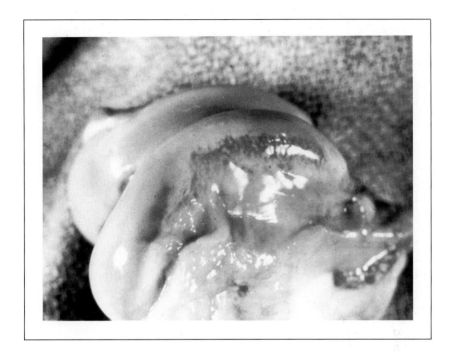

Overview

Cartilage forms a critical component of all synovial joints. It provides a smooth, low friction gliding surface that has surprising resilience and stiffness to compression. It demonstrates exceptional ability to distribute loads and remarkable durability. Loss of cartilage function leads to pain, decreased mobility, and, in some instances, deformity and instability; therefore, it is essential to improve understanding of the causes of cartilage damage and methods of restoring cartilage function following injury.

The capacity of cartilage to provide normal synovial joint function depends on the mechanical properties of the extracellular matrix. Chondrocytes create the macromolecular framework of this matrix from three classes of molecules: collagens, proteoglycans, and noncollagenous proteins. Interaction between these macromolecules and the tissue fluid provides cartilage with many of its specialized mechanical properties. The concentration and organization of the collagens, proteoglycans, noncollagenous proteins, and water influence the tensile, compression, shear, and permeability of the tissue. Alterations in the matrix, such as increased hydration, disruption of the collagen fibrillar network, and disaggregation or loss of proteoglycans, which may occur following joint injuries, adversely alter the mechanical properties of the articular cartilage.

Two recent bioengineering advances have helped increase understanding of synovial joint articular surfaces. First, an accurate constitutive model has been developed that describes the deformation, stress-strain, flow, and fluid pressurization behaviors in articular cartilage.

This biphasic theory has helped describe the deformational behavior of articular cartilage with remarkable accuracy. The second advance, analytical stereophotogrammetry, has provided quantitative maps of entire articulating surfaces. It can describe the detailed anatomy of the joint surface in mathematical terms so that geometrically precise finite element models of the joints can be developed. Furthermore, these mathematical maps make it possible to calculate the curvatures at every point in the joint surface and the congruence between articulating joint surfaces at any joint position.

Closed mechanical injuries to synovial joints caused by twisting, direct blows, indirect impact loading, and joint instability can alter the composition and structure of articular cartilage. These alterations lead to loss of the critical mechanical properties and may lead to disabling osteoarthritis. Experimental studies demonstrate that excessive joint loading may cause three types of articular cartilage damage: (1) loss of matrix macromolecules, (alteration of the macromolecular framework or cell injury without visible tissue disruption); (2) disruption of articular cartilage alone (chondral fractures and flaps); and (3) disruption of articular cartilage and subchondral bone (osteochondral fractures). Joint instability may be associated with any of these three types of cartilage damage. Understanding of the clinical mechanisms, natural history, and optimal treatment of cartilage injuries resulting from closed mechanical trauma or instability is limited, at least partially, because of the difficulty in defining the tissue damage.

The potential for cartilage repair following some types of closed mechanical injuries or in unstable joints remains uncertain, but the available evidence suggests that chondrocytes can repair certain types of tissue damage caused by closed mechanical trauma or joint instability. It is not yet clear what types of mechanical trauma or joint instability exceed the natural reparative capacity of the chondrocytes.

Methods that may help restore articular surfaces following damage that exceeds the capacity of the tissue to heal itself include use of growth factors and cell technologies such as mesenchymal cell transplantation and allograft replacement. Growth factors stimulate cell migration, proliferation, and differentiation in cartilage defects. Chondroprogenitor cells can be isolated, stimulated to proliferate in culture, and then implanted into cartilage defects where they will form new cartilage. Irreversibly damaged articular surfaces can be successfully replaced with carefully matched osteochondral allografts. Although all of these methods have the potential to restore or improve synovial joint function following injury, further study is needed to develop and define their optimal clinical value.

Chapter 4

Anatomic Form and Biomechanical Properties of Articular Cartilage of the Knee Joint

Van C. Mow, PhD
Gerard A. Ateshian, PhD
Anthony Ratcliffe, PhD

Introduction

Knee function involves many complex extra-articular biomechanical interactions between muscles and anatomic structures surrounding the joint,[1-6] as well as many intra-articular interactions.[7-20] These intra-articular interactions involve the contact mechanics between highly curved articular cartilage, and between the meniscus and the articular cartilage of the femoral condyles and the tibial plateaus.[7,8,21-30] In general, very high loads are experienced at the patellofemoral joint[8,12,17] and at the femoro-menisco-tibial articulation.[4,7,10] These high loads are sustained by the articular cartilage and the smooth, nearly frictionless articular surface.[31-33] The subchondral bone and cancellous bone also play major roles in providing load support and normal knee function.[34-40] The stability of the knee is provided primarily by ligamentous constraints and secondarily by the menisci.[2,6,15,41-45] The remarkably smooth, nearly frictionless performance of diarthrodial joints, in particular the knee, is due in large part to the mechanical properties of articular cartilage and the anatomic form of the joint, with each joint having a structure specifically suited for its function. Alterations in cartilage and ligament biomechanical properties, in the anatomic form of the joint, and in muscular action around the joint can cause pathologic processes to be initiated, which lead to cartilage destruction, and perhaps to osteoarthritis.[46-52]

This chapter provides a discussion of two major bioengineering advances that have occurred over the past decade, leading toward a complete description of diarthrodial joints (the knee being just one example) for biomechanical investigations. First, an accurate constitutive theory, the biphasic theory for soft hydrated tissues, has been developed to describe the deformation, stress-strain, flow, and fluid pressurization behaviors in articular cartilage.[21,24,27,28,53-55] This constitutive theory, which relates tissue stresses and strains, is based on the general mixture theory developed by Truesdell and

Noll,[56] and applied to incompressible binary mixtures by Mow and associates[53] and Bowen.[57] The biphasic theory makes two assumptions: (1) Both the collagen-proteoglycan of the extracellular matrix (solid phase) and the water (fluid phase) of the tissue are intrinsically incompressible. (2) The frictional drag of interstitial fluid flow through the porous-permeable solid matrix is the dominant physical mechanism responsible for the experimentally observed viscoelastic creep and stress-relaxation behaviors of soft hydrated tissues such as articular cartilage and meniscus. This biphasic theory describes these deformational behaviors of articular cartilage and meniscus with remarkable accuracy.

Second, an optical method, analytical stereophotogrammetry (SPG), has been developed to provide a quantitative map with very low measurement uncertainties (25 to 90 microns) of the entire articulating surface of large and small diarthrodial joints.[58-64] This method provides the means to describe the detailed anatomy of any joint surface in a mathematical form so that geometrically precise finite element models of joints can be developed. These mathematical maps can also be used to calculate in a defined and quantitative manner the curvatures at every point on the joint surface as well as the congruence between the two articulating surfaces. In addition, this method has now been used to obtain similar quantitative maps of the subchondral bone surface so that entire cartilage thickness maps of the patella, femoral condyles, and tibial plateaus have been developed.[58] These capabilities provide the basis for more realistic models in future finite element analyses of diarthrodial joints, in general, and of knees, in particular.

In order to understand the biomechanics of the knee joint, it is necessary to know the material properties of articular cartilage on the relevant articulating surfaces, as well as the topography and congruence of the two surfaces. The following sections focus on the biomechanics of the patellofemoral joint. The femoro-menisco-tibial articulation involves analysis of a three-body contact problem in which highly complex anatomic forms are lined with biphasic materials of varying thickness. No solution to this type of problem is currently available. Clearly, this problem will be the focus of much future research on the biomechanics of the knee. In this chapter, our limited objective is to describe, in a quantitative manner, the anatomy of the patellar and the femoral groove cartilages, and the biphasic material properties of these two tissues. Finally, we shall describe the articulation process at the patellofemoral joint, based on this type of fundamental information.

Anatomy of the Articular Layers of the Knee Joint

Topography

Recently, topography and thickness maps of the knee (femur, tibia, patella, and meniscus) have been precisely determined[58] using the SPG method originally developed by Selvik[64] and Ghosh,[60] and extended by Huiskes and associates,[61] and Ateshian and associates.[58,65] Essentially, this optical technique is based on the concept that three-dimensional spatial coordinates of a joint surface can be mathematically calculated from two high-quality two-dimensional (2-D) photographic images, a stereogram, of the surface using both perspective and projective geometry. Precision landmarks are located on a calibration frame surrounding the joint in a laboratory coordinate system, and a fine grid is projected with a high intensity light source onto the featureless curved articular surface. The 2-D points in the plane of each stereogram are then recorded in a digital format, using a precision digitizer, and transferred to a computer. Appropriate mathematical surfaces are fitted through the data providing a continuous description of the cartilage layer surface.[62,65] Figure 1, *left*, shows a wireframe representation of the cartilage surface of a typical patella, femur, and tibial plateau, and Figure 1, *right*, shows a shaded model of these same surfaces.

From this mathematical format,[59,65] it is possible to look at their curvature characteristics. The curvature at a given point on a surface is a measure of its concavity, convexity, or flatness in a small region around that point. In other words, the curvature characterizes the shape of the surface in that region. Figure 2 depicts a graphic definition of the curvature of the planar curve C. If the circle tangent to C at the given point x has its first and second derivatives equal to those of the curve, then it is called the osculating circle at x. The radius ρ of this circle is called the radius of the curvature, and its reciprocal $\kappa = 1/\rho$ is known as the curvature of the curve C at the point x. When $\kappa = 0$, the curve is flat in the neighborhood of x; conversely, if κ becomes very large (as ρ tends to zero), the curve is said to have a cusp at the point x. This definition can be extended to the case of a surface with some additional considerations, as shown in Figure 3. Consider a plane perpendicular to a surface S (shaded area) at a point x, which intersects the surface along a curve C. Then the curvature of the surface in the direction of that plane is equal to the curvature κ of the curve C at x. Suppose now that we rotate this plane around the normal **n** to the surface to some new position (Fig. 3), then a new intersection curve C will be defined. This new curve C will have a curvature κ that is different than in the original direction. (If the intersecting plane passes through the center of a sphere, then the curvature for any plane must remain the same.) As the plane completes a rotation around **n**, that is, 360 degrees, there will be one direction along which κ assumes a maximum value κ_{max}, and another direction along which it will assume a minimum value κ_{min}. Interestingly, these two directions will always be perpendicular to each other.[66] The curvatures κ_{min} and κ_{max} are known as principal curvatures, and the directions along which they occur are called principal directions of curvature. These quantities represent intrinsic geometric properties of a surface that do not depend on the direction along

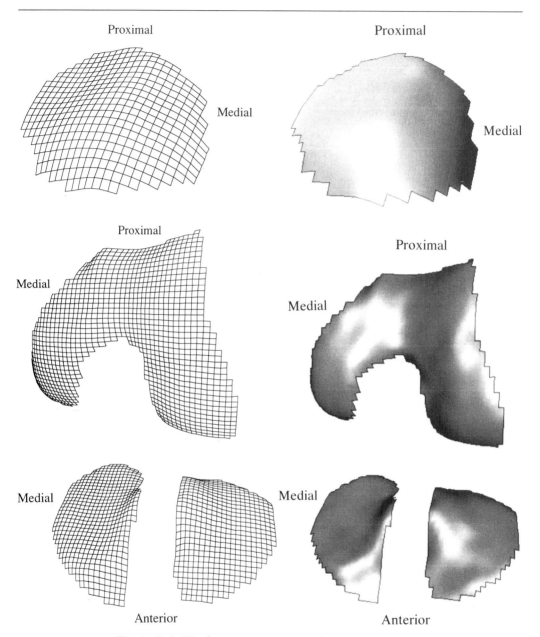

Fig. 1 *Left, Wireframe representation of the cartilage surface of a typical patella, femur, and tibial plateau. Right, Shaded model of same surfaces.*

which they are viewed by an observer. If the value of κ in a given direction is positive, the surface is convex along that direction, that is, the center of the osculating circle is opposite to the direction of the outward normal **n**. If κ is negative, the surface is concave. The

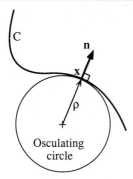

Fig. 2 *Graphic definition of the curvature of a planar curve C.*

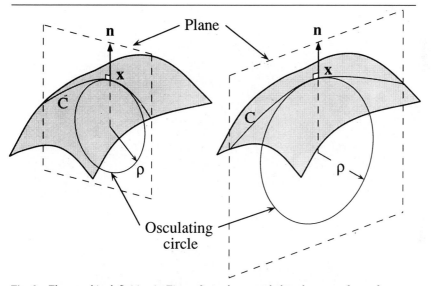

Fig. 3 *The graphic definition in Figure 2 can be extended to the case of a surface.*

flatness of a surface is provided by the root-mean-square measure κ_{rms} given by the simple formula

$$\kappa_{rms} = \sqrt{\frac{\kappa^2_{min} + \kappa^2_{max}}{2}}$$

When $\kappa_{rms} = 0$ at some point x, the surface is perfectly flat in the neighborhood of that point (because both κ_{max} and κ_{min} must be zero). Conversely, high values of κ_{rms} indicate a sharp change in the shape of the surface in that region. Figure 4 shows the variation of κ_{rms} across typical patella, femur, and tibial plateau articular surfaces. The midsagittal ridge of the patella is immediately apparent from these curvature maps, where a sharp increase of κ_{rms} across the ridge can be observed (the strip of dark color) spanning the surface

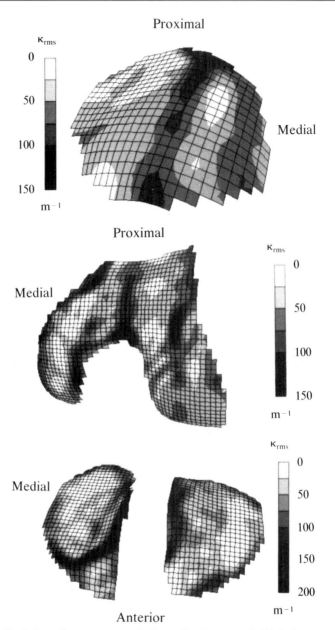

Fig. 4   *Variation of κ_{rms} across typical patella, femur, and tibial plateau articular surfaces.*

from its proximal to distal aspects. Similar ridges can be observed on the distal femoral surface. A depression is also visible along the midsagittal section of the trochlea.

The congruence of a joint, such as the patellofemoral joint, is a function of both the topography and curvature characteristics of

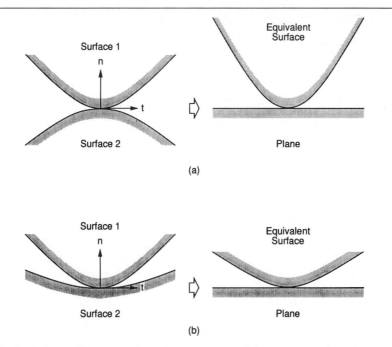

Fig. 5 *It is possible to represent the congruence of the contact region of two articular surfaces by a mathematically equivalent geometric system of a "surface-on-plane."*

both its opposing articulating surfaces, as well as their relative spatial position and orientation for a given joint angle. It is commonly understood that a congruent joint has close-fitting surfaces; however, this favorable relationship may not be maintained throughout the range of motion of the joint. The concept of equivalent surfaces can be used to quantify congruence for any given joint position (Fig.5). The congruence of the contact region of two articular surfaces is represented by a mathematically equivalent geometric system of a "surface-on-plane," in which the new equivalent surface is defined as the difference in the profiles of the two original surfaces in the contacting region. The congruence of the joint at the original contact region is then defined by the principal curvatures of this equivalent surface. It is then straightforward to compare congruence at various joint positions because all comparisons are made relative to a fixed planar reference. In essence, this method indicates that it is not the absolute topography of the joint surfaces that determines congruence, but rather the relative topography of these surfaces. Thus, a spherical ball and socket of identical radii are just as congruent as two flat surfaces.

Figure 6, *top*, shows an SPG representation of a patellofemoral joint at 30 degrees of flexion; Figure 6, *center*, shows typical midsagittal (left) and midhorizontal (right) sections of this joint; and

61

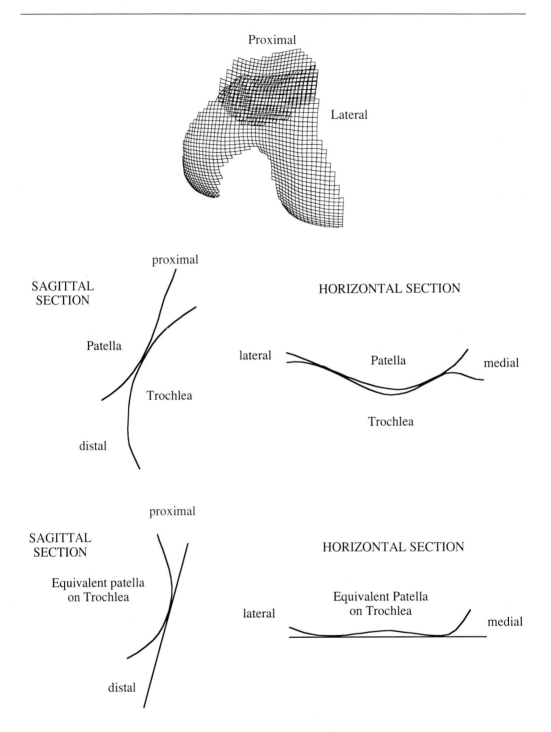

Proximal

Lateral

SAGITTAL
SECTION

proximal

Patella

Trochlea

distal

HORIZONTAL SECTION

lateral

Patella

medial

Trochlea

SAGITTAL
SECTION

proximal

Equivalent patella
on Trochlea

distal

HORIZONTAL SECTION

Equivalent Patella
on Trochlea

lateral

medial

Fig. 6 *Top, SPG representation of a patellofemoral joint at 30 degrees of flexion.* **Center,** *Typical midsagittal (left) and midhorizontal (right) sections of this joint.* **Bottom,** *Equivalent system for these same sections.*

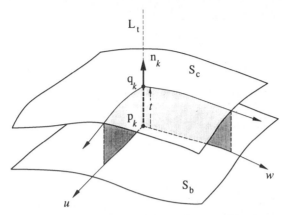

Fig. 7   *Cartilage thickness at a point is defined by the length of the segment between the bone and cartilage surfaces, such that the segment is perpendicular to the bone surface at that point. (Reproduced with permission from Ateshian GA, Soslowsky LJ, Mow VC: Quantitation of articular surface topography and cartilage thickness in knee joints using stereophotogrammetry. J Biomech 1991;24:761-776.)*

Figure 6, *bottom*, shows the equivalent system for these same sections, for the same joint flexion angle. These figures clearly indicate that the patellofemoral joint is more congruent in the horizontal plane than in the sagittal plane. Similar curves may be plotted and compared for various flexion angles. We envision that future biomechanics studies on the knee joint will use this type of technology to provide more precision to knee biomechanical models.

Cartilage Thickness

After the three-dimensional topography of the articular surface of a joint is measured using our SPG system, the cartilage layer may be dissolved using a mild solution of sodium hypochlorite to expose the underlying subchondral bone surface. This surface has also been quantified using our SPG system, and then cartilage thickness maps were determined by calculating the perpendicular distance between the bone and cartilage surfaces (Fig. 7).[58] These maps provide a direct visual and quantitative description of the spatial variation of cartilage thickness over an entire joint, as shown for the patella, distal femur, and tibial plateau in Figure 8. A pattern of cartilage thickening along the midhorizontal section of the patella is consistently observed in all normal patellar specimens, and is more pronounced on the lateral side where thicknesses may reach 6 to 7 mm. The trochlea also demonstrates thicker cartilage relative to the anterior condyles, although thicknesses are not as high as in the opposing patellar articular surface. On the tibial plateau, as observed earlier by McLeod and associates,[67] cartilage is thickest in those areas not covered by the menisci. Furthermore, we have computed the mean, minimum, and maximum cartilage thickness values for each

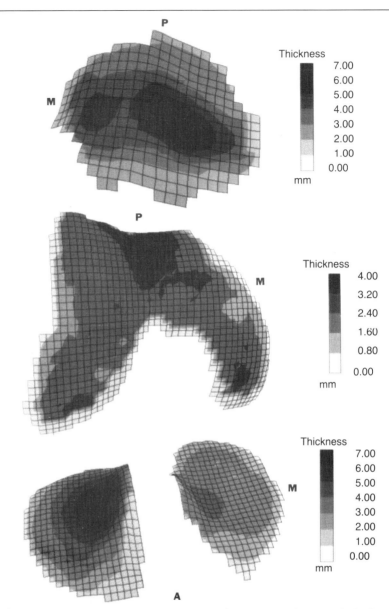

Fig. 8 *Cartilage thickness maps of a typical patella, distal femur and tibial plateau (P = proximal, M = medial, A = anterior). (Reproduced with permission from Ateshian GA, Soslowsky LJ, Mow VC: Quantitation of articular surface topography and cartilage thickness in knee joints using stereophotogrammetry. J Biomech 1991;24:761-776.)*

surface (Table 1). For example, the mean cartilage thickness on the lateral tibial compartment (3.51 mm) is greater than on the medial compartment (2.42 mm). These new findings of rapid changes of cartilage thickness over the patella, femoral condyles, trochlea, and tibial plateaus·provide cogent evidence for a reexamination of previous calculations and results based on uniform thickness models. In

Table 1 Anatomic data for the patella, femur, tibial plateau, and meniscus (average ± standard deviation)

Joint surface	n	Surface area (cm²)	Cartilage Thickness (mm)			Coeff. of var. (%)
			Mean	Minimum	Maximum	
Patella	12	10.7 ± 1.6	3.33 ± 0.39	0.89 ± 0.31	5.91 ± 0.87	33 ± 11
Femur*	3	29.5 ± 2.5	1.99 ± 0.12	0.16 ± 0.06	3.61 ± 0.30	29 ± 1
Tibial plateau	12	22.5 ± 2.4	2.92 ± 0.52	0.35 ± 0.27	6.25 ± 0.85	44 ± 8
Lateral tibial plateau	12	10.7 ± 1.1	3.51 ± 0.87	0.95 ± 1.20	6.25 ± 0.85	39 ± 13
Medial tibial plateau	12	11.8 ± 1.6	2.42 ± 0.61	0.56 ± 0.43	4.46 ± 1.04	33 ± 9
Lateral meniscus	12	5.6 ± 1.2	NA**	NA	NA	NA
Medial meniscus	12	5.5 ± 1.4	NA	NA	NA	NA

*Excluding posterior aspect of the condyles.
**NA: not applicable.
(Reproduced with permission from Ateshian GA, Soslowsky LJ, Mow VC: Quantitation of articular surface topography and cartilage thickness in knee joints using stereophotogrammetry. *J Biomech* 1991;24:761-776.)

the future, for stress and strain calculations, variation of cartilage thickness over the joint surface will have to be incorporated in finite element modeling of the knee.

The Biphasic Theory for Articular Cartilage

Articular Cartilage Composition

The biphasic theory assumes that there are two distinct phases in cartilage: a fluid phase composed of water and electrolytes, and a solid phase that includes collagen fibrils, proteoglycans, and other glycoproteins.[28,53,54] In general, water consists of 60% to 85% of the wet weight of cartilage,[21,68-71] while collagen accounts for another 15% to 22%.[71-73] The collagen network provides the high tensile stiffness and strength of the tissue.[74-80] Intramolecular and intermolecular covalent crosslinks within the collagen fibrils function to maintain the cohesiveness of this network. The large proteoglycans (aggrecan) of articular cartilage are macromolecules composed of a protein core to which are attached a number of chondroitin sulfate (CS) and keratan sulfate (KS) glycosaminoglycan chains.[81-83] These molecules contribute significantly to the mechanical and physicochemical properties of cartilage.[21,54,69-71,84-87] Indeed, the close spacing between negatively charged carboxyl and sulfate groups of the CS and KS chains leads to significant Donnan osmotic pressure and charge-to-charge repulsive forces that are fundamental mechanisms in cartilage swelling. The total number of these charged groups in the tissue is measured in terms of a fixed charge density (FCD). The FCD in cartilage determines the total counter-ion concentration within the interstitium via the Donnan equilibrium distribution law, which in turn governs the Donnan osmotic pressure for cartilage.[69,70,88] It has been recently shown that the Donnan osmotic pressure and charge-to-charge repulsion may contribute up to 50% of the overall compressive stiffness of cartilage.[89]

The large proteoglycans of articular cartilage (aggrecan) bind very specifically to hyaluronate via the G1 domain of the protein core. This noncovalent binding is stabilized by a separate link protein, forming a very stable ternary complex.[71,90-93] In this way proteoglycan molecules can bind to a chain of hyaluronate, forming macromolecular complexes within the collagen network and distributed throughout the depth of the articular cartilage.[94,95] The formation of this highly stable proteoglycan-link protein-hyaluronate complex provides a mechanism by which the proteoglycans are essentially immobilized within the cartilage matrix, thereby maintaining the biochemical composition and material properties of the articular cartilage. Disruption of this mechanism, for example by enzymatic degradation of the protein core of the proteoglycan and/ or link protein, can rapidly result in loss of proteoglycans from the cartilage matrix[96] leading to cartilage degradation. Furthermore, recent rheologic studies have shown that the complex structure of the proteoglycans enhances their capacity to form molecular networks[97,98] that stabilize the organization of the extracellular matrix. The heterogeneity of the distribution of proteoglycans and collagen through the cartilage, and their complex molecular organization undoubtedly contribute to the overall mechanical function of the cartilage. However these parameters have not yet been included in a mathematical model of cartilage.

Biphasic Properties of Cartilage

When cartilage is subjected to loads, its response varies as a function of time. Under compression, this time-dependence is largely due to the flow of interstitial fluid through the porous-permeable collagen-proteoglycan solid matrix. The motion of the fluid is resisted by a diffusive drag that is controlled by the pore size of the porous solid matrix, which, in turn, is controlled by the organization of the collagen meshwork and proteoglycan molecular organization. The presence of glycosaminoglycan chains on the proteoglycan molecules is believed to be a major factor responsible for retarding interstitial fluid flow.[99] In order to model the response of cartilage from basic thermodynamic and continuum mechanics principles, it is essential to account for both the collagen-proteoglycan solid phase and the interstitial fluid phase of the tissue. The biphasic theory for hydrated soft tissues has been used successfully to model the compressive flow-dependent creep and stress-relaxation behaviors of articular cartilage.[21,24,28,53,55,100] In this theory, the total stress σ^T in cartilage is separated into two parts:

$$\sigma^T = \sigma^s + \sigma^f$$

where σ^s is the stress acting on the solid phase and σ^f is the stress acting on the fluid phase. In the tissue, these stresses depend on the interstitial fluid pressure p and the interstitial fluid velocity through the porous-permeable solid phase of the tissue. To illustrate how the

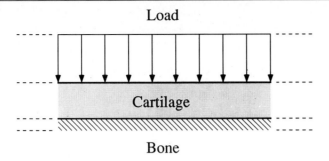

Fig. 9   *One-dimensional analysis of cartilage in compression.*

tissue might function, consider a one-dimensional analysis of the tissue in compression (Fig. 9). In this simple problem, the total stress acting on the tissue is equal to

$$\sigma^T = -p + H_A\epsilon$$

where H_A is called the aggregate modulus (the one-dimensional compressive modulus) and represents a measure of the compressive stiffness of the solid matrix of cartilage, and ϵ is the compressive strain in the solid matrix. The aggregate modulus can be measured at equilibrium where there is no fluid flow, that is, when the frictional drag force of fluid flow is zero, and the pressure is zero. In the theory, the fluid stress σ^f is directly proportional to the pressure p in the tissue, and is given by $\sigma^f = -\phi^f p$ where the proportionality constant ϕ^f is simply the tissue porosity (volume of water/total volume), which is approximately 75% in human knee cartilage.

The solid stress consists of the remaining pressure component, $(1 - \phi^f)p$, as well as all deformational effects due to the strain ϵ: $\sigma^s = -(1 - \phi^f)p + H_A\epsilon$. Thus, the fluid and solid stresses satisfy both of the equations above.

If the tissue is immersed in a fluid under hydrostatic pressure, a special form of the one-dimensional problem, then by virtue of incompressibility there will be no deformation of the solid matrix, that is, $\epsilon = 0$. Under this circumstance, the fluid stress is $\sigma^f = -\phi^f p$, and the solid stress is $\sigma^s = -(1 - \phi^f)p$. In other words, under hydrostatic loading, approximately 75% of the total stress is supported by the fluid phase and 25% by the solid phase. This situation applies for highly congruent joints, and typically during the first few seconds after load application when there is likely to be a thin layer of synovial joint fluid between the articulating surfaces.

In another extreme case, if the tissue pressure p is zero (no interstitial fluid flow), then $\sigma^f = 0$ and $\sigma^s = H_A\epsilon$. Under this circumstance, all of the applied stress must be supported by the collagen-proteoglycan solid matrix. This case applies to experiments when the cartilage specimen is loaded in compression by a rigid porous-

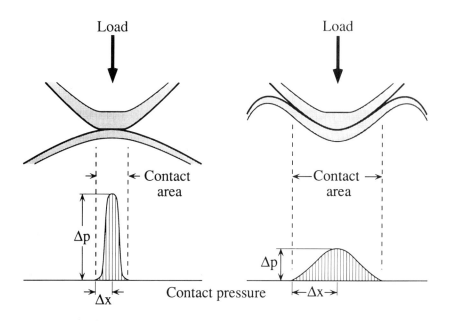

Fig. 10   *Left, Incongruent joint contact.* **Right,** *Congruent joint contact.*

permeable filter and allowed to creep to equilibrium when the movement of interstitial fluid inside the tissue has completely stopped. Typically, this occurs after a period of several hundreds or thousands of seconds of continuous loading. Therefore, the aggregate modulus H_A, which is an intrinsic material property of cartilage, governs the amount of strain in the tissue for given applied stress. This situation could occur in very incongruent joints where the interstitial fluid may flow unimpeded from the highly stressed contact region or when joint loading is maintained for long periods of time.

The speed of fluid flow w relative to the solid matrix in any direction x is given by $w = -k\Delta p/\phi^f\Delta x$. Here, Δp represents the pressure drop over a distance Δx within the tissue and k is the permeability. The quantity $\Delta p/\Delta x$ is often called the pressure gradient. A pressure gradient may exist in all three spatial directions, and it is highly sensitive to the geometry of the articular surfaces and the stresses acting in the region of contact. In an incongruent joint, the pressure gradient along a tangential direction to the surfaces will be high because the contact region will be small, and the pressure will decrease rapidly from its peak value at the center of the contact region to a zero value at its periphery, causing a high fluid velocity in that direction (Fig. 10, *left*). Conversely, in a congruent joint, the pressure gradient will be small (Fig. 10, *right*), and the resulting fluid velocity will be small in that direction. Under these circumstances, there will be a delay in the transmission of the load from the fluid phase to the solid phase as compared to an incongruent joint.

The other term that controls the magnitude of w is the permeability k of the cartilage. Its effect on the fluid velocity is the same as that of the pressure gradient, ie, low permeability cartilage will keep a significant portion of the total load on its fluid phase for a longer time than high permeability cartilage. Articular cartilage has another very important property regarding permeability. In 1976, Mansour and Mow[101] used a direct permeability experiment to demonstrate that cartilage permeability decreases with increasing compressive strain. This was subsequently verified independently in a series of biphasic creep and stress-relaxation experiments, which produced a very good match between theory and data.[28,54,102] The physiologic implication of this strain-dependent permeability effect is to retard fluid flow in the highly-stressed regions of the tissue, thus maintaining the benefit of fluid pressurization and load support in cartilage.

In an isotropic biphasic material, an axially loaded tissue specimen under compression will expand laterally, both as a result of lateral fluid exudation and pore compression. After the movement of interstitial fluid has stopped (ie, the tissue has reached equilibrium conditions), the lateral expansion is due only to pore compression and will depend on a quantity v_s known as Poisson's ratio. Poisson's ratio is related to the ratio of the lateral (expansion) strain over the axial (compressive) strain at equilibrium. If $v_s = 0$, the tissue does not expand laterally at equilibrium; this means that the change in tissue volume as a result of pore compression is exactly equal to the volume of water that has exuded from the tissue. Conversely, $v_s = 0.5$ indicates that the lateral tissue expansion is such that no change in tissue volume has occurred, even though the tissue dimensions may have changed. This is known as the incompressibility condition, and one of its consequences is that pore volume will not change and relative fluid flow will not occur. From indentation tests, the Poisson ratio of articular cartilage has been determined to range from 0 to 0.4.[24,103] In addition, Athanasiou and associates[24] found that Poisson's ratio for human articular cartilage is much lower than for other species. It could be that human articular cartilage requires the transport of more interstitial fluid because the tissue is compressed. At present, we know of no physiologic reasons why this should be the case, other than the possible role in the transport of nutrients.

From the above discussion, we see that an appreciation of the biphasic nature of articular cartilage is fundamental to an understanding of how the issue supports loads in knee joints. The biphasic material properties of articular cartilage—aggregate modulus H_A, Poisson's ratio v_s, and permeability k—emerge as fundamental intrinsic properties of the tissue that govern its compressive behavior under load. These properties may differ from one articular surface to another, as well as from site to site within the same articular layer. In the following section, we shall describe how these material properties of knee joint cartilage are determined.

Material Properties and Biochemical Composition of Human Knee Joint Cartilage

The biphasic indentation method was used to determine simultaneously the three biphasic material properties of cartilage in situ on the patella, femur, and tibial plateau of human knee joints.[24,103-105] In this experiment, the joint surface, while immersed in a physiologic saline solution containing enzymatic inhibitors, is indented with a small, flat, rigid, porous-permeable indenter tip under a constant load. By measuring the time-dependent biphasic creep behavior of the tissue under the indenter, H_A, k, and ν_s may be obtained using a curve-fitting procedure. This procedure, which determines the values of the material properties, produced data that agreed with the theoretical solution for the indentation problem, as predicted by the biphasic constitutive theory.

Seventeen cadaveric human knee joints, from subjects 18 to 42 years of age, were used in this study; all were normal on visual examination. Four sites were tested on the patella, on the proximal and distal aspects of each of the medial and lateral facets, and five sites were tested on the distal femur, three along the proximal trochlea and two along the distal trochlea (Fig. 11). On each patella and femur these sites were grouped into two regions that correspond to the contact regions of the knee joint at 30 and 90 degrees of flexion. The mean value of the aggregate modulus for all patellar sites was found to be 0.42 MPa, while the corresponding value for the femur was 0.62 MPa (Fig. 12, *top*), which indicates that femoral cartilage is stiffer than patellar cartilage (P<0.001). The difference was also found to be more accentuated in those regions of the patellofemoral groove corresponding to contact areas at 90 degrees of flexion, as compared to 30 degrees of flexion. Furthermore, the permeability of patellar cartilage was measured to be almost 90% higher than that of femoral cartilage, and this difference was also highly significant (Fig. 12, *bottom*). Thus, under similar loading conditions, water would flow faster in patellar cartilage than in femoral cartilage, thereby transmitting load to the solid phase within a shorter amount of time. No statistical differences between the two surfaces were found for Poisson's ratio. In the regions corresponding to 90 degrees of flexion, the thickness of cartilage was found to be higher in the patella than in the femur, as can also be observed from the typical cartilage thickness maps of Figure 8.

The data also showed that the aggregate modulus and Poisson's ratio do not vary significantly from site to site within the patella or the femur when observed separately. However, permeability within the patella was significantly higher on the distal lateral facet compared to the other facets tested on this surface. Similarly, cartilage from the anterior femoral groove demonstrated significantly higher

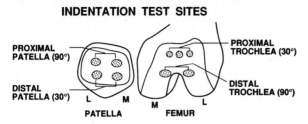

Fig. 11   *Indentation test sites on the patella and distal femur.*

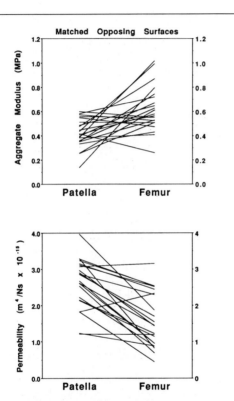

Fig. 12   *Patellar versus trochlear cartilage material properties for all specimens: Top, Aggregate modulus, H_A; Bottom, Permeability.*

permeability than that from the posterior groove or condyles. In this sample of specimens, there was no correlation between material properties and age.

Biochemical composition results show that water content was significantly higher in patellar cartilage where it averaged 76%, than in femoral cartilage where it was 73%. Conversely, no regional differences in water content were observed within each of these surfaces. Furthermore, the concentration of proteoglycan was lower in the

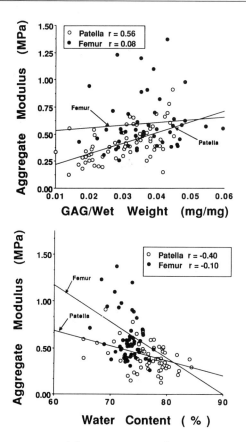

Fig. 13 *Top, Aggregate modulus versus proteoglycan content. **Bottom**, Aggregate modulus versus water content.*

patella (3% of the wet weight) than in the femur (3.6%). However, the collagen content was not appreciably different in the cartilage from these two surfaces. Comparison of the composition of the cartilage from different sites of the femur and patella showed that on the patella, the distal lateral facet had lower collagen and higher proteoglycan contents than other regions. No significant variation of composition was detected for different sites on the femur.

By plotting data from the material properties of cartilage as a function of biochemical composition, it is possible to study the relationship between the biochemical composition and the biomechanical properties of the tissue. Figure 13, *top* and *bottom*, displays the aggregate modulus data as compared with proteoglycan content and water content, respectively. A correlation is found between H_A and proteoglycan content for patellar cartilage (r = 0.56) but not for femoral cartilage (r = 0.08). Similarly, the aggregate modulus correlates weakly with water content in the patella (r = 0.40) but not in the femur (r = 0.10). For the patellar cartilage, this finding is similar to that reported by Armstrong and Mow in 1982.[21]

Discussion

Knee cartilage may be subjected to continuous load, such as during standing, or intermittent load, such as during walking or running. It may also be subjected to sudden impact, either through a hard heel strike or from a direct blow to the patella. Each of these loading modes results in a different mechanical environment in the joint and, consequently, a different tissue response. Thus, articular cartilage is subjected to a wide variety of conditions where it is required to function in an optimal way to prevent or minimize potential damage to its collagen-proteoglycan extracellular solid matrix or chondrocytes. This optimal function actually exists as a result of the biphasic nature of cartilage. When load is applied across two articular surfaces separated by a layer of synovial fluid, a major component of this load is carried by interstitial water, which may constitute 80% of the tissue by weight. As described above, most of this water is free to move inside the tissue at a rate that is proportional to the tissue permeability. While cartilage has a high water content, its permeability is very low, thus preventing fluid from quickly squeezing out of a loaded region. Consequently, the transmission to the solid phase of that portion of the applied load supported by the fluid phase is also occurring at a very slow rate, typically on the order of minutes. If the patella is subjected to an impact load with a duration of a few milliseconds,[22,30] the collagen-proteoglycan solid matrix stress at the articular surface (for a porosity of 75%) is only 25% of the total impacting stress. During walking phase, a particular region of knee cartilage is subjected to loads only during short intermittent periods. This allows fluid that has squeezed out of that region during loading to be replenished as the tissue recovers. Indeed, some of the fluid that escapes the loaded region may flow into the adjacent region, which is about to be loaded.

The permeability of patellar cartilage is higher than that of the femur. When the patellar surface comes into contact with the trochlea, the amount of load being applied on each surface is the same according to Newton's 3rd law of action and reaction. However, because of the mismatch in their permeabilities, load transmission from fluid to solid will occur faster in the patella than in the trochlea, thus resulting in higher deformations in the collagen-proteoglycan solid matrix of patellar cartilage. Furthermore, because of the small size (the proximal to distal length) of the patella relative to the trochlea, a given region of patellar cartilage will be loaded for a longer time than a region of trochlear cartilage during the same walking cycle. This means that the collagen-proteoglycan solid matrix of patellar cartilage will always deform more than that of trochlear cartilage. Also, this will reduce the recovery time of patellar cartilage and its ability to re-imbibe its lost fluid. All of these factors may

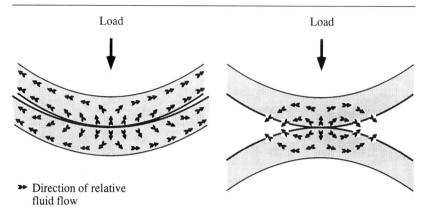

Load   Load

➤➤ Direction of relative
fluid flow

Fig. 14   *Fluid flow pattern in a congruent joint (**left**), and incongruent joint
(**right**).*

lead to fatigue failure of the patellar collagen-proteoglycan solid matrix at a rate that is greater than on the trochlea.

Thus, an essential loadbearing component of cartilage during
physiologically realistic time periods is the interstitial water, and the
effectiveness of this mechanism is contingent on preventing fluid
from flowing out of the loaded region too fast. While permeability
controls the interstitial fluid flow rate within cartilage, it is joint
congruence that determines the amount of fluid that escapes cartilage through its surface at the periphery of the contact region. A
highly congruent joint has a large contact area at the interface between its articular surfaces, thus preventing interstitial fluid from
quickly escaping through the surfaces by forcing it to travel a large
distance inside the cartilage where permeability is very low (Fig. 14,
left). An incongruent joint, however, has a small contacting region
that can quickly be circumscribed by the interstitial fluid in its effort
to seek a path of least resistance to flow (Fig. 14, *right*). Furthermore, incongruent contact leads to high-pressure gradients in cartilage, which further increase the rate at which fluid will escape the
region of cartilage loading (Fig. 10). (High-pressure gradients at the
articular surface also result in high-shear stresses at the cartilage-
subchondral bone interface.)[106] In the patellofemoral joint, the horizontal plane exhibits good congruence while the sagittal plane
reveals an incongruent contact. Hence, the highest pressure gradients will occur along the sagittal direction, which will also be the
predominant direction of interstitial fluid flow.

Just as fluid may escape through the articular surfaces of an incongruent joint, it may also flow towards the deep zone of the cartilage layer. In a thin cartilage layer, the biphasic theory shows that
the pressure distribution across the cartilage thickness is approximately uniform, and most of the fluid will flow either sideways or
across the surface. However, in a thick cartilage layer, the pressure

in the deep zone will typically be lower than that at the surface zone. This principle can be better understood in the case of a very thick cartilage layer where, very far from the surface, the pressure will tend to zero. Thus, in thick cartilage layers there is an additional path by which fluid can flow from high-pressure to low-pressure regions (Fig. 14). In this instance, again, because cartilage is generally thicker on the patella (Fig. 8), load transfer from fluid phase to solid phase of cartilage will occur at a higher rate in the patella than in the trochlea.

The collagen-proteoglycan extracellular matrix of cartilage provides the solid phase support. The collagen fibrous structure and proteoglycan fixed-charge density control the permeability of this solid phase. As fluid flows through cartilage, it generates a diffusive drag load that is resisted by the stiffness of the solid phase. When fluid flows out of a loaded region, the load becomes progressively more supported by the collagen-proteoglycan extracellular matrix. This load transfer from the fluid phase to the solid phase increases the collagen-proteoglycan matrix deformation in proportion to the aggregate modulus of the tissue. Patellar cartilage, which has a lower modulus than femoral cartilage, will again experience higher deformation for the same applied stress.

Although correlations can be obtained between material properties of articular cartilage and its biochemical composition (water, collagen, and proteoglycan contents), these are usually far from ideal. It is, therefore, apparent that other compositional and/or structural parameters, not yet determined, play important roles in imparting the mechanical properties. Collagen cross-linking, type IX collagen, quantitatively minor proteoglycans, and structural organization of the collagen fibrils may all contribute.

Some studies indicate that the rate of proteoglycan synthesis and release differs significantly when cartilage is under hydrostatic pressure (when the applied load is most supported by the fluid) as opposed, for example, to unidirectional compressive stresses (when the load has been transferred to the solid phase). Clearly, the differences in the intrinsic mechanical properties of cartilage between the patella and the trochlea not only have biomechanical functional implications but also have physiologic implications. Thus, the pathophysiologic implications of the differences in the intrinsic properties of cartilage from these two joint surfaces must be further explored in future studies on patellofemoral joint biomechanics and on chondromalacia of patellar cartilage.

Summary

The biomechanics of knee joint articular surfaces can be studied by analyzing the material properties and biochemical composition of the cartilage as well as the anatomy of the cartilage layers. By combining these elements with a basic understanding of the fundamentals of fluid transport in soft tissues, it is possible to describe the various mechanisms that govern the stress and strain environment of the joint. This information may lead to a better understanding of knee joint pathophysiology and possibly to the process of degenerative joint disease. For the patellofemoral joint, many of the results described above point to the higher vulnerability of patellar versus trochlear cartilage. This may partly explain the higher incidence of degenerative changes in the patella, which has been extensively reported in the literature.[107] A more detailed analysis of the biomechanics of this joint would integrate these anatomic and material data into a more accurate finite element model of the joint, which could then provide precise spatial and temporal variations of pressure, stress, strain, deformation, and fluid velocity across the entire joint articulating surfaces. The methodology outlined in this chapter is applicable for any diarthrodial joint. In our laboratory, work is also in progress using this technology on the study of the glenohumeral joint and the thumb carpometacarpal joint.[65,108]

Acknowledgment

This work was sponsored by a grant from the Bristol-Myers Squibbs Center of Excellence for Orthopaedic Research.

References

1. Andriacchi TP, Mikosz RP: Musculoskeletal dynamics, locomotion and clinical applications, in Mow VC, Hayes WC (eds): *Basic Orthopaedic Biomechanics.* New York, Raven Press, 1991, pp 51-92.

2. Butler DL, Noyes FR, Grood ES: Ligamentous restraints to anterior-posterior drawer in the human knee: A biomechanical study. *J Bone Joint Surg* 1980;62A:259-270.

3. Cappozzo A, Figura F, Marchetti MJ: The interplay of muscular and external forces in human ambulation. *J Biomech* 1976;9:35-43.

4. Morrison JB: The mechanics of the knee joint in relation to normal walking. *J Biomech* 1970;3:51-61.

5. Steindler A: A historical review of the studies and investigations made in relation to human gait. *J Bone Joint Surg* 1953;35A:540-542, 728.

6. Woo SL, Gomez MA, Akeson WH: The time and history: Dependent viscoelastic properties of the canine medial collateral ligament. *J Biomech Eng* 1981;103:293-298.

7. Ahmed AM, Burke DL: *In-vitro* measurement of static pressure distribution in synovial joints: Part I: Tibial surface of the knee. *J Biomech Eng* 1983;105:216-225.

8. Ahmed AM, Burke DL, Yu A: *In-vitro* measurement of static pressure distribution in synovial joints: Part II: Retropatellar surface. *J Biomech Eng* 1983;105:226-236.

9. Brown TD, Shaw DT: A technique for measuring instantaneous *in vitro* contact stress distributions in articular joints. *J Biomech* 1982;15:329-333.

10. Brown TD, Shaw DT: *In vitro* contact stress distribution on the femoral condyles. *J Orthop Res* 1984;2:190-199.

11. Fukubayashi T, Kurosawa H: The contact area and pressure distribution pattern of the knee: A study of normal and osteoarthrotic knee joints. *Acta Orthop Scand* 1980;51:871-879.

12. Huberti HH, Hayes WC: Patellofemoral contact pressures: The influence of Q-angle and tendofemoral contact. *J Bone Joint Surg* 1984;66A:715-724.

13. Kettelkamp DB, Jacobs AW: Tibiofemoral contact area: Determination and implications. *J Bone Joint Surg* 1972;54A:349-356.

14. King D: The function of semilunar cartilages. *J Bone Joint Surg* 1936;18:1069-1076.

15. Levy IM, Torzilli PA, Warren RF: The effect of medial meniscectomy on anterior-posterior motion of the knee. *J Bone Joint Surg* 1982;64A:883-888.

16. MacConaill MA: Function of intra-articular fibrocartilages, with special reference to knee and inferior radio-ulnar joints. *J Anat* 1932;66: 210-227.

17. Matthews LS, Sonstegard DA, Henke JA: Load bearing characteristics of the patello-femoral joint. *Acta Orthop Scand* 1977;48:511-516.

18. Seedhom BB: Transmission of the load in the knee with special reference to the role of the menisci: Part I. *Eng Med* 1979;8:207-218.

19. Seedhom BB, Hargreaves DJ: Transmission of the load in the knee joint with special reference to the role of the menisci: Part II. *Eng Med* 1979;8:220-228.

20. Walker PS, Erkman MJ: The role of the menisci in force transmission across the knee. *Clin Orthop* 1975;109:184-192.

21. Amstrong CG, Mow VC: Variations in the intrinsic mechanical properties of human articular cartilage with age, degeneration, and water content. *J Bone Joint Surg* 1982;64A:88-94.

22. Amstrong CG, Mow VC, Wirth CR: Biomechanics of impact-induced microdamage to articular cartilage: A possible genesis for chondromalacia patella, in Finerman G (ed): *Symposium on Sports Medicine: The Knee*. St. Louis, CV Mosby, 1985, pp 70-84.

23. Arnoczky S, Adams ME, DeHaven K, et al: Meniscus, in Buckwalter JA Jr, Woo SL-Y (eds): *Injury and Repair of the Musculoskeletal Soft Tissues*. Park Ridge, IL, American Academy of Orthopaedic Surgeons, 1988, pp 487-537.

24. Athanasiou KA, Rosenwasser MP, Buckwalter JA, et al: Interspecies comparison of In Situ intrinsic mechanical properties of distal femoral cartilage. *J Orthop Res* 1991;9:330-340.

25. Fithian DC, Kelly MA, Mow VC: Material properties and structure-function relationships in the menisci. *Clin Orthop* 1990;252:19-31.

26. Huiskes R, Blankevoort L: The relationship between knee motion and articular surface geometry, in Mow VC, Ratcliffe A, Woo SL-Y (eds): *Biomechanics of Diarthrodial Joints*. New York, Springer-Verlag, 1990, vol II, pp 269-286.

27. Kwan MK, Lai WM, Mow VC: A finite deformation theory for cartilage and other soft hydrated connective tissues: I. Equilibrium results. *J Biomech* 1990;23:145-155.

28. Mow VC, Hou JS, Owens JM, et al: Biphasic and quasilinear viscoelastic theories for hydrated soft tissues, in Mow VC, Ratcliffe A, Woo SL-Y, *Biomechanics of Diarthrodial Joints*. New York, Springer-Verlag, 1990, vol I, pp 215-260.

29. Proctor CS, Schmidt MB, Whipple RR, et al: Material properties of the normal medial bovine meniscus. *J Orthop Res* 1989;7:771-782.

30. Thompson RC Jr, Oegema TR, Lewis JL, et al: Osteoarthrotic changes after acute transarticular load: An animal model. *J Bone Joint Surg* 1991;73A:990-1001.

31. Mow VC, Soslowsky LJ: Friction, lubrication, and wear of diarthrodial joints, in Mow VC, Hayes WC (eds): *Basic Orthopaedic Biomechanics.* New York, Raven Press, 1991, pp 245-292.

32. Dowson D, Jin Z: An analysis of micro-elastohydrodynamic lubrication in synovial joints considering cyclic loading and entraining velocities, in Dowson D, Taylor CM, Godet M, et al (eds): *Fluid Film Lubrication— Osborne Reynolds Centenary.* Amsterdam, Elsevier, 1987, pp 375-386.

33. Dowson D: Bio-tribology of natural and replacement synovial joints, in Mow VC, Ratcliffe A, Woo SLY (eds): *Biomechanics of Diarthrodial Joints.* New York, Springer-Verlag, 1990, vol II, pp 305-345.

34. Bourne RB, Finlay JB, Papadopoulos P, et al: The effect of medial meniscectomy on strain distribution in the proximal part of the tibia. *J Bone Joint Surg* 1984;66A:1431-1437.

35. Burstein AH, Reilly DT, Martens M: Aging of bone tissue: Mechanical properties. *J Bone Joint Surg* 1976;58A:82-86.

36. Carter DR, Hayes WC: The compressive behavior of bone as a two-phase porous structure. *J Bone Joint Surg* 1977;59A:954-962.

37. Goldstein SA: The mechanical properties of trabecular bone: Dependence on anatomic location and function. *J Biomech* 1987;20:1055-1061.

38. Odgaard A, Pedersen CM, Bentzen SM, et al: Density changes at the proximal tibia after medial meniscectomy. *J Orthop Res* 1989;7:744-753.

39. Radin EL, Parker HG, Pugh JW, et al: Response of joints to impact loading: III: Relationship between trabecular microfractures and cartilage degeneration. *J Biomech* 1973;6:51-57.

40. Reilly DT, Burstein AH, Frankel VH: The elastic modulus for bone. *J Biomech* 1974;7:271-275.

41. Grood ES, Suntay WJ, Noyes FR, et al: Biomechanics of the knee-extension exercise: Effect of cutting the anterior cruciate ligament. *J Bone Joint Surg* 1984;66A:725-734.

42. Woo SL, Orlando CA, Gomez MA, et al: Tensile properties of the medial collateral ligament as a function of age. *J Orthop Res* 1986;4: 133-141.

43. Markolf KL, Bargar WL, Shoemaker SC, et al: The role of joint load in knee stability. *J Bone Joint Surg* 1981;63A:570-585.

44. Markolf KL, Gorek JF, Kabo JM, et al: New insights into load bearing functions of the anterior cruciate ligament, in Mow VC, Ratcliffe A, Woo SL-Y (eds): *Biomechanics of Diarthrodial Joints.* New York, Springer-Verlag, 1990, vol I, pp 155-175.

45. Shoemaker SC, Markolf KL: The role of the meniscus in the anterior-posterior stability of the loaded anterior cruciate-deficient knee. *J Bone Joint Surg* 1986;68A:71-79.

46. Altman RD, Tenenbaum J, Latta L, et al: Biomechanical and biochemical properties of dog cartilage in experimentally induced osteoarthritis. *Ann Rheum Dis* 1984;43:83-90.

47. Brandt KD, Mankin HJ: Etiopathogenesis of osteoarthritis. *J Rheum* 1987;13:1127-1160.

48. Eyre DR, McDevitt CA, Billingham ME, et al: Biosynthesis of collagen and other matrix proteins by articular cartilage in experimental osteoarthrosis. *Biochem J* 1980;188:823-837.

49. McDevitt CA, Muir H: Biochemical changes in the cartilage of the knee in experimental and natural osteoarthritis in the dog. *J Bone Joint Surg* 1976;58B:94-101.

50. McDevitt C, Gilbertson E, Muir H: An experimental model of osteoarthritis: Early morphological and biochemical changes. *J Bone Joint Surg* 1977;59B:24-35.

51. Mow VC, Setton LA, Ratcliffe A, et al: Structure-function relationships for articular cartilage and effects of joint instability and trauma on cartilage function, in Brandt KD (ed): *Cartilage Changes in Osteoarthritis*. Indianapolis, IN, University of Indiana Press, 1990, pp 22-42.

52. Setton LA, Mow VC, Muller FJ, et al: Comparison of tensile and swelling properties of disuse and Pond-Nuki osteoarthritic knee cartilage. *Trans Orthop Res Soc* 1991;16:358.

53. Mow VC, Kuei SC, Lai WM, et al: Biphasic creep and stress relaxation of articular cartilage in compression: Theory and experiments. *J Biomech Eng* 1980;102:73-84.

54. Mow VC, Holmes MH, Lai WM: Fluid transport and mechanical properties of articular cartilage: A review. *J Biomech* 1984;17:377-394.

55. Spilker RL, Suh JK, Mow VC: Effects of friction on the unconfined compressive response of articular cartilage: A finite element analysis. *J Biomech Eng* 1990;112:138-146.

56. Truesdell C, Noll W: The nonlinear field theory of mechanics, in Flügge S (ed): *Handbuck der Physik*. Berlin, Springer-Verlag, 1965, vol III, p 3.

57. Bowen RM: Incompressible porous media models by use of the theory of mixtures. *Int J Eng Sci* 1980;18:182-185.

58. Ateshian GA, Soslowsky LJ, Mow VC: Quantitation of articular surface topography and cartilage thickness in knee joints using stereophotogrammetry. *J Biomech* 1991;24:761-776.

59. Ateshian GA, Mow VC: B-Spline surface-fitting method for articular surfaces of diarthrodial joints. *J Biomech Eng*, in press.

60. Ghosh SK: A close-range photogrammetric system for 3-D measurements and perspective diagramming in biomechanics. *J Biomech* 1983;16:667-674.

61. Huiskes R, Kremers J, de Lange A, et al: Analytical stereophotogrammetric determination of three-dimensional knee-joint geometry. *J Biomech* 1985;18:559-570.

62. Scherrer PK, Hillberry BM: Piecewise mathematical representation of articular surfaces. *J Biomech* 1979;12:301-311.

63. Scherrer PK, Hillberry BM, Van Sickle D: Determinating the in-vivo areas of contact in the canine shoulder. *J Biomech Eng*1979b;101:271-278.

64. Selvik G: A roentgen stereophotogrammetric method for the study of the kinematics of the skeletal system, PhD thesis. Lund, Sweden, University of Lund, 1974.

65. Ateshian GA, Rosenwasser MP, Mow VC: Curvature characteristics and congruence of the thumb carpometacarpal joint. *J Biomech*, in press.

66. Eisenhart LP: *A Treatise on the Differential Geometry of Curves and Surfaces*. New York, Ginn & Co, 1909.

67. McLeod WD, Moschi A, Andrews JR, et al: Tibial plateau topography. *Am J Sports Med* 1977;5:13-18.

68. Mankin HJ, Thrasher AZ: Water content and binding in normal and osteoarthritic human cartilage. *J Bone Joint Surg* 1975;57A:76-80.

69. Maroudas A: Biophysical chemistry of cartilaginous tissues with special reference to solute and fluid transport. *Biorheology* 1975;12:233-248.

70. Maroudas A: Physicochemical properties of articular cartilage, in Freeman MAR (ed): *Adult Articular Cartilage*. Tunbridge Wells, England, Pitman Medical, 1979, pp 215-290.

71. Muir H: Proteoglycans as organizers of the intercellular matrix. *Biochem Soc Trans* 1983;11:613-622.

79

72. Buckwalter JA, Hunziker E, Rosenberg L, et al: Articular cartilage: Composition and structure, in Woo SL-Y, Buckwalter JA (eds): *Injury and Repair of the Musculoskeletal Soft Tissues*. Park Ridge, IL, American Academy of Orthopaedic Surgeons, 1988, pp 405-425.

73. Eyre DR: Collagen: Molecular diversity in the body's protein scaffold. *Science* 1980;207:1315-1322.

74. Akizuki S, Mow VC, Müller F, et al: Tensile properties of human knee joint cartilage: I. Influence of ionic conditions, weight bearing, and fibrillation on the tensile modulus. *J Orthop Res* 1986;4:379-392.

75. Akizuki S, Mow VC, Muller F, et al: Tensile properties of human knee joint cartilage: II. Correlations between weight bearing and tissue pathology and the kinetics of swelling. *J Orthop Res* 1987;5:173-186.

76. Kempson GE, Muir H, Pollard C, et al: The tensile properties of the cartilage of human femoral condyles related to the content of collagen and glycosaminoglycans. *Biochim Biophys Acta* 1973;297:456-472.

77. Roth V, Mow VC: The intrinsic tensile behavior of the matrix of bovine articular cartilage and its variation with age. *J Bone Joint Surg* 1980;62A:1102-1117.

78. Schmidt MB, Schoonbeck JM, Mow VC, et al: The relationship between collagen crosslinking and the tensile properties of articular cartilage. *Trans Orthop Res Soc* 1987;12:134.

79. Schmidt MB, Mow VC, Chun LE, et al: Effects of proteoglycan extraction on the tensile behavior of articular cartilage. *J Orthop Res* 1990;8:353-363.

80. Woo SL, Akeson WH, Jemmott GF: Measurements of nonhomogeneous, directional mechanical properties of articular cartilage in tension. *J Biomech* 1976;9:785-791.

81. Hascall VC: Proteoglycans: The chondroitin sulfate/keratan sulfate proteoglycan of cartilage, ISI Atlas of Science. *Biochemistry* 1988;1:189-199.

82. Heinegård D, Oldberg A: Structure and biology of cartilage and bone matrix noncollagenous macromolecules. *FASEB J* 1989;3:2042-2051.

83. Doege K, Rhodes C, Sasaki M, et al: Molecular biology of cartilage proteoglycan (aggrecan) and link protein, in Sandell LJ, Boyd CD (eds): *Extracellular Matrix Genes*. San Diego, Academic Press, 1990, pp 137-155.

84. Hardingham TE, Muir H, Kwan MK, et al: Viscoelastic properties of proteoglycan solutions with varying proportions present as aggregates. *J Orthop Res* 1987;5:36-46.

85. Hascall VC: Interaction of cartilage proteoglycans with hyaluronic acid. *J Supramol Structure* 1977;7:101-120.

86. Mow VC, Zhu W, Lai WM, et al: The influence of link protein stabilization on the viscometric properties of proteoglycan aggregate solutions. *Biochim Biophys Acta* 1989;992:201-208.

87. Mow VC, Zhu W, Ratcliffe A: Structure and function of articular cartilage and meniscus, in Mow VC, Hayes WC (eds): *Basic Orthopaedic Biomechanics*. New York, Raven Press, 1991, pp 143-198.

88. Donnan FG: The theory of membrane equilibria. *Chemical Rev* 1924;1:73-90.

89. Lai WM, Hou JS, Mow VC: A triphasic theory for the swelling and deformational behaviors of articular cartilage. *J Biomech Eng* 1991;113:245-258.

90. Heinegård D, Hascall VC: Aggregation of cartilage proteoglycans. 3. Characteristics of the proteins isolated from trypsin digests of aggregates. *J Biol Chem* 1974;249:4250-4256.

91. Hardingham TE, Muir H: The specific interaction of hyaluronic acid with cartilage proteoglycans. *Biochim Biophys Acta* 1972;279:401-405.

92. Ratcliffe A, Hardingham T: Cartilage proteoglycan binding region and link protein: Radioimmunoassays and the detection of masked determinants in aggregates. *Biochem J* 1983;213:371-378.

93. Pottenger LA, Lyon NB, Hecht JD, et al: Influence of cartilage particle size and proteoglycan aggregation on immobilization of proteoglycans. *J Biol Chem* 1982;257:11479-11485.

94. Ratcliffe A, Fryer PR, Hardingham TE: The distribution of aggregating proteoglycans in articular cartilage: Comparison of quantitative immunoelectron microscopy with radioimmunoassay and biochemical analysis. *J Histochem Cytochem* 1984;32:193-201.

95. Stockwell RA, Scott JE: Distribution of acid glycosaminoglycans in human articular cartilage. *Nature* 1967;215:1376-1378.

96. Ratcliffe A, Tyler JA, Hardingham TE: Articular cartilage cultured with Interleukin 1: Increased release of link protein, hyaluronate-binding region and other proteoglycan fragments. *Biochem J* 1986;238:571-580.

97. Zhu WB, Mow VC: Viscometric properties of proteoglycan solutions at physiological concentrations, in Mow VC, Ratcliffe A, Woo SL-Y (eds): *Biomechanics of Diarthrodial Joints.* New York, Springer-Verlag, 1990, vol I, pp 313-344.

98. Zhu W, Lai WM, Mow VC: The density and strength of proteoglycan-proteoglycan interaction sites in concentrated solutions. *J Biomech* 1991;24:1007-1018.

99. Comper WB, Zamparo O: Hydraulic conductivity of polymer matrices. *Biophys Chem* 1989;34:127-135.

100. Brown TD, Singerman RJ: Experimental determination of the linear biphasic constitutive coefficients of human fetal proximal femoral chondroepiphysis. *J Biomech* 1986;19:597-605.

101. Mansour JM, Mow VC: The permeability of articular cartilage under compressive strain and at high pressures. *J Bone Joint Surg* 1976;58A:509-516.

102. Holmes MH: Finite deformation of soft tissue: Analysis of a mixture model in uni-axial compression. *J Biomech Eng* 1986;108:372-381.

103. Mow VC, Gibbs MC, Lai WM, et al: Biphasic indentation of articular cartilage: II. A numerical algorithm and an experimental study. *J Biomech* 1989;22:853-861.

104. Froimson MI, Ratcliffe A, Mow VC: Patellar cartilage mechanical properties vary with site and biochemical composition. *Trans Orthop Res Soc* 1989;14:150.

105. Mak AF, Lai WM, Mow VC: Biphasic indentation of articular cartilage: I. Theoretical analysis. *J Biomech* 1987;20:703-714.

106. Armstrong CG: An analysis of the stresses in a thin layer of articular cartilage in a synovial joint. *Eng Med* 1986;15:55-61.

107. Radin EL, Martin RB, Burr DB, et al: Effects of mechanical loading on the tissues of the rabbit knee. *J Orthop Res* 1984;2:221-234.

108. Soslowsky LJ, Flatow EL, Bigliani LU, et al: Articular geometry of the glenohumeral joint. *Clin Orthop*, in press.

Chapter 5

Mechanical Injuries of Articular Cartilage

Joseph A. Buckwalter, MD

Normal synovial joint function depends on the smooth, low friction gliding surface provided by articular cartilage. Although it is at most only a few millimeters thick, articular cartilage has surprising stiffness to compression and resilience, and exceptional ability to distribute loads, thereby minimizing peak stresses on subchondral bone. Perhaps most important, it has remarkable durability, providing normal joint function for 80 years or more in many people. Yet, excessive joint loading can damage articular cartilage, causing loss of joint motion, instability, deformity, and pain.

Articular surface injuries resulting from open joint injuries including osteochondral fractures, penetrating injuries, and dislocations can be diagnosed easily; however, open injuries probably occur much less frequently than closed injuries of articular cartilage (injuries that do not penetrate or expose the interior of the joint). Experimental work shows that excessive joint loading and direct blunt joint trauma subject articular cartilage to intense compression and shear forces, which can damage the cartilage matrix and cells, altering the cartilage mechanical properties without disrupting the tissue, or which can fracture or rupture the cartilage matrix.[1-4] Clinical observations suggest that progressive cartilage degeneration follows these injuries in at least some patients. Less frequently, acute closed injuries fracture cartilage and the underlying bone.[5-14]

The clinical presentations, frequencies, and natural histories of cartilage injuries caused by mechanical forces are less well understood than those of injuries to the other musculoskeletal tissues including bone, tendon, ligament, and muscle. The clinical mechanisms of cartilage injuries have not been well defined. Closed articular surface injuries are difficult, if not impossible, to detect by physical examination, and plain radiographs do not directly show cartilage injuries. Magnetic resonance imaging cannot, at present, provide clear demonstrations of cartilage injuries, and sensitive clinically applicable measures of cartilage mechanical function do not currently exist. Therefore, no reliable, clinically useful method currently exists for detecting articular surface injuries that do not cause visible disruption of the tissue. Injuries that do cause tissue disruption currently can reliably be evaluated only by direct inspection during arthroscopy or arthrotomy.[15-17]

Arthroscopic examinations of injured joints suggest that closed articular surface injuries occur frequently. One group of surgeons examined arthroscopically 85 knees with traumatic hemarthrosis but absent or negligible ligamentous instability. In 20% of these knees they found chondral fractures or an articular surface defect.[15] In many patients, cartilage injuries occur in association with injuries to other synovial joint tissues, including menisci, ligaments, joint capsule, and synovium.[15] In these people, the cartilage injury may be overlooked, and even when the cartilage injury is identified, its effects are difficult to distinguish from the effects of the injuries to the other tissues.[3,4]

Advances in understanding mechanical injuries to articular surfaces and the frequency and outcome of these injuries, and in developing better methods of diagnosing and treating cartilage injuries depend on knowledge of the types of cartilage injury and the response of the synovial tissues to these injuries. In this chapter I discuss the differences among closed mechanical injuries of articular cartilage, define three types of closed mechanical injury to articular cartilage, and discuss the response of the synovial joint to these injuries.

Differences in Mechanical Injuries of Articular Cartilage

Mechanical injuries of articular cartilage differ in the extent and type of tissue damage and in the response of the tissues to the injury. Joint trauma can damage the matrix macromolecular framework and cells without causing mechanical disruption of the tissue, or it can fracture or rupture the cartilage matrix, causing visible splits in the articular surface.[2,5-8,18-22] Because cartilage lacks blood vessels, damage to the cartilage alone does not cause inflammation. If an injury disrupts cartilage and subchondral bone, the damage to bone blood vessels causes inflammation and initiates the fracture-healing process.[4] The clot and repair tissue from the bone can then fill the articular cartilage defect and follow the sequence of inflammation, repair, and remodeling in the same way as the repair tissue in ligaments. Unlike the repair tissue in ligaments, the repair tissue that fills cartilage defects initially differentiates toward articular cartilage rather than toward dense fibrous tissue.[3,4]

Differences in type of tissue damage separate mechanical injuries of cartilage into three types:[2,4,23-25] (1) disruption or alteration of the macromolecular framework, loss of matrix macromolecules, or cell injury without visible tissue disruption; (2) disruption of articular cartilage alone (chondral fractures); and (3) mechanical disruption of articular cartilage and subchondral bone (osteochondral fractures). Each of these types of cartilage damage presents a different

Table 1 Closed mechanical injuries to articular cartilage

Injury Type	Clinical Presentation	Tissue Response	Potential for Healing
Damage to matrix and/or cells without visible disruption of the articular surface	No known symptoms Direct inspection of the articular surface and current clinical imaging methods cannot detect this type of injury. This type of injury presumably can alter the mechanical properties of the tissue.	Synthesis of new matrix macromolecules Cell proliferation?	If the basic matrix structure remains intact and enough viable cells remain, the cells can restore the normal tissue composition. If the matrix and/or cell population sustains significant damage or if the tissue sustains further damage, the lesion may progress.
Cartilage disruption (cartilage fractures or ruptures)	May cause mechanical symptoms, synovitis, and joint effusions	No fibrin clot formation or inflammation Synthesis of new matrix macromolecules and cell proliferation, but new tissue does not fill the cartilage defect	Depending on the location and size of the lesion and the structural integrity, stability, and alignment of the joint, the lesion may or may not progress.
Cartilage and bone disruption (osteochondral fractures)	May cause mechanical symptoms, synovitis, and joint effusions	Formation of a fibrin clot, inflammation, invasion of new cells, and production of new tissue	Depending on the location and size of the lesion and the structural integrity, stability, and alignment of the joint, the lesion may or may not progress.

problem for repair and stimulates a different response (Table 1),[23] but the categories overlap. Progressive loss of matrix macromolecules or disruption of the organization of the matrix macromolecular framework eventually results in mechanical disruption of the tissue; mechanical disruption of the cartilage and bone may release tissue factors that stimulate matrix degradation and loss of matrix macromolecules.

Cartilage Injury Without Tissue Disruption

Experimental work shows that acute or repetitive blunt trauma can damage cartilage, causing a decrease in matrix proteoglycan concentration and possibly altering the collagen meshwork and injuring chondrocytes. This damage can occur without visible tissue disruption.[1-3,19-22,24,26] Other causes of this type of cartilage injury include traumatic or surgical disruption of the synovial membrane that leaves the articular surface exposed, prolonged joint immobilization, some medications, joint irrigation with some types of fluids, and synovial inflammation.[3,4,20,24,25,27-29] The intensity and type of cartilage loading that can cause tissue damage without visible disruption have not been well defined.[2] Physiologic levels of joint loading do not appear to cause cartilage injury; however, impact loading above that associated with normal activities, but less than that necessary to produce cartilage disruption, can cause alterations of the cartilage matrix.[20]

Maintenance of normal cartilage structure, composition, and function requires a minimal level of joint loading and motion. Increased joint loading and motion, up to a certain level, may increase cartilage matrix synthesis relative to matrix degradation. In dogs, increased loading of a limb, resulting from cast immobilization of the opposite limb or moderate running exercise (4 km/day), increased cartilage glycosaminoglycan concentration and thickness.[30] Yet, strenuous running (20 km/day) reduced cartilage thickness and glycosaminoglycan concentration in normal joints, suggesting that loading and motion above a certain level may adversely affect articular cartilage. Disturbances in the neuromuscular control of joints or such joint abnormalities as articular surface incongruities or ligamentous instability presumably increase loading of at least some regions of the articular surface, thereby increasing the probability of cartilage damage.[2,31]

Damage to the cartilage matrix without tissue disruption has not been studied extensively, but experimental evidence shows that loss of proteoglycans or alteration of their organization (in particular, a decrease in proteoglycan aggregation) occurs before other signs of significant matrix injury. The loss of proteoglycans may be caused by increased degradation or decreased synthesis of the molecules.[3,4,24,27-29] Significant loss of matrix proteoglycans decreases cartilage stiffness and increases its hydraulic permeability.[25,32] These alterations may cause greater loading of the remaining macromolecular framework, including the collagen fibrils, thereby increasing the vulnerability of the tissue to further damage from impact loading.[25]

In addition to loss of proteoglycans, these injuries may cause other matrix abnormalities such as distortions of the collagen fibril meshwork or disruptions of the collagen fibril-proteoglycan relationships, and they may injure chondrocytes. Alterations in the cartilage matrices of dogs following impact loading that did not visibly disrupt the tissue included cartilage swelling, increased cartilage collagen fibril diameter, and disturbances of the relationships between collagen and proteoglycans.[20] Presumably, these changes represent more severe matrix damage than a decrease in proteoglycan concentration.

Although experimental studies show that cartilage damage may occur without visible disruption of the tissue, currently there is neither a clinically applicable method of detecting such alterations in cartilage matrix composition as decreased proteoglycan concentration or increased water concentration, nor is there a reliable, accurate, clinically applicable method of measuring cartilage mechanical properties. When probing the articular surface, surgeons sometimes find regions of apparent "softening" that may result from alterations in the matrix; however, it is not known if cartilage "softening" progresses to matrix disruption.

The ability of chondrocytes to sense changes in matrix composition and synthesize new molecules allows them to repair damage to the macromolecular framework. Available evidence suggests that following a loss of proteoglycans, the chondrocytes increase synthesis of these macromolecules, restoring matrix concentration of proteoglycans toward normal and, as a result, returning the material properties of the matrix toward normal. Matrix repair, following significant depletion of proteoglycans, may require many weeks and possibly months.[4,27-29]

If the cells do not repair significant matrix macromolecular abnormalities, or if the loss of matrix molecules progresses, the tissue will deteriorate. It is not clear at what point this type of injury becomes irreversible and leads to progressive loss of articular cartilage. Presumably, the chondrocytes can restore the matrix if the loss of matrix proteoglycans does not exceed what the cells can rapidly produce, if the fibrillar collagen meshwork remains intact, and if enough chondrocytes remain viable.[3,25] When these conditions are not met, the cells cannot restore the matrix, the chondrocytes will be exposed to excessive loads, and the tissue will degenerate.

For these reasons, insults that cause this type of articular cartilage injury, including immobilization, exposure of articular cartilage, and inflammation, should be minimized. Because this type of matrix macromolecular injury may temporarily increase the vulnerability of cartilage to mechanical injury, minimizing the intensity of impact loading of cartilage following severe blunt trauma, prolonged immobilization, or inflammation appears advisable.

Chondral Fractures

Impact loading, twisting, and direct blows to synovial joints occur frequently, especially during vigorous activity. The resulting compression or shear forces applied to an articular surface can rupture the cartilage matrix producing chondral fissures, flaps, or fractures.[5,6,8,10-13,18,33,34]

Disrupting normal articular cartilage with a single impact requires substantial force. A study of human articular cartilage subjected to blunt trauma showed that articular cartilage could withstand impact loads of up to 25 N/mm² (25 MPa) without apparent damage. Impact loads exceeding this level caused chondrocyte death and matrix fissures.[21] Repo and Finlay[21] suggested that reaching a stress level that could cause cartilage damage required a force greater than that necessary to fracture the femur. In another study, Haut[35] measured the pressure on human patellofemoral articular cartilage during impact loading and found that impact loads less than the level necessary to fracture bone caused stresses greater than 25 MPa in some regions of the articular surface. With the knee flexed 90 degrees, 50% of the load necessary to cause a bone fracture produced joint pressures greater than 25 MPa over nearly 20% of the patellofemoral joint. At 70% of the bone fracture load, pressures on nearly 35% of the contact area of the patellofemoral joint exceeded 25 MPa, and at 100% of the bone fracture load, 60% of the patellofemoral joint pressures exceeded 25 MPa. These results suggest that impact loads can disrupt cartilage without fracturing bone.

Results from other investigations show that repetitive impact loads split articular cartilage matrix and initiate progressive cartilage degeneration.[19,36] Cyclic loading of human cartilage samples in vitro caused surface fibrillation,[36] and periodic impact loading of bovine metacarpophalangeal joints in vitro combined with joint motion caused degeneration of articular cartilage.[26] Repeated overuse and peak overloading of rabbit joints in vivo caused articular cartilage damage including formation of chondrocyte clusters, fibrillation of the matrix, thickening of subchondral bone, and penetration of subchondral capillaries into the calcified zone of articular cartilage.[19] The extent of cartilage damage appeared to increase with longer periods of repetitive overloading, and deterioration of the cartilage continued after the excessive loading stopped. This latter finding suggests that some cartilage damage is not immediately visible.

Repetitive loading also disrupted the tissue in an investigation of cartilage plugs; the severity of the damage increased with increases in the load and the number of loading cycles.[22] Two hundred and fifty cycles of a 1,000-psi compression load caused surface abrasions, 500 cycles produced primary fissures penetrating to calcified cartilage, and 1,000 cycles produced secondary fissures extending from the primary fissures. After 8,000 cycles, the fissures coalesced and undermined cartilage fragments. Higher loads caused similar changes with fewer cycles. The results of these experiments suggested that repetitive loading can cause both propagation of vertical cartilage fissures from the joint surface to calcified cartilage and extension of oblique fissures into areas of intact cartilage, extending the damage and creating cartilage flaps and free fragments.

Clinical diagnosis of chondral fractures is difficult.[12,13] Because cartilage lacks innervation, injuries limited to cartilage do not cause pain directly. Therefore, the most common symptoms of chondral fractures include locking, catching, or giving way of the joint or a joint effusion. Arthroscopy, currently the best method of evaluating chondral injuries, can show chondral damage that cannot be detected by other methods.[5,8,9,15-17,34,37,38] Important variables in the arthroscopic classification of acute and chronic chondral lesions include the condition of the articular surface and the depth, diameter, and locations of the damage.[16]

Articular cartilage fissures, flaps, and free fragments similar to those produced experimentally by single and repetitive impact loads have been identified in clinical studies.[5-8] In some patients, the cartilage damage may have resulted from acute impact loading of the articular surface or twisting movements of the joint;[5,6,10,12,13,34] in other patients, the cartilage damage may have resulted from repetitive loading. Other joint injuries, including rupture of the anterior cruciate ligament and meniscal tears, frequently occur in association with the cartilage damage.

The lack of blood vessels and of cells that can repair significant tissue defects limits the response of cartilage to injury.[3,4,24,25,39-41] Because cartilage lacks blood vessels, these injuries do not cause hemorrhage, fibrin clot formation, or inflammation. Undifferentiated mesenchymal cells cannot migrate to the site of injury and then proliferate, differentiate, and synthesize a new matrix at that site. The local response to injury depends entirely on chondrocytes. Chondrocytes do not migrate through the matrix to the site of injury; they respond to tissue injury by proliferating and increasing the synthesis of matrix macromolecules near the injury.[3,4,24,25] Yet, the newly synthesized matrix and proliferating cells do not fill the tissue defect, and the chondrocytes' increased proliferative and synthetic activity ceases soon after injury.

Current treatments of chondral fractures and flaps include debridement of the cartilage edges, debridement of the cartilage and abrasion of exposed subchondral bone, and replacement of cartilage fragments with tissue adhesives.[12,13,18,34,42,43] It is not clear which treatment provides the best results or if any of these treatments produce better results than removing loose cartilage fragments and leaving the defect site untreated.

Osteochondral Fractures

In addition to chondral fractures, closed-joint injuries can cause fractures that extend through the cartilage into the subchondral bone.[5-8,10-14,34] Chondral and osteochondral fractures may result from similar impact and twisting joint injuries, but they tend to occur in different age groups.[5-8] Chondral fractures generally occur in skeletally mature people, while osteochondral fractures typically occur in skeletally immature people or young adults. This difference may result from age-related changes in the mechanical properties of the articular surface, including the uncalcified cartilage, the calcified cartilage zone, and the subchondral bone, or it may result from age-related differences in activities that cause joint injuries.

Large osteochondral fractures can be treated by reduction and mechanical fixation of the fragments. If the fracture is not treated soon after the injury, the fragments will remodel, making accurate reduction difficult, and the articular surface may begin to deteriorate.[7] Experimental work indicates that the best results are produced by immediate anatomic reduction and rigid stabilization of osteochondral fractures. In a study of intra-articular fractures of the distal femur in rabbits, anatomically reduced cartilage fractures stabilized by compression fixation of the bone fracture healed with apparently normal articular cartilage,[44] but inadequately reduced and adequately reduced fractures that were not stabilized by compression fixation healed with fibrocartilage.

Unlike injuries limited to cartilage, fractures that extend into subchondral bone cause hemorrhage and fibrin clot formation and activate the inflammatory response. Experimental studies of osteochondral defects have clarified the complex sequence of vascular and cellular events that follow acute loss of a region of articular cartilage and underlying subchondral bone.[3,24,25,39-41,45-52] Soon after injury, blood escaping from blood vessels in the damaged bone forms a hematoma that temporarily fills the injury site. Fibrin forms within the hematoma, and platelets bind to fibrillar collagen and establish hemostasis. A continuous fibrin clot fills the bone defect and extends for a variable distance into the cartilage defect. Platelets within the clot release vasoactive mediators and growth factors or cytokines (small proteins that influence multiple cell functions including migration, proliferation, differentiation, and matrix synthesis), including transforming growth factor beta (TGF-β) and platelet-derived growth factor (PDGF).[4] Bone matrix also contains growth factors, including TGF-β, bone morphogenic protein, PDGF, insulin-like growth factor I (ILG-I), ILG-II, and possibly others. Release of these growth factors may have an important role in the repair of osteochondral defects. In particular, the growth factors probably stimulate vascular invasion and migration of undifferentiated cells into the clot and influence the proliferative and synthetic activities of those cells.

Shortly after entering the tissue defect, the undifferentiated mesenchymal cells proliferate and synthesize a new matrix. Within two weeks of injury, some mesenchymal cells assume the rounded form of chondrocytes and begin to synthesize a matrix that contains type II collagen and a relatively high concentration of proteoglycans.[3,4,24,25] These mesenchymal cells produce regions of hyaline-like cartilage in the chondral and bone portions of the defect. In many osteochondral defects, the regions of hyaline-like cartilage first appear next to the exposed bone matrix, leaving the central region of the defect filled with more fibrous tissue (J. A. Buckwalter, M. Olmstead, unpublished observations).

Six to eight weeks after injury, the repair tissue within the chondral region of most experimental osteochondral defects contains many chondrocyte-like cells in a matrix consisting of type II collagen, proteoglycans, some type I collagen, and noncollagenous proteins (J. A. Buckwalter, M. Olmstead, unpublished observations). The cells in the bone portion of the defect produce immature bone, fibrous tissue, and hyaline-like cartilage.

Six months after injury, the mesenchymal cells have repaired the bone defect with a tissue that consists primarily of bone, although it also contains some regions of fibrous tissue, small blood vessels, and hyaline cartilage. In contrast, repair tissue rarely fills the chondral portions of large osteochondral defects. In animal experiments, repair tissue filled about two thirds of the total volume of the chondral portion and more than 95% of the total volume of the bone portion of large osteochondral defects.[4,24] Moreover, the tissue in the chondral portion of the defect differs significantly in composition from the tissue in the bone portion of the same defect (J. A. Buckwalter, M. Olmstead, unpublished observations). The chondral repair tissue contains no bone or blood vessels and has a significantly higher proportion of hyaline-like cartilage. The composition and structure of the chondral repair tissue are usually between those of hyaline cartilage and fibrocartilage, and it rarely replicates the elaborate structure of normal articular cartilage. The differences in the repair tissue in the chondral and bony parts of the same defect show how the environment in the two regions causes the same repair cells to produce different types of tissue. It is not clear whether the important differences in environment are mechanical, biological, electrical, or a result of unknown factors.

Occasionally, the cartilage repair tissue persists unchanged or progressively remodels to form a functional joint surface. However, within a year or less, the chondral repair tissue in most large osteochondral injuries begins to show evidence of depletion of matrix proteoglycans, fragmentation and fibrillation, increasing collagen content, and loss of chondrocyte-like cells.[3,4,24,25,50,52] The remaining cells often assume the appearance of fibroblasts as the surrounding matrix comes to consist primarily of densely packed collagen fibrils. This fibrous tissue usually fragments and often disintegrates, leaving areas of exposed bone.[3,24,25,52]

The inferior mechanical properties of cartilage repair tissue may be responsible for its frequent deterioration.[25] In several experimental studies, repair tissue that successfully filled osteochondral defects was found to lack the stiffness of normal articular cartilage. Cartilage repair tissue formed in rabbit metatarsophalangeal joint arthroplasties deformed more easily and took longer to recover from deformation than normal articular cartilage.[53] Cartilage repair tissue formed in pig joints swelled more in Ringer's solution than normal cartilage and had greater permeability and less stiffness on compression than normal cartilage.[54] In addition, chondral repair cartilage in primate osteochondral defects was more permeable and less stiff on compression than normal articular cartilage.[55]

The differences between the mechanical properties of repair cartilage and those of normal cartilage and the frequent deterioration of repair cartilage may be caused by differences in matrix composition and organization.[25] The increased swelling of repair cartilage may result from a lack of organization or weakness of the collagen fibril meshwork. Microscopic studies of repair cartilage support this suggestion; the orientation of the collagen fibrils in even the most hyaline-like cartilage repair tissue does not follow the pattern seen in normal articular cartilage.[25] In addition, lack of organization of the macromolecules, insufficient concentrations of some macromolecules, or the presence of molecules like type I collagen that may interfere with the assembly of a normal cartilage matrix may prevent the repair tissue cells from establishing normal relationships between matrix macromolecules, particularly, the relationship between cartilage proteoglycans and the collagen fibril network. The decreased stiffness and increased permeability of the repair cartilage matrix may increase loading of the macromolecular framework during joint use, resulting in progressive structural damage to the matrix collagen and proteoglycans. The repair chondrocytes would then be exposed to excessive loads, further compromising their ability to restore the matrix.

Clinical experience and experimental results suggest that the success of chondral repair in osteochondral injuries may depend to some extent on the severity of the injury, as measured by the volume of tissue or surface area of cartilage injured, and on the age of the injured individual.[4] Smaller osteochondral defects that do not alter joint function heal more predictably than larger defects that may change the loading of the articular surface.[4,24,48] Age-related differences in healing of chondral and osteochondral injuries have not been thoroughly investigated; however, bone heals more rapidly in children than in adults, and the articular cartilage chondrocytes in skeletally immature animals show a better proliferative response to injury and synthesize larger proteoglycan molecules than those from mature animals.[4,56-59] Furthermore, a growing synovial joint can remodel the articular surface to decrease the mechanical abnormalities created by a chondral or osteochondral defect.

Summary

Direct blunt trauma, twisting, or impact loading of a joint can damage articular cartilage without disrupting the surrounding soft tissues, and some mechanical injuries of articular cartilage lead to progressive degeneration of the joint surface. Understanding of the mechanisms, natural history, and optimal treatment of these cartilage injuries is limited, at least partially because of the difficulty in defining the tissue damage; but arthroscopic examination of injured joints shows that visible articular surface disruption occurs frequently in association with other joint injuries. According to data from experimental studies, excessive joint loading causes three types of articular cartilage damage: (1) loss of matrix macromolecules, alteration of the macromolecular framework, or cell injury without visible tissue disruption; (2) disruption of articular cartilage alone (chondral fractures and flaps); and (3) disruption of articular cartilage and subchondral bone (osteochondral fractures).

Loss or alteration of the organization of matrix macromolecules can change the mechanical properties of cartilage and may make the tissue more vulnerable to further mechanical injury. Data from experimental studies indicate that if a cartilage injury decreases proteoglycan aggregation or the tissue proteoglycan concentration, the chondrocytes can usually replace lost matrix macromolecules as long as the fibrillar collagen meshwork of the matrix remains intact and enough cells remain viable. Other data suggest that repetitive excessive loading weakens the cartilage macromolecular framework before visible matrix disruption occurs. These observations may help explain the frequently reported association between joint instability and deterioration of the articular cartilage. That is, joint instability causes repetitive excessive loadings of some regions of the articular surface, which lead to decreased proteoglycan aggregation and depletion of matrix proteoglycans, thereby increasing matrix permeability and decreasing matrix stiffness. These changes increase loading of the matrix collagen fibril meshwork, which eventually fails, and visible matrix fissures appear.

Disruption of cartilage alone stimulates proliferation and matrix synthesis by the chondrocytes surrounding the injury, but this response does not persist and the cells do not migrate into the tissue defect or fill the defect with new matrix. The natural history of these injuries is not well understood, but clinical experience suggests that large lesions in load-bearing areas of the articular surface cause symptoms and may progress. Current treatments of chondral fractures and flaps do not predictably restore the articular surface.

Injuries that extend through cartilage into the subchondral bone cause hemorrhage and inflammation followed by repair that fills the bone defect and a variable portion of the cartilage defect with new cells and matrix. Six months after most osteochondral injuries, mesenchymal cells have filled the bone defect with a tissue consisting primarily of bone and some fibrous tissue, small blood vessels, and hyaline cartilage. In contrast, the chondral portions of large osteochondral defects are rarely filled completely with repair tissue. The repair tissue in the chondral portion of the defect differs significantly in composition from the repair tissue in the bone portion of the same defect; the chondral repair tissue contains no bone or blood vessels and has a significantly higher proportion of hyaline-like cartilage. Usually, chondral repair tissue has a composition and structure intermediate between that of hyaline cartilage and that of fibrocartilage.

Occasionally, the cartilage repair tissue persists unchanged or progressively remodels to form a functional joint surface, but within a year or less, the chondral repair tissue in most large osteochondral injuries loses matrix proteoglycans and cells with the appearance of chondrocytes, the collagen content increases, and the matrix fibrillates and fragments. The remaining cells assume the appearance of fibroblasts as the surrounding matrix comes to consist primarily of densely packed collagen fibrils. This fibrous tissue often disintegrates, leaving areas of exposed bone.

Although they probably occur frequently and may have significant consequences, cartilage injuries caused by mechanical forces are not as well understood as injuries to the other musculoskeletal tissues. Advances that will help improve diagnosis and treatment of these injuries include better understanding of the effects of acute and repetitive loadings of joints, development of clinically applicable methods of measuring cartilage mechanical properties, and methods of stimulating regeneration of articular cartilage in chondral and osteochondral injuries.

References

1. Armstrong CG, Mow VC, Wirth CR: Biomechanics of impact-induced microdamage to articular cartilage: A possible genesis for chondromalacia patella, in Finerman G (ed): *Symposium on Sports Medicine: The Knee*. St. Louis, CV Mosby, 1985, pp 70-84.
2. Mow VC, Setton LA, Ratcliff A, et al: Structure-function relationship of articular cartilage and the effects of joint instability and trauma on cartilage, in Brandt KD (ed): *Cartilage Changes in Osteoarthritis*. Indianapolis, IN, Indiana University School of Medicine, 1990, pp 22-42.
3. Buckwalter JA, Rosenberg L, Coutts R, et al: Articular cartilage: Injury and repair, in Woo SL, Buckwalter JA (eds): *Injury and Repair of the Musculoskeletal Soft Tissues*. Park Ridge, IL, American Academy of Orthopaedic Surgeons, 1988, pp 465-482.
4. Buckwalter JA, Cruess RL: Healing of musculoskeletal tissues, in Rockwood CA Jr, Green DP, Bucholz RW (eds): *Rockwood and Green's Fractures in Adults*, ed 3. Philadelphia, JB Lippincott, 1991, pp 181-222.
5. Johnson-Nurse C, Dandy DJ: Fracture-separation of articular cartilage in the adult knee. *J Bone Joint Surg* 1985;67B:42-43.
6. Kennedy JC, Grainger RW, McGraw RW: Osteochondral fractures of the femoral condyles. *J Bone Joint Surg* 1966;48B:436-440.
7. Matthewson MH, Dandy DJ: Osteochondral fractures of the lateral femoral condyle: A result of indirect violence to the knee. *J Bone Joint Surg* 1978;60B:199-202.
8. Bradley J, Dandy DJ: Osteochondritis dissecans and other lesions of the femoral condyles. *J Bone Joint Surg* 1989;71B:518-522.
9. DeHaven KE: Diagnosis of acute knee injuries with hemarthrosis. *Am J Sports Med* 1980;8:9-14.
10. Hopkinson WJ, Mitchell WA, Curl WW: Chondral fractures of the knee: Cause for confusion. *Am J Sports Med* 1985;13:309-312.
11. Milgram JW, Rogers LF, Miller JW: Osteochondral fractures: Mechanisms of injury and fate of fragments. *AJR* 1978;130:651-658.
12. O'Donoghue DH: Chondral and osteochondral fractures. *J Trauma* 1966;6:469-481.
13. O'Donoghue DH: Chondral and osteochondral fractures, in O'Donoghue DH (ed): *Treatment of Injuries to Athletes*. Philadelphia, WB Saunders, 1984, pp 76-85.
14. Rosenberg NJ: Osteochondral fractures of the lateral femoral condyle. *J Bone Joint Surg* 1964;46A:1013-1026.
15. Noyes FR, Bassett RW, Grood ES, et al: Arthroscopy in acute traumatic hemarthrosis of the knee: Incidence of anterior cruciate tears and other injuries. *J Bone Joint Surg* 1980;62A:687-695.
16. Noyes FR, Stabler CL: A system for grading articular cartilage lesions at arthroscopy. *Am J Sports Med* 1989;17:505-513.
17. Gillquist J, Hagberg G: Findings at arthroscopy and arthrography in knee injuries. *Acta Orthop Scand* 1978;49:398-402.
18. Buckwalter JA, Drez DA, Garrett WW, et al: Articular surface injuries: Meeting Abstracts, in *Symposia of Instructional Courses*. Presented at the Sixteenth Annual Meeting of the American Orthopaedic Society for Sports Medicine, Sun Valley, ID, July 16, 1990, pp 55-56.

19. Dekel S, Weissman SL: Joint changes after overuse and peak overloading of rabbit knees in vivo. *Acta Orthop Scand* 1978;49:519-528.

20. Donohue JM, Buss D, Oegema TR, et al: The effects of indirect blunt trauma on adult canine articular cartilage. *J Bone Joint Surg* 1983;65A:948-957.

21. Repo RU, Finlay JB: Survival of articular cartilage after controlled impact. *J Bone Joint Surg* 1977;59A:1068-1076.

22. Zimmerman NB, Smith DG, Pottenger LA, et al: Mechanical disruption of human patellar cartilage by repetitive loading in vitro. *Clin Orthop* 1988;229:302-307.

23. Buckwalter JA, Mow VC: Sports injuries to articular cartilage, in Drez D, Delee J (eds): *Orthopaedic Sports Medicine: Principles and Practice*. Philadelphia, WB Saunders, in press.

24. Buckwalter JA, Rosenberg LA, Hunziker EB: Articular cartilage: Composition, structure, response to injury, and methods of facilitation repair, in Ewing JW (ed): *Articular Cartilage and Knee Joint Function: Basic Science and Arthroscopy*. New York, Raven Press, 1990, pp 19-56.

25. Buckwalter JA, Mow VC: Cartilage repair in osteoarthritis, in Moskowitz RW, Howell DS, Goldberg VM, et al (eds): *Osteoarthritis: Diagnosis and Management*, ed 2. Philadelphia, WB Saunders,1992, pp 71-107.

26. Radin EL, Paul IL: Response of joints to impact loading: I. In vitro wear. *Arthritis Rheum* 1971;14:356-362.

27. Palmoski M, Perricone E, Brandt KD: Development and reversal of a proteoglycan aggregation defect in normal canine knee cartilage after immobilization. *Arthritis Rheum* 1979;22:508-517.

28. Palmoski MJ, Brandt KD: Running inhibits the reversal of atrophic changes in canine knee cartilage after removal of a leg cast. *Arthritis Rheum* 1981;24:1329-1337.

29. Palmoski MJ, Brandt KD: Proteoglycan aggregation in injured articular cartilage: A comparison of healing lacerated cartilage with osteoarthritic cartilage. *J Rheum* 1982;9:189-197.

30. Kiviranta I: *Joint Loading Influences on the Articular Cartilage of Young Dogs*, ed 1. Kuopio, Finland, University of Kuopio, 1987, p 91.

31. Mow VC, Bigliani LU, Flatow EL, et al: The role of joint instability in joint inflammation and cartilage deterioration: A study of the glenohumeral joint, in Leadbetter WB, Buckwalter JA, Gordon SL (eds): *Sports Induced Inflammation: Clinical and Basic Science Concepts*. Park Ridge, IL, American Academy of Orthopaedic Surgeons, 1990, pp 337-355.

32. Mow VC, Rosenwasser MP: Articular cartilage: Biomechanics, in Woo SL, Buckwalter JA (eds): *Injury and Repair of the Musculoskeletal Soft Tissues*. Park Ridge, IL, American Academy of Orthopaedic Surgeons, 1988, pp 427-463.

33. Visuri T, Kuusela T: Fixation of large osteochondral fractures of the patella with fibrin adhesive system: A report of two operative cases. *Am J Sports Med* 1989;17:842-845.

34. Terry GC, Flandry F, Van Manen JW, et al: Isolated chondral fractures of the knee. *Clin Orthop* 1988;234:170-177.

35. Haut RC: Contact pressures in the patellofemoral joint during impact loading on the human flexed knee. *J Orthop Res* 1989;7:272-280.

36. Weightman BO, Freeman MA, Swanson SA: Fatigue of articular cartilage. *Nature* 1973;244:303-304.

37. Johnson LL: Diagnostic arthroscopy in clinical practice, in Johnson LL (ed): *Diagnostic and Surgical Arthroscopy: The Knee and Other Joints*. St. Louis, CV Mosby, 1981, pp 69-96.

38. Johnson LL: Chondral conditions, in Johnson LL (ed): *Diagnostic and Surgical Arthroscopy: The Knee and Other Joints*. St. Louis, CV Mosby, 1981, pp 338-351.

39. Mankin HJ: The reaction of articular cartilage to injury and osteoarthritis: Part I. *N Engl J Med* 1974;291:1285-1292.

40. Mankin HJ: The reaction of articular cartilage to injury and osteoarthritis: Part II. *N Engl J Med* 1974;291:1335-1340.

41. Mankin HJ: Current concepts review: The response of articular cartilage to mechanical injury. *J Bone Joint Surg* 1982;64A:460-466.

42. Kaplonyi G, Zimmerman I, Frenyo AD et al: The use of fibrin adhesive in the repair of chondral and osteochondral injuries. *Injury* 1988;19:267-272.

43. Farkas TA, Kaplonyi GL, Melly AI, et al: Healing of cartilage wounds with auto-fibrin glueing. *Trans Orthop Res Soc* 1989;14:544.

44. Mitchell N, Shepard N: Healing of articular cartilage in intra-articular fractures in rabbits. *J Bone Joint Surg* 1980;62A:628-634.

45. Bennett GA, Bauer W: Further studies concerning the repair of articular cartilage in dog joints. *J Bone Joint Surg* 1935;17:141-150.

46. Calandruccio RA, Gilmer WS Jr: Proliferation, regeneration, and repair of articular cartilage of immature animals. *J Bone Joint Surg* 1962;44A:431-455.

47. Campbell CJ: The healing of cartilage defects. *Clin Orthop* 1969;64:45-63.

48. Convery FR, Akeson WH, Keown GH: The repair of large osteochondral defects: An experimental study in horses. *Clin Orthop* 1972;82:253-262.

49. DePalma AF, McKeever CD, Subin DK: Process of repair of articular cartilage demonstrated by histology and autoradiography with tritiated thymidine. *Clin Orthop* 1966;48:229-242.

50. Furukawa T, Eyre DR, Koide S, et al: Biochemical studies on repair cartilage resurfacing experimental defects in the rabbit knee. *J Bone Joint Surg* 1980;62A:79-89.

51. Meachim G, Roberts C: Repair of the joint surface from subarticular tissue in the rabbit knee. *J Anat* 1971;109:317-327.

52. Mitchell N, Shepard N: The resurfacing of adult rabbit articular cartilage by multiple perforations through the subchondral bone. *J Bone Joint Surg* 1976;58A:230-233.

53. Coletti JM, Akeson WH, Woo SL-Y: A comparison of the physical behavior of normal articular cartilage and the arthroplasty surface. *J Bone Joint Surg* 1972;54A:147-160.

54. Whipple RR, Gibbs MC, Lai WM, et al: Biphasic properties of repaired cartilage at the articular surface. *Trans Orthop Res Soc* 1985;10:340.

55. Athanasiou KA: Biomechanical assessment of articular cartilage healing and interspecies variability, thesis. New York, Columbia University, 1988.

56. Buckwalter JA, Kuettner KE, Thonar EJ-M: Age-related changes in articular cartilage proteoglycans: electron microscopic studies. *J Orthop Res* 1985;3:251-257.

57. Buckwalter JA, Rosenberg LC, Ungar R: Age related changes in link protein function. *Orthop Trans* 1989;13:258.

58. Buckwalter JA, Rosenberg LC: Electron microscopic studies of cartilage proteoglycans. *Elec Microsc Rev* 1988;1:87-112.

59. Thonar EJ, Buckwalter JA, Kuettner KE: Maturation-related differences in the structure and composition of proteoglycans synthesized by chondrocytes from bovine articular cartilage. *J Biol Chem* 1986;261:2467-2474.

Chapter 6

Response of Articular Cartilage to Instability

Victor M. Goldberg, MD
Roland W. Moskowitz, MD
Charles J. Malemud, PhD
Joseph Mansour, PhD

Articular cartilage is a complex tissue, uniquely constructed to withstand significant joint pressure generated by normal daily activities.[1-10] The cellular components, chondrocytes, are embedded in a supersaturated matrix that is 60% to 80% water. This high water content is a critical factor in determining the material properties of the tissue. The major macromolecules of cartilage include collagens, proteoglycans, and noncollagenous proteins or glycoproteins. Aggrecan, a large, aggregating, chondroitin sulfate proteoglycan, is a central component necessary for load transmissions and for providing a low-friction joint surface.[11] Aggrecan forms a noncovalent bond with hyaluronic acid to create large masses. This interaction is stabilized by a glycoprotein called link protein. The collagen network is critical in maintaining the integrity of the articular cartilage.[3,12-15]

For some time it was believed that cartilage was a relatively inactive tissue capable of a minimal response to injury. The synthetic activity of chondrocytes was thought to be depressed, because the half-life of proteoglycan was measured at greater than 300 days, and that of collagen at greater than 1,500 days. Reports of recent studies of articular cartilage physiology in normal and diseased joints as well as in vitro organ and cell culture investigations have indicated that chondrocytes are actively involved in the maintenance of physiologic concentrations of proteoglycan and collagen.[6,9,10,16-18] This suggests that chondrocytes may have the metabolic capacity to repair cartilage matrix following an injury causing joint instability.

There has been significant work to delineate the response of cartilage to injury. Injuries to articular cartilage that fail to penetrate to subchondral bone usually are not repaired.[19-21] Full-thickness defects that expose the underlying subchondral bone appear to repair with variable tissue types. Results of extensive animal studies have corroborated clinical evidence and show that articular cartilage has a limited capacity for repair.[22,23] The response of articular cartilage to joint instability is manifested by altered biomechanics, in terms of altered joint loads and abnormal kinematics that result in biologic abnormalities leading to cartilage destruction. Results from previous studies have indicated that there is a minimum level of abnormal joint load that results from instability; this level is prerequisite to chondrocyte necrosis and matrix abnormalities.[6,24,25] These processes may be defined in terms of injury to the cells or to the existing matrix.

The anatomic and biochemical changes reported after induction of experimental instabilities are quite consistent with those observed in early osteoarthritis in humans.[26-28] Within the first few weeks after surface injury, swelling of the articular surface is seen. A concomitant increase in hexuronic acid and water content and an alteration in the interaction between proteoglycans and collagen result.[26,27,29] Donohue and associates[30] and Radin and associates[31-36] have indicated from their animal studies of impact trauma that there is early cellular activity with an increase in cell proliferation as well as synthesis of proteoglycans and collagens. A repair response may be seen, which depends on the extent of instability and articular cartilage damage.[37-40]

The general consensus is that the nature of the cartilage response to injury depends on the depth of the cartilage defect.[19,41] Superficial lesions appear to have a response similar to that of the early lesions described in osteoarthritis.[42,43] Anatomic changes include disruption of the collagen fibers in the superficial zone, the formation of clefts and fissures, and chondrocyte necrosis. There appears to be a loss of matrix proteoglycan, although the overall collagen content remains constant. In an effort to repair surface damage, adjacent chondrocytes proliferate and form clusters around the injured surface. Proteoglycan synthesis is increased; however, little functional repair is seen. Full-thickness lesions do undergo a repair process, but the tissue response is variable and the functionality of the repair is suspect.[44-46]

Because clinical instability is so difficult to quantify, animal models are useful to define the changes seen in articular cartilage after joint instability develops. In the prevalent models studied, instability was induced by the resection of one or more ligaments with or without partial or complete meniscectomies.[22,23] Findings from these studies of chronic injuries were similar to findings previously described for acute injuries. Surface fibrillation, ulceration, and fissuring occur; chondrocyte dysfunction and rapid matrix changes, including proteoglycan depletion and collagen abnormalities, are seen. Osteophyte development appears to be an early consequence of joint instability, without concomitant articular cartilage erosion in many of these models.[27,47-49] The force that alters the function of ligaments and menisci results in proliferation and migration of pluripotential cells that form osteophytes.

The response of the articular cartilage to an unstable joint depends on the regulation of chondrocyte repair mechanisms. Although data from previous studies point to the extracellular matrix as the primary structure resisting compressive, tensile, and shearing forces,[1-3,15,50] little is known about the mechanical force transduction of chondrocytes. The mechanical instability of the joint clearly provides stimuli that affect chondrocyte metabolism.

Chondrocyte metabolic regulation has been investigated under different in vitro mechanical circumstances.[51-54] DNA synthesis was stimulated when hydrostatic pressure above 80 g/cm^2 was applied to chondrocytes. Increases in cyclic adenosine monophosphate (cAMP) and chondrocyte proteoglycan synthesis obtained by applying intermittent compressive forces to cartilage explants have been reported. Other data indicate that increased hydrostatic pressure causes a decrease in adenylate cyclase, which can have an inhibitory effect on collagen synthesis.[52] A better understanding of the response of cellular receptors to mechanical environments is essential to the understanding of articular cartilage response to joint instability. These experimental models not only have increased understanding of joint instability, but also have been used to study the pathophysiology of osteoarthritis, a consequence of significant unchecked joint instability. Although observations from these animal studies, including the time of disease induction and the anatomic, biochemical, and biomechanical changes in articular cartilage are useful, they must be viewed with caution because of species differences and the relevance of the findings to human disease. The remainder of this chapter will discuss the outcomes in two models of instability: anterior cruciate resection in dogs and partial medial meniscectomy in rabbits.

Animal Models

Resection of the anterior cruciate ligament in the dog results in a significant joint instability that leads to deterioration of articular cartilage.[13,26,27,55-59] Anatomic studies of the articular cartilage after anterior cruciate ligament resection demonstrated early softening, fibrillation, and erosions, most prominent on the uncovered area of the medial tibial plateau. Osteophyte formation was prominent and present on the femoral condyles as early as two weeks after surgery (Fig. 1). The osteophytes progressively increased in number and size with involvement of all surfaces. Detailed studies, using fluorochrome microangiography and microradiography, of the sequence of osteophyte development provided data that indicated the prevalence of these osteophytes at the marginal zone where the synovial membrane intersected with fibrocartilage.[27]

Osteophyte formation began with the deposition of new mineral surrounding the existing femoral cortex, and with a concomitant increase in vascularity. An increase in bone turnover in the entire distal femur was seen. Remodeling of these osteophytes, with the deposition of new bone and resorption of old material, continued throughout the period of observation. Deep cartilage clefts and erosions were seen histologically in all areas, with a significant loss of

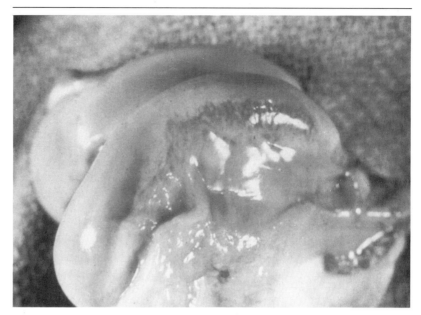

Fig. 1 *Photograph of the distal femoral condyle of a dog after anterior cruciate ligament resection, demonstrating peripheral osteophyte formation.*

metachromatic staining in the severely fibrillated areas. Cellular density increased, with cell clones becoming quite abundant. This increase in cellular density appeared to be present in the deeper layers, suggesting a hypertrophic regenerative remodeling of articular cartilage in response to these abnormal mechanical stresses.

Biochemical changes in the dog model were seen in all regions of the cartilage and appeared to begin prior to any anatomically observable degenerative lesions.[13,60] These changes include an increase in tissue hydration, more easily extracted proteoglycans, and a higher galactosamine-glucosamine molar ratio. The number of proteoglycan subunits increased while proteoglycan aggregates were smaller. These results suggest that chondrocytes were synthesizing the proteoglycans usually seen in immature articular cartilage as a response to the altered mechanical state of joint instability. Similar changes have been shown after anterior or posterior cruciate ligament transection in other species.[22,23] In all of these models, osteophyte formation is a prominent occurrence and is present either on the tibial plateaus or femoral condyles.

The induction of knee joint instability in a rabbit or dog model that resects one third to one half of the anterior aspect of the medial meniscus and leads to experimental osteoarthritis has been studied in our laboratory by Moskowitz and associates.[28,48,61-65] Gross pathologic lesions seen in the first three weeks after surgery include pitting and ulceration, fissuring, and cyst formation, which is seen primarily on the medial femoral condyle. Osteophytes occur early and are prominent not only on the medial femoral condyle, but also

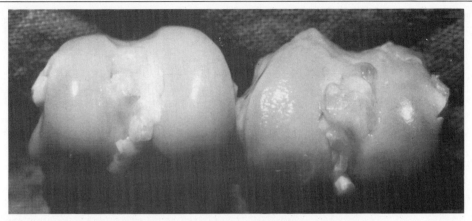

Fig. 2   *Photograph of the distal femoral condyle of a rabbit after medial meniscectomy, demonstrating formation of osteophytes, ulceration, and erosion on the right. The normal condyle is on the left. (Reproduced with permission from Moskowitz RW: Osteoarthritis: Studies with experimental models.* Arthritis Rheum *1977;20:S104-S108.)*

on the inner aspect of the medial tibial plateau. Interestingly, when meniscal regeneration was seen, cartilage degeneration was limited, suggesting the importance of joint instability in the deterioration of articular cartilage. Pitting and ulceration were also more common in those animal models where the knees were exercised (Fig. 2). Synovitis and proliferating pannus were seen in the peripheral aspect of the joint.

Osteophyte formation, an early finding in the partial meniscectomy model,[48] was present in over three fourths of the animals at four weeks after surgery. Increased thickness of the synovial and perichondrial/periosteal layer with concomitant cell proliferation was seen (Fig. 3). The high cellular activity seen at the joint periphery preceded the quick vascular responses. The formation of osteophytes is a predominant feature that suggests that joint instability initially may result in articular cartilage hypertrophy and increased activity in an attempt to repair the damage.

Histopathologic findings in this model included early chondrocyte cloning followed by evidence of chondrocyte degeneration, prominent fissure formation, fibrillation, and loss of cartilage. Metachromatic staining was significantly reduced, especially in the zones of gross ulceration (Fig. 4). Viable chondrocytes in focal areas appeared to be surrounded by intense metachromasia, a possible attempt to repair the insult to articular cartilage. These fibrillated lesions progressed and resulted in the absence of cartilage in many areas of the medial femoral condyle.

Autoradiographic techniques were used to assess metabolic activity in this model after in vivo intra-articular injections of ^{3}H-glycine, ^{35}sulfate, and ^{3}H-thymidine.[62] An increase in proteoglycan and protein synthesis was seen during the entire 12-week study period. Cell

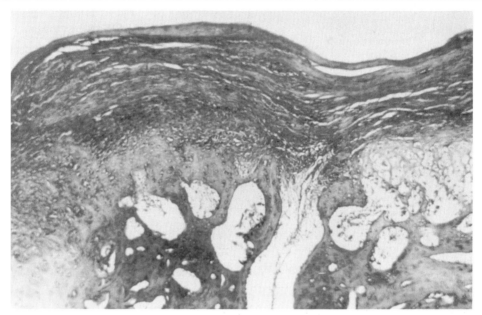

Fig. 3   *Osteophyte formation on a knee with a partial meniscectomy, 4 weeks after surgery. Synovial and periosteal thickening, proliferation, and increased vascularity are prominent. Intramembranous ossification is demonstrated (hematoxylin-eosin, x 30). (Reproduced with permission from Moskowitz RW, Goldbert VM: Studies of osteophyte pathogenesis in experimentally induced osteoarthritis.* J Rheumatol *1987;14:311-320.)*

replication in cartilage was seen early, but later diminished to control levels despite the progression of degeneration. Other investigators, using in vivo measurements for collagen synthesis after the injection of ^{3}H-proline, suggested that there was an increase in collagen synthesis, mostly type II.[14]

Different results were seen in ex vivo studies involving control, sham-operated, and partially meniscectomized rabbit cartilage incubated with [35]sulfate in short-term organ cultures.[28] Proteoglycan synthesis was reduced throughout the entire experiment, and no differences were seen between the medial tibial plateau and tibial osteophytes. Other metabolic variables such as protein and DNA synthesis were not increased in proportion to the development of the disease pathology. These contradictory outcomes may result from the lack of in vivo cues and signaling necessary for chondrocyte response. Although quantitative increases in proteoglycans have not been demonstrated in these culture techniques, significant differences have been defined qualitatively.[65] These studies showed that the newly synthesized proteoglycan was not in the form of proteoglycan aggregates, and reaggregation studies with proteoglycan monomer and exogenous hyaluronic acid confirmed this result. Further, the loss of these aggregates was seen whether the cartilage was removed from the ulcer, or located around the ulcer, or whether it was distant and normal-appearing.

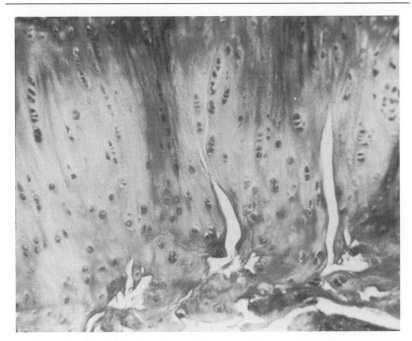

Fig. 4   *Histopathologic section of cartilage from the proximal tibia of a rabbit, 6 weeks after partial meniscectomy. Fibrillation, prominent fissure formation, and chondrocyte clones are seen (hematoxylin-eosin, x 40).*

Proteoglycan is more readily extractable from knee cartilage after partial meniscectomy. Studies of the endogenous proteoglycan monomer in the cartilage from control and meniscectomized animals showed that the weight average sedimentation coefficient of the macromolecule (15S) did not differ between the two groups (Table 1). These newly synthesized proteoglycan monomers also appear to possess a hyaluronic acid binding region, although free hyaluronic acid from articular cartilage of meniscectomized animals aggregated poorly with proteoglycan monomers. These studies clearly showed that proteoglycan disturbances exist in articular cartilage after joint stability induced by partial medial meniscectomy.

Mechanical changes of the femoral condyle after partial medial meniscectomy have been studied recently using an indentation technique described by Mow and Lai.[66] The indentation depth and cartilage thickness were measured on four sites of the femoral condyle, including areas that were not grossly ulcerated. Areas that were pitted or fibrillated demonstrated a higher compliance (softer) than noninvolved areas. Pitted areas were significantly softer when compared with all other regions. These increases in compliance must be compared with the normal aging process of rabbit articular cartilage.[67] Data from these latter studies indicate a stiffening of articular cartilage. These data are in contrast to those reported by Altman

Table 1 Weight average sedimentation constants for the total proteoglycan, individual monomer, and aggregate profiles

| A1 Preparation From | Weight Average Sedimentation Coefficient—S$_w$ | | | |
| | Frozen* | | | Fresh+ |
	Total	Monomer	Aggregate	Total
Tibia control	29.0	15.0 (68%)	59 (32%)	
Femur normal control	27.0	15.5 (75%)	62 (25%)	29.0
Femur condyle (ulcer)	15.0	15.0 (100%)	(0%)	14.3
Femur condyle (rim)	15.6	15.6 (100%)	(0%)	
Femur condyle (far from rim)	14.7	14.7 (100%)	(0%)	14.6

*Average of duplicate determinations on 4 to 6 pools.
+ Duplicate determinations on 1 pool.
(Reproduced with permission from Moskowitz RW, Howell DS, Goldberg VM, etal: Cartilage proteoglycan alterations in an experimentally induced model of rabbit osteoarthritis. *Arthritis Rheum* 1979;22:155-163.)

and associates,[68] who noted an increase in cartilage stiffness after anterior cruciate resection in the dog. Further studies are necessary to clearly define the mechanical outcomes of articular cartilage after joint instability and its correlation with biochemical changes.

Combined procedures, which involve the excision of the collateral ligaments, cruciate ligaments, and menisci, have been studied and result in marked joint instability.[23,54,69-72] Rapid degeneration of the articular surface was produced and was characterized by cellular degeneration, delamination of the superficial cartilage layers, fissures, fibrillation, and significant loss of matrix metachromasia. An ineffective attempt at cellular proliferation with the formation of cell clusters was seen in many areas. Osteophytes were not as prominent in these models. Increased DNA synthesis was observed as measured by ^{3}H-thymidine uptake. In all of these models of joint instability, when some form of stabilization was introduced or when the meniscus regenerated, the degenerative changes were muted and in some circumstances reversed.[37,38,73-75] These results provide further indication of the potential reparative capabilities of articular cartilage.

Summary

Clearly, the ultimate effect of significant joint instability on articular cartilage is osteoarthritis. The abnormal forces generated by the unstable joint produce changes in articular cartilage, but they do not always lead to progressive loss of cartilage. This potential stabilization of cartilage regions suggests that there are mechanisms of repair that are not well understood. However, it has been documented that the trauma associated with instability may lead to alterations in joint congruity, which in itself is a major contributor to the development and/or progression of osteoarthritic lesions. When the threshold limit for joint instability is reached, altered contact stresses and diminished contact areas lead to osteoarthritic changes. Although partially documented, this phenomenon is not completely understood. When this threshold is reached, the changes that have been noted include surface fibrillation, depletion of proteoglycan, and alteration of the collagen-fibrillar network. These changes are associated with increased hydration and reduction in the tensile stiffness of cartilage. Osteophyte formation is an early observation and appears to be an attempt of the joint to repair the damage. Chondrocytes multiply and orient themselves in clones, around which an increase in metachromatic straining is seen. Type II collagen synthesis is usually increased, but type IX synthesis is not concomitantly increased. Although proteoglycan loss is seen early, later total proteoglycan content remains unchanged in spite of increased proteoglycan synthesis. The molecular structure of proteoglycan is abnormal and aggregation appears to decrease. The chondrocyte is significantly influenced by the trauma associated with instability. However, the relationship of cell changes to matrix abnormalities is not well defined. Reparative mechanisms in the cell are activated, including increases in rough endoplastic reticulum production, mitotic activity, and synthesis of proteoglycan and collagen. Concomitantly, there is an increase in production of prostaglandin and synthesis of proteolytic enzymes, which result in matrix destruction.

The response of articular cartilage to instability and trauma is highly variable, and the changes observed vary temporally and in their extent, depending on the level of trauma and instability. Further, aging of cartilage may play an important role in its response to trauma and instability. The varying response of chondrocytes to instability may play a central role in the arrest and reversal of the degenerative lesions, depending on the response of the cells to the abnormal environment. The role of instability and trauma in the development of osteoarthritic changes in cartilage can be clarified by a thorough understanding of the relationships between matrix, structure and function, and chondrocyte response.

References

1. Akizuki S, Mow VC, Muller F, et al: Tensile properties of human knee joint cartilage: I. Influence of ionic conditions, weight bearing, and fibrillation on the tensile modulus. *J Orthop Res* 1986;4:379-392.

2. Akizuki S, Mow VC, Muller F, et al: Tensile properties of human knee joint cartilage. II. Correlations between weight bearing and tissue pathology and the kinetics of swelling. *J Orthop Res* 1987;5:173-186.

3. Askew MJ, Mow VC: The biomechanical function of the collagen ultrastructure of articular cartilage. *J Biomech Eng* 1978;100:105-115.

4. Clarke IC: Articular cartilage: A review and scanning electron microscope study. 1. The interterritorial fibrillar architecture. *J Bone Joint Surg* 1971;53B:732-750.

5. Hardingham T, Bayliss M: Proteoglycans of articular cartilage: Changes in aging and in joint disease. *Semin Arthritis Rheum* 1990;20(suppl 1):12-33.

6. Malemud CJ, Hering TM: Regulation of chondrocytes in osteoarthrosis, in Adolphe M (ed): *Biological Regulation of Chondrocytes*. Boca Raton, FL, CRC Press, 1992, pp 295-319.

7. Markolf KL, Mensch JS, Amstutz HC: Stiffness and laxity of the knee: The contributions of the supporting structures: A quantitative *in vitro* study. *J Bone Joint Surg* 1976;58A;583-594.

8. Redler I, Zimny ML: Scanning electron microscopy of normal and abnormal articular cartilage and synovium. *J Bone Joint Surg* 1970;52A:1395-1404.

9. Roughley PJ: Changes in cartilage proteoglycan structure during ageing: Origin and effects: A review. *Agents Actions* 1986;18(suppl):19-29.

10. Shuckett R, Malemud CJ: Proteoglycans synthesized by chondrocytes of human nonarthritic and osteoarthritic cartilage. *Proc Soc Exp Biol Med* 1989;190:275-281.

11. Woessner JF Jr: Matrix metalloproteinases and their inhibitors in connective tissue remodeling. *FASEB J* 1991;5:2145-2154.

12. Myers ER, Hardingham TE, Billingham MEJ, et al: Changes in the tensile and compressive properties of articular cartilage in a canine model of osteoarthritis. *Trans Orthop Res Soc* 1986;11:231.

13. Pelletier J-P, Martel-Pelletier J, Altman RD, et al: Collagenolytic activity and collagen matrix breakdown of the articular cartilage in the Pond-Nuki dog model of osteoarthritis. *Arthritis Rheum* 1983;26: 866-874.

14. Eyre DR, McDevitt CA, Billingham MEJ, et al: Biosynthesis of collagen and other matrix proteins by articular cartilage in experimental osteoarthrosis. *Biochem J* 1980;188:823-837.

15. Maroudas AI: Balance between swelling pressure and collagen tension in normal and degenerate cartilage. *Nature*, 1976;260:808-809.

16. Malemud CJ: Changes in proteoglycans in osteoarthritis: Biochemistry, ultrastructure and biosynthetic processing. *J Rheumatol* 1991;18(suppl 27):60-62.

17. Cheung HS, Cottrell WH, Stephenson K, et al: *In vitro* collagen biosynthesis in healing and normal rabbit articular cartilage. *J Bone Joint Surg* 1978;60A:1076-1081.

18. Cheung HS, Lynch KL, Johnson RP, et al: *In vitro* synthesis of tissue-specific type II collagen by healing cartilage: I. Short-term repair of cartilage by mature rabbits. *Arthritis Rheum* 1980;23:211-219.

19. Mankin HJ: Current concepts review: The response of articular cartilage to mechanical injury. *J Bone Joint Surg* 1982;64A:460-466.

20. Meachim G: The effect of scarification on articular cartilage in the rabbit. *J Bone Joint Surg* 1963;45B:150-161.

21. Ghadially FN, Thomas I, Oryschak AF, et al: Long-term results of superficial defects in articular cartilage: A scanning electron microscope study. *J Pathol* 1977;121:213-217.

22. Moskowitz RW: Experimental models of osteoarthritis, in Moskowitz RW, Howell DS, Goldberg VM, et al (eds): *Osteoarthritis: Diagnosis and Management*. Philadelphia, WB Saunders, 1984, pp 109-128.

23. Moskowitz RW: Models of osteoarthritis, in Moskowitz RW, Howell DS, Goldberg VM, et al (eds): *Osteoarthritis: Diagnosis and Management*. Philadelphia, WB Saunders, 1992.

24. Armstrong CG, Mow VC, Wirth CR: Biomechanics of impact-induced microdamage to articular cartilage: A possible genesis for chondromalacia patella, in Finerman G (ed): American Academy of Orthopaedic Surgeons *Symposium on Sports Medicine: The Knee*. St. Louis, CV Mosby, 1985, pp 70-84.

25. Hoch DH, Grodzinsky AJ, Koob TJ, et al: Early changes in material properties of rabbit articular cartilage after meniscectomy. *J Orthop Res* 1983;1:4-12.

26. McDevitt CA, Muir H: Biochemical changes in the cartilage of the knee in experimental and natural osteoarthritis in the dog. *J Bone Joint Surg* 1976;58B:94-101.

27. McDevitt C, Gilbertson E, Muir H: An experimental model of osteoarthritis; early morphological and biochemical changes. *J Bone Joint Surg* 1977;59B:24-35.

28. Malemud CJ, Goldberg VM, Moskowitz RW: Pathological, biochemical and experimental therapeutic studies in meniscectomy models of osteoarthritis in the rabbit: Its relationship to human joint pathology. *Br J Clin Pract* 1986;40(suppl):21-31.

29. Lust G, Pronsky W, Sherman DM: Biochemical and ultrastructural observations in normal and degenerative canine articular cartilage. *Am J Vet Res* 1972;33:2429-2440.

30. Donohue JM, Buss D, Oegema TR Jr, et al: The effects of indirect blunt trauma on adult canine articular cartilage. *J Bone Joint Surg* 1983;65A:948-957.

31. Radin EL, Paul IL: Response of joints to impact loading: I. In vitro wear. *Arthritis Rheum* 1971;14:356-362.

32. Radin EL, Parker HG, Pugh JW, et al: Response of joints to impact loading: 3. Relationship between trabecular microfractures and cartilage degeneration. *J Biomech* 1973;6:51-57.

33. Radin EL, Paul IL, Lowy M: A comparison of the dynamic force transmitting properties of subchondral bone and articular cartilage. *J Bone Joint Surg* 1970;52A:444-456.

34. Radin EL, Ehrlich MG, Chernack R, et al: Effect of repetitive impulsive loading on the knee joints of rabbits. *Clin Orthop* 1978;131:288-293.

35. Radin EL, Martin RB, Burr DB, et al: Effects of mechanical loading on the tissues of the rabbit knee. *J Orthop Res* 1984;2:221-234.

36. Radin EL: Aetiology of osteoarthrosis. *Clin Rheum Dis* 1976;2:509-522.

37. Cox JS, Nye CE, Schaefer WW, et al: The degenerative effects of partial and total resection of the medial meniscus in dogs' knees. *Clin Orthop* 1975;109:178-183.

38. Elmer RM, Moskowitz RW, Frankel VH: Meniscal regeneration and postmeniscectomy degenerative joint disease. *Clin Orthop* 1977;124:304-310.

39. Reimann I: Experimental osteoarthritis of the knee in rabbits induced by alteration of the load-bearing. *Acta Orthop Scand* 1973;44:496-504.

40. Sandy JD, Adams ME, Billingham ME, et al: In vivo and in vitro stimulation of chondrocyte biosynthetic activity in early experimental osteoarthritis. *Arthritis Rheum* 1984;27:388-397.

41. Mankin HJ, Brandt KD, Shulman LE: Workshop on etiopathogenesis of osteoarthritis: Proceedings and recommendations. *J Rheumatol* 1986;13:1130-1160.

42. Brandt K: *Cartilage Changes in Osteoarthritis.* Indianapolis, Indiana University School of Medicine, 1990.

43. Furukawa T, Eyre DR, Koide S, et al: Biochemical studies on repair cartilage resurfacing experimental defects in the rabbit knee. *J Bone Joint Surg* 1980,62A:79-89.

44. Mitchell N, Shepard N: The resurfacing of adult rabbit articular cartilage by multiple perforations through the subchondral bone. *J Bone Joint Surg* 1976;58A:230-233.

45. Salter RB, Simonds DF, Malcolm BW, et al: The biological effect of continuous passive motion on the healing of full-thickness defects in articular cartilage. *J Bone Joint Surg* 1980;62A:1232-1251.

46. Mow VC, Howell DS, Buckwalter JA: Structure-function relationships of articular cartilage and the effects of joint instability and trauma on cartilage function, in Brandt K (ed): *Cartilage Changes in Osteoarthritis*. Indianapolis, Indiana University School of Medicine, 1990, pp 22-42.

47. Gilbertson EM: Development of periarticular osteophytes in experimentally induced osteoarthritis in the dog: A study using microradiographic, microangiographic, and fluorescent bone-labelling techniques. *Ann Rheum Dis* 1975;34:12-25.

48. Moskowitz RW, Goldberg VM: Studies of osteophyte pathogenesis in experimentally induced osteoarthritis. *J Rheumatol* 1987;14:311-320.

49. Marshall JL: Periarticular osteophytes: Initiation and formation in the knee of the dog. *Clin Orthop* 1969;62:37-47.

50. Ahmed AM, Burke DL: In-vitro measurement of static pressure distribution in synovial joints: Part 1: Tibial surface of the knee. *J Biomech Eng* 1983;105:216-225.

51. DeWitt MT, Handley CJ, Oakes BW, et al: *In vitro* response of chondrocytes to mechanical loading: The effect of shot term mechanical tension. *Connect Tissue Res* 1984;12:97-109.

52. Lippiello L, Kaye C, Neumata T, et al: In vitro metabolic response of articular cartilage segments to low levels of hydrostatic pressure. *Connect Tissue Res* 1985;13:99-107.

53. Van Kampen GPJ, Veldhuijzen JP, Kuijer R, et al: Cartilage response to mechanical force in high-density chondrocyte cultures. *Arthritis Rheum* 1985;28:419-424.

54. Colombo C, Butler M, O'Bryne E, et al: A new model of osteoarthritis in rabbits: I. Development of knee joint pathology following lateral meniscectomy and section of the fibular collateral and sesamoid ligaments. *Arthritis Rheum* 1983;26:875-886.

55. Carney SL, Billingham ME, Muir H, et al: Demonstration of increased proteoglycan turnover in cartilage explants from dogs with experimental osteoarthritis. *J Orthop Res* 1984;2:201-206.

56. Carney SL, Billingham MEJ, Muir H, et al: Structure of newly synthesised (^{35}S)-proteoglycans and (^{35}S)-proteoglycan turnover products of cartilage explant cultures from dogs with experimental osteoarthritis. *J Orthop Res* 1985;3:140-147.

57. McDevitt CA, Billingham MEJ, Muir H: *In-vivo* metabolism of proteoglycans in experimental osteoarthritic and normal canine articular cartilage and the invertebral disc. *Semin Arthritis Rheum* 1981;11(suppl 1):17-18.

58. Pelletier JP, Martel-Pelletier J: Neutral-proteoglycan-degrading protease activity in the early cartilage lesions of experimental osteoarthritis. *Trans Orthop Res Soc* 1985;10:128.

59. Pond MJ, Nuki G: Experimentally-induced osteoarthritis in the dog. *Ann Rheum Dis* 1973;32:387-388.

60. Pelletier JP, Martel-Pelletier J, Malemud CJ: Canine osteoarthritis: Effects of endogenous neutral metalloproteoglycanases on articular cartilage proteoglycans. *J Orthop Res* 1988;6:379-388.

61. Mayor MB, Moskowitz RW: Metabolic studies in experimentally-induced degenerative joint disease in the rabbit. *J Rheumatol* 1974;1: 17-23.

62. Moskowitz RW, Goldberg VM, Malemud CJ: Metabolic responses of cartilage in experimentally induced osteoarthritis. *Ann Rheum Dis* 1981;40:584-592.

63. Moskowitz RW: Osteoarthritis: Studies with experimental models. *Arthritis Rheum* 1977;20:S104-S108.

64. Moskowitz RW, Davis W, Sammarco J, et al: Experimentally induced degenerative joint lesions following partial meniscectomy in the rabbit. *Arthritis Rheum* 1973;16:397-405.

65. Moskowitz RW, Howell DS, Goldberg VM, et al: Cartilage proteoglycan alterations in an experimentally induced model of rabbit osteoarthritis. *Arthritis Rheum* 1979;22:155-163.

66. Mow VC, Lai WM: Recent developments in synovial joint biomechanics. *Soc Ind Appl Math Rev* 1980;22:275-317.

67. Matsuura T, Mansour J, Goldberg VM: Indentation testing of rabbit distal femoral cartilage. *ADM* Biomechanics Symposium 1991;120: 157-160.

68. Altman RD,Tenenbaum J, Latta L, et al: Biomechanical and biochemical properties of dog cartilage in experimentally induced osteoarthritis. *Ann Rheum Dis* 1984;43:83-90.

69. Butler M, Colombo C, Hickman L, et al: A new model of osteoarthritis in rabbits: III. Evaluation of anti-osteoarthritic effects of selected drugs administered intra-articularly. *Arthritis Rheum* 1983;26:1380-1386.

70. Colombo C, Butler M, Hickman L, et al: A new model of osteoarthritis in rabbits: II. Evaluation of anti-osteoarthritic effects of selected antirheumatic drugs administered systemically. *Arthritis Rheum* 1983;26:1132-1139.

71. Floman Y, Eyre DR, Glimcher MJ: Induction of osteoarthrosis in the rabbit knee joint: Biochemical studies on the articular cartilage. *Clin Orthop* 1980;147:278-286.

72. Hulth A, Lindberg L, Telhag H: Experimental osteoarthritis in rabbits. Preliminary report. *Acta Orthop Scand* 1970;41:522-530.

73. Moon MS, Chung IS: Degenerative changes after meniscectomy and meniscal regeneration. *Int Orthop* 1988;12:17-19.

74. Shapiro F, Glimcher MJ: Induction of osteoarthrosis in the rabbit knee joint: Histologic changes following meniscectomy and meniscal lesions. *Clin Orthop* 1980;147:287-295.

75. Tapper EM, Hoover NW: Late results after meniscectomy. *J Bone Joint Surg* 1969;51A:517-526.

Chapter 7

Cell-Based Technologies for Cartilage Repair

Arnold I. Caplan, PhD
Tatsuhiko Goto, MD
Shigeyuki Wakitani, MD
Steven J. Pineda, MD
Stephen E. Haynesworth, PhD
Victor M. Goldberg, MD

Introduction

Cartilage is a simple yet complex tissue. It is simple because it is made by one cell type, the chondrocyte, unlike most tissues such as nerve, vascular, immune, or connective, which contain other cell types. It is complex because it is composed predominantly of an unusual extracellular matrix and a large amount of water. The macromolecules of the extracellular matrix provide the tissue with tensile strength (in the form of collagen) and resiliency (in the form of proteoglycans). The collagen fibers form a scaffold, and the proteoglycan structures hold water; together these macromolecules cause water to be forced out of cartilage upon loading, with a resilient return to the cartilage's original shape upon unloading.[1,2] The voluminous extracellular matrix, the relatively acellular tissue, and the isolation of the tissue from systemic influence (no vasculature or nerves) create a situation in which turnover is extremely slow and self-repair unlikely. Some molecular turnover can be matched by the steady but relatively slow synthesis of new macromolecules and, indeed, some have speculated that this slow replacement phenomenon is responsible for slow, age-related changes that eventually result in tissue failure in the elderly.[3,4] However, significant damage to cartilage, such as a simple tear, does not self-repair; while in a tissue with a high turnover rate, such as skin, lung, or gut, these lesions rapidly self-repair.

A key element of successful tissue repair is the acute inflammatory process, which involves access to adequate, systemically supplied macrophages to remove the dead and injured tissue; these phagocytic cells subsequently prepare the site for colonization by reparative/regeneration cells. In most cases, the reparative cells are naturally present and are usually responsible for the cell-mediated turnover of the tissue. Thus, tissues with naturally high turnover rates also exhibit relatively rapid repair. Because of its isolation from systemic regulation, its extremely low turnover rate, and its low to normal metabolism and synthesis, cartilage is not equipped for self-repair.

When injuries or defects are deep enough to penetrate the subchondral bone, access to systemic influence is possible via the bleeding wound (vascular subchondral bone). In young animals, the pathway from the subchondral bone and marrow spaces can direct cells of sufficient repair potential to the injury site.[5,6] In some instances of full-thickness defects, substantial or complete repair/regeneration can be observed. Clearly, the optimal repair strategy would be to attract or transplant reparative cells into the cartilage defect and thereby ensure repair.

However, it must be stressed here that even a simple cut over a limited section of cartilage is not repaired. Discontinuity of cartilage extracellular matrix usually is not bridged by reparative tissue or matrix, nor is there an observed, substantial increase in the macromolecules synthesized by adjacent chondrocytes. Thus, superficial discontinuities are not repaired, and because of mechanical and other factors, such wounds often enlarge, fragment, and eventually progress to form large, degenerative lesions that compromise the tissue and, thus, joint function. Because no curative treatment exists for such damage, these lesions progress until pain and/or lack of mobility forces the patient to elect total joint arthroplasty with prosthetic replacement.

Cartilage Repair

Historically, the attempts to surgically repair or totally replace large joints dates back to the turn of the century;[7-9] other approaches soon followed.[10-13] The isolation and cryopreservation of chondrocytes initiated several attempts at cellular repair of cartilage defects.[14-17] To effect repair, the damaged tissue must be removed to make way for reparative cells. Concomitant with the removal of damaged tissue by macrophages and other resorptive cells is the release of powerful bioactive molecules that chemically attract reparative cells and cause these newly arrived cells to undergo mitotic expansion to fill the void created by the phagocytic cells. In the case of cartilage tissue damage, the matrix appears to contain natural inhibitors of vascular and macrophage invasion. Thus, the damaged tissue must be excavated surgically, and the reparative cells added manually.

These reparative cells can be delivered by at least two different approaches. Some investigators have introduced complex tissues, such as periosteum[18,19] or perichondrium,[20] which are known to have chondroprogenitor cells as a minor component. This complex tissue can thus be attacked by phagocytic cells, resulting in the release of the progenitor cells and their mitotic expansion into the cartilaginous defect. Such surgical implantation requires that the damaged cartilage be removed and the subchondral bone penetrated to ensure access to systemic factors and phagocytic progenitors.

The repair observed in these cases is never complete because it is likely that some fibrous tissue progenitors also expand in the repair site and diminish the amount of cartilage that could form.

The other approach is to add a full complement of reparative chondrogenic cells in an appropriate delivery vehicle that takes up the entire volume of the defect. The advantage of this approach is that in situ mitotic expansion by the reparative cells is not necessary. Several types of cell preparations have been used, including embryonic or adult allogeneic chondrocytes, and several delivery vehicles have been explored, with collagen or fibrin being the most popular.[21-23] Before formally evaluating these approaches, the questions "What is a chondrocyte?" and "Where do they come from?" must be addressed.

Chondrocytic Lineages

A chondrocyte is a cell that produces the unique and voluminous extracellular matrix of cartilage. This matrix is composed of collagen (predominantly type II), proteoglycans (predominately the large, aggregating chondroitin-keratan sulfate proteoglycan), non-collagenous matrix proteins, and water. All chondrocytes are not equal; chondrocytes in different anatomic regions may make different matrices or respond differently to specific cytokines or growth factors. Clearly, chondrocytes that produce cartilage at the articular surface of the knee are different from spinal (disk) chondrocytes. Chondrocytes at the surface are very different from those in the same tissue at locations that are deeper by only a few cell diameters into the cartilaginous tissue;[24,25] such differences reflect the differences in mechanical, nutritional, and functional environments within the articular cartilage. These micro site-specific biochemical differences are comparable to the molecular differences observed as mature chondrocytes develop sequentially from chondroprogenitor cells.

The sequential molecular expression pattern observed during cartilage development represents a lineage (Fig. 1)[26-29] comparable to that observed in other tissue or cell developmental processes,[30,31] notably hematopoiesis.[32] Such a lineage implies that several important principles are related to optimal cell-based therapies for cartilage repair/regeneration. For example, what cytokines or growth factors are required to allow a cell to transit from one lineage developmental stage to the next? What factors control modulation of expression, causing articular surface chondrocytes and deeper chondrocytes to make functionally different matrices? A more complicated problem is how to inhibit lineage transit to ensure that some chondrocytes never become hypertrophic while encouraging other chondrocytes to become hypertrophic, so that subchondral bone can re-form in a full-thickness defect. By recognizing that a chondrogenic lineage exists, we also appreciate the molecular and cellular complexity of the control of cartilage development and repair.

CHONDROGENIC LINEAGE

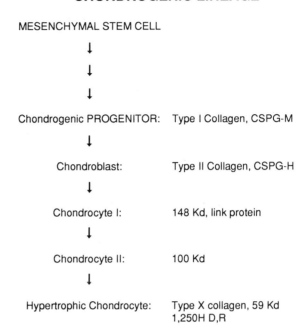

MESENCHYMAL STEM CELL

↓

↓

↓

Chondrogenic PROGENITOR: Type I Collagen, CSPG-M

↓

Chondroblast: Type II Collagen, CSPG-H

↓

Chondrocyte I: 148 Kd, link protein

↓

Chondrocyte II: 100 Kd

↓

Hypertrophic Chondrocyte: Type X collagen, 59 Kd
1,250H D,R

Fig. 1 *A proposed sequential lineage map based on the published studies[26] previously discussed.[30,31] The pluripotential mesenchymal stem cell (MSC) is proposed to go through a number of phenotypic changes to generate chondro-committed cells, which then progress through the lineage. Lineage progress is marked by the appearance of stage-specific macromolecules as listed on the right. The hypertrophic chondrocyte can exist indefinitely, but it usually expires and is directly replaced by vascular and marrow elements and eventually bone.[27-29] CSPG = chondroitin sulfate proteoglycan; 148, 100, and 59kD refer to cartilage proteins; $1,25(OH)_2D_3R$ = the receptor for 1,25 dehydroxy vitamin D_3.*

Mesenchymal Stem Cells

Because chondrogenic lineage is comparable to the hematopoietic sequence, there is a possibility that a stem cell exists, which gives rise to a variety of mesenchymatous tissues such as bone, cartilage, ligament, and tendon. Studies done in our laboratory have recently provided strong evidence for an osteogenic lineage,[33-35] and, in the past, we have worked with embryonic limb mesenchymal cells that seem to be able to commit to either a chondrogenic or osteogenic pathway, depending on the local environment.[36-38] Friedenstein,[39] Owen,[40] Bab and associates,[41] Budenz and Bernard,[42] and others[43,44] have clearly documented that bone marrow contains such osteo-chondral progenitor cells. Recently, we have reported isolating an osteochondral progenitor cell from either marrow or long bone peri-osteum; these cells may be pluripotent mesenchymal stem cells (MSCs) (Fig. 2).[45-52] Importantly, we have developed the technology

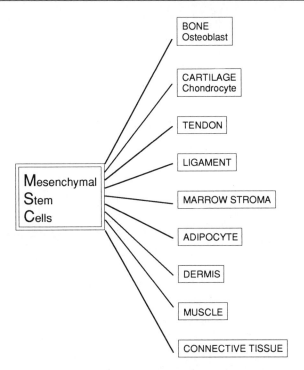

Fig. 2   *The mesenchymal stem cell (MSC) found in the bone marrow or periosteum of adults is proposed to be capable of establishing separate and distinct lineages, which result in cells that can produce different mesenchymatous tissues. Our studies have clearly documented that such MSCs can give rise to cartilage or bone.[45-52]*

for isolating and mitotically expanding these MSCs so that, from a relatively few cells in the initial isolate, we have been able to generate millions of autologous MSCs. In 7 to 10 days after in vivo implantation of these purified, culture-expanded progenitor cells in porous ceramic cubes[45,50] or by direct subcutaneous injections,[46] high levels of cartilage and/or bone tissue can be observed at the implantation sites. These observations indicate that we can obtain relatively large amounts of osteochondral progenitors that can be made available for implantation in a cartilage repair model.

Cell Therapy

Several technical approaches to facilitate cartilage repair have been attempted with various levels of success.[18-23] The more successful of these attempts involved encasing allogeneic embryonic or mature chondrocytes in a delivery matrix prior to implantation into full-thickness articular cartilage defects in mature animals. This approach is based on complete surgical removal of the host's cartilaginous/subchondral bone tissue with replacement by chondrocytes

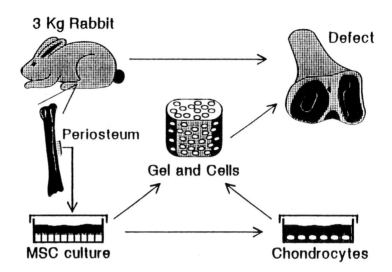

Fig. 3 *Cartilage repair protocols are diagrammed: Autologous periosteal- or marrow-derived mesenchymal stem cells (MSCs) are isolated and cell culture expanded. These cells are either directly incorporated into a collagenous delivery vehicle (gel) or stimulated to differentiate into chondrocytes in the culture dish. The MSC-derived chondrocytes or allogeneic-cultured chondrocytes can likewise be incorporated into a delivery vehicle. Properly encased cells are delivered to a full-thickness defect (6 x 3 x 3 mm) in the medial aspect of the distal femoral condyle of the original donor rabbit (S. Wakitani, T. Goto, V.M. Goldberg, et al, unpublished data, 1992). Repair is monitored at one, three, and six months by both histologic and mechanical analyses.[53,54]*

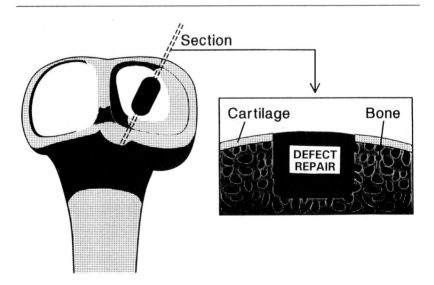

Fig. 4 *A section through the full-thickness defect created in Figure 3. The relationships between the normal cartilage and bone and the defect are diagrammed.*

capable of immediately synthesizing cartilaginous extracellular matrix. A factor not addressed, but of interest, is whether sternal, rib, or articular cartilage chondrocytes behave in a similar manner in these repair motifs.

As a variant of these approaches, we have directly compared the implantation (Figs. 3 and 4)[53,54] of rabbit allogeneic articular chondrocytes (Fig. 5) with that of autologous bone marrow- or periosteal-derived MSCs (Fig. 6), into a large (6 x 3 x 3 mm) defect (S. Wakitani, T. Goto, S.J. Pineda, et al, unpublished data, 1992).[53] The use of MSCs is based on the assumption that systemic or local bioactive factors will be available to induce the entrance of these progenitor cells into the chondrogenic lineage, to accelerate the transit of the cells below the subchondral bone-cartilage interface into the hypertrophic stage so that vascular and marrow replacement can occur, and to inhibit the articular chondrocytes from transit into the hypertrophic stage. If such local factors are not available or if their concentration is too low, then in vitro exposure of these agents to MSCs will be required with subsequent transplantation of these factor-stimulated cells into the defect.

Figure 4 is a diagram of the histologic sections shown in Figures 5 and 6. Both of the samples seen in Figures 5 and 6 were from animals sacrificed one month after implantation and are representative of this time interval (S. Wakitani, T. Goto, V.M. Goldberg, et al, unpublished data, 1992). The focus of interest here is the fact that both the allogeneic, mature chondrocytes and MSC-derived chondrocytes have initially made a reparative cartilage that fills the entire full-thickness defect. The MSC-derived cartilage is being replaced by osseous tissue below the subchondral bone-cartilage junction, while no apparent change is observed in the mature chondrocyte implant. One interpretation of this observation is that the defect limited to subchondral bone releases sufficient quantities of the appropriate cytokines/growth factors to induce the MSCs to become chondrocytes and to further stimulate these cells to transit rapidly to the hypertrophic stage. This hypertrophic cartilage is then replaced by vasculature and host-derived MSCs, which differentiate into osteoblasts and make the new subchondral bone. Clearly, these same intrinsic factors do not appear to affect the already mature chondrocytes placed into a comparable defect. Other observations that are not shown in these figures also indicate that periosteum- and bone marrow-derived MSCs behave similarly in the first month in a full-thickness defect.

Evaluation of the mechanical properties of the reparative cartilage and histologic or biochemical analysis are essential. Such analyses are now underway[54] with the preliminary observation that reparative cartilage with a histologically healthy appearance is correlated with cartilage that is mechanically similar to normal cartilage in that joint. Such determinations have been conducted in specimens from one-, three-, and six-month postimplantation surgeries. Attempts have not yet been made to evaluate the effects of constant

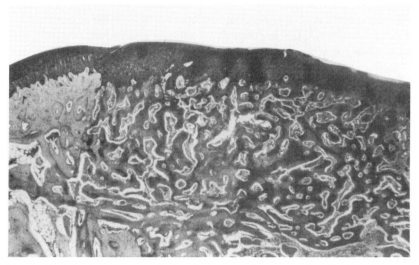

Fig. 5 *Histologic section, as depicted in Figure 4, one month following the implantation of marrow-derived MSCs into the full-thickness defect. The regenerated cartilage is observed above the newly formed subchondral bone. This new bone is more dense than the surrounding host bone, which facilitates identification of the original defect.*

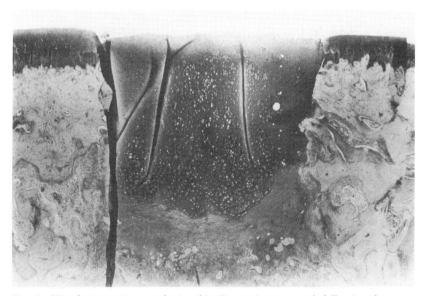

Fig. 6 *Histologic section, as depicted in Figure 4, one month following the implantation of allogeneic chondrocytes into the full-thickness defect. The chondrocytes have produced a rich cartilage extracellular matrix throughout the depth of the defect.*

passive motion or gradual weightbearing on the success of this implantation repair.

Future Cell Therapy

Based on our current state of knowledge, it is difficult to imagine that a cytokine/growth factor can be identified and effectively delivered to the impervious articular cartilage to stimulate repair; such a factor has not been found. Given this point of view, it seems more reasonable to explore the surgical implantation of reparative tissue. Several other investigators have considered the transplantation of allogeneic cartilage and of cartilage with its own adjacent subchondral bone; long-term tissue integration and immunocompatibility must also be considered. Alternately, the transplantation of autologous, culture-expanded MSCs offers several advantages, including immunocompatibility, high cytokine/growth factor sensitivity, and availability; however, several ethical/legal factors must be considered. The availability of cell culture-expanded MSCs makes possible the design of autologous cell-based therapies, which will require surgeons to acquire new skills and will herald an era of physician-controlled, patient-specific, hospital-delivered tissue regeneration.

Summary

The natural repair of any tissue is keyed to the mechanisms that regulate various aspects of tissue turnover. Tissues with high turnover and repair rates are usually connected systemically to facilitate the sequential delivery of resorptive or phagocytic cells to the turnover/repair site. Such resorptive events lead to the release of bioactive agents that both attract and mitotically expand reparative cells, which eventually occupy the volume of the excavated tissue. Eventually the reparative cells differentiate and integrate into the host tissue, resulting in regeneration of the injured tissue. Articular cartilage is unique in its isolation from systemic influences and its lack of nonchondrogenic cells (vascular, neural, or immune). Thus, repair of cartilage requires surgical excavation of the site into the subchondral bone to remove the injured tissue and to expose the site to systemic influences. In addition, because of the paucity of reparative cells near cartilage, it is essential to deliver an enriched population of reparative cells directly into the repair site. The approach used in this laboratory is to isolate autologous chondroprogenitor cells and expand such cells in cell culture for implantation into large, full-thickness articular defects. The delivery of these progenitor cells has several advantages over that of mature chondrocytes, including their superior ability to respond to different microenvironmental changes throughout the depth of the defect.

Acknowledgments

We are deeply grateful to our colleagues who directly contributed to the research efforts reviewed here, especially Scott P. Bruder, PhD, Haruhiko Nakahara, MD, and James E. Dennis, MS. We also gratefully acknowledge support of NIH grants AR37726 and AR40990.

References

1. Hassell JR, Kimura JH, Hascall VC: Proteoglycan core protein families. *Ann Rev Biochem* 1986;55:539-567.

2. Kuettner KE, Schleyerbach R, Hascall VC (eds): *Articular Cartilage Biochemistry*. New York, Raven Press, 1986.

3. Caplan AI, Fiszman MY, Eppenberger HM: Molecular and cell isoforms during development. *Science* 1983;221:921-927.

4. Caplan AI: Cartilage. *Sci Am* 1984;251:84-94.

5. Furukawa T, Eyre DR, Koide S, et al: Biochemical studies on repair cartilage resurfacing experimental defects in the rabbit knee. *J Bone Joint Surg* 1980;62A:79-89.

6. Buckwalter JA, Rosenberg LC, Hunziker EB: Articular cartilage: Composition, structure, response to injury, and methods of facilitating repair, in Ewing JW (ed): *Articular Cartilage and Knee Joint Function: Basic Science and Arthroscopy*. New York, Raven Press, 1990, pp 19-56.

7. Lexer E: Substitution of whole or half joints from freshly amputated extremities by free plastic operation. *Surg Gynecol Obstet* 1908;6: 601-607.

8. Judet H: Essai sur la greffe des tissue articulaires. *Comptes rendus des seances de l'Academie des Sciences* 1908;146:600-603.

9. Lexer E: Joint transplantations and arthroplasty. *Surg Gynecol Obstet* 1925;40:782-809.

10. Herndon CH, Chase SW: The fate of massive autogenous and homogenous bone grafts including articular surfaces. *Surg Gynecol Obstet* 1954;98:273-290.

11. Langer F, Gross AE: Immunogenicity of allograft articular cartilage. *J Bone Joint Surg* 1974;56A:297-304.

12. Lane JM, Brighton CT, Ottens HR, et al: Joint resurfacing in the rabbit using an autologous osteochondral graft. *J Bone Joint Surg* 1977;59A:218-222.

13. Goldberg VM, Heiple KG: Experimental hemijoint and whole-joint transplantation. *Clin Orthop* 1983;174:43-53.

14. Smith AU: Survival of frozen chondrocytes isolated from cartilage of adult mammals. *Nature* 1965;205:782-784.

15. Chesterman PJ, Smith AU: Homotransplantation of articular cartilage and isolated chondrocytes. *J Bone Joint Surg* 1968;50B:184-197.

16. Bentley G, Greer RB III: Homotransplantation of isolated epiphyseal and articular cartilage chondrocytes into joint surfaces of rabbits. *Nature* 1971;230:385-388.

17. Bentley G, Smith AU, Mukerjhee R: Isolated epiphyseal chondrocyte allografts into joint surfaces. *Ann Rheum Dis* 1978;37:449.

18. O'Driscoll SW, Salter RB: The repair of major osteochondral defects in joint surfaces by neochondrogenesis with autogenous osteoperiosteal grafts stimulated by continuous passive motion: An experimental investigation in the rabbit. *Clin Orthop* 1986;208:131-140.

19. O'Driscoll SW, Keeley FW, Salter RB: Durability of regenerated articular cartilage produced by free autogenous periosteal grafts in major full-thickness defects in joint surfaces under the influence of continuous passive motion. *J Bone Joint Surg* 1988;70A:595-606.

20. von Schroeder HP, Billings E, Amiel D, et al: The use of demineralized bone and rib perichondrium composite grafts for the repair of full-thickness articular defects. *Trans Orthop Res Soc* 1990;15:346.

21. Itay S, Abramovici A, Nevo Z: Use of cultured embryonal chick epiphyseal chondrocytes as grafts for defects in chick articular cartilage. *Clin Orthop* 1987;220;284-303.

22. Wakitani S, Kimura T, Hirooka A, et al: Repair of rabbit articular surfaces with allograft chondrocytes embedded in collagen gel. *J Bone Joint Surg* 1989;71B:74-80.

23. Grande DA, Pitman MI, Peterson L, et al: The repair of experimentally produced defects in rabbit articular cartilage by autologous chondrocyte transplantation. *J Orthop Res* 1989;7:208-218.

24. Aydelotte MB, Kuettner KE: Differences between subpopulations of cultured bovine articular chondrocytes: I. Morphology and cartilage matrix production. *Connect Tissue Res* 1988;18:205-222.

25. Aydelotte MB, Greenhill RR, Kuettner KE: Differences between subpopulations of cultured bovine articular chondrocytes: II. Proteoglycan metabolism. *Connect Tissue Res* 1988;18:223-234.

26. Franzen A, Heinegard D, Solursh M: Evidence for sequential appearance of cartilage matrix proteins in developing mouse limbs and in cultures of mouse mesenchymal cells. *Differentiation* 1987;36: 199-210.

27. Pechak DG, Kujawa MJ, Caplan AI: Morphology of bone development and bone remodeling in embryonic chick limbs. *Bone* 1986;7:459-472.

28. Caplan AI, Pechak D: The cellular and molecular embryology of bone formation, in Peck WA (ed): *Bone and Mineral Research*. New York, Elsevier, 1987, pp 117-184.

29. Caplan AI: Cartilage begets bone versus endochondral myelopoiesis. *Clin Orthop* 1990;261:257-267.

30. Caplan AI: Regenerating tissues in adults, in Goldberg VM (ed): *Controversies of Total Knee Arthroplasty*. New York, Raven Press, 1991, pp 249-252.

31. Caplan AI: Mesenchymal stem cell-mediated cartilage and bone repair, in Davidovitch Z (ed): *The Biological Mechanisms of Tooth Movement and Craniofacial Adaptation*. EBSCO, in press.

32. Metcalf D: *The Hematopoietic Colony Stimulating Factors*. Amsterdam, Elsevier, 1991.

33. Bruder SP, Caplan AI: First bone formation and the dissection of an osteogenic lineage in the embryonic chick tibia is revealed by monoclonal antibodies against osteoblasts. *Bone* 1989;10:359-375.

34. Bruder SP, Caplan AI: Osteogenic cell lineage analysis is facilitated by organ cultures of embryonic chick periosteum. *Dev Biol* 1990;141: 319-329.

35. Bruder SP, Caplan AI: Terminal differentiation of osteogenic cells in the embryonic chick tibia is revealed by a monoclonal antibody against osteocytes. *Bone* 1990;11:189-198.

36. Caplan AI: Bone development and repair: *Bioessays* 1987;6:171-175.

37. Osdoby P, Caplan AI: Osteogenesis in cultures of limb mesenchymal cells. *Dev Biol* 1979;73:84-102.

38. Caplan AI, Syftestad G, Osdoby P: The development of embryonic bone and cartilage in tissue culture. *Clin Orthop* 1983;174:243-263.

39. Friedenstein AJ: Stroma mechanisms of bone marrow: Cloning in vitro and retransplantation in vivo, in Thienfelder S (ed): *Immunobiology of Bone Marrow Transplantation*. Berlin, Springer-Verlag, 1980, pp 19-29.

40. Owen M: Marrow stromal stem cells: *J Cell Sci Suppl* 1988;10:63-76.

41. Bab I, Passi-Even L, Gazit D, et al: Osteogenesis in in vivo diffusion chamber cultures of human marrow cells. *Bone Miner* 1988;4:373-386.

42. Budenz RW, Bernard GW: Osteogenesis and leukopoiesis within diffusion-chamber implants of isolated bone marrow subpopulations. *Am J Anat* 1980;159:455-474.

43. Bruder SP, Gazit D, Passi-Even L, et al: Osteochondral differentiation and the emergence of stage-specific osteogenic cell-surface molecules by bone marrow cells in diffusion chambers. *Bone Miner* 1990;11: 141-151.

44. Beresford JN: Osteogenic stem cells and the stromal system of bone and marrow. *Clin Orthop* 1989;240:270-280.

45. Goshima J, Goldberg VM, Caplan AI: The osteogenic potential of culture-expanded rat marrow mesenchymal cells assayed in vivo in calcium phosphate ceramic blocks. *Clin Orthop* 1991;262:298-311.

46. Nakahara H, Bruder SP, Goldberg VM, et al: In vivo osteochondrogenic potential of cultured cells derived from the periosteum. *Clin Orthop* 1990;259:223-232.

47. Nakahara H, Watanabe K, Sugrue SP, et al: Temporal and spatial distribution of type XII collagen in high cell density culture of periosteal-derived cells. *Dev Biol* 1990;142:481-485.

48. Goshima J, Goldberg VM, Caplan AI: The origin of bone formed in composite grafts of porous calcium phosphate ceramic loaded with marrow cells. *Clin Orthop* 1991;269:274-283.

49. Nakahara H, Goldberg VM, Caplan AI: Culture-expanded human periosteal-derived cells exhibit osteochondral potential in vivo. *J Orthop Res* 1991;9:465-476.

50. Haynesworth SE, Goshima J, Goldberg VM, et al: Characterization of cells with osteogenic potential from human marrow. *Bone* 1992;13: 81-88.

51. Nakahara H, Bruder SP, Haynesworth SE, et al: In vitro differentiation of bone and hypertrophic cartilage from periosteal-derived cells. *Exp Cell Res* 1991;195:492-503.

52. Caplan AI: Mesenchymal stem cells. *J Orthop Res* 1991;9:641-650.

53. Pineda SJ, Pollack A, Stevenson S, et al: A semiquantitative scale for histological grading of articular cartilage repair. *Acta Anat*, in press.

54. Matsuura T, Mansour J, Goldberg VM, et al: Mechanical properties of rabbit articular cartilage after partial meniscectomy. *Trans Ortop Res Soc* 1991;16:76.

Chapter 8

Fresh Small Fragment Osteochondral Allografts Used for Posttraumatic Defects in the Knee Joint

Allan E. Gross, MD, FRCS (C)
Richard J. Beaver, MD, FRACS
Mohammed N. Mahomed, MD

Introduction

The use of bone allografts in orthopaedic surgery dates back to 1908 when Lexer first published his results.[1,2] Since then, interest in the use of bone allografts has steadily increased over the years; initially, however, their use was limited to limb salvage in cases of severe trauma such as war injuries. Techniques and knowledge in the areas of immunology and transplantation improved with time, and the applications of bone allografts increased.

In the 1970s, advances were made in the diagnosis and chemo-therapeutic treatment of bone tumors, making it possible to perform limb salvage surgery rather than amputation in patients afflicted with such tumors. Large defects created by en bloc resection of bone tumors would require reconstruction with either large implants, allografts, or combinations of implants and allografts (bioimplants).

In the 1970s and 1980s, there was renewed interest in implantation of bone allografts. With the increasing popularity of total joint arthroplasties, revision procedures became more prevalent. As it became necessary to restore bone stock in order to insert a new implant, it was discovered that allograft bone could be used for this purpose.

The increased demand for osteochondral allografts encouraged several investigators[3-5] to implant allografts during the 1970s, with promising results. This led to the establishment of large, institutional bone banks that facilitated further research into the biology of osteochondral allografts.

The repair of osteoarticular defects in the joints of relatively young, active patients is difficult, and only a limited number of options are presently available to deal with this problem: (1) arthroplasty, which reestablishes joint function but is presently unacceptable in this patient population because of the high stresses placed on the joint; (2) arthrodesis, which results in a relatively pain-free joint but yields a less than ideal level of function; and (3) fresh

Table 1 A list of those diagnoses for which fresh osteochondral allografts have been performed in the knee joint.

Diagnosis	Number of Cases*	Exclusions
Trauma	92	7
Osteoarthritis	18	1
Osteonecrosis	7	
Osteochondritis dissecans	10	
Total	127	8

*Those cases performed for reconstruction of defects following resection of tumors are not included in this review.

small-fragment osteochondral allograft implantation, which results in both a pain-free joint and good range of motion while allowing some time before knee arthroplasty is necessary. Therefore, a more biologic method of replacing articular cartilage and subchondral bone is preferable in these patients.

The University of Toronto's Orthopaedic Transplant Program, which began in 1971, is the largest program of its kind in the world and has four major components: (1) deep frozen allograft bone, used in general orthopaedic procedures such as grafting bone cavities; (2) fresh small-fragment osteochondral allografts, used for articular surface replacement of traumatic defects; (3) deep frozen allograft bone, used for bone stock replacement in revision arthroplasty surgery; and (4) deep frozen large-fragment allograft bone, used for limb salvage after en bloc excision of bone tumors.

Initially, fresh osteochondral allograft procedures were performed for a variety of diagnoses, including unicompartmental osteoarthritis, spontaneous osteonecrosis of the knee, steroid-induced osteonecrosis of the knee, osteochondritis dissecans, and posttraumatic defects. After reviewing our first 100 cases, we recognized that the best results were obtained in restoring cartilage and bone to traumatically-induced defects. Osteochondritis dissecans was believed to be only a relative indication to implantation of fresh allografts; both osteoarthritis and osteonecrosis were considered as relative contraindications.[6-9] A summary of the various diagnoses for which fresh osteochondral allografts have been inserted in the knee joint is shown in Table 1. The effects of certain selection criteria such as age, sex, and anatomic site of the graft were also analyzed to deduce their importance on allograft survival. We also decided to compare the clinical performance of the unipolar grafts with that of the bipolar grafts, which were thought to perform poorly.[10]

Based on our results, we now use osteochondral allografts primarily for unicompartmental posttraumatic defects in the knees of patients younger than 50 years of age. As of July 1, 1991, of the 187 operations using fresh allografts, 127 have been performed for traumatic defects about the knee. We have also implanted four grafts for elbow joint defects, three for femoral head defects, and four for talus defects, but our discussion here will focus on posttraumatic defects of the knee joint.

124

Graft Acquisition, Planning, and Implantation

Preoperative Planning

The following points are important to remember before surgery: (1) It is essential to correct joint malalignment prior to or simultaneously with the implantation of the allograft. (2) Attempts to correct malalignment using the height of the allograft lead to a high incidence of graft failure.[7,8,11] (3) Varus deformities are corrected with proximal tibial valgus osteotomy. (4) Valgus deformities are corrected with distal femoral varus osteotomy; this technique has been discussed in other publications.[12]

Harvesting of Allografts

The donors are located by the Multiple Organ Retrieval and Exchange program (M.O.R.E.) of Toronto. The fresh osteochondral allografts are acquired according to procedures established by the American Association of Tissue Banks.[13-15] In addition, the donor must be younger than 30 years old to ensure maximum cartilage quality. The graft is procured under strict aseptic precautions, within 24 (preferably 12) hours of donor death. The entire donor joint, including the joint capsule and ligaments, is excised. Cultures for bacteria, fungi, and mycobacteria are obtained. The joint is then immersed in sterile Ringer's solution containing 1 g of cefazolin and 50,000 units of bacitracin per liter. The joint is sealed with sterile adhesive plastic in a sterile container. This container is triple wrapped in towels and sterile plastic bags and stored at a temperature of 4 C until it is ready to be used. There is no histocompatibility testing, and no immunosuppression is used.

The appropriate recipient is selected only on the basis of sex and approximate sizing of the donor allograft. The recipient is notified as soon as a donor has been located and comes to the hospital immediately; the allograft is always implanted into the recipient within 12 to 24 hours of graft procurement.

Preparation and Implantation of Allografts

Two operating teams are usually employed: one to prepare the allograft, and the other to perform any realignment procedure and prepare the recipient bed.

Whenever possible, a midline longitudinal anterior incision is used and, depending on the site of the joint defect, either a medial or lateral parapatellar arthrotomy is performed. After arthrotomy, the meniscus is inspected. If possible, the host meniscus is preserved or repaired; if not, a meniscectomy is performed and a donor meniscus implanted with the allograft. In the case of a tibial allograft, the meniscus is left attached to the donor plateau and sutured to the capsule of the recipient. Similarly, if a femoral allograft is used, the

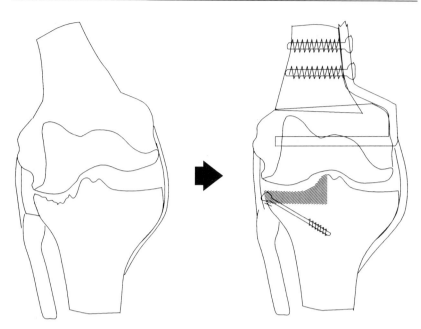

Fig. 1 *An osteoarticular defect in the weightbearing portion of the lateral tibial plateau producing genu valgum deformity corrected by fresh osteochondral allograft of the tibial plateau. The allograft has been unloaded by a distal femoral varus osteotomy. (Reproduced with permission from Beaver RJ, Mahomed M, Backstein D, et al: Fresh osteochondral allografts for post-traumatic defects in the knee.* J Bone Joint Surg *1992;74B:105-110.)*

capsular attachments of the meniscus to the femoral allograft are retained and the meniscus is sutured to the host capsule using absorbable suture material.

The most common scenario is a defect in the weightbearing portion of the lateral tibial plateau, producing a genu valgum deformity. In this case, the damaged articular surface of the tibia is resected and "squared off" down to healthy, bleeding, cancellous bone. The corresponding segment of the donor joint is resected and trimmed to match the defect in the recipient. The valgus deformity is corrected by a distal femoral varus osteotomy in order to unload the allograft, thereby reducing the chance of graft failure (Fig. 1). If a meniscus is to be implanted as well, three or four absorbable mattress sutures are placed in the periphery of the meniscus and affixed to the capsule of the host. These sutures are not tied until after fitting of the graft.

The allograft is rigidly fixed to the tibia with 4.0-mm AO spongiosa screws. It is important to place the screws well away from the articular cartilage, in a site not likely to cause impingement problems (Fig. 1). Closure is performed over suction drains. An example of lateral tibial plateau fresh allografts is shown in Figure 2.

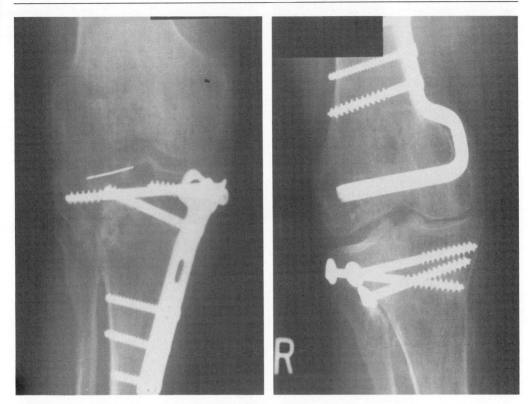

Fig. 2   *Case 1:* **Left**, *Anteroposterior radiograph of the right knee of a 55-year-old woman with a malunited lateral tibial plateau fracture.* **Right**, *Three years following transplantation, the allograft has completely united to the host with minimal subsidence.*

In those cases in which there is a varus deformity of the knee with destruction of the medial femoral condyle, a proximal tibial valgus osteotomy with osteochondral allograft replacement of the medial femoral condyle is performed (Fig. 3). The surgical technique is similar to that previously outlined. The specific techniques for proximal tibial valgus osteotomy have been well described.[16-19] It has been the practice at Mount Sinai Hospital to perform a closing wedge osteotomy 2 cm distal to the knee joint, with a concomitant evaluation of the tibial tubercle (Maquet procedure) as described by Putnam and associates in 1985.[20]

It is often possible to obtain sufficient exposure of the medial femoral condyle by a medial parapatellar approach and subluxation of the patella without complete dislocation. As with the tibial plateau graft, considerable care is given to obtaining an accurate press-fit of the allograft and rigid fixation of the graft using AO screws. An example of a medial femoral condylar fresh allograft is shown in Figure 4.

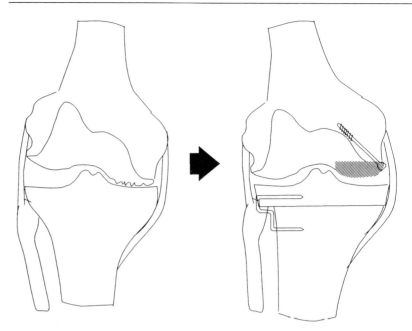

Fig. 3 *An osteoarticular defect in the weightbearing portion of the medial femoral condyle producing genu varum deformity corrected by fresh allograft to the femoral condyle. The allograft is unloaded by proximal tibial valgus osteotomy. (Reproduced with permission from Beaver RJ, Mahomed M, Backstein D, et al: Fresh osteochondral allografts for post-traumatic defects in the knee. J Bone Joint Surg 1992;74B:105-110.)*

A bipolar graft is one in which both the tibial and femoral condyles on one side of the joint are replaced, whereas a unipolar graft is one in which only one condyle, tibial or femoral, is replaced. No cases of patellofemoral replacement are included.

Postoperative Management

Continuous passive motion of the operated knee is instituted immediately in the recovery room because this technique is believed to prevent the formation of intra-articular adhesions and to optimize cartilage nutrition. Immediate mobilization is possible only because of the rigidity of the fixation between graft and host bone. Patients are mobilized without bearing weight as soon as suction drains are removed. Partial weightbearing is maintained for at least one year by the application of an ischial-bearing long leg orthosis.

Collection of Clinical Data

We reviewed 127 cases of fresh osteochondral allograft procedures performed for posttraumatic defects in the knee. Where possible, each patient's knee score was calculated using a modified knee

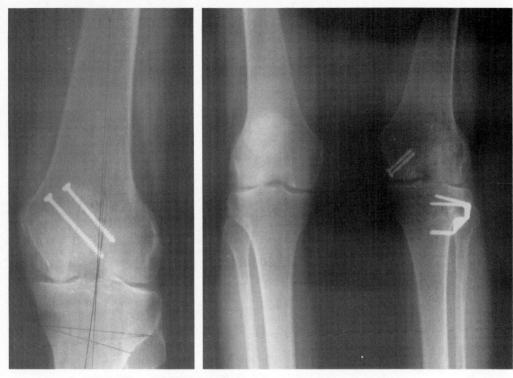

Fig. 4   *Case 2:* ***Left***, *Radiograph of the right knee of a 33-year-old woman with a traumatic defect in the weightbearing portion of the medial femoral condyle.* ***Right***, *The knee is seen 4.5 years following replacement of the medial femoral condyle with a fresh osteochondral allograft and proximal tibial valgus osteotomy.*

rating system of The Hospital for Special Surgery (Table 2). If the knee score could not be obtained, the patient was contacted by telephone and answered a questionnaire that assessed the clinical success of the operation. This review process was purely clinical, and no attempt was made to incorporate radiologic appearances in the knee rating. Twenty-five patients were assessed by phone questionnaire. Failure was defined as an increment in the postoperative knee score of less than 10 points, any need for revision operations apart from removal of hardware, or a statement by the patient that the knee was worse than before the allograft procedure. An attempt was made to accurately define the time when the allograft failed.

Seven patients were excluded because they could not be contacted by telephone and had insufficient data in their files for calculation of knee scores. The demographics of the excluded patients did not significantly differ from those of the other patients. Patients who were inaccessible by telephone but whose data were complete until the time of last review were regarded as lost to follow-up, and

Table 2 The Hospital for Special Surgery modified knee rating system.

Description	Measure	Points	Comment
Subjective		(60)	
Pain	None	35	
	Mild	28	
	Moderate	21	Occasional analgesics
	Severe	14	Regular analgesics
	At rest	0	
Instability	None	10	
	Occasional	7	
	Moderate	4	Decreased activity
	Severe	0	Requires braces
Walking aids	None	5	
	Cane	3	
	Crutches	2	
	Canes	1	
	Walker	0	
Walking distance	1 mile or more	10	
	1 to 5 blocks	6	
	1 block	3	
	Inside the house	1	
	Confined to bed	0	
Objective		(40)	
Flexion contracture	None	10	
	5 degrees	7	
	5 to 10 degrees	4	
	10 to 20 degrees	2	
	> 20 degrees	0	
Flexion	> 120 degrees	20	
	90 to 120 degrees	15	
	45 to 90 degrees	8	
	<45 degrees	0	
Effusion	None	10	
	Moderate	5	
	Severe	0	
Total (subjective and objective for normal knee)		100	

their data were included in the survivorship analysis only up until the time of last review, at which time they were withdrawn from the study. There were 16 patients in the posttraumatic group who were lost to follow-up. There were five deaths resulting from causes unrelated to the surgery, and the data of these patients were treated the same as that of the patients who were lost to follow-up.

Results

Life-table analysis according to the technique of Kaplan and Meier[21] was performed on the group of patients who received fresh osteochondral allografts for posttraumatic defects in the knee joint. Ninety-two grafts were implanted in 91 patients (51 men, 40 women) with an average follow-up of 68 months (median 79 months, range 4 to 174 months) and average age of 41.9 years (median age 46 years, range 17 to 75 years). The age distribution of the posttraumatic group is shown in Figure 5. Thirteen patients are known to have

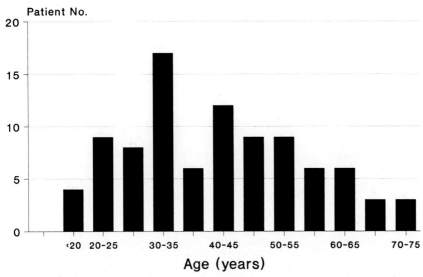

Fresh Osteochondral Allografts
Age Distribution

Fig. 5 *Age distribution of patients undergoing fresh osteochondral allografts for posttraumatic defects of the knee joint. (Reproduced with permission from Beaver RJ, Mahomed M, Backstein D, et al: Fresh osteochondral allografts for post-traumatic defects in the knee.* J Bone Joint Surg *1992;74B:105-110.)*

undergone revision surgery of the knee. Of these, four had unicompartmental bipolar grafts, eight had lateral plateau replacement, and one had a medial plateau replacement. A breakdown of the revision procedures is shown in Table 3, a list of postoperative complications is shown in Table 4, and a distribution of failed grafts is shown in Figure 6. Because continuous passive motion is now part of the postoperative regimen, stiffness is no longer perceived as a complication.

Actuarial survivorship analysis revealed that 75% of cases were still rated clinical successes five years after transplantation. The percentage of successes at 10 and 14 years was approximately 64% (Fig. 7). Log-rank analysis was used to compare the survival rates of unipolar grafts to those of bipolar grafts, and a statistically significant trend toward an improved success rate was seen in the unipolar grafts (two-tailed $p = 0.09$). The optimum success rates were found in the group who had received unipolar allografts for posttraumatic defects, with the percentage of cases rated as successful 5 years after transplantation (76%) falling to 69% at 10 years and to 67% at 14 years (Fig. 8). A comparison of male and female patients (Fig. 9) showed no statistically significant difference between the clinical success rate for each sex (two-tailed $p = 1.00$). Similarly, there was no statistically significant difference (two-tailed $p = 0.49$) between

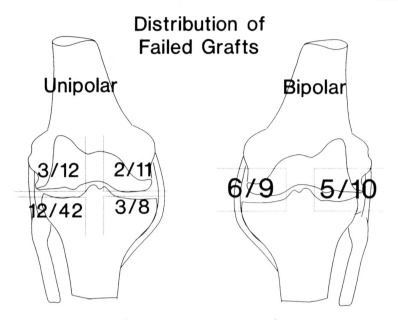

Fig. 6 *Distribution of failed unipolar and bipolar osteochondral allografts. (Reproduced with permission from Gross AE: Use of fresh allografts for traumatic joint defects, in Czitrom A, Gross AE (eds):* Allografts in Orthopaedic Practice. *Baltimore, Williams & Wilkins, 1992, p 74.)*

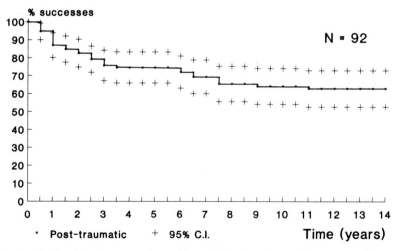

Fig. 7 *Kaplan-Meier survivorship analysis of fresh grafts in all patients with posttraumatic defects. (Reproduced with permission from Beaver RJ, Mahomed M, Backstein D, et al: Fresh osteochondral allografts for post-traumatic defects in the knee.* J Bone Joint Surg *1992;74B:105-110.)*

Table 3 Revision procedures known to have been performed on patients with fresh osteochondral allografts for posttraumatic defects in the knee.

Procedure	No.
Total knee arthroplasty	6
Arthrodesis	3
Retransplant	3
Curettage and drilling	1
Total	13

Table 4 Postoperative complications

Complication	No.
Stiffness requiring manipulation	3
Reflex sympathetic dystrophy	1
Wound hematoma	1
Rupture of the patellar tendon	1
Respiratory	2
Total	8

the clinical success rate for those grafts implanted in the tibia as compared with those implanted in the femur (Fig. 10), nor for those grafts implanted on the medial side of the joint as compared with the lateral side of the joint (Fig. 11) (two-tailed p = 1.00). The success rate of fresh grafts was compared in patients 60 years old or older and patients younger than 60. There was a statistically significant trend toward an improved success rate in the younger group of patients (two-tailed p = 0.08), but it is worth noting that the number of bipolar grafts was greater in the older group (6 of 12) than in the younger group (13 of 67), indicating more advanced degenerative changes in the older group (Fig. 12).

In a follow-up study of the fresh osteochondral allografts we implanted for posttraumatic defects of the knee, 55 grafts were examined radiographically;[8] 54 of these had sufficient radiographs for the assessment of bony collapse and cartilage space. The joint space was well preserved in 30 grafts, reduced in 10 grafts, and arthritic or ablated in 14 grafts. Most of the grafts showed a collapse of 1 to 3 mm, with 15 grafts collapsing between 4 to 5 mm; only 1 graft collapsed completely.

Alignment of the osteochondral allografts was assessed using 3-foot standing radiographs of the patients in a weightbearing position. For lateral compartment allografts, the ideal alignment is a femorotibial axis of 0 degrees. For medial compartment allografts, the ideal alignment is considered to be 10 or more degrees of valgus. Of the 55 cases studied, only 44 had films appropriate for assessment of alignment. Of these, ideal alignment was observed in 16, eight of whom had undergone earlier osteotomies, and suboptimal alignment was observed in 28, nine of whom had undergone previous osteotomies.

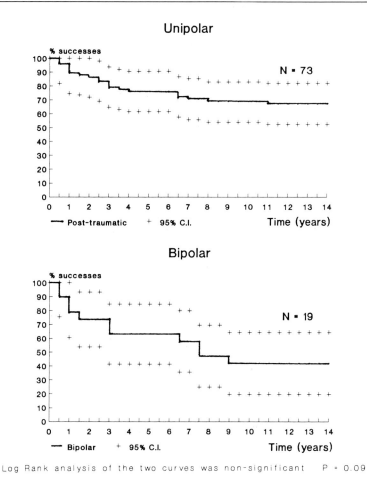

Fig. 8 *Survivorship analysis of fresh unipolar versus bipolar grafts performed for posttraumatic defects. (Reproduced with permission from Beaver RJ, Mahomed M, Backstein D, et al: Fresh osteochondral allografts for posttraumatic defects in the knee. J Bone Joint Surg 1992;74B:105-110.)*

Discussion

To ensure long-term survival of fresh osteochondral allografts, three criteria must be met: (1) The transplanted chondrocytes must remain viable. (2) These chondrocytes must continue producing sufficient proteoglycan and collagen to provide mechanical support for the chondrocytes. (3) Subchondral bone support should be maintained. In 1983, Jimenez and Brighton[22] described a biomechanical and biochemical study of fresh femoral condylar allografts in rabbits. They found 56% good to excellent histologic grades in the articular cartilage one year after transplantation. In 1988, Oakeshott and associates[11] indirectly assessed chondrocyte viability histologically and with electron microscopy in 18 failed fresh osteochondral grafts. They found that 66% of the failed grafts had viable chondrocytes.[11]

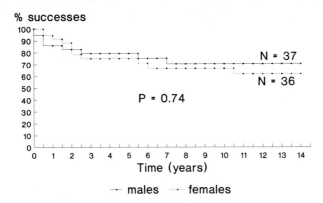

Fig. 9   *Comparison of success rate in men and women. All p values are two-tailed. (Reproduced with permission from Beaver RJ, Mahomed M, Backstein D, et al: Fresh osteochondral allografts for post-traumatic defects in the knee.* J Bone Joint Surg *1992;74B:105-110.)*

In 1989, Stevenson[23] reported a canine study comparing fresh and frozen osteochondral allografts in antigen matched and antigen mismatched groups. According to the study, even when using advanced cryopreservative techniques, chondrocyte survival was only 40% to 50% in the frozen allografts, and the cartilage markedly degenerated. In contrast, the chondrocytes in the antigenically mismatched, fresh allografts retained viability and cartilage thickness. Although freezing the allograft somewhat lessened the immune response to the allograft, the severe damage to the cartilage rendered this advantage ineffective.

In 1990, Czitrom and associates[24] reported chondrocyte viability in biopsies of fresh osteochondral allografts obtained from patients between 1 and 6 years after transplantation. They found that, when assessed by $^{35}SO_4$ and ^3H-cytidine autoradiography, the percentage of viable chondrocytes ranged from 69% to 99% in three osteochondral allografts that were studied at 12, 24, and 41 months after transplantation, and that the chondrocytes were producing proteoglycan.[24,25] In a graft that had been implanted 6 years previously, 37% of chondrocytes were viable and actively producing proteoglycan. This was the first direct observation of the viability of articular cartilage in humans after allotransplantation.

The present survivorship study demonstrates that fresh osteochondral allograft procedures, when performed for posttraumatic unipolar defects of the knee joint, produce clinically successful results in 76% of cases at five years after transplantation and in 67% of cases at 14 years. Calculation of 95% confidence intervals about the survivorship curves supports the success of these results. Compared with unipolar grafts, bipolar grafts have a lower success rate at all time periods. Although this difference is not statistically signif-

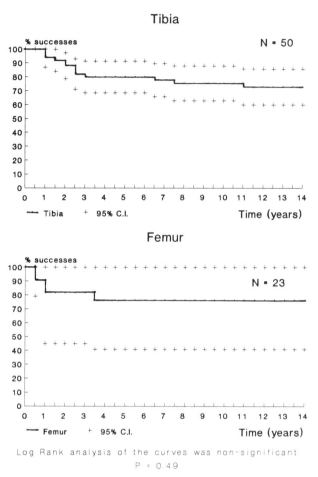

Fig. 10 *Comparison of fresh grafts performed in the tibia with those performed in the femur. (Reproduced with permission from Beaver RJ, Mahomed M, Backstein D, et al: Fresh osteochondral allografts for post-traumatic defects in the knee.* J Bone Joint Surg *1992;74B:105-110.)*

icant, our present approach is to perform these operations before secondary changes on the opposing pole necessitate a bipolar graft.

In 1989, Zukor and associates[6,7] reported on a radiographic analysis of this same group of patients. They found that the radiographic joint space was preserved or slightly reduced in the majority of the cases of fresh osteochondral allografts for several years following transplantation.

It is apparent, therefore, that human chondrocytes, when implanted as a fresh composite osteochondral allograft, can survive for prolonged periods, but these cells seem to deteriorate slowly over time. The reason for this is unclear, but it may be related to adequacy of graft fixation and stability,[21] mechanical overloading of the graft,[11] immunologic assault on link-protein and proteoglycan

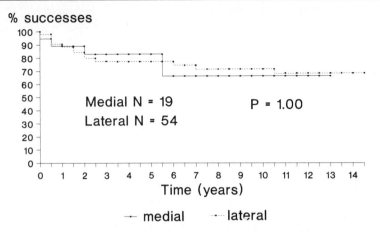

Fig. 11 *Comparison of fresh grafts performed on the medial side of the knee joint with those on the lateral side. (Reproduced with permission from Beaver RJ, Mahomed M, Backstein D, et al: Fresh osteochondral allografts for post-traumatic defects in the knee.* J Bone Joint Surg *1992;74B:105-110.)*

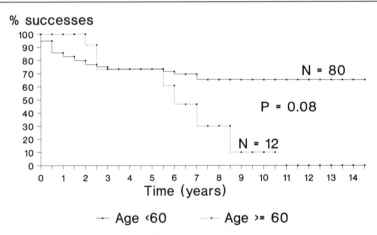

Fig. 12 *Comparison of grafts performed in patients younger than 60 years of age with those in patients aged 60 years or older. (Reproduced with permission from Beaver RJ, Mahomed M, Backstein D, et al: Fresh osteochondral allografts for post-traumatic defects in the knee.* J Bone Joint Surg *1992;74B:105-110.)*

monomer by host synovium,[26] or poor fit between the graft and the host, producing incongruence.[27]

The role of the immune response in the incorporation and survival of fresh osteochondral allografts is important. The fact that bone provokes an immune response is undisputed. In 1975, Langer and associates[28] demonstrated a positive lymphocyte migration assay following transplantation of fresh osteochondral allografts, indicating a cell-mediated immune response to allogenic bone; this response may be stimulated by specific antigen-presenting cells derived from the graft bone marrow.[29] Less important sources of bone antigen may be osteoclasts, osteoblasts, and their precursors, but the main source is the bone marrow. The cell-mediated immune response is the main cause of experimental bone graft rejection.[29] However, there was no case in our series where complete rejection of the allograft could be implicated in graft failure.

In 1988, Oakeshott and associates[11] studied 18 cases of failed fresh osteochondral allografts and found that the graft bone was not viable; the necrotic bone was eventually replaced by creeping substitution. Every graft that had been in place for more than 44 months underwent complete bony substitution. It is likely that the slight but nonprogressive subsidence that had been seen in these grafts is caused by loading of the relatively softened allograft bone during the revascularization phase of creeping substitution. It is between 2 and 3 years after the transplant that the graft appears to become most prone to subsidence.[11] The reason for the delay in revascularization may be that the immune response significantly delays the incorporation of the bone graft and its subsequent replacement by host bone. This would also explain the poor clinical and radiologic results found in those cases where joint malalignment had not been corrected, thereby leading to overloading of the grafted compartment.[6,7,11]

Although isolated chondrocytes in tissue culture are subject to immune assault as are other cells, it appears that their surrounding matrix protects them from the ingress of immunocompetent cells, thereby making them immunoprivileged.[30] This is in agreement with the previously mentioned studies on retrieved fresh osteochondral allografts[11,23] and explains the retention of the radiographic joint space for many years in the successful cases.

The long-term survival and function of meniscal allografts has not yet been convincingly demonstrated in humans; however, very promising arthroscopic appearances have been seen in the menisci transplanted in association with fresh osteochondral allografts at Mount Sinai Hospital. Successful survival and apparent function have been observed up to 8.5 years after transplantation.[31] Long-term analysis of retrieved menisci will be invaluable in determining their role in this type of surgery; their role in cartilage nutrition and redistribution of joint contact forces is well accepted and it would seem prudent to preserve or replace them as required.[31]

We strongly believe that, on the basis of this unrivaled experience with fresh osteochondral allografts, biomechanical factors are much more important in the long-term success of these grafts than are the theoretical risks of graft rejection. Close attention must be paid to the selection of the patient, the correction of coexisting joint malalignment, and the rigid internal fixation of the allograft to the host. Under no circumstances should the height of the graft be used to correct malalignment; a minimum graft thickness of 1 cm is recommended.

Although there is a learning curve with these procedures, we believe that these techniques are well within the capabilities of most orthopaedic surgeons experienced in knee joint arthroplasty, providing they have access to a modern tissue retrieval service. These procedures are truly conservative because bone stock and cartilage are restored and minimal host tissue is removed. Should the cartilage fail, future revision surgery is facilitated by the improvement in bone stock. The potential benefits to active and productive patients who would probably otherwise choose prosthetic arthroplasty or arthrodesis are evident. We believe that these benefits greatly outweigh the logistic difficulties involved in implantation of fresh osteochondral allografts.

In the future, progress in the field of cryopreservation may make it possible to store bone and cartilage for prolonged periods and still maintain chondrocyte viability and function. Until this occurs, it is our opinion that implantation of fresh osteochondral allografts to correct major defects in weightbearing joints will continue to be the best solution to these difficult problems.

Summary

Ninety-two fresh osteochondral allografts were implanted in 91 patients with posttraumatic osteoarticular defects of the knee joint. These patients have been prospectively followed since 1972, and long-term survival was analyzed. The overall success rate was 75% at 5 years, 64% at 10 years, and 63% at 14 years. Unipolar grafts, which involve only one surface of the compartment, were compared with bipolar grafts, which involve both surfaces. The unipolar grafts had a lower rate of failure, with 76% survival at 5 years, 69% at 10 years, and 67% at 14 years. When considering other factors that might affect the survival of the fresh osteochondral allografts, the influence of the anatomic location of the graft, patient sex, and patient age was calculated. Neither the location of the allograft nor the sex of the patient had any meaningful impact on allograft survival. However, allograft longevity increased in patients younger than 60 years of age. The best indication for the use of unipolar fresh osteochondral allografts is for posttraumatic defects in relatively young, active patients. Joint malalignment should be corrected to achieve best results.

The following points can be concluded from the studies presented in this chapter: (1) Fresh osteochondral allografts are preferable to stored allografts in the replacement of large, posttraumatic articular defects in the knee. (2) The best results for these grafts occur in relatively young patients with traumatically induced defects of the articular surface of the knee joint. (3) Immunologic rejection of the allograft does not appear to occur. (4) It is essential to correct alignment of the limb prior to or simultaneous with implantation of the allograft. (5) Rigid internal fixation of the allograft is vital. (6) Bipolar and bicompartmental allografts perform poorly. (7) Continuous passive motion immediately after surgery, while not essential to the success of the procedure, appears to diminish the incidence and severity of knee stiffness after surgery. It is not clear, however, whether it improves short-term or long-term chondrocyte survival. (8) Implantation of meniscal allografts appears to be associated with excellent functional results and biomechanically is to be recommended when the host meniscus is unsalvageable. (9) Chondrocyte survival and continued function has been directly observed after fresh osteochondral transplantation.

References

1. Lexer E: Substitution of whole or half joints from freshly amputated extremities by free plastic operation. *Surg Gynecol Obstet* 1908; 6:601-607.

2. Lexer E: Joint transplantations and arthroplasty. *Surg Gynecol Obstet* 1925;40:782-809.

3. Volkov M: Allotransplantation of joints. *J Bone Joint Surg* 1970;52B: 49-53.

4. Ottolenghi CE: Massive osteo and osteo-articular bone grafts: Technic and results of 62 cases. *Clin Orthop* 1972;87:156-164.

5. Parrish FF: Allograft replacement of all or part of the end of a long bone following excision of a tumor: Report of twenty-one cases. *J Bone Joint Surg* 1973;55A:1-22.

6. Zukor DJ, Gross AE: Osteochondral allograft reconstruction of the knee, part 1: A review. *Am J Knee Surg* 1989;2:139-149.

7. Zukor DJ, Oakeshott RD, Gross AE: Osteochondral allograft reconstruction of the knee, part 2: Experience with successful and failed fresh osteochondral allograft. *Am J Knee Surg* 1989;2:182-191.

8. McDermott AGP, Langer F, Pritzker KPH, et al: Fresh small-fragment osteochondral allografts: Long-term follow-up study on first 100 cases. *Clin Orthop* 1985;197:96-102.

9. Locht RC, Gross AE, Langer F: Late osteochondral allograft resurfacing for tibial plateau fractures. *J Bone Joint Surg* 1984;66A: 328-335.

10. Zukor DJ, Paitich B, Oakeshott RD, et al: Reconstruction of post-traumatic articular surface defects using fresh small-fragment osteochondral allografts, in Aebi M, Regazzoni P (eds): *Bone Transplantation*. Berlin, Springer-Verlag, 1989, pp 293-305.

11. Oakeshott RD, Farine I, Pritzker KPH, et al: A clinical and histologic analysis of failed fresh osteochondral allografts. *Clin Orthop* 1988;233:283-294.

12. McDermott AGP, Finklestein JA, Farine I, et al: Distal femoral varus osteotomy for valgus deformity of the knee. *J Bone Joint Surg* 1988;70A:110-116.

13. Friedlaender GE, Mankin HJ: Guidelines for the banking of musculoskeletal tissues. *Am Assoc Tissue Banks Newsletter* 1979;3:21.

14. Tomford WW, Mankin HJ: Cadaver bone procurement, in Fawcett KJ, Barr AR (eds): *Tissue Banking*. Arlington, VA, American Association of Tissue Banks, 1987, pp 97-107.

15. Tomford WW, Mankin HJ, Friedlaender GE, et al: Methods of banking bone and cartilage for allograft transplantation, in Fawcett KJ, Barr AR (eds): *Tissue Banking*. Arlington, VA, American Association of Tissue Banks, 1987, pp 241-247.

16. Jackson JP, Waugh W, Green JP: High tibial osteotomy for osteoarthritis of the knee. *J Bone Joint Surg* 1969;51B:88-94.

17. Coventry MB: Osteotomy about the knee for degenerative and rheumatoid arthritis. Indications, operative technique and results. *J Bone Joint Surg* 1973;55A:23-48.

18. Maquet PJ: *Biomechanics of the Knee*. Berlin, Springer-Verlag, 1976.

19. Maquet PGJ: The treatment of choice in osteoarthritis of the knee. *Clin Orthop* 1985;192:108-112.

20. Putnam MD, Mears DC, Fu FH: Combined Maquet and proximal tibial valgus osteotomy. *Clin Orthop* 1985;197:217-223.

21. Kaplan EL, Meier P: Nonparametric estimation from incomplete observations. *J Am Stat Assoc* 1958;53:457-481.

22. Jimenez SA, Brighton CT: Experimental studies on the fate of transplanted articular cartilage, in Friedlaender GE, Mankin HJ, Sell KW (eds): *Osteochondral allografts: Biology, Banking, and Clinical Applications*. Boston, Little Brown, 1983, pp 73-79.

23. Stevenson S, Dannucci GA, Sharkey NA, et al: The fate of articular cartilage after transplantation of fresh and cryopreserved tissue-antigen-matched and mismatched osteochondral allografts in dogs. *J Bone Joint Surg* 1989;71A:1297-1307.

24. Czitrom AA, Keating S, Gross AE: The viability of articular cartilage in fresh osteochondral allografts after clinical transplantation. *J Bone Joint Surg* 1990;72A:574-581.

25. Czitrom AA, Langer F, McKee N, et al: Bone and cartilage allotransplantation: A review of 14 years of research and clinical studies. *Clin Orthop* 1986;208:141-145.

26. Yablon IG: Immune responses to matrix components, in Friedlaender GE, Mankin HJ, Sell KW (eds): *Osteochondral Allografts: Biology, Banking, and Clinical Applications*. Boston, Little Brown, 1983, pp 165-174.

27. Rodrigo JJ: The problem of fit in osteocartilaginous allografts, in Friedlaender GE, Mankin HJ, Sell KW (eds): *Osteochondral Allografts: Biology, Banking, and Clinical Applications*. Boston, Little Brown, 1983, pp 249-255.

28. Langer F, Czitrom A, Pritzker KPH, et al: The immunogenicity of fresh and frozen allogeneic bone. *J Bone Joint Surg* 1975;57A:216-220.

29. Czitrom AA, Axelrod T, Fernandes B: Antigen presenting cells and bone allotransplantation. *Clin Orthop* 1985;197:27-31.

30. Langer F, Gross AE: Immunogenicity of allograft articular cartilage. *J Bone Joint Surg* 1974:56A:297-304.

31. Zukor DJ, Cameron JC, Brooks PJ, et al: The fate of human meniscal allografts, in Ewing JW (ed): *Articular Cartilage and Knee Joint Function: Basic Science and Arthroscopy*. New York, Raven Press, 1990, pp 147-152.

Future Directions

There is a clear need for new investigations of the structure, composition, function, and biomechanical properties of articular cartilage, the response of articular cartilage to mechanical injuries, and the methods of treating cartilage injuries. Clinical and experimental studies show that closed mechanical injuries to articular cartilage and the resulting joint instability alter the composition and structure of the articular cartilage. This alteration causes loss of essential mechanical properties, pain, and loss of motion. In some instances, progressive deformity and instability ensue; many patients with these problems develop disabling osteoarthritis.

During the past decade, substantial progress has been made in a variety of focused areas of cartilage mechanics and biology. Based on these basic scientific advances, clear opportunities exist to apply basic scientific knowledge to clinical problems. To do so, scientists from different disciplines in biology and biomechanics must work with clinicians to develop strategies that will translate new scientific information into clinical practice.

Specific investigations should be carried out in articular cartilage biomechanics, closed mechanical injuries of articular cartilage, joint instability, and methods of repairing or replacing articular cartilage surfaces.

Articular Cartilage Biomechanics

Currently, we have limited understanding of the interactions of cartilage macromolecules and the contributions of these macromolecules to the mechanical properties of cartilage. We need better high-resolution, three-dimensional models of the molecular structure of the cartilage matrix and better understanding of the homeostatic mechanisms and changes associated with aging in normal articular cartilage.

Develop methods of creating three-dimensional models of synovial joint articular surfaces in vivo.

The shapes or contours of joint surfaces and the congruency of opposing joint surfaces make a critical contribution to normal joint function, including joint stability. Three-dimensional models of joint surfaces created from in vitro stereophotogrammetry have helped explain how loads are distributed in diarthrodial joints, but in vivo models would have greater value. Three-dimensional (3-D) in vivo anatomic models of diarthrodial joints could be developed using magnetic resonance imaging (MRI) and compared with models developed using precise in vitro techniques such as stereophotogrammetry. This approach would make it possible to determine in vivo contact areas from MRI and to understand the pathomechanics of diarthrodial joints in general, and the patellofemoral, glenohumeral, and tibiofemoral joints in particular. It would also make it possible to determine the evolution or changes in joint shape as a result of aging or disease, using precise curvature mapping techniques.

Determine the compositional, ultrastructural, and structural parameters that play important roles in providing articular cartilage mechanical properties.

Correlations between material properties of articular cartilage and its biochemical composition usually fall short of explaining the relationships between the composition and mechanical properties of cartilage. Collagen cross-linking, type IX collagen, quantitatively minor proteoglycans, and the ultrastructural and structural organization of the cartilage matrix may all contribute to the mechanical properties of articular cartilage. One common characteristic of osteoarthritic and disuse changes in cartilage is the change in water content. Because the aggregate modulus of cartilage often correlates with water content, this and other, as yet to be determined, compositional parameters may be used to study the onset of osteoarthritic or disuse changes, and their effect on the mechanics of the joint.

Determine biaxial mechanical properties of articular cartilage.

The variation in articular cartilage tensile and compressive material properties as a function of depth from the articular surface show that articular cartilage is inhomogeneous and anisotropic, but no studies have examined the biaxial mechanical properties of articular cartilage through direct experimentation. Such studies would shed additional light on the functional role of the articular surface and the effect of collagen fiber orientation or cartilage split lines on the tissue's mechanical behavior.

Determine the structural and mechanoelectrochemical forces that control articular cartilage hydration.

The tissue fluid makes an essential contribution to the mechanical properties of articular cartilage, and an alteration in cartilage hydration is among the first changes associated with degeneration of the tissue. Donnan osmotic pressure and chemical expansion stress contribute to the normal swelling properties of cartilage. Removal of the surface zone of articular cartilage alters the swelling and mechanical responses of the tissue. Early degenerative lesions in cartilage are characterized by an increased tissue hydration and surface fibrillation. Thus, the stiffness and strength of the collagen-rich surface zone may play a role in controlling the degree of cartilage hydration. To understand how articular cartilage degenerates, it is important to learn how this surface zone functions as a barrier or membrane against this swelling effect and to explore the fundamental mechanoelectrochemical forces that control tissue hydration.

Develop better 3-D, finite-element models of articular cartilage and diarthrodial joints.

Recent studies indicate that the two articulating surfaces of a joint often have very different intrinsic material properties. This is clearly documented for the human patellofemoral joint; the patellar properties appear to be inferior to those of the trochlea from the standpoint of load carriage within the tissue. The discovery of this mismatch or asymmetry of tissue properties of mating surfaces of a joint has profoundly altered our perception of joint contact mechanics and of stresses and strains existing within the tissue during articulation. This situation must be analyzed further in order to understand joint pathophysiology. For example, complete characterization of the material properties of femoral and tibial cartilage as well as meniscus would make it possible to develop 3-D analytical and finite element models of three-body soft, hydrated tissue contact, including the effects of synovial fluid lubrication on the tibiofemoral joint.

Joint Instability and Closed Mechanical Injuries of Articular Cartilage

We have limited understanding of how mechanical forces damage articular cartilage, the functional consequences of this damage, the ability of injured cartilage to heal, and the effects of treatments. Gaining this understanding will depend on development of better methods of evaluating cartilage function and cartilage injuries in vivo.

Develop methods of measuring in vivo cartilage loads in stable and unstable joints.

Acute and repetitive impact loads and chronic alterations in loads on articular cartilage resulting from joint instability presumably cause cartilage degeneration. A method of measuring cartilage loads in vivo could help define the mechanisms of closed injuries to articular cartilage and clarify the relationship between knee instability and cartilage degeneration.

Develop methods of measuring in vivo cartilage mechanical properties.

Experimental studies show that loss or alteration of cartilage matrix macromolecules, especially proteoglycans, changes cartilage mechanical properties. These changes may make the tissue more vulnerable to injury, initiate progressive deterioration of the tissue, or be corrected spontaneously. A reliable method of measuring cartilage mechanical properties in vivo would make it possible to identify this type of cartilage injury and determine its natural history as well as to investigate methods of treatment. Correlation of in vivo mechanical properties of articular cartilage with imaging studies like MRI might make it possible to conduct systematic clinical studies of alterations in articular cartilage caused by impact loading and joint instability without directly testing the cartilage properties.

Investigate the healing and remodeling of articular cartilage following impact loading.

Experimental work shows that acute and repetitive impact loading of articular cartilage causes cartilage injury that varies from loss of matrix proteoglycans to disruption of the matrix. The natural history and potential for repair of these injuries remain poorly understood. Models of acute and chronic chondral and osteochondral injuries would help define the mechanisms of articular surface injuries and the intrinsic mechanics of healing, thereby making it possible to test methods of treating cartilage injury or preventing cartilage degeneration. Development of the methods of measuring in vivo cartilage mechanical properties discussed above would make it possible to conduct long-term studies of cartilage healing and remodeling following impact loading.

Define the relationship between joint instability and articular cartilage degeneration.

Clinical studies and experimental models of cartilage degeneration show that ligamentous instability of the knee often precedes the development of degenerative joint disease, but the relationship between them has not been well defined. For example, the mechanisms of cartilage degeneration in unstable joints remain poorly understood, the effect of instability varies among individuals (for example, degeneration of the articular cartilage rapidly develops among some individuals with unstable joints and may not develop in others), and the degree and/or duration of instability that can be expected to cause joint degeneration have not been defined. Investigation of the relationship between joint instability and cartilage degeneration will require methods of measuring static and kinetic joint instability and methods of detecting the response of articular cartilage to changes in joint stability in addition to the methods discussed above. It will also be important to define the degree or threshold of joint instability and the duration of instability that cause irreversible cartilage degeneration.

Investigate the cartilage repair response in unstable joints.

Experimental evidence shows that joint instability can stimulate a repair response within the articular cartilage and may stimulate remodeling of the joint surface. Other work suggests that restoring joint stability may slow or prevent progression of cartilage degeneration or possibly even allow repair of some types of cartilage damage. These capacities for repair of articular cartilage in unstable joints need to be investigated.

Methods of Repairing or Replacing Articular Cartilage

We need to develop and assess new methods of facilitating cartilage healing. In particular, we need to devise more objective assessments of the success of currently used surgical procedures and to develop new clinical therapies. Progress needs to be made in understanding the underlying mechanisms of healing after mechanical injury and in defining conditions associated with nonhealing of articular cartilage. Major emphasis should be given to surgical and nonsurgical manipulations that will promote healing and to systematic clinical follow-up studies.

Investigate methods of stimulating healing of articular surface damage including chondral defects and osteochondral fractures.

Arthroscopic examinations show that chondral injuries and osteochondral fractures frequently occur in normal joints. If a significant portion of the articular surface is lost, these injuries can lead to pain and loss of joint function. The natural history of many of these lesions is not clear, but clinical experience indicates that large, deep cartilage defects in load-bearing areas cause symptoms and may progress. Methods of regenerating or replacing the articular surface could restore joint function. The value of current treatments of these injuries is uncertain, but none of them stimulates formation of a new articular surface. New methods that may improve healing of these lesions include use of growth factors and cell transplants.

Define the mechanoelectrochemical factors that control the transformation of chondroprogenitor cells into chondrocytes.

One requirement for healing of chondral and osteochondral injuries is a population of cells that can function as chondrocytes. Experimental work shows that some mesenchymal cells have the potential to develop into chondrocytes that can synthesize a cartilaginous matrix. Although the steps in the differentiation of mesenchymal cells into chondrocytes have been defined, the factors that control differentiation have not. Defining these factors would include (1) identification of chondroprogenitors, (2) characterization of their stages of differentiation by protein and proteoglycan synthesis or synovial receptors, and (3) identification of differentiation factors that act on the cells to stimulate progression from one

stage to the next. For example, we need to know what factors trigger the expression of hypertrophic chondrocyte-specific molecules on exposure to mature chondrocytes and what biologic and mechanical factors stimulate chondrogenes that would facilitate healing of cartilage defects by implanting cells.

Identify sources for chondroprogenitor cells that can be used for cartilage healing.

Previous work shows that mesenchymal stem cells capable of forming cartilage can be isolated from bone marrow and periosteum. Are there other sources for these pluripotential cells? For example, could stem cells be harvested from peripheral blood or skin?

Develop optimal delivery vehicles for chondroprogenitor cells or chondrocytes for implantation into cartilage defects.

Mesenchymal cells and chondrocytes can be implanted into cartilage and osteochondral defects and will form cartilage. The optimal methods of implanting and maintaining the cells in the defects need to be defined.

Develop models in vivo and in vitro to investigate the intrinsic ability of articular cartilage chondrocytes to proliferate, migrate into areas of injury, and synthesize extracellular matrix.

Experimental work suggests that under carefully controlled conditions articular cartilage chondrocytes can proliferate, migrate into cartilage defects, and synthesize a new matrix. Methods of stimulating repair of chondral defects by chondrocytes could have considerable value in the treatment of articular surface damage.

Determine the effect of growth factors and cytokines on the response of articular cartilage to injury.

Chondrocytes and other mesenchymal cells can respond to growth factors and cytokines by proliferating, migrating, and synthesizing new matrix. The potential of using these factors to stimulate cartilage repair needs to be investigated further in both in vitro and in vivo models of cartilage injury.

Investigate the effects of extrinsic factors, including subchondral bone injury, synovial fluid, intra-articular hemorrhage, and synovial inflammation, on the response of articular cartilage to injury.

Cartilage injuries rarely, if ever, occur in isolation. It will be important to determine the effect on cartilage healing of associated injuries and the environment of the synovial joint.

Investigate the effects of systemic and metabolic influences, sex, and ethnic differences on chondrocyte proliferation, migration, and matrix synthesis and on the proliferation, migration, and differentiation of chondroprogenitor cells.

It is not clear how systemic and metabolic factors including age-related changes, osteoporosis, diabetes, and other endocrine abnormalities influence the potential for healing of articular surfaces by chondrocytes or chondroprogenitor cells. It also is not clear if articular cartilage healing differs between men and women and among different ethnic groups.

Investigate methods of using cartilage and osteochondral grafts to replace damaged articular surfaces.

Clinical experience shows that fresh and preserved cartilage allografts can replace limited areas of damaged articular cartilage. It is not clear what types of grafts produce the best results. For example, it is not clear whether vascularized grafts or nonviable grafts that retain their mechanical properties offer the greater potential for successfully replacing damaged articular surfaces.

Develop methods to ensure that repair cartilage or transplanted cartilage integrates molecularly, ultrastructurally, and mechanically with host cartilage.

Several studies of osteochondral repair tissue and osteochondral grafts show that repair tissue or grafts may fail to heal along with the surrounding tissue. Repair or graft tissue that fills a chondral or osteochondral defect may fail to restore a functional articular surface if it fails to become integrated with the surrounding tissue. Therefore, identifying mechanical and biologic factors that stimulate integration of repair tissue or grafts with surrounding tissues will be an important part of successful healing of articular cartilage damage.

147

Section Three
Meniscus

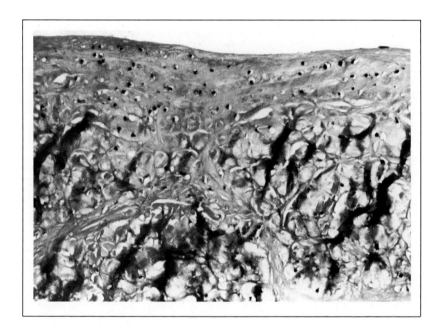

Overview

The menisci, once thought to be the functionless vestiges of intra-articular muscle attachments, are now known to serve a crucial role in the complex biomechanics of knee joint function. The fact that meniscal injury and meniscectomy may result in early osteoarthrosis of the knee serves as the impetus to advance our knowledge of this structure with regard to its basic biomechanics, kinematics, and reparative qualities. Also, efforts are being made to substitute the meniscus with allograft and prosthetic replacements.

Each meniscus is composed of fibrocartilaginous lamellae interposed between the tibia and femur. It is firmly attached along the tibial spine and has variable peripheral attachments. The amplitude and direction of meniscal translation during knee joint motion are directed by a host of factors including femorotibial bony geometry, meniscal capsular and ligamentous attachments, and collateral and cruciate ligament kinematics.

The ultrastructure of the meniscus is biphasic. The solid phase includes an extracellular matrix with a sparse population of cells, which is made up primarily of circumferentially oriented type I collagen fibers. Fibrochondrocytes, elastins, proteoglycans, and other collagenous and noncollagenous proteins complete the solid phase of the matrix. The fluid phase consists of water electrolytes. The biphasic model of the meniscus describes its viscoelastic nature and its ability to respond to compression, tension, and shear. The circumferential collagen fibers, as well as radial tie fibers, dictate the loadbearing function of the meniscus.

To understand the kinematics of the menisci, it is important to explore basic knee joint motion. The crossed, four-bar linkage of the cruciate ligaments and the collateral ligaments provides restraints to joint motions in all six degrees of freedom. The medial meniscus is constrained in the posterior corner by the posterior oblique ligament and demonstrates a 2.3-fold smaller posterior translation than the lateral meniscus during flexion of the knee. In addition, the menisci deform and maintain congruity with the articulating surfaces of the femur and tibia during flexion.

Injury of the meniscus can occur in isolation or in association with other joint injuries. While repair of the meniscus dates back over 100 years, the advent of the arthroscope and a thorough understanding of the meniscal vascular supply have allowed successful repair to occur. The vascular supply of the meniscus, derived from the perimeniscal capillary plexus of the genicular arteries, penetrates 30% of the peripheral medial meniscus and 25% of the lateral. While repair is often limited to the peripheral region, a variety of techniques including vascular access channels, synovial abrasion, and exogenous fibrin clot incorporation are used for avascular meniscal repair. In general, peripheral longitudinal tears not involving disruption of the body of the meniscus are amenable to repair. Other tear patterns require careful consideration before repair is attempted. While surgical technique for repairing a meniscal tear varies, common elements include a careful arthroscopic examination, protection of the posterior neurovascular structures, and debridement of the meniscal rim and capsular bed. Current techniques include inside-out and outside-in arthroscopic repair. Results are promising for repair of meniscus tears in both the vascularized and central avascular portions of the meniscus.

When the native meniscal tissue is not fit for repair, an alternative to total excision is meniscal replacement. Previously, attempts were made to replace menisci with autografts composed of fascia lata, fat pad, and various ligaments. Although they supported the ingrowth of fibrochondrocytes, the grafts became fibrotic and were biomechanically unable to provide sufficient joint stability, shock absorption, and load transmission to prevent arthritic degeneration of the joint.

The most common method of meniscal replacement is allograft transplantation. Factors that must be considered for allograft transplantation include potential antigenicity of the graft, preservation and/or secondary sterilization, and the ability of the graft to maintain, or reestablish, its viability, structure, composition, and function. Allografts are currently preserved by cryopreservation, deep freezing, or lyophilization. Deep freezing and lyophilization provide secondary sterilization of the graft and a longer shelf life, but graft cells do not survive. Menisci that have a viable cell population when transplanted do not appear to elicit a significant immunologic response within the joint, and low level gamma irradiation has not been shown to adversely affect biomaterial properties of the allograft. Lyophilized menisci demonstrate altered remodeling. Clinically, meniscal transplantation is still in its infancy and results are variable.

Prosthetic replacements have produced less than optimal results because of difficulties in duplicating the size, shape, and physical and biomechanical properties of the normal meniscus. The complex structure, composition, and function of the meniscus make it virtually impossible to replicate. Synthetic meniscal replacements have been composed primarily of Teflon, polyester, and carbon fibers. Several problems associated with these composites include adhesions, inflammatory reaction, synovitis, and articular cartilage degeneration. Xenograft meniscal replacements have not been studied because not enough is known about size, immunologic, biochemical, and biomechanical compatibility with human menisci. Reconstituted bioresorbable collagen meniscal scaffolds have been examined recently. Positive attributes of this technique include the ability to influence the rate of resorption, the immunogenicity of the scaffold, and the shape/size configuration of the scaffold. Subtotal meniscectomy with replacement with bioresorbable scaffold allows significant meniscal regeneration while providing stability in the interim period. Early results in animals are encouraging; however, extensive study is required before clinical investigation.

Chapter 9

Biomechanics and Kinematics of Meniscus

Freddie H. Fu, MD
William O. Thompson, MD

Introduction

The menisci, once thought to be the functionless vestiges of intra-articular muscle attachments, are now known to serve a crucial role in the complex biomechanics of normal knee joint function.[1]

Recent advances in microscopy, biochemistry, bioengineering, and image processing have significantly expanded our knowledge of the form and function of these vital structures within the knee. This chapter provides a thorough review of the functional anatomy, composition, material properties, biomechanics, and kinematics of the meniscus.

Functional Anatomy

The menisci are two crescent-shaped fibrocartilaginous lamellae that have been regarded functionally as extensions of the tibia.[2-4] Anatomically, the menisci act to deepen the articular fossae of the tibia for the reception of the femoral condyles.[5-8] Each meniscus covers roughly the peripheral two thirds of its corresponding tibial plateau. At the periphery, the meniscus is thick, convex, and attached to the internal joint capsule. Triangular in cross section, it tapers to a thin, freely mobile edge centrally. The proximal surface of the meniscus is concave and in intimate contact with each femoral condyle, while the distal surface is relatively flat and rests on the head of the tibia (Fig. 1).[4] A recently developed finite-element model has shown that the triangular cross section of the meniscus is important to determination of the stresses and strains developed within the meniscus during function.[9,10]

Medial Meniscus

The medial meniscus has a semilunar shape, is approximately 3.5 cm long, is narrow anteriorly, and broadens posteriorly. The width

153

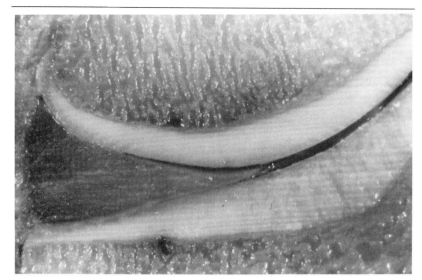

Fig. 1   *Frontal section of the medial compartment of a human knee illustrating the articulation of the meniscus with the femoral condyles and tibia. (Reproduced with permission from Warren R, Arnoczky SP, Wickiewicz TL: Anatomy of the knee, in Nicholas JA, Hershman EB (eds):* The Lower Extremity and Spine in Sports Medicine. *St. Louis, CV Mosby, 1986, vol 1, pp 657-694.)*

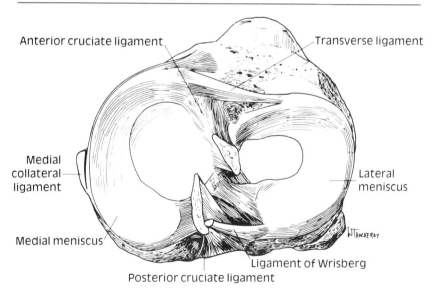

Fig. 2   *Drawing of a human tibial plateau demonstrates the position and attachments of the medial meniscus (MM) and the lateral meniscus (LM). ACL, anterior cruciate ligament; PCL, posterior cruciate ligament. (Reproduced with permission from Warren R, Arnoczky SP, Wickiewicz TL: Anatomy of the knee, in Nicholas JA, Hershman EB (eds):* The Lower Extremity and Spine in Sports Medicine. *St. Louis, CV Mosby, 1986, vol 1, pp 657-694.)*

of the medial meniscus, when measured radially along the tibia, is 7.7 mm at the anterior horn, 9.6 mm at its midpoint, and 10.6 mm at

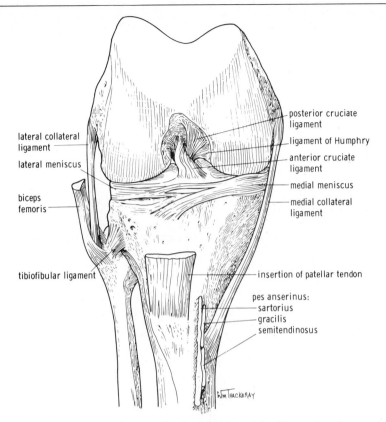

Fig. 3 *Frontal drawing of a partially dissected knee joint illustrating the anterior horn attachment of the medial meniscus. (Reproduced with permission from Insall JN: Anatomy of the knee, in Insall JN (ed):* Surgery of the Knee. *New York, Churchill Livingstone, 1984, pp 1-20.)*

the posterior horn (Fig. 2).[11] The anterior horn is attached to the intercondylar fossa of the tibia in front of the origin of the anterior cruciate ligament (Fig. 3); this attachment can be rather modest, within the realm of normal variation.[12] In addition, the transverse ligament of the knee connects the anterior horn of the medial meniscus with the lateral meniscus. The posterior horn is attached firmly to the posterior intercondylar fossa in front of the base of the posterior cruciate ligament.

Capsular Attachments

The peripheral attachment of the medial meniscus is quite complex (Fig. 4).[13] Posterior to the deep medial collateral ligament, the posterior oblique fibers of the superficial medial collateral ligament combine with the joint capsule and with the tendon sheath of the semimembranosus to form the posteromedial capsule. According to Kaplan,[14] the meniscus receives a portion of the semimembranosus through the capsular attachments; this observation has been dis-

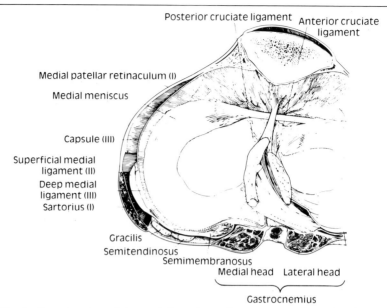

Posterior cruciate ligament   Anterior cruciate ligament

Medial patellar retinaculum (I)

Medial meniscus

Capsule (III)

Superficial medial ligament (II)

Deep medial ligament (III)

Sartorius (I)

Gracilis

Semitendinosus

Semimembranosus

Medial head   Lateral head

Gastrocnemius

Fig. 4   *Superior view of the medial meniscus demonstrating the order of attachments in the intercondylar notch. Also shown is the attachment of the medial meniscus to the medial collateral ligament and the arrangement of the three fascial layers on the medial aspect of the knee. (Reproduced with permission from Warren R, Arnoczky SP, Wickiewicz TL: Anatomy of the knee, in Nicholas JA, Hershman EB (eds):* The Lower Extremity and Spine in Sports Medicine. *St. Louis, CV Mosby, 1986, vol 1, pp 657-694.)*

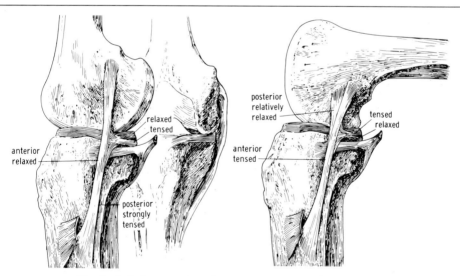

relaxed

tensed

anterior relaxed

posterior strongly tensed

posterior relatively relaxed

tensed relaxed

anterior tensed

Fig. 5   *Left, In extension, the posterior margin of the medial collateral ligament is tense and the anterior border relatively relaxed. Proximal anterior fibers are drawn underneath the posterior fibers. (Reproduced with permission from Insall JN: Anatomy of the knee, in Insall JN (ed):* Surgery of the Knee. *New York, Churchill Livingstone, 1984, pp 1-20.) Right, With flexion, the posterior oblique fibers of the superficial medial collateral ligament become more tense.*

puted by others.[15] Elsewhere around the periphery, the thin, lax capsule attaches the medial meniscus to the femur proximally and to the tibia a few millimeters distal to the articular surface through the coronary ligament, which is the tibial portion of the posteromedial capsule.

Functionally, the posterior oblique fibers of the superficial medial collateral ligament act to limit posterior translation of the meniscus during knee flexion.[16] In extension, these fibers are lax and lie partly beneath the anterior parallel fibers (Fig. 5, *left*), becoming tense during flexion (Fig. 5, *right*).

Lateral Meniscus

The lateral meniscus is nearly circular and covers a large portion of the tibial plateau. It has a fairly consistent tibial width, which is 10.2 mm at the anterior horn, 11.6 mm at the midpoint, and 10.6 mm at the posterior horn.[11] Along the intercondylar eminence the menis-cal attachments are much closer together than for the medial menis-cus. The anterior horn is firmly attached to the intercondylar fossa, lateral and posterior to the base of the anterior cruciate ligament. The posterior horn usually has a dual attachment, with its anterior portion attached to the intercondylar eminence of the tibia just in front of the posterior rim of the medial meniscus and its posterior portion attached to the femur by the meniscofemoral ligaments. The circumference of the meniscus is attached by a lax capsule, the coronary ligament, to the articular margins of the femur and tibia except at the popliteal hiatus (Fig. 6). Posterolaterally, the meniscus is attached by the popliteus tendon and receives an aponeurotic insertion from the upper half of the popliteus muscle into its poste-rior convexity (Fig. 7).[17] The arcuate ligament is also firmly attached towards its upper end to the posterior arch of the lateral meniscus. Unlike the medial meniscus, the lateral meniscus has no firm tibial or femoral peripheral attachments (lateral collateral ligament), ac-counting, in part, for its increased mobility.

Meniscofemoral Ligaments of Wrisberg and Humphrey

Two small accessory ligaments arise from the posterior horn of the lateral meniscus in close proximity to the posterior cruciate liga-ment (PCL). Once thought to be the third cruciate ligament,[18] these divisions are the anterior and posterior meniscofemoral ligaments of Humphrey and Wrisberg, respectively (Fig. 7). They pass anteriorly and posteriorly to the PCL as they insert into the lateral aspect of the medial femoral condyle.

The presence of these ligaments is variable; conflicting results have been reported for several recent studies.[12,19] Heller and Langman[12] noted the presence of the anterior or posterior menis-cofemoral ligament, with equal incidence, in 99 (71%) of the 140 specimens studied, and the presence of both meniscofemoral liga-

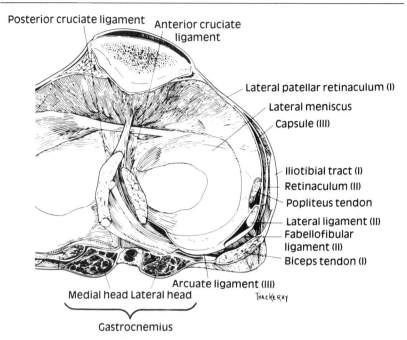

Posterior cruciate ligament   Anterior cruciate
ligament

Lateral patellar retinaculum (I)
Lateral meniscus
Capsule (III)

Iliotibial tract (I)
Retinaculum (II)
Popliteus tendon
Lateral ligament (II)
Fabellofibular
ligament (II)
Biceps tendon (I)

Arcuate ligament (III)
Medial head Lateral head
Gastrocnemius

THACKERAY

Fig. 6 *Superior view of the lateral meniscus demonstrating the three fascial layers on the lateral aspect of the knee. (Reproduced with permission from Warren R, Arnoczky SP, Wickiewicz TL: Anatomy of the knee, in Nicholas JA, Hershman EB (eds):* The Lower Extremity and Spine in Sports Medicine. *St. Louis, CV Mosby, 1986, vol 1, pp 657-694.)*

ments in eight (6%) knees. Friederich and O'Brien[19] were able to demonstrate one or both meniscofemoral ligaments in 100% of 50 specimens examined. Both ligaments were present in 44 knees (88%), an isolated ligament of Humphrey was present in two knees (4%), and a solitary ligament of Wrisberg was present in the remaining four knees (8%). The ligament of Humphrey may be up to one third the size of the PCL, while the ligament of Wrisberg can approach half the diameter of the PCL.[12]

These accessory ligaments increase the congruity between the meniscotibial socket and the lateral femoral condyle. This occurs primarily during weightbearing and knee flexion with the foot firmly fixed, as in the stance of a skier. Because the lateral and medial collateral ligaments are somewhat lax, the PCL serves as the main restraint of anterior movement of the femur on the tibia. The resultant anterior movement of the femur tightens the meniscofemoral ligament and draws the posterior horn of the lateral meniscus anteromedially.[12] During flexion, the ligament of Humphrey becomes increasingly tense and acts to stabilize the posterior horn of the lateral meniscus.[19] Conversely, the ligament of Wrisberg provides meniscal stability during knee extension (Fig. 8). During internal rotation of the femur on a fixed tibia, the meniscofemoral ligaments become slack. During external rotation of the femur on the tibia (for

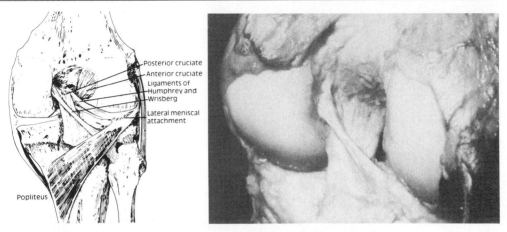

Fig. 7   *Left, Posterior view demonstration of the popliteus muscle origin and partial insertion into the posterior rim of the lateral meniscus.* **Right,** *Anatomic dissection depicting the PCL and posterior meniscofemoral ligament of Wrisberg. (Reproduced with permission from Warren R, Arnoczky SP, Wickiewicz TL: Anatomy of the knee, in Nicholas JA, Hershman EB (eds):* The Lower Extremity and Spine in Sports Medicine. *St. Louis, CV Mosby, 1986, vol 1, pp 657-694.)*

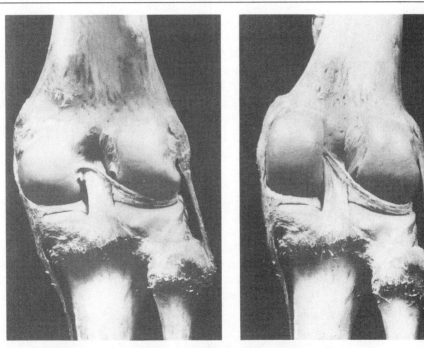

Fig. 8   *Dissected specimen* **(left)** *at 30 degrees of flexion and* **(right)** *at full extension. The terminal screwing home of the medial femoral condyle is apparent, while the lateral femoral condyle does not display substantial articular surface posteriorly* **(right)**. *During final extension the ligament of Wrisberg undergoes its definitive tensioning, drawing the posterior rim of the lateral meniscus in an anterior direction. (Reproduced with permission from Müller W:* The Knee: Form, Function, and Ligament Reconstruction. *Berlin, Springer-Verlag, 1983, pp 8-115.)*

example, during the "unlocking" of the knee at the beginning of flexion), the posterior horn is drawn anteromedially by the ligament of Humphrey. This movement in isolation would place the posterior lateral meniscus at risk of crush injury by the lateral femoral condyle. Fortunately, the simultaneous contraction of the popliteus muscle through its aponeurotic attachment acts to draw the posterior horn of the lateral meniscus downward and backward, thereby preventing the posterior meniscus from being crushed between the femoral condyle and the tibial plateau.[17] This system thus acts to provide "controlled" meniscal excursion as the popliteus muscle rotates the tibia internally during the initiation of knee flexion.

Parsons[20] demonstrated that the presence and configuration of the lateral meniscus, popliteus muscle, and meniscofemoral ligament complex were associated with an animal's ability to generate rotatory movements about the knee. Animals in which sudden rotation is vital to survival have no posterior horn tibial attachments; the meniscus is held primarily by the meniscofemoral ligaments and the popliteus muscle. On the other hand, Cheiroptera Pteropus (fruit bats), which lack any rotational ability about the knee joint, have knees that lack menisci, popliteus muscles, or a meniscofemoral ligament.

Ultrastructure

Similar to articular cartilage, the fibrocartilaginous meniscus performs many highly specialized functions, including load bearing,[21-39] shock absorption,[40-43] joint stabilization,[14,44-46] and joint lubrication.[10,41,47,48] These functions are dependent on its tissue composition and architecture.[3,10,39,49,50]

Composition

The meniscus is a hydrated fibrocartilage composed of a dense extracellular matrix and a sparse population of cells. The matrix is composed primarily of a fluid phase consisting of water and electrolytes (74% wet weight) and a solid phase composed of collagens, proteoglycans, elastins, and noncollagenous proteins (26% wet weight). Because the meniscus is anisotropic its description depends on the anatomic area under consideration.[51,52]

Cells   The major type of cell in the meniscus is the so-called fibrochondrocyte;[6,53,54] the sparse population of these cells is surrounded by the "territorial" or "pericellular" matrix.[53,55] In articular cartilage, this matrix has been described as a delicate meshwork that surrounds the chondrocyte. Additionally, the territorial matrix is surrounded by a 2 to 4-micron thick territorial region, which consists of collagen fibrils.[5,55] A high concentration of proteoglycans and pericellular collagen fibrils acts to protect the fibrochondrocyte locally from damage caused by mechanical stress.[56-60]

Collagens   Collagens constitute roughly 75% of the dry weight of meniscal tissue. Type I collagen, the predominant form, makes up more than 90% of the collagen content and is the primary structural component in the meniscus;[61,62] other collagens in the meniscus include types II, III, V, and VI.[63] Fibrillar collagens, such as types I, II, III, and V have tensile properties.[64] Recent evidence indicates that type VI collagen may serve as an intermolecular adhesive protein as well as a cell attachment protein.[62]

Superficially, the collagen fibers are randomly oriented with some predilection toward a radial direction.[41,61,65] In the deep, internal portion of the meniscus, collagen fibers are oriented primarily circumferentially. Large fascicles, measuring approximately 50 to 150 microns in diameter, are continuous with the anterior and posterior ligamentous horns that firmly anchor the meniscus to the tibial plateau. In addition, Bullough and associates[66] have described radially-oriented fibers in the deep portion of the meniscus. Although the exact role of these fibers is as yet poorly defined, it has been suggested that they may aid in collagen fiber bundle recruitment under conditions of circumferential tensile loading. The radially oriented fibers also may resist shearing along these bundles as they move relative to one another.[67] The distribution and orientation of radial tie fibers is inhomogeneous; radial fibers found in the posterior medial meniscus are larger, more numerous, and display a higher degree of horizontal orientation. These characteristics correlate with an increased radial tensile stiffness and strength found in the posterior medial meniscus.[68]

Elastins   The meniscal elastic fibers consist of two entities: elastin and elastin fibers.[69] Elastin is present in human meniscal tissue in small amounts, typically less than 0.6%.[70] Mechanically, elastin resembles rubber in that it can withstand high tensile strain without fracture, and regain its original resting dimensions following the removal of the deforming force. Therefore, it has been suggested that elastin acts to help the meniscus recover its original shape once the applied load decreases[71] or that elastin confers added resilience to an otherwise stiff collagenous structure.[9]

Proteoglycans   Proteoglycans make up only about 1% of the wet weight of the meniscus. Quantitatively, large, aggregating proteoglycans contribute the most to the material properties of the meniscus.[72-74] The glycosaminoglycan chains of the proteoglycan define many of its physical properties. Repeating disaccharide units containing sulfate (SO_4) and carboxyl (COOH) groups are capable of ionization in free solution as well as in vivo. These groups can accumulate a high-fixed-charge density as well as contributing significant charge-charge repulsive forces. These interactions provide meniscal tissue with several properties, including compressive stiffness, Donnan osmotic pressure, tissue hydration equilibrium, and shear stiffness. The fixed negative charge of the proteoglycan molecule

acts to support a high degree of tissue hydration in articular cartilage, which is important in compressive stiffness.[13,42,43,45,54,75-77]

Electrostatic interactions between positively charged groups
aside collagen fibrils and the negatively charged groups of proteoglycans contribute to the overall function of the meniscus.[78] Although osmotic pressure is a known contributor to cartilaginous
compressive stiffness, studies indicate that, theoretically, the intrinsic stiffness of the proteoglycan and collagen molecules contributes
more than Donnan forces with regard to tissue compressive stiffness.[58,67,79-84]

Shear stiffness is governed by the proteoglycans' ability to expand the extracellular matrix, thereby resisting high tensile stresses
produced in shear.[58,64,79,81,85] The concentration of proteoglycan in
the circumferential direction does not vary considerably. However,
the concentration increases radially toward the inner aspect.[86] The
significance of this finding is unclear at present.

Noncollagenous Proteins   In addition to type VI collagen, two
other adhesion proteins are identified: thrombospondin and fibronectin. These two proteins may be important in tissue repair, cell
movement, and metastasis.[85]

Material Properties

Biphasic Modeling

Mechanically, the meniscus is best understood using the biphasic
finite element model of soft, hydrated tissues developed by Mow
and associates.[59,72,83] The solid phase is made up of the extracellular
matrix, and the fluid phase consists of interstitial fluid and electrolytes. The solid phase, a fiber-reinforced matrix, is porous and permeable; the fluid phase, in turn, as a function of hydraulic forces and
matrix compression, controls the deformation properties of the meniscus.[58,80] Although each component of the model is assumed to be
incompressible, the meniscus as a whole undergoes compression
with loading because the fluid phase can flow out of the tissue.
When the meniscus is deformed by the action of a constant compressive or tensile load, the time-dependent creep and stress-relaxation viscoelastic responses are governed by frictional drag of the
fluid phase through the solid, porous matrix. Additionally, the flow-
independent response in shear of the solid matrix may be a result of
molecular relaxation of long-chain polymers, seen as proteoglycans
and collagen.[87] This phenomenon dictates the dynamic response of
the meniscus.

Fluid flow and pressurization of the meniscus have been shown to
be important in load carriage, energy dissipation, and viscoelasticity
within the knee joint.[88] The physical properties of the components of
the matrix, such as collagen, are also vital to the mechanical function of the meniscus.

Recently, the biphasic finite element model has been expanded to include the influence of dissolved electrolytes. Lai and associates have developed a triphasic model that includes Donnan osmotic pressures and physicochemical swelling effects.[58,89,90]

Hoop Stress

The circumferential collagen fiber arrangement of the meniscus makes this tissue much stiffer in the circumferential direction when compared with other orientations. Assuming the articulating surfaces of the meniscus are frictionless, a load transmitted onto the meniscus acts perpendicular to the femoral surface and, thus, is composed of a vertical and a radial component. The radial component of the load tends to extrude the meniscus toward the periphery of the joint. The considerable tensile stiffness of the circumferential collagen bundles, together with the strong anterior and posterior ligamentous tibial attachments, act to resist this extrusive force. This tensile stress, which develops during loading, is often called a hoop stress. The radial wedge shape and near frictionless femoral-tibial articulation act to convert the compressive loads across the knee into tensile loads acting parallel to the primarily circumferentially arranged collagen bundles.

Several investigators have examined the strength and stiffness of bovine and human meniscal tissue in vitro.[41,49,51,91] Posterior bovine meniscal specimens have been shown to be significantly stiffer under tension than anterior specimens, and circumferential specimens are stiffer under tension than radial specimens. These observations hold true for deep meniscal samples, but not for samples from the surface.[41,51,91] Circumferential specimens have been shown to have up to 100 times greater tensile stiffness than radially-oriented specimens. These studies support the idea that the meniscus is a highly complex tissue, displaying anisotropy as well as inhomogeneity. Additionally, the central and posterior regions of human meniscal tissue display the weakest tensile stiffness as compared with the anterior or lateral regions.

In addition to the large hoop stresses acting on it, the meniscus is subjected to significant radial stresses and strains. These forces are applied only to the sparse radial tie fibers. Using a recently developed finite element model, investigators have predicted larger radial stresses and strains in the internal portion of the meniscus.[88,92] The distribution of these stresses and strains implies that lesions, such as a bucket-handle tear, are caused by such forces.[52]

Load-bearing Function

Clinical and biomechanical data accrued over the past several decades suggest that one of the most important roles of the meniscus is as a load-bearing member of the knee.[93] In that regard, meniscectomy has been shown to alter the pattern and distribution of static load transmission across the knee joint. Peak stresses increase, a greater stress concentration develops, and the knee displays a decreased shock absorption following total meniscectomy.

Fairbank[32] provided the first evidence of a direct load-bearing function of the meniscus. In a classic investigation, he roentgenographically demonstrated an increase in degenerative changes within the articular surface of the knee following meniscectomy. Several methods, including radiologic techniques, casting compression, pressure sensitive film, and micro-indentation transducers, have been used to demonstrate the contact area and peak stress distribution in normal and abnormal menisci.[27-39] As described above, forces acting at the surface of the meniscus are converted into radial and axial vectors. The circumferential arrangement of the collagen fascicles translates force applied during weightbearing into a radial extrusive force, which is resisted by the large tensile hoop stress that develops within the meniscus. Through this mechanism approximately 40% to 50% of the load is applied across the knee in extension. This load-bearing increases to 85% at 90 degrees of flexion.

Joint Stabilization

The meniscus contributes to the stability of the knee joint.[14,44-46] Several studies have shown the meniscus to contribute little to the anteroposterior stability of the knee when the cruciate ligaments are intact. However, the meniscus does prevent anterior tibial subluxation on the femur in the anterior cruciate ligament-deficient knee. The meniscal ligamentous interaction is discussed in detail in a subsequent section.

Kinematics of the Meniscus

The human knee is perhaps the most complex diarthrodial joint in the body; its kinematics are governed by articular geometry and ligamentous, capsular, meniscal, and muscular constraints. Several models exist that describe the movements of the cruciate and collateral ligaments through a range of motion. The kinematics of these ligaments affect the kinematics of the meniscus.

To explore the kinematics of the meniscus it is necessary to appreciate the six degrees of freedom in which the femur moves in relation to the tibia.[94,95] Any general displacement of the tibia relative to the femur can be illustrated using an orthogonal coordinate system (Fig. 9). The possible translations along the three orthogonal axes include: anteroposterior, mediolateral, and proximodistal translation. The corresponding rotations about the same axes are: varus-valgus, flexion-extension, and internal-external rotation.

The Crossed Four-bar Linkage

The primary movement of the knee is flexion-extension. This movement, unlike that of a simple hinge, consists of a varying mix-

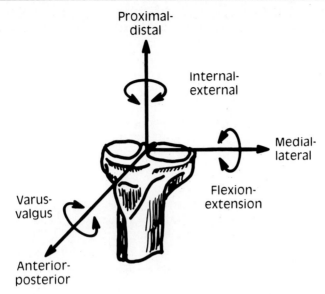

Fig. 9 *Any general displacement of the tibia relative to the femur can be described using an illustrated orthogonal coordinate system. The six degrees of freedom are three translations: anteroposterior, mediolateral, and proximodistal. The three rotations about these axis are: varus-valgus, flexion-extension, and internal-external. (Reproduced with permission from Torzilli PA: Biomechanical analysis of knee stability, in Nicholas JA, Hershman EB (eds):* The Lower Extremity and Spine in Sports Medicine. *St. Louis, CV Mosby, 1986, vol 1, p. 729.)*

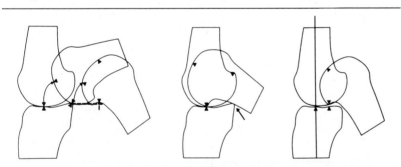

Fig. 10 *Both isolated and combined rolling and gliding movements of the femoral condyle. With only rolling motion (left), the femur rolls off the tibial plateau well before the completion of knee flexion; with only gliding motion (center) the femur is checked by the posterior lip of the tibial plateau before full flexion is achieved; combined rolling and gliding of the femoral condyles (right) allows a full range of motion. Closed arrowheads are changing contact points between the femoral condyle and tibial plateau. (Reproduced with permission from Shapeero LG, Dye SF, Lipton MJ, et al: Functional dynamics of the knee joint by ultrafast, cine-CT.* Invest Radiol *1988;23:118-123.)*

ture of rolling and gliding. If only rolling (flexion-extension rotation without anteroposterior translation) occurred, the femoral condyle would roll off the tibial plateau long before flexion was completed

(Fig. 10, *left*). Conversely, if gliding (anteroposterior translation without flexion-extension rotation) were the principle movement, the posterior margin of the femur would strike the posterior tibial plateau before the completion of full flexion (Fig. 10, *center*). Therefore, for a normal range of motion, a mixture of rolling and gliding must occur (Fig. 10, *right*). Looking at this complex rotation, including automatic initial and terminal rotation as well as voluntary rotation, as if it were in a single, sagittal plane makes it simple to demonstrate and understand how the femoral condyle rolls and glides simultaneously on the tibial plateau.

The basic kinematic principle of motion in the knee can be demonstrated by a mechanical system described by a crossed four-bar linkage.[7,93,96-99] The crossed four-bar system, as described by Müller,[100] consists of a sheet of drawing paper on which two rods are linked at one end. The two hinge points must lie on a line that intersects the long axis at a 40 degree angle through one of the points. This angle corresponds to the angle formed between the intercondylar roof, the intersection of proximal attachment sites of the cruciates, and the vertical long axis of the femur. One of the crossed rods is longer than the other, with length ratios similar to those of the cruciate ligaments. The distal free ends are linked by a movable bar, representing the tibial plateau. This bar forms the coupler that, when taken through its various positions, defines multiple tangents that delineate a curve (Fig. 11, *top)*. The coupler envelope curve (Fig. 11, *center and bottom*) defined by this system resembles the sagittal contour of the posterior femoral condyle. This model holds true only for knee motion in the sagittal plane without any rotational component.

The coupler model easily demonstrates the obligatory shift in femorotibial contact during knee flexion. The exact ratio of rolling to gliding changes throughout flexion. Rolling predominates during early flexion with the gliding component increasing during flexion to the point where the femoral condyles glide on the tibial plateau at full flexion. Shapeero and associates[99] report an overall rolling to gliding ratio of approximately 1:1 for the medial condyle and nearly 1:4 for the lateral condyle. The lateral condyle was found to move 2.3 times farther on the tibial plateau than its medial counterpart.

Burmester Curves

As the crossed four-bar linkage depicts the motion of the cruciate ligaments, the Burmester curve depicts that of the collateral ligaments of the knee.[96-98,101] The collateral ligament function consists of two third-order curves, designated the pivot cubic and the vertex cubic (Fig. 12). The Burmester curve is fundamental to the proper medial collateral ligament (MCL) insertion and function. If a straight line is drawn from a point on the vertex cubic through the crossing point P of the crossed four-bar linkage to a corresponding point on the pivot cubic, the two points approximate circular paths

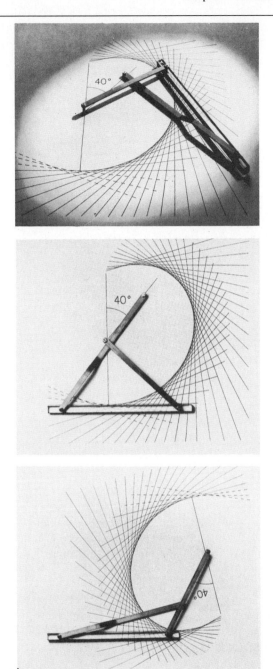

Fig. 11 *Model of a crossed four-bar linkage showing phases in the movement (representing increasing femoral flexion) of the crossed four-bar linkage with the coupler (representing the tibial plateau) as a fixed member. The cruciate ligaments are represented by rigid rods that are hinged on a line set at a 40 degree angle to a given perpendicular. The tibial plateau is represented by the coupler, consisting of a rectangular plastic bar. (Reproduced with permission from Müller W:* The Knee: Form, Function, and Ligament Reconstruction. *Berlin, Springer-Verlag, 1983, pp 8-115.)*

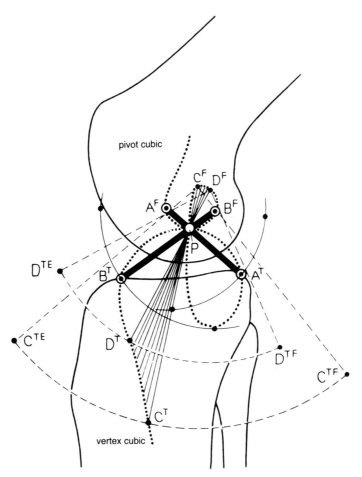

Fig. 12 *Burmester curve, the theoretical course of the MCL. The crossed four-bar linkage and the Burmester curve share a common intersection labeled point P. (Reproduced with permission from Müller W:* The Knee: Form, Function, and Ligament Reconstruction. *Berlin, Springer-Verlag, 1983, pp 8-115.)*

when the femorotibial linkage is moved, and their respective distance relative to one another remains essentially constant.

In application of this construct, it is apparent at 43 degrees of flexion, if several points of the pivot cubic loop are connected through center P with the corresponding limb of the vertex cubic, an approximation of the MCL is obtained in both length and form. This arrangement is also considered to be a type of crossed four-bar linkage. The fibrous strands always intersect at the pole[96-98,101] of the transverse flexion axis and radiate outward like spokes of a wheel (Fig. 13). Therefore, the larger number of collagenous fibers that constitute the MCL do not all fall on the ideal Burmester line. In this situation, critical overtension of the ligament fibers can occur after

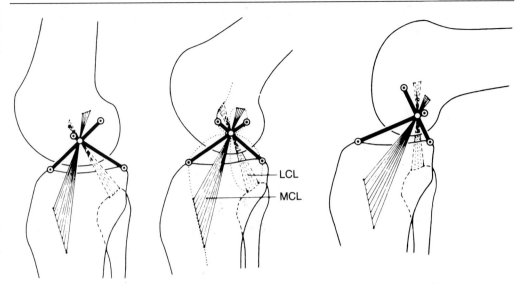

Fig. 13 *The cruciate ligaments are represented by the crossed four-bar linkage, and the MCL and LCL by the principles of the Burmester curve. All elements intersect at the crossing point of the four-bar linkage. The crossing point can be maintained in extension (**left**) and in flexion (**center** and **right**) and probably also represents the point where the flexion axis crosses the femur. (Reproduced with permission from Müller W:* The Knee: Form, Function, and Ligament Reconstruction. *Berlin, Springer-Verlag, 1983, pp 8-115.)*

90 degrees of flexion. However, at this flexion angle there is an automatic internal rotation with increasing varus, which decreases the valgus-external rotation of early flexion. This involves relaxation of the lateral collateral ligament at the onset of flexion, with relative tension maintained on the cruciate ligaments and with internal rotation serving to partially unload the MCL and avoid excess tensioning of the ligament.

The interactions of the cruciate ligaments, collateral ligaments, and disparate femoral condyles produce a phenomenon known as the "screw home mechanism." In the last 20 degrees of extension, the knee automatically rotates 15 degrees internally, while the reverse occurs at the onset of flexion. This mechanism is believed to be caused by the outer edge of the medial condyle bearing surface in the form of an annular sector of 50 to 60 degrees and is controlled by the cruciate linkage. The lateral femoral condyle demonstrates significantly greater translation during extension-flexion.

Measuring Meniscal Kinematics

The kinematics of the menisci during an extension-flexion arc requires further study. In the initial studies,[102-104] the menisci were observed directly to describe displacement during flexion. In each study, the knee was dissected down to and including the joint capsule, leaving the menisci, the cruciate ligament, and the collateral ligaments intact. The menisci were visually examined for displacement and deformation. Unfortunately, the femoral condyles obscured much of the meniscal surface, restricting assessment to the exposed, nonarticular segments. Bylski,[105] using single planar roentgenography, examined the effects of compression, rotation, and translation on meniscal displacement through the first 30 degrees of flexion.

Advances in radiographic technique, such as computed tomography (CT) and magnetic resonance imaging (MRI), allow for the kinematic analysis of an intact joint. Indirect imaging has been used to avoid the limitations of dissection. Cardiac cine CT has been used to assess the change in femorotibial contact points during flexion in the intact cadaver knee.[99] Unfortunately, CT cannot adequately resolve soft tissue adjacent to bone because of a beam-hardening artifact, making it deficient for the description of meniscal dynamics.[106,107] Multiplanar imaging and processing, such as three-dimensional (3-D) reconstruction, allows the researcher to effectively dissect the knee, isolate the menisci, and study their dynamics without altering joint kinematics.

As shown, the motion of menisci is influenced by the capsular, muscular, and ligamentous attachments, as well as by tibial and femoral articular configurations and knee joint biomechanics. By following the principles of the crossed four-bar linkage, Burmester's curve, and automatic rotation, it is possible to predict the motion of the menisci quite reasonably. These kinematic constraints mandate an obligatory posterior translation of the femorotibial contact during flexion. Additionally, with automatic rotation, the lateral femoral condyle describes a wide arc along the tibial plateau during flexion and demonstrates greater posterior translation than the medial femoral condyle.[108]

Meniscal Excursion   A 3-D kinematic meniscal MRI model has been created in intact, undissected, nonweightbearing cadaveric knee joints.[108,109] The high soft-tissue contrast resolution and its noninvasive and multiplanar capabilities make MRI the ideal medium with which to study meniscal kinematics.

Our imaging technique is outlined below. We obtained serial MRI images using previously described techniques.[108-111] The MRI data were transferred to a computer for 3-D reconstruction using a region of interest and threshold technique, and 3-D images were obtained (Fig. 14), which could be rotated to view the menisci in any plane desired.

In addition, representative sagittal MR images were linked together on the computer and viewed in a cinematic format to visualize tibial excursion of the menisci. The differential movement of the anterior and posterior horns was measured along the tibial plateau and recorded. The measurements were averaged and a mean excursion value was obtained. The resultant 3-D meniscal images were

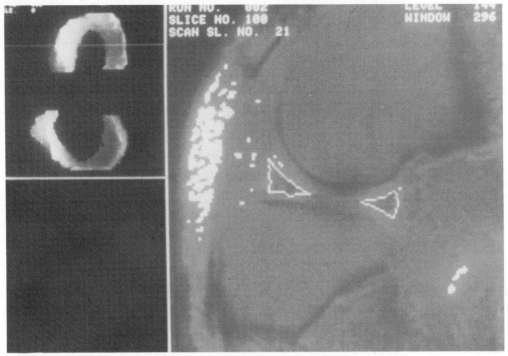

Fig. 14 *Sample parasagittal M image with region of interest outline and corresponding 3-D reconstruction image. (Reproduced with permission from Fu F, Thompson WO: Motion of the meniscus during knee flexion, in Mow VC, Arnoczky SP, Jackson DW (eds):* Knee Meniscus: Basic and Clinical Foundations. *New York, Raven Press, 1992, pp 75-89.)*

also displayed in cinematic format and viewed dynamically to assess deformation.

The mean meniscal excursion was defined as the average antero-posterior displacement of the anterior meniscal horn and the posterior meniscal horn along the tibial plateau in the midcondylar, parasagittal plane. The medial meniscal excursion was 5.1 ± 0.96 mm and the mean lateral meniscal excursion was 11.2 ± 3.27 mm. The ratio of medial to lateral excursion was 1:2.3 ± 0.86 and was statistically significant. This displacement is clearly visualized by sagittal MRI and 3-D reconstruction imaging (Figs. 15-18). The classic investigation of Brantigan and Voshell[102] revealed the meniscal excursion to be roughly 2 mm medially and 1 cm laterally. DePalma,[103] using a similar technique, reported an average 0.3 cm posterior displacement for the medial meniscus and 0.9 cm for the lateral meniscus during an extension-flexion arc. The range of values obtained was marked and felt to reflect the individual articular geometry of each specimen. However, the lateral femoral condyle and meniscus consistently displayed a significantly greater posterior translation than the medial. It is surprising that results of the studies

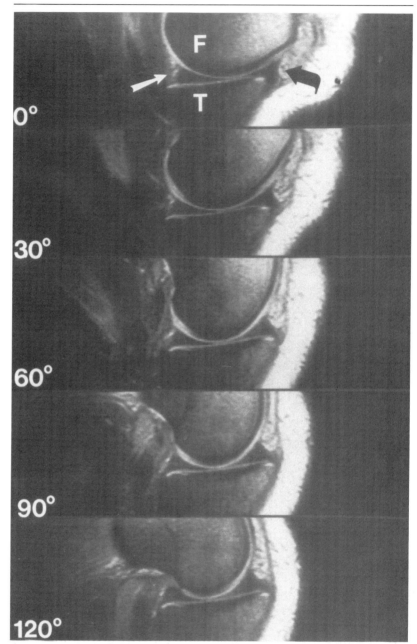

Fig. 15   *Parasagittal magnetic resonance images through the medial femoral condyle obtained at 30-degree increments from 0 to 120 degrees of flexion. F, femur; T, tibia; black arrow, anterior meniscal horn; white arrow, posterior meniscal horn. (Reproduced with permission from Thompson WO, Thaete FL, Fu FH, et al: Tibial meniscal dynamics using three-dimensional reconstruction of magnetic resonance images. Am J Sports Med 1991;19:210-216.)*

that examined the menisci via dissection[102-104] were not markedly different from results of the study of intact specimens.[108]

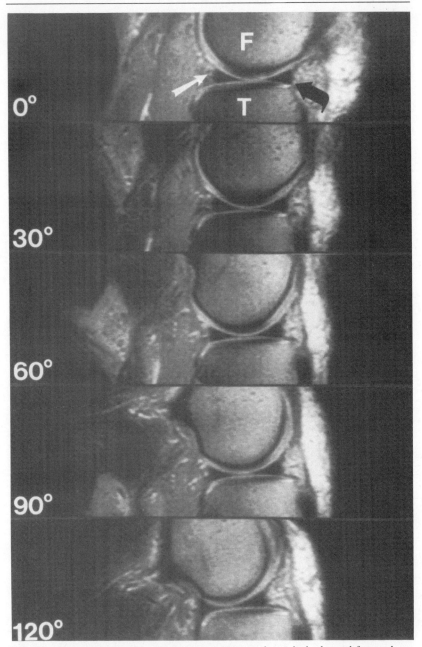

Fig. 16 *Parasagittal magnetic resonance images through the lateral femoral condyle obtained at 30-degree increments from 0 to 120 degrees of flexion. F, femur; T, tibia; black arrow, anterior meniscal horn; white arrow, posterior meniscal horn. (Reproduced with permission from Thompson WO, Thaete FL, Fu FH, et al: Tibial meniscal dynamics using three-dimensional reconstruction of magnetic resonance images. Am J Sports Med 1991;19:210-216.)*

A segmental analysis of both menisci has also been performed.[108] The mean posterior horn excursion when compared with the mean

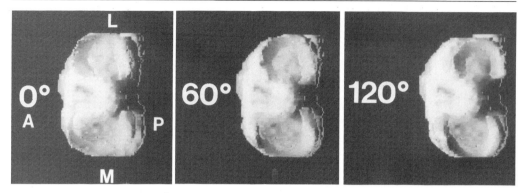

Fig. 17 *Superior 3-D meniscal images in 60-degree increments from 0 to 120 degrees of flexion. A, anterior; P, posterior; L, lateral. (Reproduced with permission from Thompson WO, Thaete FL, Fu FH, et al: Tibial meniscal dynamics using three-dimensional reconstruction of magnetic resonance images.* Am J Sports Med *1991;19:210-216.)*

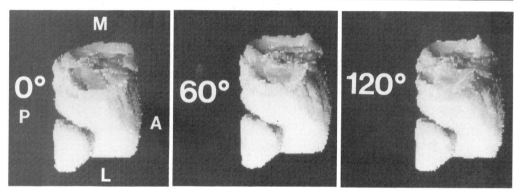

Fig. 18 *Lateral 3-D meniscal images in 60-degree increments from 0 to 120 degrees of flexion. A, anterior; P, posterior; M, medial; L, lateral. (Reproduced with permission from Thompson WO, Thaete FL, Fu FH, et al: Tibial meniscal dynamics using three-dimensional reconstruction of magnetic resonance images.* Am J Sports Med *1991;19:210-216.)*

anterior horn excursion of the same side was statistically smaller in both menisci. The ratio of mean posterior horn excursion to mean anterior horn excursion was 1:2.4 ± 0.81 medially and 1:1.3 ± 0.23 laterally. These results are shown diagrammatically in Figure 19. The menisci demonstrate a marked difference in translation during passive extension and flexion, with the posterior horns exhibiting less displacement than the anterior horns during flexion (Figs. 20 and 21). This limitation of motion is most marked in the posterior medial corner. The posterior horn of the medial meniscus is constrained medially by its attachment to the tibial plateau via the meniscotibial portion of the posterior oblique ligament fibers, as well as by the articular geometry of the femoral condyle and con-

MEAN MENISCAL EXCURSION (mm)

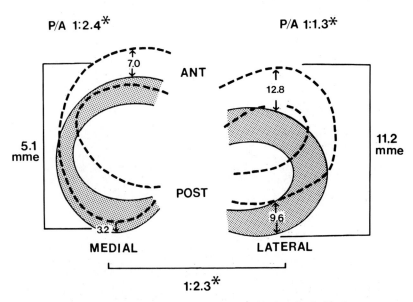

Fig. 19 *Diagram of mean meniscal excursion along the tibial plateau. Ant, anterior; post, posterior; mme, mean meniscal excursion; P/A, ratio of posterior to anterior meniscal translation during flexion; *, p <0.05 by student's t-test analysis (Reproduced with permission from Thompson WO, Thaete FL, Fu FH, et al: Tibial meniscal dynamics using three-dimensional reconstruction of magnetic resonance images. Am J Sports Med 1991;19:210-216.)*

cave tibial plateau. The anterior horns are, in general, less restrained bilaterally than the posterior horn.

A study by DePalma,[103] which analyzes various phases of knee flexion, indicates the majority of lateral meniscal displacement occurs after 5 to 7 degrees of knee flexion have been achieved. In contrast, the medial meniscus is quiescent until 17 to 20 degrees of flexion. Also, the medial meniscus begins translation at 70 degrees as the posterior horn is ". . .gripped firmly between the posterior flare of the femoral condyle and the tibial plateau,"[103] while the lateral meniscus continues its posterior excursion until the completion of flexion. This observation is quite reasonable on consideration of the lateral compartment anatomy. The lack of posterior bony opposition from the convex femoral condyle and tibial plateau, an unconstrained peripheral meniscal margin, and close central tibial attachments allow the lateral meniscus a wide range of excursion.[108]

Motion During Rotation   The knee demonstrates a significantly greater rotation of the lateral compartment as compared with the medial; the excursion of the menisci reflect this fact. Ruetsch and

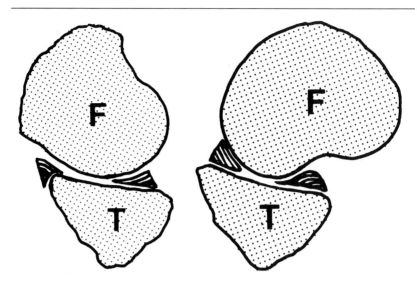

Fig. 20   *Diagram of the midcondylar, sagittal position of the medial meniscus in extension (**left**) and at 120 degrees of flexion (**right**). F, femur; T, tibia. (Reproduced with permission from Fu F, Thompson WO: Motion of the meniscus during knee flexion, in Mow VC, Arnoczky SP, Jackson DW (eds):* Knee Meniscus: Basic and Clinical Foundations. *New York, Raven Press, 1992, pp 75-89.)*

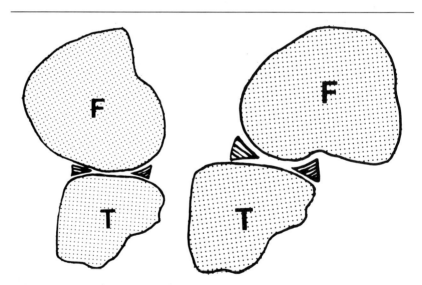

Fig. 21   *Diagram of the midcondylar, sagittal position of the lateral meniscus in extension (**left**) and at 120 degrees of flexion (**right**). F, femur; T, tibia. (Reproduced with permission from Fu F, Thompson WO: Motion of the meniscus during knee flexion, in Mow VC, Arnoczky SP, Jackson DW (eds):* Knee Meniscus: Basic and Clinical Foundations. *New York, Raven Press, 1992, pp 75-89.)*

Morscher[112] show an average rotation range of 36 degrees at 90 degrees of knee flexion. Of this 36 degrees, external rotation consists of 21 degrees, while internal rotation contributes 15 degrees. The

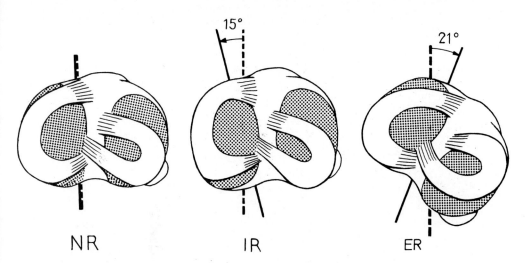

Fig. 22   *Range of internal and external rotation with associated meniscal movement on the tibial plateau. The average range of 15 degrees of internal rotation and 21 degrees of external rotation correspond to measurements of Ruetsch and Morscher. (Reproduced with permission from Müller W:* The Knee: Form, Function, and Ligament Reconstruction. *Berlin, Springer-Verlag, 1983, pp 8-115.)*

range of values in this study is impressive, varying from 27 to 54 degrees of total rotation. External rotation ranges from 14 to 29 degrees and internal rotation between 9 and 29 degrees. The menisci are displaced markedly by these rotations, with the lateral meniscus again showing the greater displacement (Fig. 22). Also, the posterior oblique fibers of the MCL limit movement of the posteromedial meniscus in rotation and increase its risk of tear injury. The marked mobility of the lateral meniscus accounts for its markedly decreased risk of tear.[108]

Meniscal Deformation   The menisci remain in constant congruity to the tibial and femoral articular surfaces throughout the full range of motion (Figs. 15 and 16) and, thus, provide additional stability to the tibiofemoral joint. The anterior horn segœents bilaterally demonstrate differing mobility compared with posterior horn segments. This differential allows the menisci to assume a decreasing radius with flexion (Figs. 17 and 18), correlating with a decreased radius of curvature of the posterior femoral condyles. The change in radius enables the menisci to maintain congruity with the articulating surfaces throughout flexion. The greatest deformation is observed in the anterior medial horn as it moves onto the tibial plateau with flexion (Fig. 18). Deformation is primarily demonstrated as increasing concavity of the superior articulating meniscal surface in response to increasing femoral flexion (Figs. 17 and 18). The anterior horn of the medial meniscus demonstrates the greatest degree of deformation. In full extension, a portion of the meniscal substance is displaced anterior to the tibial plateau margin (Figs. 15, *top* and 18, *left*). The collateral ligaments can also be seen attached to the inferior margins of both anterior horns. These ligaments are redundant in extension and become taut during flexion (Figs. 15 and 16).

Summary

The human knee menisci are important to proper knee joint function. An appreciation of their anatomic attachments is necessary both when planning meniscectomy or repair, and in transplantation surgery. The medial meniscus has been shown to be constrained in the posteromedial corner. The lateral meniscus is relatively more mobile, and its movement is controlled by the meniscofemoral ligaments and the popliteus muscle. The medial meniscus is more subject to traumatic rupture than is the lateral. The menisci act to fill the void created by the incongruous femoral condyles and tibial plateau and, thereby, enhance joint stability. The menisci also act as guides to facilitate the automatic rotation that occurs during an extension-flexion arc.

Various models have been developed, including the biphasic anisotropic composite, that now allow mathematical predictions of meniscal response to load, shear, and strain. Through these models reconstruction, replacement, and total knee-joint biomechanics can be explored further.

References

1. Sutton JB: *Ligaments: Their Nature and Morphology*. London, MK Lewis & Co, 1897.

2. Arnoczky SP, Adams ME, DeHaven K, et al: Meniscus, in Woo SL-Y, Buckwalter J (eds): *Injury and Repair of the Musculoskeletal Soft Tissues*. Park Ridge, IL, American Academy of Orthopaedic Surgeons, 1988, pp 487-537.

3. Bullough PG, Vosburgh F, Arnoczky SP, et al: The menisci of the knee, in Insall JN (ed): *Surgery of the Knee*. New York, Churchill Livingstone, 1984, pp 135-146.

4. Warren R, Arnoczky SP, Wickiewicz TL: Anatomy of the knee, in Nicholas JA, Hershman EB (eds): *The Lower Extremity and Spine in Sports Medicine*. St. Louis, CV Mosby, 1986, vol 1, pp 657-694.

5. Clark CR, Ogden JA: Development of the menisci of the human knee joint: Morphological changes and their potential role in childhood meniscal injury. *J Bone Joint Surg* 1983;65A;538-547.

6. Ghadially FN, Thomas I, Yong N, et al: Ultrastructure of rabbit semilunar cartilages. *J Anat* 1978;125:499-517.

7. Huson A: Biomechanische probleme des kniegelenkes. *Orthopaede* 1974;3:119-129.

8. Insall JN: Anatomy of the knee, in Insall JN (ed): *Surgery of the Knee*. New York, Churchill Livingstone, 1984, pp 1-20.

9. Hukins DWL: Properties of spinal materials, in Jayson MIV (ed): *The Lumbar Spine and Back Pain*, ed 3. Edinburgh, Churchill Livingstone, 1987, pp 138-160.

10. Mow VC, Fithian DC, Kelly MA: Fundamentals of articular cartilage and meniscus biomechanics, in Ewing JW (ed): *Articular Cartilage and Knee Joint Function: Basic Science and Arthroscopy*. New York, Raven Press, 1990, pp 1-18.

11. Ferrer-Roca O, Vilalta C: Lesions of the meniscus: Part I. Macroscopic and histologic findings. *Clin Orthop* 1980;146:289-300.

12. Heller L, Langman J: The menisco-femoral ligaments of the human knee. *J Bone Joint Surg* 1964;46B:307-313.

13. Warren LF, Marshall JL: The supporting structures and layers on the medial side of the knee: An anatomical analysis. *J Bone Joint Surg* 1979;61A:56-62.

14. Kaplan EB: Some aspects of functional anatomy of the human knee joint. *Clin Orthop* 1962;23:18-29.

15. Last RJ: The popliteus muscle and the lateral meniscus. *J Bone Joint Surg* 1950;32B:93-99.

16. Palmer I: On the injuries to the ligaments of the knee joint: A clinical study. *Acta Chir Scanda* 1938, Supplement 53.

17. Last RJ: Some anatomical details of the knee joint. *J Bone Joint Surg* 1948;30B:683-688.

18. Poirier P, Charpy A: *Traite d'Anatomie Humaine: Tome 1*. Paris, Masson, 1899.

19. Friederich NF, O'Brien WR: Functional anatomy of the meniscofemoral ligaments. Presented at the Fourth Congress of the European Society of Knee Surgery and Arthroscopy, Stockholm, Sweden, June 1990.

20. Parsons FG: The joints of mammals compared with those of man: A course of lectures delivered at the Royal College of Surgeons of England: Part II. Joints of the hind limb. *J Anat Physiol* 1900;34: 301-323.

21. Allen PR, Denham RA, Swan AV: Late degenerative changes after meniscectomy. *J Bone Joint Surg* 1984;66B:666-671.

22. Burr DB, Radin EL: Meniscal function and the importance of meniscal regeneration in preventing late medial compartment osteoarthrosis. *Clin Orthop* 1982;171:121-126.

23. Cox JS, Cordell LD: The degenerative effects of medial meniscus tears in dogs' knees. *Clin Orthop* 1977;125:236-242.

24. Cox JS, Nye CE, Schaefer WW, et al: The degenerative effects of partial and total resection of the medial meniscus in dogs' knees. *Clin Orthop* 1975;109:178-183.

25. Gould JD, Torzilli PA, Adams TC, et al: The effect of lateral meniscectomy on knee motion. *Trans Orthop Res Soc* 1984;9:25.

26. Radin EL, de Lamotte F, Maquet P: Role of the menisci in the distribution of stress in the knee. *Clin Orthop* 1984;185:290-294.

27. Ahmed AM, Burke DL: In-vitro measurement of static pressure distribution in synovial joints: Part I. Tibial surface of the knee. *J Biomech Eng* 1983;105:216-225.

28. Baratz ME, Fu FH, Mengato R: Meniscal tears: The effect of meniscectomy and of repair on intraarticular contact areas and stress in the human knee: A preliminary report. *Am J Sports Med* 1986;14:270-275.

29. Baratz ME, Rehak DC, Fu FH, et al: Peripheral tears of the meniscus: The effect of open versus arthroscopic repair on intraarticular contact stresses in the human knee. *Am J Sports Med* 1988;16:-6.

30. Bourne RB, Finlay JB, Papadopoulos P, et al: The effect of medial meniscectomy on strain distribution in the proximal part of the tibia. *J Bone Joint Surg* 1984;66A:1431-1437.

31. Brown TD, Shaw DT: In vitro contact stress distribution on the femoral condyles. *J Orthop Res* 1984;2:190-199.

32. Fairbank TJ: Knee joint changes after meniscectomy. *J Bone Joint Surg* 1948;30B:664-670.

33. Fukubayashi T, Kurosawa H: The contact area and pressure distribution pattern of the knee: A study of normal and osteoarthrotic knee joints. *Acta Orthop Scand* 1980;51:871-879.

34. Kettelkamp DB, Jacobs AW: Tibiofemoral contact area: Determination and implications. *J Bone Joint Surg* 1972;54A:349-356.

35. Maquet PG, Van de Berg AJ, Simonet JC: Femorotibial weightbearing areas. *J Bone Joint Surg* 1975;57A:766-771.

36. Seedhom BB, Hargreaves DJ: Transmission of the load in the knee joint with special reference to the role of the menisci: Part II. Experimental results, discussion and conclusions. *Eng Med* 1979;8: 220-228.

37. Seedhom BB, Dowson D, Wright V: *The Load-Bearing Function of the Menisci in the Knee Joint.* Amsterdam, Exerpta Medica, 1974 (International Congress Series No. 324).

38. Seedhom BB: Transmission of the load in the knee joint with special reference to the role of the menisci: Part I. Anatomy, analysis and apparatus. *Eng Med* 1979;8:207-219.

39. Shrive NG, O'Connor JJ, Goodfellow JW: Load-bearing in the knee joint. *Clin Orthop* 1978;131:279-287.

40. Krause WR, Pope MH, Johnson RJ, et al: Mechanical changes in the knee after meniscectomy. *J Bone Joint Surg* 1976;58A:599-604.

41. Proctor CS, Schmidt MB, Whipple RR, et al: Material properties of the normal medial bovine meniscus. *J Orthop Res* 1989;7:771-782.

42. Voloshin AS, Wosk J: Shock absorption of meniscectomized and painful knees: A comparative in vivo study. *J Biomed Eng* 1983;5: 157-161.

43. Walker PS, Erkman MJ: The role of the menisci in force transmission across the knee. *Clin Orthop* 1975;109:184-192.

44. Hsieh HH, Walker PS: Stabilizing mechanisms of the loaded and unloaded knee joint. *J Bone Joint Surg* 1976;58A:87-93.

45. Levy IM, Torzilli PA, Warren RF: The effect of medial meniscectomy on anterior-posterior motion of the knee. *J Bone Joint Surg* 1982;64A:883-888.

46. Shoemaker SC, Markolf KL: The role of the meniscus in the anterior-posterior stability of the loaded anterior cruciate-deficient knee. *J Bone Joint Surg* 1986;68A:71-79.

47. DeHaven KE: The role of the meniscus, in Ewing JW (ed): *Articular Cartilage and Knee Joint Function: Basic Science and Arthroscopy.* New York, Raven Press, 1990, pp 103-115.

48. MacConaill MA: The function of intra-articular fibrocartilages, with special reference to the knee and inferior radio-ulnar joints. *J Anat* 1932;66:210-227.

49. Fithian DC, Kelly MA, Mow VC: Material properties and structure-function relationships in the menisci. *Clin Orthop* 1990;252:19-31.

50. Myers ER, Zhu W, Mow VC: Viscoelastic properties of articular cartilage and meniscus, in Nimni ME (ed): *Collagen: Chemistry, Biology and Biotechnology.* Boca Raton, FL, CRC Press, 1988, vol II, pp 268-288.

51. Whipple RR, Wirth CR, Mow VC: Anisotropic and zonal variations in the tensile properties of the meniscus. *Trans Orthop Res Soc* 1985;10:367.

52. Fithian DC, Zhu W, Ratcliffe A, et al: Exponential law representation of tensile properties of human meniscus. London, *Proc Mech Eng Bioeng* 1989, pp 89-90.

53. Ghadially FN, Lalonde JM, Wedge JH: Ultrastructure of normal and torn menisci of the human knee joint. *J Anat* 1983;136:773-791.

54. Webber RJ, Harris MG, Hough AJ Jr: Cell culture of rabbit meniscal fibrochondrocytes: Proliferative and synthetic response to growth factors and ascorbate. *J Orthop Res* 1985;3:36-42.

55. Ghadially FN: *Fine Structure of Synovial Joints: A Text and Atlas of the Ultrastructure of Normal and Pathological Articular Tissues.* London, Butterworths, 1983.

56. Guilak F, Ratcliffe A, Mow VC: The stress-strain environment around a chondrocyte: A finite element analysis of cell-matrix interactions, in Goldstein SA (ed): *Advances in Bioengineering.* New York, ASME, 1990, pp 395-398.

57. Guilak F, Ratcliffe A, Hunziker EB, et al: Finite element modeling of articular cartilage chondrocytes under physiological loading conditions. *Trans Orthop Res Soc* 1991;16:366.

58. Maroudas A: Physicochemical properties of articular cartilage, in Freeman MAR (ed): *Adult Articular Cartilage.* Tunbridge Wells, England, Pitman Medical, 1979, p 215.

59. Mow VC, Lai WM, Hou JS: A triphasic theory for the swelling properties of hydrated charged soft biologic tissues. *Appl Mech Rev* 1990;43(part 2):134-141.

60. Mulholland R: Lateral hydraulic permeability and morphology of articular cartilage, in Ali SY, Elves MW, Leabeck DH (eds): *Normal and Osteoarthritic Cartilage.* London, Institute of Orthopaedics, 1974, pp 268-288.

61. Aspden RM, Yarker YE, Hukins DW: Collagen orientations in the meniscus of the knee joint. *J Anat* 1985;140:371-380.

62. McDevitt CA, Webber RJ: The ultrastructure and biochemistry of meniscal cartilage. *Clin Orthop* 1990;252:8-18.

63. Clarke IC: Articular cartilage: A review and scanning electron microscope study: II. The territorial fibrillar architecture. *J Anat* 1974;118:261-280.

64. Cheung HS: Distribution of type I, II, III and V in the pepsin solubilized collagens in bovine menisci. *Connect Tissue Res Soc* 1987;16:343-356.

65. Yasui K: Three dimensional architecture of normal human menisci. *J Jpn Orthop Assoc* 1978;52:391.

66. Bullough PG, Miunuera L, Murphy J, et al: The strength of the menisci of the knee as it relates to their fine structure. *J Bone Joint Surg* 1970;52B:564-570.

67. Mow VC, Whipple RR: The biology and mechanical properties of cartilage and menisci, in American Academy of Orthopaedic Surgeons Committee on Basic Sciences: *Williamsburg Seminar 1984: Resources for Basic Science Educators.* Park Ridge, American Academy of Orthopaedic Surgeons, 1984, pp 165-197.

68. Skaggs DL, Mow VC: Function of radial tie fibers in the meniscus. *Trans Orthop Res Soc* 1990;15:248.

69. Ross R: The electric fiber. *J Histochem Cytochem* 1973;21:199-208.

70. Peters TJ, Smillie IS: Studies on the chemical composition of the menisci of the knee joint with special reference to the horizontal cleavage lesion. *Clin Orthop* 1972;86:245-252.

71. Ghosh P, Taylor TKF: The knee joint meniscus: A fibrocartilage of some distinction. *Clin Orthop* 1987;224:52-63.

72. Mow VC, Holmes MH, Lai WM: Fluid transport and mechanical properties of articular cartilage: A review. *J Biomech* 1984;17:377-394.

73. Hardingham TE, Muir H, Kwan MK, et al: Viscoelastic properties of proteoglycan solutions with varying proportions present as aggregates. *J Orthop Res* 1987;5:36-46.

74. Mow VC, Zhu W, Lai WM, et al: The influence of link protein stabilization on the viscometric properties of proteoglycan aggregate solutions. *Biochim Biophys Acta* 1989;992:201-208.

75. Maroudas A, Urban JPG: Swelling pressures of cartilaginous tissues, in Mourdas A, Holborrow EJ (eds): *Studies in Joint Disease.* Tunbridge Wells, England, Pitman Medical, 1980, pp 87-116.

76. Walker PS, Hajek JV: The load-bearing area in the knee joint. *J Biomech* 1972;5:581-589.

77. Wang CJ, Walker PS: Rotatory laxity of the human knee joint. *J Bone Joint Surg* 1974;56A:161-170.

78. Hayes WC, Bodine AJ: Flow-independent viscoelastic properties of articular cartilage matrix. *J Biomech* 1978;11:407-419.

79. Armstrong CG, Mow VC: Biomechanics of normal and osteoarthrotic articular cartilage, in Wilson PD, Straub LR (eds): *Clinical Trends in Orthopaedics.* New York, Thieme-Stratton, 1982, pp 189-197.

80. Linn FC, Sokoloff L: Movement and composition of interstitial fluid of cartilage. *Articular Rheum* 1965;8:481-494.

81. Maroudas A: Biophysical chemistry of cartilaginous tissues with special reference to solute and fluid transport. *Biorheology* 1975;12:233-248.

82. Mow VC, Lai WM: Recent developments in synovial joint biomechanics. *SIAM Rev* 1980;22:275.

83. Mow VC, Kuei SC, Lai WM, et al: Biphasic creep and stress relaxation of articular cartilage in compression: Theory and experiments. *J Biomech Eng* 1980;102:73-84.

84. Mow VC, Lai WM, Holmes MH: Advanced theoretical and experimental techniques in cartilage research, in Huiskes R, van Campen DH, de Wijn JR (eds): *Biomechanics: Principles and Applications.* The Hague, Martinus Nijhoff, 1982, pp 47-74.

85. McDevitt CA, Miller RR, Spindler KP: The cells and cell matrix interactions of the meniscus, in *Knee Meniscus: Basic and Clinical Foundations.* New York, Raven Press, 1992, pp 29-36.

86. Eyre DR, Wu JJ: Collagen of fibrocartilage: A Distinctive molecular phenotype in bovine meniscus. *FEBS Lett* 1983;158:265-270.

87. Mow VC, Ratcliffe A, Chern KY, et al: Structure and function relationships of the menisci of the knee, in Mow VC, Arnoczky SW, Jackson DW (eds): *Knee Meniscus: Basic and Clinical Foundations.* New York, Raven Press, 1992, pp 37-58.

88. Spilker RL, Donzelli PS: A biphasic finite element model of the meniscus for stress-strain analysis, in Mow VC, Arnoczky SW, Jackson DW (eds): *Knee Meniscus: Basic and Clinical Foundations.* New York, Raven Press, 1992, pp 91-106.

89. Lai WM, Hou JS, Mow VC: A triphasic theory for the swelling and deformational behaviors of articular cartilage. *J Biomech Eng* 1991;113:245-258.

90. Lai WM, Hou JS, Mow VC: A triphasic theory for cartilage swelling. *Proc Biomech Symp*, ASMA, AMD 1989;98:33-36.

91. Whipple RR, Wirth CR, Mow VC: Mechanical properties of the meniscus, in Spilker RL (ed): *Advances in Bioengineering*. New York, ASME, 1984, pp 32-33.

92. Spilker RL, Donzelli PS, Mow VC: A Transversely isotropic finite cement model of the meniscus. *J Biomech Eng*, in press.

93. Kapandji IA: *The Physiology of the Joints*. Edinburgh, Churchill Livingstone, 1970, vol II.

94. Grood ES, Suntay WJ: A joint coordinate system for the clinical description of three-dimensional motions: Application to the knee. *J Biomech Eng* 1983;105:136-144.

95. Blankevoort L, Huiskes R, de Lange A: The envelope of passive knee joint motion. *J Biomech* 1988;21:705-720.

96. Menschik A: The basic kinematic principle of the collateral ligaments, demonstrated on the knee joint, in Chapchal G (ed): *Injuries of the Ligaments and Their Repair: Hand—Knee—Foot*. Stuttgart, Georg Thieme, 1977, pp 9-16.

97. Menschik A. Mechanik des Kniegelenkes: II. Teil: Schlussrotation. *Z Orthop* 1975;113:388-400.

98. Menschik A: Mechanik des Kniegelenkes: Teil 3. Sailer, Wein, 1974.

99. Shapeero LG, Dye SF, Lipton MJ, et al: Functional dynamics of the knee joint by ultrafast, cine-CT. *Invest Radiol* 1988;23:118-123.

100. Müller W: *The Knee: Form, Function, and Ligament Reconstruction*. Berlin, Springer-Verlag, 1983, pp 8-115.

101. Menschik A: The basic kinematic principle of the collateral ligaments, demonstrated on the knee joint, in Chapchal G (ed): *Injuries of the Ligaments and Their Repairs: Hand—Knee—Foot*. Stuttgart, Georg Thieme, 1977, pp 9-16.

102. Brantigan OC, Voshell AF: The mechanics of the ligaments and menisci of the knee joint. *J Bone Joint Surg* 1941;23A:44-66.

103. DePalma AF: *Diseases of the Knee: Management in Medicine and Surgery*. Philadelphia, JB Lippincott, 1954, p 6.

104. Shaer H: *Der Meniskusschaden*. Leipzig, Georg Thieme, 1938, pp 10-15.

105. Bylski DI: *In situ* measurement of meniscal mechanics in human knee joints, thesis. Ann Arbor, University of Michigan, 1986.

106. Ghelman B: Meniscal tears of the knee: Evaluation by high-resolution CT combined with arthrography. *Radiology* 1985;157:23-27.

107. Passariello R, Trecco F, de Paulis F, et al: Meniscal lesions of the knee joint: CT diagnosis. *Radiology* 1985;157:29-34.

108. Thompson WO, Thaete FL, Fu FH, et al: Tibial meniscal dynamics using three-dimensional reconstruction of magnetic resonance images. *Am J Sports Med* 1991;19:210-216.

109. Fu F, Thompson WO: Motion of the meniscus during knee flexion, in Mow VC, Arnoczky SP, Jackson DW (eds): *Knee Meniscus: Basic and Clinical Foundations*. New York, Raven Press, 1992, pp 75-89.

110. Beltran J, Noto AM, Mosure JC, et al: The knee: Surface-coil MR imaging at 1.5 T1. *Radiology* 1986;159:747-751.

111. Burk DL Jr, Kanal E, Brunberg JA, et al: 1.5-T surface-coil MRI of the knee. *AJR* 1986;147:293-300.

112. Ruetsch H, Morscher E: Measurement of the rotatory stability of the knee joint, in Chapchal G (ed): *Injuries of the Ligaments and Their Repair*. Stuttgart, Georg Thieme, 1977, pp 116-122.

Chapter 10

Meniscal Repair

Kenneth E. DeHaven, MD
Steven P. Arnoczky, DVM

Introduction

Meniscal repair is not a new concept; Annandale[1] published the first report on this topic over a century ago. However, the significance of this event went unrecognized by the medical community. In the 1930s, King[2,3] reintroduced the concept of meniscal repair in his classic experimental studies demonstrating the functional significance of the menisci as well as the healing ability of meniscal lesions within the peripheral vascular border. At the same time, Palmar[4] advocated including the meniscus in repairs of severe injury, where the collateral ligaments were avulsed from the peripheral rim of the meniscus. This same approach and its efficacy were also reported somewhat later by Price and Allen.[5]

However, the concept of preservation and repair of the meniscus still did not achieve widespread application because of the common beliefs that meniscal tears would produce significant articular damage and were incapable of healing, and that total excision not only relieved the clinical symptoms but also gave the best chance for regeneration of a new meniscus.[6,7]

During the 1960s and 1970s and part of the 1980s, however, there was an increasing awareness of the importance of preserving the meniscus. Several laboratory studies more clearly defined the importance of the meniscus in force transmission,[8-17] stability,[18-25] and shock absorption.[26-29] During this same period, the frequently disappointing late clinical results of total meniscectomy were documented,[30-34] confirming Fairbanks' classic observations published in 1948.[35] In addition, there were reports of improved clinical results from partial, as compared with total, meniscectomy.[34,36-39]

Therefore, the next logical step became obvious: If preserving some of the meniscus was good, preserving all of it should produce even better results. Meniscal repair thus emerged as an increasingly accepted clinical approach during the 1970s and 1980s as open and arthroscopic repair techniques were developed. The concurrent

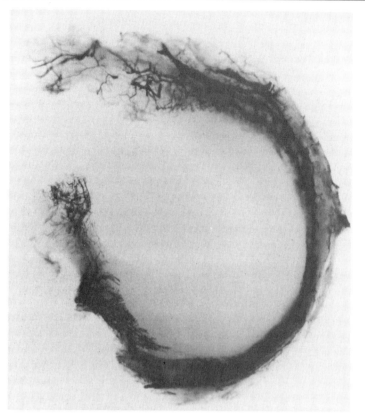

Fig. 1 *Superior aspect of a medial meniscus after vascular perfusion with India ink and tissue clearing with a modified Spalteholz technique. Note the vascularity at the periphery of the meniscus as well as the anterior and posterior attachments. (Reproduced with permission from Arnoczky SP, Warren RF: Microvasculature of the human meniscus.* Am J Sports Med *1982;10:90-95.)*

development and emergence of arthroscopy and arthroscopic surgery not only have paralleled but also have contributed significantly to meniscal repair. By providing precise diagnosis and frequently definitive therapy, along with decreased morbidity and improved cosmesis, arthroscopy has become an integral aspect of meniscal evaluation and treatment.

Basic Science of Meniscal Repair

While Thomas Annandale was credited with performing the first surgical repair of a torn meniscus in 1883,[1] it was not until 1936 when King[2] published his classic experiment on meniscal healing in dogs, that the actual biologic limitations of meniscal healing were presented. King demonstrated that in order for meniscal lesions to heal, they must be in contact with the peripheral blood supply.

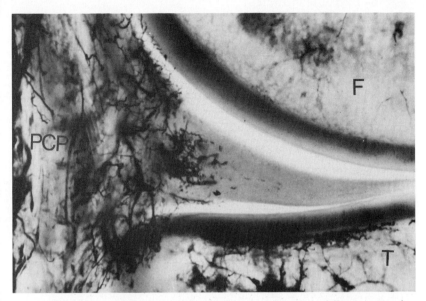

Fig. 2   *Frontal section of the medial compartment of the knee following vascular injection and tissue clearing. Branching radial vessels from the peromeniscal capillary plexus (PCP) penetrate the peripheral border of the medial meniscus. F = femur, T = tibia. (Reproduced with permission from Arnoczky SP, Warren RF: Microvasculature of the human meniscus. Am J Sports Med 1982;10:90-95.)*

Vascular Anatomy of the Meniscus

The vascular supply to the medial and lateral menisci of the knee originates predominantly from both the medial and lateral genicular arteries (both inferior and superior branches).[40] Branches from these vessels give rise to a perimeniscal capillary plexus within the synovial and capsular tissues of the knee joint. This plexus is an arborizing network of vessels that supplies the peripheral border of the meniscus about its attachments to the joint capsule (Fig. 1). These perimeniscal vessels are arranged in a predominantly circumferential pattern, with radial branches directed toward the center of the joint (Fig. 2). Anatomic studies have shown that the degrees of peripheral vascular penetration is 10% to 30% of the width of the medial meniscus, and 10% to 25% of the width of the lateral meniscus. The middle genicular vessel also supplies vessels to the menisci through the vascular synovial covering of the anterior and posterior horn attachments. These synovial vessels penetrate the horn attachments and give rise to smaller vessels that enter the meniscal horns for a short distance and end in terminal capillary loops.

A small portion of vascular synovial tissue also is present throughout the peripheral attachment of the medial and lateral menisci on both the femoral and tibial articular surfaces. This synovial fringe extends for a short distance over the articular surfaces of the menisci and does not contribute vessels to the meniscus itself, but greatly contributes to the reparative response of the meniscus.

Vascular Response to Injury

The vascular supply of the meniscus is an essential element in determining its potential for repair. Of equal importance is the ability of this blood supply to support the inflammatory response characteristic of wound repair. Clinical and experimental observations have demonstrated that the peripheral meniscal blood supply is capable of producing a reparative response similar to that observed in other connective tissues.[41-44]

Following injury within the peripheral vascular zone, a fibrin clot, rich in inflammatory cells, is formed. Vessels from the perimeniscal capillary plexus proliferate through this fibrin scaffold, accompanied by the proliferation of undifferentiated mesenchymal cells. Eventually, the lesion is filled with a cellular, fibrovascular scar tissue that glues the wound edges together and appears continuous with the adjacent normal meniscal fibrocartilage. Vessels from the perimeniscal capillary plexus, as well as a proliferative vascular pannus from the synovial fringe, penetrate the fibrous scar to provide a marked inflammatory response (Fig. 3).[41]

Experimental studies have shown that radial lesions of the meniscus extending to the synovium are completely healed with fibrovascular scar tissue by 10 weeks (Fig. 4).[41] The development of this scar into normal-appearing fibrocartilage, however, takes several months. It should be stressed that the initial strength of this repair tissue, as compared with the normal meniscus, is thought to be minimal.[44] Further studies are required to determine the biomechanical properties of this repair tissue.

When examining injured menisci for potential repair, lesions are often classified by the location of the tear relative to the blood supply of the meniscus and the vascular appearance of the peripheral and central surfaces of the tear. The so-called RED-RED tear (peripheral capsular detachment) has a functional blood supply on the capsular and meniscal side of the lesion and obviously has the best prognosis for healing. The RED-WHITE tear (meniscal rim tear through the peripheral vascular zone) has an active peripheral blood supply, while the central (inner) surface of the lesion is devoid of functional vessels (Fig. 5). Theoretically, these lesions should have sufficient vascularity to heal by the aforementioned fibrovascular proliferation. The WHITE-WHITE tears (meniscal lesion completely in the avascular zone) have no blood supply and cannot heal.[2,43]

Although meniscal repair has generally been limited to the peripheral vascular area of the meniscus (RED-RED and RED-WHITE tears), a significant number of lesions occur in the central, avascular portion of the meniscus (WHITE-WHITE tears). Experimental and clinical observations have shown that these lesions are incapable of healing and have thereby provided the rationale for partial meniscectomy.[2,41,43] In an effort to extend the level of repair into these avascular areas, techniques have been explored that provide vascu-

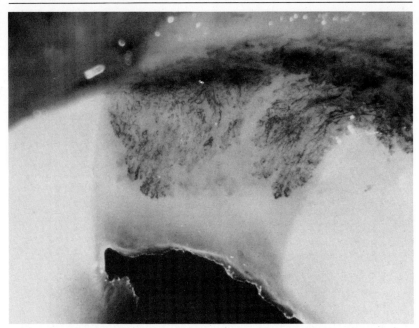

Fig. 3   *A healing radial tear in the medial meniscus of a dog six weeks following injury. The lesion is healing with fibrovascular scar tissue. Note the proliferative vascular pannus from the synovial fringe over the surface of the repair. (Reproduced with permission from Arnoczky SP, Warren RF: Microvasculature of the human meniscus.* Am J Sports Med *1982;10:90-95.)*

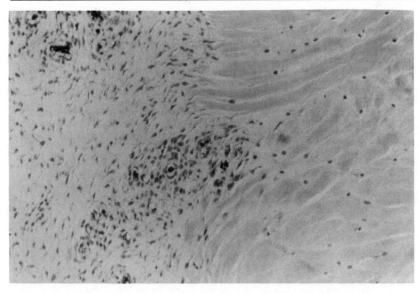

Fig. 4   *Photomicrograph of a healing dog meniscus at the junction of the fibrovascular scar and the normal adjacent meniscal tissue (hematoxylin-eosin, x 100). (Reproduced with permission from Arnoczky SP, Warren RF: Microvasculature of the human meniscus.* Am J Sports Med *1982;10:90-95.)*

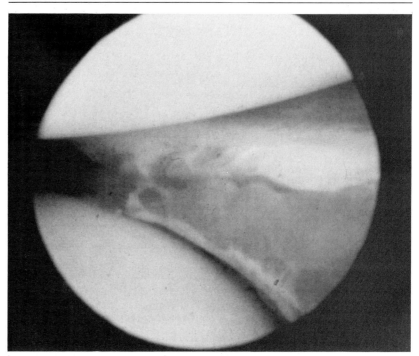

Fig. 5   *Arthroscopic view of a peripheral tear of a human meniscus. Note the vascular granulation tissue present at the margin of the lesion. This would be classified as a RED-WHITE tear. Also note the proliferation of the synovial fringe over the femoral surface of the meniscus. (Reproduced with permission from Arnoczky SP, Torzilli PA: Cartilage biology, in Hunte LY, Funk FJ Jr (eds):* Rehabilitation of the Injured Athlete. *St. Louis, CV Mosby, 1984, pp 148-209.)*

larity to the WHITE-WHITE tears. These techniques include vascular access channels and synovial abrasion.[41,45]

Results of experimental studies have indicated that if a lesion in the avascular portion of the meniscus is connected to the peripheral blood supply via a vascular access channel, these lesions can heal normally.[2,41,42] However, because the creation of a large enough vascular access channel may disrupt the normal peripheral architecture of the meniscus, other methods of vascular ingrowth have been proposed.[46] These include the creation of vascular tunnels, pedicle grafts of synovium, and synovial abrasion.[45,46] The latter technique involves the stimulation of the synovial fringe on both the femoral and tibial articular surfaces of the meniscus.[45] This is intended to produce a vascular pannus that will migrate into the lesion and hopefully support a reparative response. Results from an experimental study have demonstrated that an exogenous fibrin clot placed into a stable lesion in the avascular portion of the meniscus can support a reparative response similar to that observed in the vascular area.[47] The clot provides potent chemotactic and mitogenic stimuli as well as a scaffold on which the cellular response is supported.[47] This technique may allow the repair of avascular lesions anywhere in the meniscus or optimize the repair of lesions in areas of marginal vascularity. Clinical studies are currently underway to determine the applicability of this repair technique.

Indications for Meniscal Repair

It is clinically useful to classify meniscal tears as either definitely suitable or questionably suitable for repair. Traumatic tears at or near the meniscosynovial junction that have not suffered major structural damage have proved to be definitely suitable for repair. These tears are typically vertical and longitudinal, greater than 8 mm in length, and located in the vascular zone[40,48] and where peripheral circumferential fibers remain in continuity within the body of the meniscus. Retears of previously repaired menisci that still meet these criteria are also suitable. Tears whose reparability is questionable include those within the avascular zone of the meniscus or where the vascularity is in doubt, those in which the body of the meniscus has been damaged, and those with disruption of all the peripheral circumferential fibers.

For lesions definitely suitable for repair, time since injury is not an important factor and can be ignored if the other criteria are successfully met. For tears classified as definitely suitable, healing enhancement techniques such as synovial abrasion, vascular access channels, or fibrin clot insertion do not appear to be necessary. However, when considering repair of questionably suitable lesions, one or more of these healing enhancement techniques should be used.

It is advantageous for both the surgeon and the patient to recognize potentially reparable meniscal tears before surgery so that both can be prepared for a possible surgical procedure that is more extensive and has different requirements for postoperative care than arthroscopic partial meniscectomy. This is particularly important in cases that do not encompass concomitant ligamentous procedures.

Preoperative data that can indicate the existence of a potentially reparable lesion include the patient's clinical profile and results from preoperative diagnostic studies. Those undergoing meniscal repair are typically young (12 to 45 years of age, average age is 21) and physically active with frequently associated anterior cruciate ligament tears (80%). Both medial and lateral menisci are involved (repair ratio is three medial to two lateral).[49]

With preoperative diagnostic studies, double contrast arthrography can be helpful by demonstrating a vertical tear at or near the periphery with little or no staining of the meniscal body (Figs. 6 and 7). Arthrography is particularly helpful for chronic cases involving the medial meniscus, but is much less accurate for the posterior peripheral zone of the lateral meniscus in chronic cases and less accurate for both menisci in acute cases. Reparable meniscal lesions can be seen with magnetic resonance imaging (MRI), but the role

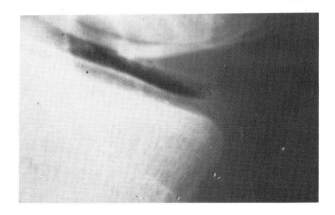

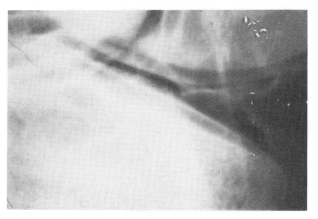

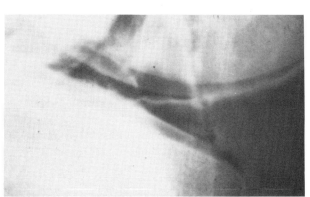

Fig. 6 *The posteromedial view of a double-contrast arthrogram demonstrating a posterior peripheral tear of the medial meniscus with no staining of the meniscal body. (Reproduced with permission from DeHaven KE, Black KP, Griffiths HJ: Open meniscus repair: Technique and two to nine year results. Am J Sports Med 1989;17: 788-795.)*

of MRI in routinely identifying reparable menisci is continuing to evolve and, at present, peripheral tears can be difficult to image.

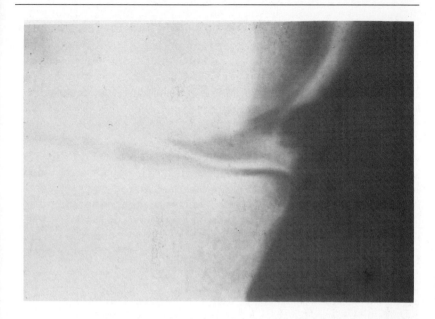

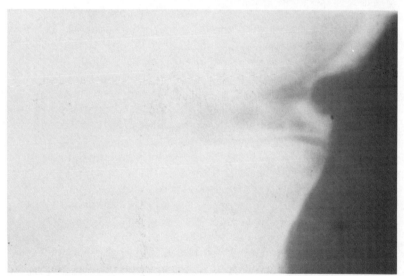

Fig. 7   *The arthrographic view of the posterior portion of the medial meniscus of another case that also demonstrates a posterior peripheral tear, but in addition has extensive staining of the meniscal body with contrast media indicating significant degeneration. (Reproduced with permission from DeHaven KE, Black KP, Griffiths HJ: Open meniscus repair: Technique and two to nine year results. Am J Sports Med 1989;17: 788-795.)*

Although preoperative information from patient profiling and diagnostic studies can identify potentially reparable tears, the final decision is based on arthroscopic evaluation. This includes careful visualization and probing to determine the exact type and length of the tear as well as its relative location to the meniscosynovial junction and whether or not it is stable. Instability is definitely present if the inner segment of the meniscus can be readily displaced. However, a peripheral tear in a tight compartment may not be readily displaced without risking damage to the meniscal body fragment. In such circumstances the length of the tear should be the determining factor (with 7 mm or longer considered unstable and less than 7 mm considered stable). These determinations require careful visualization and probing from anterior approaches, as well as posterior visualization whenever necessary to define the situation (routinely for the medial compartment of the meniscus and in selective instances for the lateral compartment). Whenever a tight compartment inhibits complete visualization of the location of the tear from an anterior approach, the ability to visualize the tear posteriorly confirms that it is sufficiently peripheral to be repaired by either open or arthroscopic techniques. However, if the tear is not easily visualized from a posterior approach, but is still considered to be reparable, an arthroscopic technique should be used.

Another essential selection factor is whether the tear is in the vascular or avascular zone of the meniscus. Bleeding at the surface of the tear is definite evidence of vascularity, and obviously an inflated pneumatic tourniquet should not be used. Conversely, an absence of bleeding at the surface of the tear is not a definitive factor because the distension pressure of the irrigating fluid can be sufficient to occlude fine capillary circulation. In the absence of bleeding, clinical judgment must be based on the location of the tear relative to the meniscosynovial junction. Based on anatomic studies,[40,41] if the tear is within 3 mm of the meniscosynovial junction, it can be considered to be vascular, while the vascularity of lesions between 3 and 5 mm is variable, and lesions greater than 5 mm are avascular. The age of the patient should also be considered, because vascular penetration has been shown to be greater in children.[50] However, it has been shown that the adult vascular pattern is already established in adolescents.[51]

The other major issue in considering suitability for repair is the extent of damage of the meniscus. Successful repair is more likely in menisci with little or no obvious damage, while menisci with extensive damage seem unlikely to provide normal mechanical function even if successful healing could be achieved. At present, no specific guidelines have been established to assist the surgeon in deciding whether or not to attempt repair of menisci with moderate degrees of structural damage.

Surgical Techniques

Principles Common to All Techniques

Certain important principles are common to all successful repair techniques. The first is a correct understanding of the nature and location of the tear by careful arthroscopic examination. The second is the use of posterior incisions to retract and protect important neurovascular structures during the repair of lesions in the posterior third of the medial or lateral meniscus. A third common element is the preparation of the meniscal rim and capsular bed. All unstable tags of tissue should be debrided from the meniscal rim and from the capsular bed. It should be emphasized, however, that stable meniscal tissue still attached to the capsule should not be removed. The fourth common principle is to freshen the surfaces of the meniscal rim and the capsular bed (including any attached portion of stable meniscal rim) with a rasp or curette. This insures vascularity on the capsular side of the repair for definitely suitable lesions, and seems to increase successful healing to the meniscal rim. The final common principle is to place as many sutures as necessary to make fixation as secure and as anatomic as possible.

Open Techniques

Open techniques for repair of peripheral meniscal lesions not associated with collateral ligament injuries, and including both acute and chronic lesions, were developed in the mid to late 1970s by DeHaven,[52] Cassidy and Shaffer,[53] Hamberg and associates,[54] and Dolan.[55] These open techniques are suitable for vertical, longitudinal tears (within 2 mm of the meniscosynovial junction) that are localized to the posterior or anterior thirds of either meniscus. Open repair is possible in tears localized to the central third (rare) or extending into the central third from anterior or posterior third lesions (more common), but extensive exposures are required, which could damage the medial or lateral collateral ligaments.

Arthroscopic Techniques

Although Ikeuchi performed the first arthroscopic meniscal repair in Tokyo in 1969,[56] orthopaedic surgeons did not take notice of this technique until Henning pioneered arthroscopic meniscal repair in the United States in 1980.[57,58] Since then, a number of individual contributions have been made.[59-69] Two basic types of arthroscopic repair have evolved, the "inside-out" techniques and the "outside-in" techniques. The "inside-out" techniques were pioneered by Henning with subsequent contributions by Clancy and Graf,[59] Rosenberg and associates,[63] and Cannon,[66] while "outside-in" techniques have been described by Johnson,[60] Warren,[62] and Morgan and Casscells.[64]

Because arthroscopic techniques permit repair of meniscal lesions that are not strictly peripheral, and which are in areas of questionable vascularity or even in the avascular zone, it is important to consider using one or more of the healing enhancement techniques such as synovial abrasion,[46] vascular access channels,[41] or fibrin clot insertion.[47] Arthroscopic surgical procedures generally have significant advantages over open techniques because of improved cosmesis (small incisions) and more rapid rehabilitation times. For meniscal repair, these advantages are negated by the need to make posterior skin incisions to prevent neurovascular complications in the posterior third repair cases and the need to delay complete rehabilitation until the healing tissue has had time for maturation. The most important advantages of arthroscopic versus open repair are the ability to repair nonperipheral tears and to treat tears of extensive length without large surgical exposures. In addition, some surgeons find the arthroscopic techniques easier to perform than the open procedures.

Postoperative Care

Important postoperative care principles for meniscal repair are (1) to provide sufficient protection during the early healing phase, and (2) to allow time for sufficient maturation of the healing response before subjecting repaired menisci to significant stresses. Initially, knees were immobilized for four to six weeks following meniscal repair, but it has been observed that limited knee motion can be permitted without adversely affecting healing rates, and most authors are permitting restricted motion (up to 80 or 90 degrees) during the first few weeks, followed by unrestricted motion.

Early weightbearing stresses were believed to be deleterious to meniscal healing. Although we have gradually liberalized range of motion following meniscus repair, the use of crutches, with minimal, partial weightbearing, is still being recommended during the first six weeks after surgery. Laboratory studies by Newman (A. Newman, unpublished data, 1990) indicate that weightbearing restrictions may not be necessary for all types of meniscal tears. Additional studies are needed to further delineate the timing and extent of weightbearing following meniscal repair.

To allow for maturation of the healing response, it is recommended that strenuous running and agility and contact stresses be avoided for at least six months following meniscal repair. However, between three and six months following repair, limited stresses such as swimming, cycling, use of a cross country ski simulator and rowing machine, and straight-line jogging can be safely undertaken if there is adequate knee motion and muscle strength.

Results

The early results of both open and arthroscopic repair have been promising, with several authors reporting healing rates of 80% or higher for tears within the vascular zone of the meniscus[49,52-55,58,63,70-72] (Figs. 8 and 9). Decreased healing rates have been reported with repair of tears increasingly distal to the meniscosynovial junction.[57,58,68] Successful healing rates of 80% to 98% have been found after repair of tears 0 to 2 mm from the meniscosynovial junction,

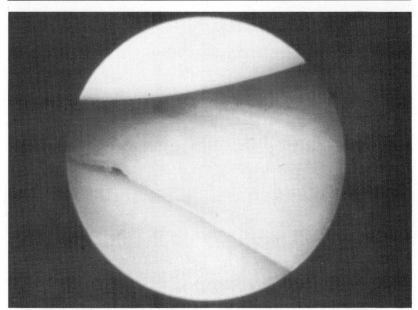

Fig. 8   *Arthroscopic appearance of repaired medial meniscus at 18 months, demonstrating excellent healing of the site of repair, and normal articular surfaces. (Reproduced with permission from DeHaven KE, Black KP, Griffiths HJ: Open meniscus repair: Technique and two to nine year results. Am J Sports Med 1989;17:788-795.)*

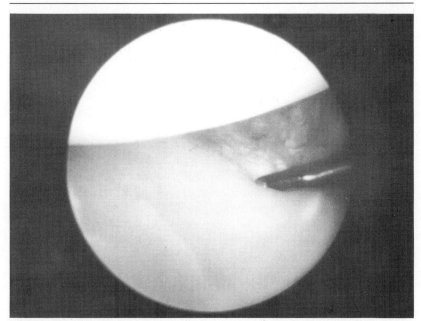

Fig. 9   *Close-up arthroscopic view of the repair site. (Reproduced with permission from DeHaven KE, Black KP, Griffiths HJ: Open meniscus repair: Technique and two to nine year results. Am J Sports Med 1989;17:788-795.)*

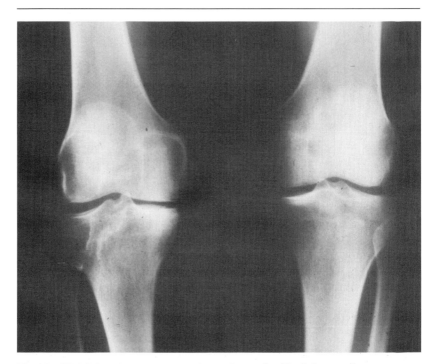

Fig. 10 *Weightbearing anteroposterior radiograph of both knees of a soccer player 7 years after anterior cruciate ligament reconstruction, partial medial meniscectomy with medial compartment narrowing, and repair of the lateral meniscus with normal lateral compartment. (Reproduced with permission from DeHaven KE, Black KP, Griffiths HJ: Open meniscus repair: Technique and two to nine year results.* Am J Sports Med *1989;17: 788-795.)*

decreasing to 65% to 79% following repairs in the 3- to 6-mm zone. Henning and associates[72] and Cannon (unpublished data, 1991) documented increased healing rates in the meniscus with synovial rasping and by adding fibrin clot to repairs in the 4- to 6-mm zone.

Investigators of the impact of tear length have reported different results. Cannon[68] reported an increased failure rate for tears over 4 cm in length, while Buseck and Noyes[71] found no difference between tears less than or greater than 2.5 cm in length. Differing results have also been reported for the effect of the age of patients at the time of repair. Buseck and Noyes[71] found no difference in failure rates for those over or under the age of 25, while Cannon[68] reported increased failure rates in patients 10 to 18 years of age.

Longer term results are available only for open repair of peripheral tears. In an average five-year follow-up study, DeHaven and associates[49] reported an 89% survival of repaired menisci, an increased incidence of retear in unstable knees (38% versus 5% in stable knees), and radiographic absence of degenerative joint changes (Fig. 10). Sommerlath and Gillquist[73] have reported similar clinical results in a seven-year follow-up study. A long-term (minimum 10 years) follow-up study (K. E. DeHaven, W. Lohrer, J. E. Lovelock, unpublished data, 1991) has documented a 79% survival rate of repaired menisci, has reconfirmed the increased incidence of meniscal retears in unstable knees (42% versus 11% in stable knees) and provides even more compelling radiographic evidence for bio-mechanical function of successful repairs. Eighty-five percent of patients with successful repairs had normal weightbearing radiographs (in extension and at 45 degrees of flexion) compared with only 43% of patients with retears who had undergone partial meniscectomy.

Although complex meniscal tears, with extensive damage to the meniscal body and complete disruption of the peripheral circumferential fibers, have reportedly healed with varying degrees of success after arthroscopic repair, there are no data at this time to indicate whether or not these healed menisci are capable of normal function.

References

1. Annandale T: An operation for displaced semilunar cartilage. *Br Med J* 1885;1:779.
2. King D: The healing of semilunar cartilages. *J Bone Joint Surg* 1936;18A:333-342.
3. King D: The function of semilunar cartilages. *J Bone Joint Surg* 1936:18A:1069-1076.
4. Palmar I: On the injuries to the ligaments of the knee joint: A clinical study. *Acta Chir Scand Suppl* 1938;81:1-282.
5. Price CT, Allen WC: Ligament repair in the knee with preservation of the meniscus. *J Bone Joint Surg* 1978;60A:61-65.
6. Smillie IS: *Injuries of the Knee Joint*. London, Churchill Livingstone, 1970.
7. Smillie IS: *Injuries of the Knee Joint*, ed 5. New York, Churchill Livingstone, 1978, pp 71-188.
8. Ahmed AM, Burke DL: In-vitro measurement of static pressure distribution in synovial joints: Part I: Tibial surface of the knee. *J Biomech Eng* 1983;105:216-225.
9. Bourne RB, Finlay JB, Papadopoulos P, et al: The effect of medial meniscectomy on strain distribution in the proximal part of the tibia. *J Bone Joint Surg* 1984;66A:1431-1437.
10. Bullough PG, Munuera L, Murphy J, et al: The strength of the menisci of the knee as it relates to their fine structure. *J Bone Joint Surg* 1970;52B:564-570.
11. Armstrong CG, Mow VC: Variations in the intrinsic mechanical properties of human articular cartilage with age, degeneration, and water content. *J Bone Joint Surg* 1982;64A:88-94.
12. Fukubayashi T, Kurosawa H: The contact area and pressure distribution pattern of the knee: A study of normal and osteoarthrotic knee joints. *Acta Orthop Scand* 1980;51:871-879.
13. Kettelkamp DB, Jacobs AW: Tibiofemoral contact area: Determination and implications. *J Bone Joint Surg* 1972;54A:349-356.
14. Mathur PD, McDonald JR, Gormley RK: A study of the tensile strength of the menisci of the knee. *J Bone Joint Surg* 1949;31A:650-654.
15. Shrive NG, Phil D, O'Connor JJ, et al: Load-bearing in the knee joint. *Clin Orthop* 1978;131:279-287.

16. Walker PS, Erkman MJ: The role of the menisci in force transmission across the knee. *Clin Orthop* 1975;109:184-192.

17. Whipple RR, Wirth CR, Mow VC: Anisotrophic and zonal variations in the tensile properties of the meniscus. *Trans Orthop Res Soc* 1985;10:367.

18. Fukubayashi T, Torzilli PA, Sherman MF, et al: An *in vitro* biomechanical evaluation of anterior-posterior motion of the knee: Tibial displacement, rotation, and torque. *J Bone Joint Surg* 1982;64A:258-264.

19. Hsieh H-H, Walker PS: Stabilizing mechanisms of the loaded and unloaded knee joint. *J Bone Joint Surg* 1976;58A:87-93.

20. Levy IM, Torzilli PA, Warren RF: The effect of medial meniscectomy on anterior-posterior motion of the knee. *J Bone Joint Surg* 1982;64A:883-888.

21. Markolf KL, Bargar WL, Shoemaker SC, et al: The role of joint load in knee stability. *J Bone Joint Surg* 1981;63A:570-585.

22. Markolf KL, Mensch JS, Amstutz HC: Stiffness and laxity of the knee: The contributions of the supporting structures: A quantitative *in vitro* study. *J Bone Joint Surg* 1976;58A:583-594.

23. Shoemaker SC, Markolf KL: The role of the meniscus in the anterior-posterior stability of the loaded anterior cruciate-deficient knee. *J Bone Joint Surg* 1986;68A:71-79.

24. Oretorp N, Gillquist J, Liljedahl SO: Long term results of surgery for non-acute anteromedial rotatory instability of the knee. *Acta Orthop Scand* 1979;50:329-336.

25. Wang C-J, Walker PS: Rotatory laxity of the human knee joint. *J Bone Joint Surg* 1974;56A:161-170.

26. Krause WR, Pope MH, Johnson RJ, et al: Mechanical changes in the knee after meniscectomy. *J Bone Joint Surg* 1976;58A:599-604.

27. Kurosawa H, Fukubayashi T, Nakajima H: Load-bearing mode of the knee joint: Physical behavior of the knee joint with or without menisci. *Clin Orthop* 1980;149:283-290.

28. Seedholm HB, Hargreaves DJ: Transmission of the load in the knee joint with special reference to the role of the menisci. *Eng Med* 1979;8:220-228.

29. Voloshin AS, Wosk J: Shock absorption of meniscectomized and painful knees: A comparative in vivo study. *J Biomed Eng* 1983;5:157-161.

30. Cox JS, Nye CE, Schaefer WW, et al: The degenerative effects of partial and total resection of the medial meniscus in dogs' knees. *Clin Orthop* 1975;109:178-183.

31. Huckell JR: Is meniscectomy a benign procedure?: A long-term follow-up study. *Can J Surg* 1965;8:254-260.

32. Jones RE, Smith EC, Reisch JS: Effects of medial meniscectomy in patients older than forty years. *J Bone Joint Surg* 1978;60A:783-786.

33. Moskowitz RW, Davis W, Sammarco J, et al: Experimentally induced degenerative joint lesions following partial meniscectomy in the rabbit. *Arthritis Rheum* 1973;16:397-405.

34. Tapper EM, Hoover NW: Late results after meniscectomy. *J Bone Joint Surg* 1969;51A:517-526, 600, 603.

35. Fairbank TJ: Knee joint changes after meniscectomy. *J Bone Joint Surg* 1948;30B:664-670.

36. O'Connor RL: *Arthroscopy*. Philadelphia, JB Lippincott,1977, pp 43-71.

37. Jackson RW, Dandy DJ: Partial meniscectomy. *J Bone Joint Surg* 1976;58B:142.

38. McGinty JB, Geuss LF, Marvin RA: Partial or total meniscectomy. *J Bone Joint Surg* 1977;59A:763-766.

39. Metcalf RW, Coward DB, Rosenberg TD: Arthroscopic partial meniscectomy: A five year follow-up study. *Orthop Trans* 1983;7:504.

40. Arnoczky SP, Warren RF: Microvasculature of the human meniscus. *Am J Sports Med* 1982;10:90-95.

41. Arnoczky SP, Warren RF: The microvasculature of the meniscus and its response to injury: An experimental study in the dog. *Am J Sports Med* 1983;11:131-141.

42. Cabaud HE, Rodkey WG, Fitzwater JE: Medial meniscus repairs: An experimental and morphologic study. *Am J Sports Med* 1981;9:129-134.

43. Arnoczky SP: Meniscus healing. *Contemp Orthop* 1985;10:31-39.

44. Arnoczky SP, Cooper DE: Meniscal repair, in Goldberg VM (ed): *Controversies of Total Knee Arthroplasty*. New York, Raven Press, 1991, pp 291-302.

45. Henning CE, Lynch MA, Clark JR: Vascularity for healing of meniscus repairs. *Arthroscopy* 1987;3:13-18.

46. Gershuni DH, Skyhar MJ, Danzig LA, et al: Experimental models to promote healing of tears in the avascular segment of canine knee menisci. *J Bone Joint Surg* 1989;71A:1363-1370.

47. Arnoczky SP, Warren RF, Spivak JM: Meniscal repair using an exogenous fibrin clot: An experimental study in dogs. *J Bone Joint Surg* 1988;70A:1209-1217.

48. Scapinelli R: Studies on the vasculature of the human knee joint. *Acta Anat (Basel)* 1968;70:305-331.

49. DeHaven KE, Black KP, Griffiths HJ: Open meniscus repair: Technique and two to nine year results. *Am J Sports Med* 1989;17: 788-795.

50. Clark CR, Ogden JA: Development of the menisci of the human knee joint. *J Bone Joint Surg* 1983;65A:538-547.

51. Arnoczky SP: Gross and vascular anatomy of the meniscus and its role in meniscal healing, regeneration and remodeling, in Mow VC, Arnoczky SP, Jackson DW (eds): *Knee Meniscus: Basic and Clinical Foundations*. New York, Raven Press, 1992, pp 1-14.

52. DeHaven KE: Peripheral meniscus repair: An alternative to meniscectomy. *J Bone Joint Surg* 1981;63B:463.

53. Cassidy RE, Shaffer AJ: Repair of peripheral meniscus tears: A preliminary report. *Am J Sports Med* 1981;9:209-214.

54. Hamberg P, Gillquist J, Lysholm J: Suture of new and old peripheral meniscus tears. *J Bone Joint Surg* 1983;65A:193-197.

55. Dolan WA, Bhaskar G: Peripheral meniscus repair: A clinical pathological study of 75 cases. *Orthop Trans* 1983;7:503-504.

56. Ikeuchi H: Surgery under arthroscopic control. *Proceedings of the Societe Internationale d'Arthroscopie* 1975:57-62.

57. Henning CE: Arthroscopic repair of meniscal tears. *Orthopedics* 1983;6:1130-1132.

58. Scott GA, Jolly BL, Henning CE: Combined posterior incision and arthroscopic intra-articular repair of the meniscus: An examination of factors affecting healing. *J Bone Joint Surg* 1986;68A:847-861.

59. Clancy WG, Graf BK: Arthroscopic meniscal repair. *Orthopedics* 1983;6:1125-1128.

60. Johnson LL: Meniscus mender II, in Johnson LL (ed): *Technical Bulletin*. Okemos, MI, Instrument Makar, Inc, 1988.

61. Barber FA, Stone RG: Meniscal repair: An arthroscopic technique. *J Bone Joint Surg* 1985;67B:39-41.

62. Warren RF: Arthroscopic meniscus repair. *Arthroscopy* 1985;1:170-172.

63. Rosenberg T, Scott S, Paulos L: Arthroscopic surgery: Repair of peripheral detachment of the meniscus. *Contemp Orthop* 1985;10:43-50.

64. Morgan CD, Casscells SW: Arthroscopic meniscus repair: A safe approach to the posterior horns. *Arthroscopy* 1986;2:3-12.

65. Hanks GA, Gause TM, Sebastianelli WJ, et al: Repair of peripheral meniscal tears: Open versus arthroscopic technique. *Arthroscopy* 1991;7:72-77.

66. Cannon WD: Arthroscopic meniscal repair as related to ligamentous instability. Presented at the American College of Surgeons Meeting, San Francisco, CA, October 1984.

67. Rosenberg TD, Scott SM, Coward DB, et al: Arthroscopic meniscal repair evaluated with repeat arthroscopy. *Arthroscopy* 1986;2:14-20.

68. Cannon WD: Arthroscopic meniscus repair, in McGinty J (ed): *Operative Arthroscopy*. New York, Raven Press, 1991, pp 237-251.

69. Johnson LL: *Arthroscopic Surgery: Principles and Practice*, ed 3. St. Louis, CV Mosby, 1986, vol 2, pp 1032-1037.

70. DeHaven KE: Meniscus repair in the athlete. *Clin Orthop* 1985;198:31-35.

71. Buseck MS, Noyes FR: Arthroscopic evaluation of meniscal repairs after anterior cruciate ligament reconstruction and immediate motion. *Am J Sports Med* 1991;19:489-494.

72. Henning CE, Clark JR, Lynch MA, et al: Arthroscopic meniscus repair with a posterior incision, in Bassett FH III (ed): American Academy of Orthopaedic Surgeons *Instructional Course Lectures, XXXVII.* Park Ridge, IL, American Academy of Orthopaedic Surgeons, 1988, pp 209-221.

73. Sommerlath K, Gillquist J: Knee function after meniscus repair and total meniscectomy: A 7-year follow-up study. *Arthroscopy* 1987;3:166-169.

Chapter 11

Meniscal Allografts

Steven P. Arnoczky, DVM

Introduction

The importance of menisci to the adequate function of the knee joint has been well documented, providing the impetus for preserving these structures whenever possible.[1-12] Although meniscal repair has become an accepted method of treatment for selected meniscal injuries, it is not applicable in every instance; partial or total meniscectomy may still be necessary. However, because of the deleterious effects of total meniscectomy on the knee joint, an alternative to total removal is being sought. One alternative would be to replace the meniscus with an allograft. Successful transplantation of a meniscal allograft, which maintains the structure, physiology, and function of the joint, may be a potential method of replacing a severely damaged meniscus and, thereby, eliminate, or at least minimize, the degenerative changes that accompany meniscectomy (Fig. 1).[1] This chapter reviews the experimental and clinical information available on the use of meniscal allografts.

Basic Science Considerations

Allograft tissues such as bone, articular cartilage, and fascia have been used in orthopaedic surgery for many years.[13-28] When allograft tissues are used as replacement materials, several factors must be considered, including (1) the potential antigenicity of the graft; (2) the method of preservation and/or secondary sterilization; and (3) the ability of the graft to maintain (or reestablish) its viability, normal biology, and normal material and functional properties within the host environment. Although a substantial amount of information is available regarding these considerations in bone and articular cartilage, experimental and clinical investigations have been undertaken only recently to explore these parameters with regard to meniscal transplantation.

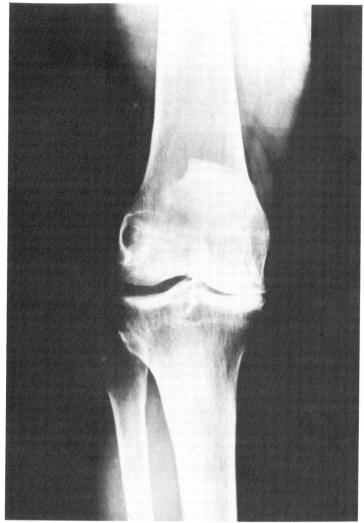

Fig. 1   *Radiograph of a knee illustrating the degenerative changes within the medial joint compartment secondary to medial meniscectomy. (Reproduced with permission from Arnoczky SP, Cooper DE: Meniscal repair, in Goldberg VM (ed):* Controversies of Total Knee Arthroplasty. *New York, Raven Press, 1991, pp 291-302).*

Antigenicity

Meniscal tissue, like articular cartilage, is thought to be an "immunologically privileged" tissue because the meniscal cells, which harbor the major histocompatibility antigens on their surface, are isolated from the host's immune system by a dense extracellular matrix.[17,24] Results of clinical and experimental studies in which fresh menisci were used alone and as components of fresh osteochondral allografts have not indicated any evidence of rejection or immunogenic response.[29-32] In addition, processed (cryopreserved, fresh-frozen, or freeze-dried) meniscal allografts did not exhibit signs of an immune response at any time after surgery.[29,31-40] However, this assessment has been limited to gross and histologic evaluation. In a study of dogs receiving anterior cruciate ligaments, antidonor leukocyte antigens were found in the synovial fluid.[28] Because there was no gross, histologic, or serologic evidence of an immune response in these animals, the effects of these local antigens are unknown. However, their presence suggests that a more critical evaluation of meniscal allografts may be necessary before the allografts' immunologic potential can be fully appreciated.

Preservation

The methods of preserving meniscal tissue are essentially the same as those for other connective tissues and include controlled-rate freezing (cryopreservation), deep-freezing, and freeze-drying (lyophilization). While results from experimental and clinical investigations have suggested that fresh menisci can be successfully used as allografts, the logistics involved in performing such transplants are substantial. These logistics include locating and preparing an appropriate recipient and performing the harvest and implantation within 12 to 18 hours. In addition, the inability to adequately screen donors for transmittable diseases within this time period may further limit the applicability of fresh-allograft implantation. Long-term preservation of meniscal allografts would allow for more complete donor screening and a potentially larger bank of meniscal sizes from which to choose.

Although these limitations exist, one possible advantage to using fresh meniscal tissue is its ability to maintain cell viability at the time of transplantation. This concept is based on the change noted in the material properties of nonviable articular cartilage after transplantation.[41,42] The desire to maintain cell viability while allowing long-term storage of tissue has led physicians to develop cryopreservation techniques that can insure cell viability after storage.

Cryopreservation techniques use a cryoprotective agent such as dimethyl sulfoxide (DMSO) or glycerol and a slow freezing rate to protect and maintain cell membrane integrity (and thus cell viability) throughout the freezing cycle. The effects of cryopreservation on meniscal tissue have been examined in several studies.[29,34,35,39,43] In one such study, Arnoczky and associates[43] demonstrated that by using DMSO and a controlled-rate freezing scheme developed for articular cartilage, 10% of the meniscal cells could remain viable after two weeks of storage. Cell viability was determined by autoradiographic evidence of S^{35} incorporation into the living cells. This viability decreased with storage time; after twelve weeks, only 3% of the cells remained viable.[43] Milton and associates,[39] using a proprietary cryopreservation technique, and Jackson and associates,[29] using a modification of the previously mentioned technique, found a 40% and 30% cell viability rate, respectively, following processing.

However, these counts were based on indirect measurements and may be artificially elevated.

Although methods of optimizing meniscal cell viability following storage are under investigation, DNA probes were used in a recent study to examine the fate of these living cells at various times after transplantation. No evidence was found of donor cells within the allograft meniscus 8 weeks after transplantation (D. W. Jackson, personal communication, 1991). The inability of the donor cells to survive in the host environment challenges the rationale of transplanting viable meniscal cells. In addition, the loss of donor cells after such a relatively short time within the host environment may reflect a cytotoxic process associated with an occult immunologic response. Obviously, more study is needed in this area to determine the role of donor cell viability in the ultimate fate of meniscal allografts.

Unlike controlled-rate freezing, deep-freezing and freeze-drying effectively kill all the cells within the donor tissue. While these preservation techniques allow the meniscus to be stored for longer periods of time, they also permit the use of secondary sterilization techniques on the tissue. Although all tissue harvesting should be done under sterile conditions, delays in procurement or questions about the health status of the donor may necessitate sterilization of the meniscus. The two most common methods of secondary sterilization are with ethylene oxide and gamma irradiation.

Ethylene oxide has been used to sterilize other connective tissues such as bone, fascia lata, and tendon. It is most commonly used in association with freeze-drying preservation techniques. Freeze-dried fascial and patellar tendon grafts sterilized with ethylene oxide have been used to reconstruct anterior cruciate ligaments; however, an increased incidence of joint effusions following their use and the presence of ethylene oxide biproducts in the joints has raised many questions regarding this sterilization technique.[44]

Gamma irradiation uses low doses of radiation from cobalt 60 to sterilize tissues. Although precise procedures and dosages have been established to assure the bactericidal action of gamma irradiation, its reliability in killing the human immunodeficiency virus without adversely affecting the material properties of the tissue is still questionable.

While deep-freezing alone or with gamma irradiation does not alter the material properties of the meniscus (modulus, tensile strength), the effect of freeze-drying and/or ethylene oxide sterilization on these parameters has not been evaluated.

Experimental studies have also been undertaken to investigate the use of meniscal allografts preserved with glutaraldehyde.[45,46] This preservation process increases the collagen cross-links of the extracellular matrix and kills the meniscal cells. Although glutaraldehyde has an unlimited shelf life and guarantees tissue sterility, the tissue shrinkage and joint effusions experienced with this type of preservation have discouraged its use.

Allograft Biology and Biomechanics

For a meniscal allograft to be a successful therapeutic modality, long-term survival and function within the knee joint are essential. Over the past several years, numerous experimental studies have been carried out to examine the biologic and biomechanical fate of meniscal allografts in animal models;[29,31,36,39,40,47] these include studies of cryopreserved, fresh-frozen, freeze-dried, and gamma irradiated meniscal allografts.

Fresh Allografts

The use of fresh meniscal allografts has been examined in two studies using a goat model.[29,35] In one study, the medial meniscus of adult goats was replaced with a fresh allograft.[29] The anterior and posterior horn attachments of the graft were left attached to bone plugs to allow for better initial fixation of the meniscal allograft. Six months after surgery, the menisci were evaluated for gross degenerative changes, proteoglycan concentration (as assessed by uronic acid), vascularity, histology, and cell viability.[29] The results demonstrated that the fresh allografts healed to the peripheral capsular tissues with complete incorporation of the bone plugs. There was no gross or histologic evidence of any type of rejection or immune response. The microvascular pattern of the transplanted graft was similar to that of the normal control and limited to the peripheral 25% of the meniscal width. The cell viability of the fresh allograft was decreased approximately 25% over normal controls, with cells in the central core being less numerous in the allograft.[29] Biochemically, the allografts had an increased (24%) water content and a decreased (50%) proteoglycan content. The authors concluded that although fresh meniscal allografts healed without incident and their gross appearance was normal after six months, the biochemical alterations observed in the extracellular matrix raise concern about the long-term biomaterial and functional properties of the transplanted tissues.[29]

In another experimental study, the use of fresh meniscal allografts resulted in a pronounced inflammatory response after three months.[35] This response was characterized by a marked lymphocytic and plasma cell infiltration that caused the meniscus to degenerate, resulting in articular cartilage destruction after seven months. This was the only study (experimental or clinical) in which results indicated a potential immunologic response to the transplantation of a viable meniscal allograft (fresh or cryopreserved).

A study in rabbits led to the conclusion that fresh meniscal allografts heal normally to the peripheral capsular tissues of the knee joint and appear normal at gross and histologic analysis at 6 and 12 months following transplantation.[32] There was no evidence of an immunologic reaction to these fresh allografts at any time during the study. Mechanical testing of these fresh allografts at 18 months

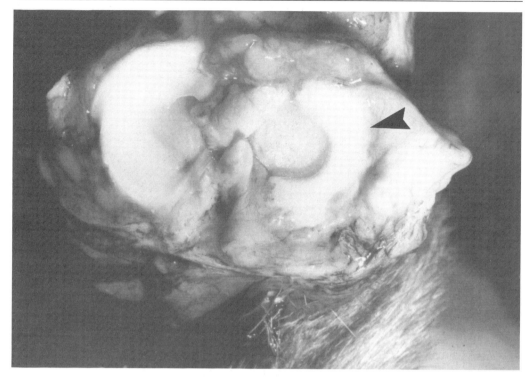

Fig. 2   *Photograph of the tibial surface of a dog's knee six months following meniscal transplantation using a cryopreserved allograft. The allograft (arrow) appears normal and completely healed to the peripheral and horn attachments. (Reproduced with permission from Arnoczky SP, Warren RF, McDevitt CA: Meniscal replacement using a cryopreserved allograft: An experimental study in the dog. Clin Orthop 1990;252:121-128.)*

revealed that the menisci were more elastic than controls and prone to deformation following prolonged compression.

Cryopreserved Allografts

Several investigators have examined the use of cryopreserved meniscal allografts in a variety of animal models.[29,34,35,39] One of the first studies involved the use of canine menisci that had been cryopreserved and stored for one week.[34] Prior evaluation of the cryopreservation process revealed that only 10% of the cells were viable at the time of transplantation.[43] The menisci healed firmly to the peripheral capsular tissues, and there was no gross or histologic evidence of an immune reaction at any time during the 6-month evaluation period (Fig. 2). However, after transplantation, only the cells on the surface of the meniscal allograft appeared viable as determined by S^{35} incorporation (Fig. 3, *top* and *bottom*). The limited weightbearing exhibited by the animals in the initial postopera-

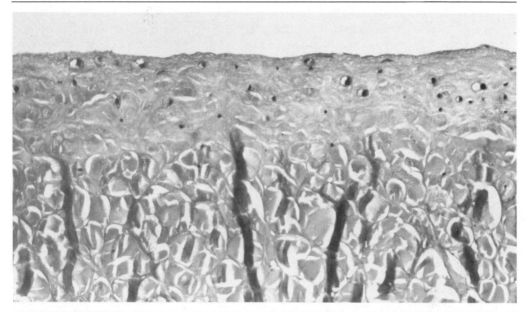
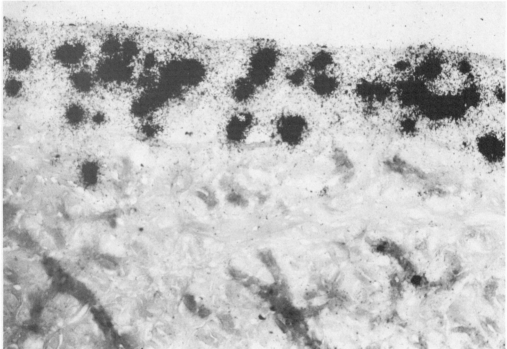

Fig. 3 *Top, Photomicrograph of a cross-section of the femoral surface of a cryopreserved meniscal allograft two weeks following transplantation. Note the limited number of cells in the surface and subsurface areas of the meniscus. **Bottom**, Autoradiograph of an adjacent section of the same meniscus showing the active uptake of radiolabeled sulfate. (hematoxylin and eosin X 100). (Reproduced with permission from Arnoczky SP, Warren RF, McDevitt CA: Meniscal replacement using a cryopreserved allograft: An experimental study in the dog. Clin Orthop 1990;252:121-128.)*

tive period may have limited diffusion of nutrients to the superficial layers of the meniscus, thus allowing only those cells in the superficial regions of the meniscus to survive.[34] However, with time, the cell population of the transplant increased and by three months the allograft had a cellular distribution and activity very similar to normal controls (Fig. 4, *top* and *bottom*). The origin of these new cells, whether from proliferation of donor cells or invasion by host cells, was not examined in this study.[34] Biochemical analysis of these transplants at six months revealed a comparable glycosaminoglycan composition between the allografts and control menisci.[34] The only major difference between the two groups is a modest increase in the proportion of dermatan sulfate in the transplanted menisci. Based on the relatively normal relative proportions of newly synthesized chondroitin and dermatan sulfate observed in the transplanted menisci, it was concluded that extensive modification of the expression of the proteoglycan phenotype did not appear to occur after transplantation.

A biomechanical evaluation of these cryopreserved allografts reveals that the transplants had approximately the same biomaterial properties (failure stress and elastic modulus) as control specimens three and six months after transplantation.[47]

Results of additional studies using cryopreserved meniscal allografts in dogs[39] and goats[29,35] have been similar in terms of peripheral capsular healing and gross and histologic appearance. In the goat study, an increase in water content and a decrease in proteoglycan content (as seen with the fresh allografts in the same study) was observed at six months.[29]

Deep Frozen Allografts

The biology of deep-frozen meniscal grafts has been investigated in dogs,[33] sheep,[36,37] and rabbits.[32] Results from these studies have shown that the acellular meniscus is invaded by host cells that appear to originate from the peripheral capsular and synovial tissues of the joint (Fig. 5). While these cells appear to proliferate and gradually invade the deeper layers of the meniscus, the core of the meniscus remains acellular at six months. Histologic alterations, characterized by a loss of normal orientation of the collagen pattern of the superficial layers of the meniscus, were evident at six months, indicating that a remodeling phenomenon may be associated with the increase in host cells in the allograft (Fig. 6, *top* and *bottom*).[33] Although no biomaterial studies of these transplants were done, the morphologic alterations observed in the collagen orientation represents a possible alteration in the material properties of the meniscus after transplantation.[33]

Results from biomechanical studies of rabbit models[32] indicated an increased elasticity in deep-frozen allografts at 18 months, while results of a similar study of sheep revealed that the tensile strength of deep-frozen meniscal grafts was less than 75% of control values at

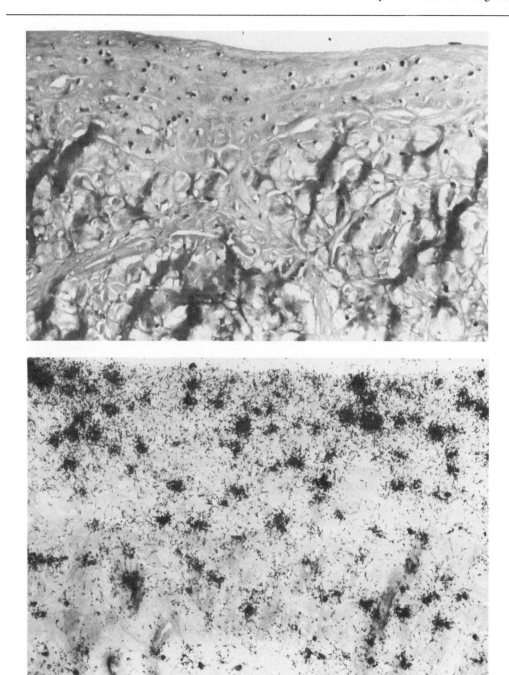

Fig. 4 *Top, Photomicrograph of a cross section of the femoral surface of a cryopreserved meniscal allograft three months following transplantation. The number and distribution of cells within the matrix is similar to that of normal controls. **Bottom**, Autoradiograph of an adjacent section of the same meniscus showing an active uptake of radiolabled sulfate by these new cells. (hematoxylin and eosin, X 100) (Reproduced with permission from Arnoczky SP, Warren RF, McDevitt CA: Meniscal replacement using a cryopreserved allograft: An experimental study in the dog. Clin Orthop 1990;252:121-128.)*

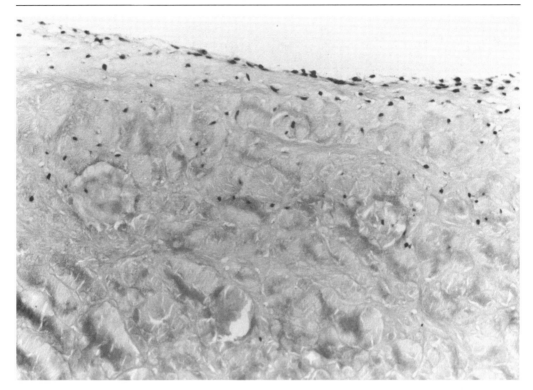

Fig. 5 *Photomicrograph of a cross section of the femoral surface of a deep-frozen meniscus one month following transplantation. Cells, apparently derived from the synovium and capsule, have migrated into the superficial and subsuperficial areas of the allograft. The deeper portions of the meniscus remain acellular at this time.*

12 and 48 weeks.[36,37] As with the fresh and cryopreserved menisci, the deep-frozen allografts readily healed to the peripheral capsular tissues, and no immunologic reactions to the deep-frozen allografts were noted in any of the studies.

Deep-frozen, Gamma Irradiated Allografts

Zukor and associates[40] used rabbit models to examine the use of deep-frozen meniscal allografts that were also subjected to 2.5 mrads of gamma irradiation as a secondary sterilization procedure. Study results led them to conclude that the radiation did not alter the biologic or biomechanical responses normally observed in deep-frozen meniscal allografts.[40]

Freeze-dried Allografts

The use of freeze-dried meniscal allografts was investigated using a goat model.[35] In this study, freeze-dried menisci healed to the peripheral capsular tissue but exhibited inconsistent degrees of cellu-

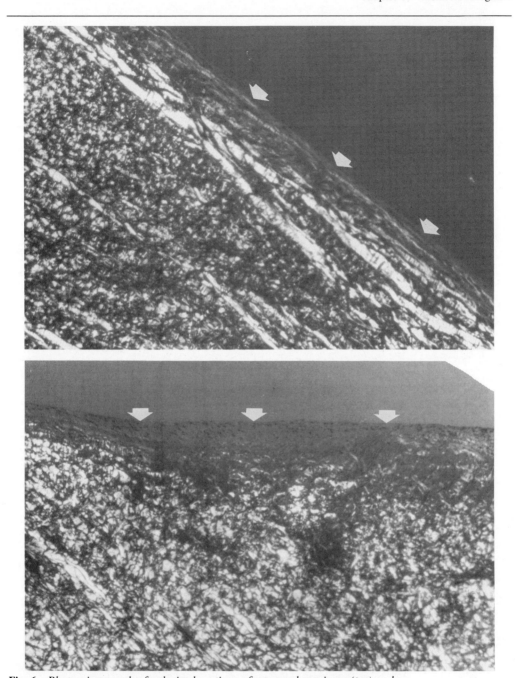

Fig. 6   *Photomicrograph of polarized sections of a normal meniscus (**top**) and a deep-frozen meniscus six months following implantation (**bottom**). Note the absence of an organized collagen pattern in the superficial and subsuperficial layers (arrows) of the deep-frozen meniscus. (Reproduced with permission from Arnoczky SP, CiCarlo EF, O'Brien SJ, et al: Cellular repopulation of deep-frozen meniscal autografts: An experimental study in the dog.* Arthroscopy, *in press.)*

lar ingrowth. In addition some degree of degeneration was found in the majority of transplants at 7 months.[35]

Freeze-dried, Gamma Irradiated Allografts

Freeze-dried, gamma irradiated menisci were transplanted into the knee joints of sheep.[36,37] The amount of radiation used was not documented. The results of the study indicated that the meniscal allografts healed to the peripheral border of the joint by six weeks.[36,37] There was marked vascular ingrowth and cellular proliferation by 12 weeks; by 24 weeks the meniscal allograft was totally vascularized, which appeared to remodel the meniscus, and by 48 weeks the shape of the allograft was altered and the meniscus appeared to shrink. Material testing of these specimens at 48 weeks revealed a tensile strength of less than 75% of control menisci.[36,37]

Although variations in animal models, methods of tissue preservation, parameters of evaluation, and testing methods make direct comparisons between studies difficult, the information obtained from these experimental investigations has provided the scientific rationale for the clinical use of meniscal allografts, and several inferences can be made from their collective results.

(1) Despite one report to the contrary, it appears that menisci transplanted with a viable cell population (fresh or cryopreserved allograft) do not elicit a significant immunologic response within the joint. (2) It appears that deep-frozen menisci become repopulated with cells from the host. This repopulation phenomenon may or may not adversely affect the biomaterial properties of the graft. (3) Gamma irradiation of deep-frozen meniscal allografts with 2.5 mrads or less does not seem to adversely affect the biologic or biomechanical remodeling of the meniscus. (4) The preservation process of freeze-drying seems to adversely affect the remodeling process of meniscal allografts.

It is apparent that additional basic science studies are needed to document the long-term functional integrity of meniscal allografts. In addition, it must be determined if a viable cell population at the time of transplantation is of any significance and, if so, what percentage of cells must be transplanted alive.

Clinical Experience

The initial clinical experience with meniscal allografts was gleaned from the results of massive proximal tibial osteochondral allografts in patients undergoing tumor resection for limb salvage.[22-24] In these cases the menisci were left attached and transplanted as part of the total allograft. Although the contribution of the meniscus to the overall clinical success of these transplants is difficult to assess, this experience suggested that meniscal transplantation was at least feasible.

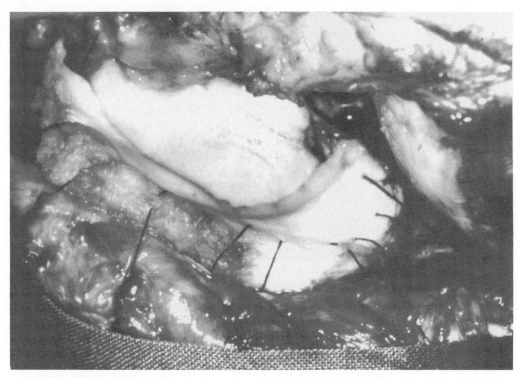

Fig. 7   *Operative photograph showing the exposure of the medial compartment of the knee and the placement of sutures in the peripheral aspect of a meniscal allograft. (Reproduced with permission from Arnoczky SP, Milachowski KA: Meniscal allografts: Where do we stand?, in Ewing JW (ed):* Articular Cartilage and Knee Joint Function: Basic Science and Arthroscopy. *New York, Raven Press, 1990, pp 129-136.)*

An indication of the fate of the meniscus when transplanted as part of an osteochondral allograft was recently reported.[32] In this study, menisci were transplanted as part of a fresh, small-fragment, osteochondral allograft of the proximal tibial plateau. Subsequent arthroscopy performed as long as 8.5 years after surgery revealed that these menisci were viable on gross and histologic evaluation. This evaluation, although limited, provided evidence that a transplanted fresh meniscal allograft was viable several years after surgery.[32] In addition, there was no evidence of rejection at the time of evaluation.[32]

These experiences have provided some of the clinical basis for the transplantation of isolated meniscal allografts.[48] The first reported use of isolated meniscal allografts came from Munich and documented the use of deep-frozen and freeze-dried meniscal allografts in 22 patients.[36,37,48] The patients in this study all had anterior cruciate ligament insufficiency, and 17 had a prior medial meniscectomy. The surgical procedure consisted of an anterior cruciate ligament

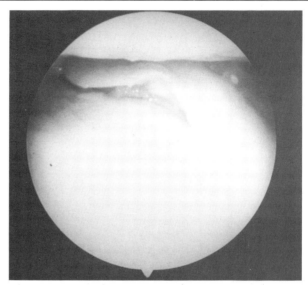

Fig. 8   *Arthroscopic photograph showing the appearance of a deep-frozen meniscal allograft 24 months following transplantation. The meniscus is firmly attached to the joint capsule at its periphery and shows no signs of degeneration. (Reproduced with permission from Arnoczky SP, Milachowski KA: Meniscal allografts: Where do we stand?, in Ewing JW (ed):* Articular Cartilage and Knee Joint Function: Basic Science and Arthroscopy. *New York, Raven Press, 1990, pp 129-136.)*

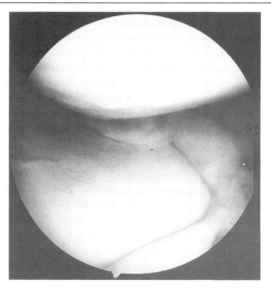

Fig. 9   *Arthroscopic photograph showing the appearance of a freeze-dried meniscal allograft 14 months following transplantation. Although the meniscus is firmly attached to the joint capsule, the meniscus has decreased in size and appears abnormal. (Reproduced with permission from Arnoczky SP, Milachowski KA: Meniscal allografts: Where do we stand?, in Ewing JW (ed):* Articular Cartilage and Knee Joint Function: Basic Science and Arthroscopy. *New York, Raven Press, 1990, pp 129-136.)*

reconstruction using the patellar tendon and a meniscal allograft (16 freeze-dried, 6 deep-frozen) (Fig. 7). After a minimum follow-up period of 24 months (range 24 to 50 months), five of the six patients with deep-frozen allografts had good to excellent clinical results as indicated by the Lysholm knee score, whereas the freeze-dried meniscal allografts were less successful with one excellent result, five good results, eight fair results, and two poor results. Subsequent arthroscopy in 19 of these patients at various intervals revealed that the menisci appeared to be healed firmly to the peripheral capsular tissues in 18 cases.[36,37,48] In one case, the meniscus failed to heal to the peripheral capsule and was removed. The report also noted that although both the deep-frozen and freeze-dried menisci appeared to shrink in size following transplantation, the shrinkage associated with the freeze-dried menisci appeared more pronounced (Figs. 8 and 9). In addition, increased synovial reactions and articular cartilage degeneration were noted in the freeze-dried transplants. These clinical findings coupled with the similar findings in an animal model suggest that freeze-drying may not be an appropriate processing method for meniscal allografts.[48]

In another clinical study, six fresh meniscal allografts (four medial, two lateral)[49] were examined after a minimum follow-up of 2 years (range 24 to 44 months). In each patient the meniscal transplant was part of an additional procedure; three patients had anterior cruciate ligament reconstructions, two patients had osteochondral allografts for defects of the lateral femoral condyle, and one patient had both an anterior cruciate ligament reconstruction and an osteochondral allograft of the lateral femoral condyle. All patients demonstrated clinical improvement after surgery; subsequent arthroscopy of four of the patients revealed normal-appearing menisci. The menisci were firmly healed to the peripheral capsular tissues and showed no evidence of shrinkage.[49]

Although the aforementioned clinical studies provide only limited insight into the efficacy of meniscal allografts, clinical experience with meniscal allografts continues to increase. However, because meniscal transplantation is usually associated with other reconstructive procedures of the knee (such as ligament reconstruction, osteochondral allograft, and osteotomy), the clinical assessment of meniscal allografts is likely to be hindered by several variables. In addition, variations in tissue processing techniques, surgical indications, and the amount of degenerative joint disease present at the time of surgery may further hinder the critical evaluation of meniscal transplantation. The surgeon and basic scientist must work together to develop prospective evaluation criteria with which to critically assess the biologic and functional fate of meniscal allografts.

References

1. Fairbanks TJ: Knee joint changes after meniscectomy. *J Bone Joint Surg* 1948;30B:664-670.

2. Krause WR, Pope MH, Johnson RJ, et al: Mechanical changes in the knee after meniscectomy. *J Bone Joint Surg* 1976;58A:599-604.

3. Kurosawa H, Fukubayashi T, Nakajima H: Load-bearing mode of the knee joint: Physical behavior of the knee joint with or without menisci. *Clin Orthop* 1980;149:283-290.

4. Levy IM, Torzilli PA, Waren RF: The effect of medial meniscectomy on anterior-posterior motion of the knee. *J Bone Joint Surg* 1982;64A:883-888.

5. Tapper EM, Hoover NW: Late results after meniscectomy. *J Bone Joint Surg* 1969;51A:517-526.

6. Ahmed AM, Burke DL: In-vitro measurement of static pressure distribution in synovial joints: Part I: Tibial surface of the knee. *J Biomech Eng* 1983;105:216-225.

7. Fukubayashi T, Kurosawa JH: The contact area and pressure distribution pattern of the knee. *Acta Orthop Scand* 1980;51:871-879.

8. Hsieh HH, Walker PS: Stabilizing mechanisms of the loaded and unloaded knee joint. *J Bone Joint Surg* 1976;58A:87-93.

9. Kettlekamp DB, Jacobs AW: Tibiofemoral contact area: Determination and implications. *J Bone Joint Surg* 1972;54A:349-356.

10. Seedholm BB, Hargreaves DJ: Transmission of the load in the knee joint with special reference to the role of the meniscus, Part II. *Eng Med* 1979;8:220.

11. Shoemaker SC, Markolf KL: The role of meniscus in the anterior-posterior stability of the loaded anterior cruciate-deficient knee. *J Bone Joint Surg* 1986;68A:71-79.

12. Walker PS, Erkman MJ: The role of the menisci in force transmission across the knee. *Clin Orthop* 1975;109:184-192.

13. Arnoczky SP, Warren RF, Ashlock MA: Replacement of the anterior cruciate ligament using a patellar tendon allograft: An experimental study. *J Bone Joint Surg* 1986;68A:376-385.

14. Aston JE, Bentley G: Repair of articular surfaces by allografts of articular and growth-plate cartilage. *J Bone Joint Surg* 1986;68B:29-35.

15. Brown KLB, Cruess RL: Bone and cartilage transplantation in orthopaedic surgery: A review. *J Bone Joint Surg* 1982;64A:270-279.

16. Campbell CJ, Ishida H, Takahashi H, et al: The transplantation of articular cartilage. *J Bone Joint Surg* 1963;45A:1579-1592.

17. Elves MW: A study of the transplantation antigens on chondrocytes from articular cartilage. *J Bone Joint Surg* 1974;56B:178-185.

18. Elves MW: Bone and cartilage grafting and organ transplantation, in Owen R, Goodfellow J, Bullough P (eds): *Scientific Foundations of Orthopaedics and Traumatology*. London, William Heinemann, 1980, pp 273-290.

19. Friedlaender GE, Strong DM, Sell KW: Studies on the antigenicity of bone: I. Freeze-dried and deep-frozen bone allografts in rabbits. *J Bone Joint Surg* 1976;58A:854-858.

20. Langer F, Czitrom A, Pritzker KP, et al: The immunogenicity of fresh and frozen allogeneic bone. *J Bone Joint Surg* 1975;57A:216-220.

21. Tomford WW, Fredericks GR, Mankin HJ: Cryopreservation of intact articular cartilage. *Trans Orthop Res Soc* 1982;7:176.

22. Lexer E: Joint transplantations and arthoplasty. *Surg Gynecol Obstet* 1925;40:782-809.

23. Mankin HJ, Gebhardt MC, Tomford WW: Use of frozen cadaveric osteoarticular allografts in the treatment of benign and malignant tumors about the knee, in Enneking WF (ed): *Limb Salvage in Musculoskeletal Oncology*. New York, Churchill Livingstone, 1987, pp 354-364.

24. Mankin HJ, Doppelt SH, Sullivan TR, et al: Osteoarticular and intercalary allograft transplantation in the management of malignant tumors of bone. *Cancer* 1982;50:613-630.

25. Minami A, Ishii S, Ogino T, et al: Effect of the immunological antigenicity of the allogeneic tendons on tendon grafting. *Hand* 1982;14:111-119.

26. Mnaymneh W, Malinin T: Massive allografts in surgery of bone tumors. *Orthop Clin North Am* 1989;20:455-467.

27. Shino K, Kawasaki T, Hirose H, et al: Replacement of the anterior cruciate ligament by an allogeneic tendon graft: An experimental study in the dog. *J Bone Joint Surg* 1984;66B:672-681.

28. Vasseur PB, Rodrigo JJ, Stevenson S, et al: Replacement of the anterior cruciate ligament with a bone-ligament-bone anterior cruciate ligament allograft in dogs. *Clin Orthop* 1987;219:268-277.

29. Jackson DW, McDevitt CA, Atwell, EA, et al: Meniscal transplantation using fresh and cryopreserved allografts: An experimental study in goats. *Trans Orthop Res Soc* 1990;15:221.

30. Keene GCR, Paterson RS, Teague DC: Advances in arthroscopic surgery. *Clin Orthop* 1987;224:64-70.

31. Zukor D, Brooks P, Gross A, et al: Meniscal allografts: Experimental and clinical study, abstract. *Orthop Rev* 1988.

32. Zukor DJ, Cameron JC, Brooks PJ, et al: The fate of human meniscal allografts, in Ewing, JW (ed): *Articular Cartilage and Knee Joint Function: Basic Science and Arthroscopy.* New York, Raven Press, 1990, pp 147-152.

33. Arnoczky SP, O'Brien SJ, DiCarlo EF, et al: Cellular repopulation of deep-frozen meniscal autografts: An experimental study in the dog. *Trans Orthop Res Soc* 1988;13:145.

34. Arnoczky SP, Warren RF, McDevitt CA: Meniscal replacement using a cryopreserved allograft: An experimental study in the dog. *Clin Orthop* 1990;252:121-128.

35. Keating EM, Malinin TI, Belchic G: Meniscal transplantation in goats: An experimental study. *Orthop Trans* 1988;13:147.

36. Milachowski KA, Weismeier K, Wirth CJ, et al: Meniscus transplantation: Experimental study and first clinical report, abstract. *Am J Sports Med* 1987;15:626.

37. Milachowski KA, Weismeier K, Erhardt W, et al: Transplantation of meniscus: An experimental study in sheep. *Sportverletzung Sportschaden* 1987;1:20-24.

38. Milachowski KA, Weismeier K, Wirth CJ: Homologous meniscus transplantation. Experimental and clinical results. *Int Orthop* 1989;13: 1-11.

39. Milton J, Flandry F, Terry G, et al: Transplantation of viable, cryopreserved menisci. *Trans Orthop Res Soc* 1990;15:220.

40. Zukor DJ, Rubins IM, Daigle MR, et al: Allotransplantation of frozen irradiated menisci in rabbits. *Trans Orthop Res Soc* 1990;15:219.

41. Brighton CT, Shadle CA, Jimenez SA, et al: Articular cartilage preservation and storage. I. Application of tissue culture techniques to the storage of viable articular cartilage. *Arthritis Rheum* 1979;22:1093-1101.

42. Black J, Shadle CA, Parsons JR, et al: Articular cartilage preservation and storage. II. Mechanical indentation of viable, stored articular cartilage. *Arthritis Rheum* 1979;22:1102-1108.

43. Arnoczky SP, McDevitt CA, Schmidt MB, et al: The effect of cryopreservation on canine menisci: A biochemical, morphologic, and biomechanical evaluation. *J Orthop Res* 1988;6:1-12.

44. Jackson DW, Windler GE, Simon TM: Intraarticular reaction associated with the use of freeze-dried, ethylene oxide-sterilized bone-patella tendon-bone allografts in the reconstruction of the anterior cruciate ligament. *Am J Sports Med* 1990;18:1-11.

45. Canham W, Stanish W: A study of the biological behavior of the meniscus as a transplant in the medial compartment of a dog's knee. *Am J Sports Med* 1986;14:376-379.

46. Powers DL, Davenport ME, Wisnewski PJ: Glutaraldehyde cross-linked meniscal allografts: Clinical, gross and histological results. *J Investigative Surg* 1988;1:249-157.

47. Schmidt MB, Arnoczky SP, Mow VC, et al: Biomechanical evaluation of cryopreserved meniscal allografts. *Trans Orthop Res Soc* 1986;11:458.

48. Arnoczky SP, Milachowski KA: Meniscal allografts: Where do we stand?, in Ewing JW (ed): *Articular Cartilage and Knee Joint Function: Basic Science and Arthroscopy*. New York, Raven Press, pp 129-136, 1990.

49. Garrett JC, Stevenson RN: Meniscal transplantation in the human knee: A preliminary report. *J Arth Rel Surg* 1991;7:57-62.

Chapter 12

Prosthetic Meniscal Replacement

William G. Rodkey, DVM
Kevin R. Stone, MD
J. Richard Steadman, MD

Introduction

In 1986, the United States National Center for Health Statistics (personal correspondence, 1990) reported that approximately 56 million office visits were made to orthopaedic surgeons annually, and that 1 in 8 of these visits (7 million) was related to knee injury or symptoms. Furthermore, approximately 1 in 9 of the knee patients (766,000) had a major knee injury. The National Center for Health Statistics also estimated that these knee problems led to 1.4 million annual arthroscopic procedures for knee pain or instability, and that 600,000 of these were directly related to meniscal problems. The Center also reported annual estimates of 160,000 total knee replacements and 500,000 osteotomies to relieve knee symptoms.

Based on these statistics alone, it is apparent that knee problems, more specifically those related to the meniscal cartilage, have great financial and personal impact on the general population of the United States. Because partial and complete excision are presently the only accepted treatments for irreparably damaged menisci, the concept of replacement with artificial material is very attractive.

Unfortunately, many factors and problems exist that preclude a simple solution to prosthetic meniscal replacement. The menisci have a unique shape and properties that have not been reproduced well in prosthetic replacements. Microscopically, the meniscus is a fibrocartilage structure that consists of well arranged, predominantly type I collagen fibers populated with meniscal fibrochondrocytes.[1] The collagen fibers are arranged in a circumferential pattern, and they appear to be stabilized by radially positioned fibers that probably act as tension rods to prevent disruption under loading (Fig. 1).[1,2] The menisci also have a very complex biochemical makeup which includes noncollagenous protein and hexosamine in addition to the collagen.[3] Moreover, there is variation in the concentration of the noncollagenous proteins in the different anatomic portions of the menisci.[4]

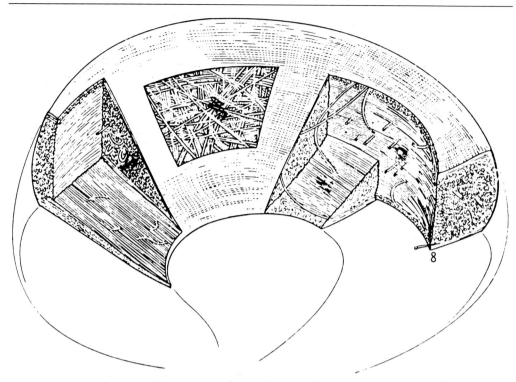

Fig. 1 *Diagram of the reconstruction of the complex fiber pattern of the meniscus. (Reproduced with permission from Bullough PG, Munuera L, Murphy J, et al: The strength of the menisci of the knee as it relates to their fine structure. J Bone Joint Surg 1970;52B:564-570.)*

The meniscus performs various biomechanical and physical functions, including shock absorption, joint stabilization, and lubrication.[1,5-7] The meniscus adds congruity to the tibial plateau so that it can better articulate with the femoral condyles. The improved congruity is directly related to increased joint stability. The menisci are attached to the tibia and the joint capsule by a complex network of ligaments and fibrous bands. The varying elasticity of these attachments gives the menisci unique mobility while restraining anterior displacement of the tibia on the femur.[8]

In summary, the extremely complex interaction of structure, composition, and function has made the meniscus virtually impossible to replicate. Without completely replacing the unique physical properties of the meniscus and its many functions, normal joint motion, function, and stability cannot be expected to be maintained.[5,7] The result of any derangement is degeneration of the joint and progressive osteoarthritis.

Previous Studies of Prosthetic Meniscal Replacement

A prosthesis is an artificial device used to replace a missing body part. A somewhat broader definition might be that a prosthesis is any substance, material, or device used to aid the performance of a natural function. If the latter definition is accepted, then prosthetic meniscal replacement might include as many as five different categories of devices—autografts, allografts, synthetic artificial material structures, xenografts, and reconstituted biologic structures.

Many different tissues have been used as autografts to replace menisci. This approach seems logical and attractive, especially because of the evidence provided by Arnoczky and associates[9] that meniscus fibrochondrocytes have the ability to migrate into collagenous tissues placed in the knee joint. They also provided proof that there was active matrix synthesis by these migrating cells. Because of these results, Milachowski and associates[10] attempted to replace menisci with autograft tissue including fascia lata, fat pad, and ligaments. These tissues were rolled into tubes, made into the shape of the meniscus, and sewn into the knee joint in place of menisci. While cellular migration appeared to occur, these transplanted tissues became fibrotic as they assumed a concave shape. For the duration of this study, there was no morphologic resemblance to the normal meniscus and more importantly, the transplanted tissues did not provide the biomechanical stability or shock absorption necessary to prevent severe arthritic and degenerative changes.

The use of allografts for prosthetic meniscal replacement has been discussed in earlier chapters of this book. Although this approach is gaining popularity and acceptance, various problems still exist, such as questions regarding biomechanical characteristics, ability of the allograft to survive during the period of cellular repopulation, incongruities of size and shape, insertion and preservation techniques, control of disease transmission, and graft shrinkage after implantation. All of these problems are being addressed by various investigators, and positive results are anticipated.

Several synthetic artificial materials have been used for the attempted replacement of meniscal cartilage.[11-14] Those that have gained the most attention include Teflon, polyester, and carbon fibers. Toyonaga and associates[11] performed total resection of the lateral meniscus in a group of dogs, then replaced the meniscus with a Teflon-net prosthesis that was folded and rolled into a cylinder and sutured to the joint capsule. Over a period of 12 months, they reported slowly progressive degeneration of the tibial articular cartilage and slight degeneration of the femoral articular cartilage. They attributed these degenerative changes to the finding that the Teflon-net substitute meniscus was forced laterally from the joint by the femoral condyle. They also reported significant adhesions between the Teflon-net substitute meniscus and the popliteal muscle that impeded knee joint motion. Chronic inflammatory cells, fibroblasts, and foreign body giant cells were seen around the Teflon-net fibers less than three months after implantation, and these cell types were still present after 12 months. Toyonaga and associates[11] concluded that Teflon is an ideal material for meniscal replacement because of its pliability, softness, and histocompatibility; its potential to protect articular cartilage; and its ability to infiltrate rapidly with migrating cells. Nonetheless, no further work on this material has been published.

Leenslag and associates[12] used a poly (L-lactide) reinforced carbon fiber material as a porous composite to replace or reconstruct the meniscus. This material provided questionable knee joint stability and did not prevent degenerative arthritis. Furthermore, interpretation of the results of Leenslag and associates'[12] study were complicated by the presence of significant synovitis, which resulted from free carbon fiber particles released within the joints. No further studies regarding the use of this material have been published. More recently, Wood and associates[13] replaced the medial meniscus of the rabbit with a polyester-carbon fiber bioprosthesis that was composed of concentrically stacked hoops of carbon fibers and sheathed by woven, high-tenacity polyester fibers. The polyester fibers were continued on either end of the bioprosthesis and used for anchorage through drill holes in the tibia. This device was placed in the knee joints of 18 rabbits for three or six months. At the time of final evaluation, the device had been displaced from its location in the majority of the knees. Carbon fiber fragmentation produced a high incidence of synovitis. Wood and associates[13] also observed a marked inflammatory response around the polyester fibers in nearly all cases, with no significant ingrowth of cells into the carbon fibers and essentially no biologic regeneration of a meniscus in any of the experimental knees. In all of these studies, the prosthetic device failed to provide the normal functional properties of the meniscus: knee joint stability, shock absorption, force transmission, and prevention of degenerative changes within the joint. In 1985, Wall[14] patented an artificial meniscus made of "pliable" materials, such as rubber or Teflon, that was reinforced with nylon or stainless steel. No other studies regarding this approach have been published.

The concept of xenograft meniscal replacement has numerous positive aspects. Meniscus is widely available from bovine, porcine, and ovine sources. However, meniscal xenografts have not been extensively reported because of a lack of information regarding sizing, biomechanical properties, and biochemical characteristics of menisci obtained from different species. (This fact is in direct contrast to the still rather common use of porcine heart valves by cardiothoracic surgeons.) The major concern in the use of xenografts is probably host rejection caused by immunogenic factors.[15] Nonetheless, such rejections normally can be avoided or at least minimized through biochemical procedures to modify the telopeptide side chains, which usually cause immunologic reactions.[15] We are presently examining some of the potential advantages, as well as problems, involving xenographic transplantation of menisci.

The use of reconstituted bioresorbable collagen structures has many positive features, including the fact that the rate of resorption can be controlled by the degree of crosslinking, the immune response can be minimized through enzymatic treatment of the collagen, and the extremely complex biochemical composition of the normal meniscus can be closely approximated in the reconstituted structure.[16] We believe this approach is one possible solution to replacement, or in this case regeneration, of the irreparably damaged meniscus.

Yannas[17] is credited with much of the original work in the development of resorbable collagen-based scaffolds. His work has led to the successful development of bioresorbable materials, which have been used as nerve conduits and skin replacements. This work served as the original stimulus and basis for the formation and development of a bioresorbable collagen-based regeneration template.

While developing our bioresorbable collagen-based regeneration template for the meniscus, we considered several factors and requirements. We developed our graft to maintain its structural integrity in the intra-articular environment for a period long enough to support cellular ingrowth, matrix formation, and maturation. We also used biochemical techniques to assure that our material would not trigger an immunologic reaction, which might cause rejection and eventual destruction of the implant. We considered the biomechanical inadequacies of many of the devices previously used for meniscal replacement, and we therefore made every effort to assure that our regeneration template would provide immediate joint stability that was comparable to that given by the normal meniscus. Finally, we designed our graft to prevent or help minimize degenerative arthritis and to relieve joint pain.

Laboratory Results With Collagen-Based Regeneration Templates

Prosthesis Fabrication

The techniques for creation of the collagen-based prosthesis were developed by Stone,[18] who also gives a detailed description of the fabrication process.[19] The collagen-based regeneration templates were formed from bovine Achilles tendons. After the tissue was trimmed and minced, it was washed with a copious amount of tap water to remove blood residue and water-soluble materials. Various acid and enzyme processes were used to purify the washed tendons. Cross-linking was then done with glycosaminoglycans and dehydrothermal techniques. Salt-soluble noncollagenous materials, lipids, and most of the telopeptides were removed by these various processes. The purified collagen fibers were then manually positioned in a mold. Final cross-linking was done with 0.2% glutaraldehyde solution, and the disk of collagen material was then rinsed repeatedly to remove residual glutaraldehyde prior to lyophilization and final dehydrothermal cross-linking by vacuum and heat.[19]

In Vitro Studies

Before implanting the collagen-based regeneration templates in any animal models, we evaluated several different prototypes in vitro in organ cultures.[16] We wanted to be sure that the collagen-based material would not be toxic to the meniscal fibrochondrocytes, and we also wanted to determine whether or not the meniscal fibrochondrocytes could be induced to migrate and penetrate the interstices of the scaffold material. By using this organ culture system, we also were able to estimate the most appropriate density of the material for cellular ingrowth and maturation.

We used an organ culture system developed by Webber and associates.[20] The source of the original tissue for this system was the menisci of mature dogs. The organ cultures with the collagen-based materials were maintained from one to six weeks.

The most important finding of these initial in vitro studies was that the material did not appear to be toxic to the meniscal fibrochondrocytes. In fact, there was a notable increase over time in the cellular migration and penetration of the meniscal fibrochondrocytes into the different prototypes of regeneration templates. The morphology of the cells that populated the scaffold material in the organ cultures was similar, but not identical, to normal meniscal fibrochondrocytes. We also observed that the material with the highest density seemed to limit the penetration of the migrating cells. Finally, the addition of fibrin and fibronectin to the collagen-based material appeared to stimulate and hasten the migration of the cells into the material.

Based on these initial results, we believed that limited in vivo studies would be necessary to confirm these preliminary findings; so we selected the prototype of material that had supported the most abundant cellular ingrowth in vitro for use in the in vivo studies.

In Vivo Studies

For the initial in vivo pilot study,[16] we performed an 80% subtotal resection of the medial meniscus in seven knee joints of immature pigs, replacing each meniscus with the prosthetic regeneration template by size-matching it to the resected tissue. These joints were then evaluated at one, three, or six weeks. To serve as controls, two joints underwent an 80% subtotal medial meniscus resection without prosthetic replacement. At the time of final evaluation, it appeared that all of the prostheses had been resorbed without any evidence of joint destruction or articular cartilage abrasion. The primary healing response in both the prosthetic menisci and the two controls was a proliferative vascular response with granulation tissue. In both the prosthetic joints and the control joints, there was early evidence of regeneration of the menisci. From this study, it was apparent that the resorption of the collagen-based regeneration template was well advanced by three weeks, and, furthermore,

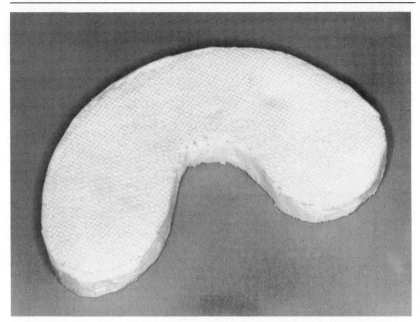

Fig. 2   *The collagen-based regeneration template trimmed and contoured in preparation for implantation into the knee joint to replace the excised meniscus.*

there is spontaneous, early regeneration of the partially resected meniscus in immature pigs.

Although this preliminary pilot study[16] answered the question of whether or not our material could be implanted without producing adverse effects, it did leave a number of unanswered questions. We were uncertain of the mechanism of resorption of the prosthetic material. From this study, it could not be determined if the material stimulated regeneration of the meniscus or if it simply did not impede the naturally-occurring regeneration of the meniscus in this particular animal model. Because this pilot study was of short duration, we also could draw no conclusion regarding the ability of this regenerated tissue to mature and function as a normal meniscus. Consequently, we elected to continue our in vivo studies in skeletally-mature dogs.[19]

We chose mature dogs as our model for several reasons. First, the canine knee joint is exquisitely sensitive to any biomechanical derangement, and any instability quickly leads to early degenerative arthritic changes.[21] Second, there is a plethora of basic science information on the canine meniscus, and it is very similar to the biology of the human meniscus.[21,22] Finally, both the canine and human menisci will regenerate only partially following subtotal resection, and the regenerated tissue typically is biomechanically not adequate to completely protect the joint from osteoarthritic changes.[5,21]

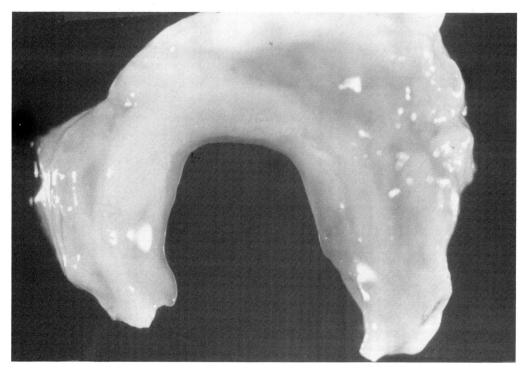

Fig. 3   *Regenerated canine meniscus three months after an 80% meniscal resection and implantation of a collagen-based template. (Reproduced with permission from Stone KR, Rodkey WG, Webber RJ, et al: Meniscal regeneration with copolymeric collagen scaffolds: In vitro and in vivo studies evaluated clinically, histologically, and biochemically.* Am J Sports Med 1992;20:104-111.)

A total of 50 knee joints in 26 dogs were subjected to an 80% subtotal resection of the medial meniscus. One of the meniscectomized joints in each of the 26 dogs then received the collagen-based regeneration template, custom-contoured to replace the resected tissue immediately following the meniscectomy (Fig. 2). Of the remaining 24 joints, 12 underwent subtotal meniscal resection alone, and 12 had the resected portion of the meniscus immediately replanted as an autograft. These joints were evaluated at three, six, nine, 12, or 27 months. At monthly intervals throughout the study, we evaluated joint stability, gait, and treadmill performance. Clinical evaluations of the dogs' gait and treadmill performance revealed a statistical trend over time in favor of the joints that had received the collagen-based regeneration templates when compared with either the resection-only controls or the autograft controls.

At final evaluation, two thirds of the prosthesis-implanted joints had a significant degree of meniscal regeneration through the collagen-based template (Fig. 3). Meniscal regeneration was almost complete in 25% of the joints that had undergone meniscal resection

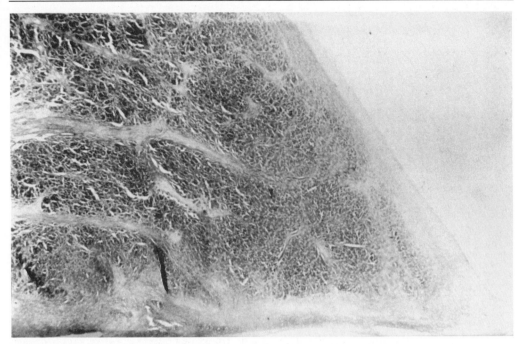

Fig. 4 *Cross-section of a canine meniscus 12 months after an 80% meniscal resection followed by implantation of a collagen-based regeneration template. The meniscus is characterized by a straight sided contour, interwoven dense collagen core, and an inner margin of fibrocartilage (Masson's trichome, x 2.5). (Reproduced with permission from Stone KR, Rodkey WG, Webber RJ, et al: Meniscal regeneration with copolymeric collagen scaffolds: In vitro and in vivo studies evaluated clinically, histologically, and biochemically. Am J Sports Med 1992;20:104-111.)*

alone. Two thirds of the immediate autograft control joints revealed complete reattachment and apparently functional menisci. The articular cartilage appeared grossly similar in the prosthesis-implanted joints, the resection-only controls, and the autograft controls. The regenerated menisci in the joints with the prosthetic material, when examined histologically, appeared mature with organized collagen bundles and viable chondrocytes in lacunae (Fig. 4).

There was a small amount of the original regeneration template still present in the two joints evaluated 27 months after implantation. Histologic staining also revealed ongoing formation of new collagen and glycosaminoglycans. Biochemical analysis indicated that the cells of the prosthesis-regenerated meniscus did not synthesize normal proteoglycans until nine months after implantation. However, normal proteoglycans were being produced at nine months, and this finding showed that fibrocartilage matrix production was within the normal range for the canine meniscus. These newly synthesized proteoglycans at nine and 12 months were similar in hydrodynamic size and chromatographic profiles when compared with the matched control menisci. We believe that these findings are significant evidence that the collagen-based regeneration template will support significant meniscal regeneration and provide enough biomechanical stability to minimize degenerative osteoarthritis in the canine knee joint.

Conclusions

Irreparable damage or loss of the meniscal cartilage of the knee is a significant clinical problem in the general population. It is well documented that loss of the meniscus rapidly leads to degenerative and osteoarthritic changes in the knee joint. Clearly, the use of a meniscal prosthesis or some other device that would support and enhance meniscal regeneration would significantly improve long-term outcome following injuries to and surgical removal of the meniscus. This chapter has reviewed some of the options that have been or might be applied to meet this challenge.

Because no adequate direct substitute for the meniscus has yet been identified, we have directed our research efforts toward the development and refinement of a collagen-based regeneration template. This template will permit the host to regenerate a near-normal meniscus that will provide the many functions required of the meniscus to maintain knee joint stability and homogeneity. This material has been subjected to a number of in vitro and in vivo laboratory studies with encouraging results. Increased efforts to further refine this material are underway.

References

1. Bullough PG, Munuera L, Murphy J, et al: The strength of the menisci of the knee as it relates to their fine structure. *J Bone Joint Surg* 1970;52B:564-570.
2. Seedholm BB, Hargreaves DJ: Transmission of the load in the knee joint with special reference to the role of the menisci. *Eng Med* 1979;8:220-228.
3. Eyre DR, Wu JJ: Collagen of fibrocartilage: A distinctive molecular phenotype in bovine meniscus. *FEBS Lett* 1983;158:265-270.
4. Ingman AM, Ghosh P, Taylor TK: Variation of collagenous and non-collagenous proteins of human knee joint menisci with age and degeneration. *Gerontologia* 1974;20:212-223.
5. Burr DB, Radin EL: Meniscal function and the importance of meniscal regeneration in preventing late medial compartment osteoarthrosis. *Clin Orthop* 1982;171:121-126.
6. Favensi JA, Shaffer JC, Mow VC: Biphasic mechanical properties of knee meniscus. *Trans Orthop Res Soc* 1983;8:57.
7. Shoemaker SC, Markolf KL: The role of the meniscus in the anterior-posterior stability of the loaded anterior cruciate-deficient knee: Effects of partial versus total excision. *J Bone Joint Surg* 1986;68A:71-79.
8. Mow VC, Holmes MH, Lai WM: Fluid transport and mechanical properties of articular cartilage: A review. *J Biomech* 1984;17:377-394.
9. Arnoczky SP, O'Brien SJ, DiCarlo EF, et al: Cellular repopulation of deep-frozen meniscal autografts: An experimental study in dogs. *Trans Orthop Res Soc* 1988;13:145.

10. Milachowski KA, Weismeier K, Wirth CJ: Homologous meniscus transplantation: Experimental and clinical results. *Int Orthop* 1989;13: 1-11.

11. Toyonaga T, Uezaki N, Chikama H: Substitute meniscus of Teflon-net for the knee joint of dogs. *Clin Orthop* 1983;179:291-297.

12. Leenslag JW, Pennings AJ, Veth RPH, et al: A porous composite for reconstruction of meniscus lesions, in Christel P, Meunier A, Lee AJC (eds): *Biological and Biomechanical Performance of Biomaterials: Advances in Biomaterials*. Amsterdam, Elsevier Science Publishers BV, 1986, vol 6, pp 147-149.

13. Wood DJ, Minns RJ, Strover A: Replacement of the rabbit medial meniscus with a polyester-carbon fibre bioprosthesis. *Biomaterials* 1990;11:13-16.

14. Wall WH: Prosthetic meniscus for the repair of joints. U.S. Patent No. 4,502,161, March 5, 1985.

15. Oliver RF, Grant RA, Kent CM: The fate of cutaneously and subcutaneously implanted trypsin purified dermal collagen in the pig. *Brit J Exp Path* 1972;53:540-549.

16. Stone KR, Rodkey WG, Webber RJ, et al: Future directions: Collagen-based prosthesis for meniscal regeneration. *Clin Orthop* 1990;252: 129-135.

17. Yannas IV: Regeneration of skin and nerve by use of collagen templates, in Nimni ME (ed): *Collagen: Biotechnology*. Boca Raton, FL, CRC Press, 1988, vol III, pp 87-115.

18. Stone KR: Prosthetic knee joint meniscal cartilage. U.S. Patent No. 4,880,429, November 14, 1989.

19. Stone KR, Rodkey WG, Webber RJ, et al: Meniscal regeneration with copolymeric collagen scaffolds: *In vitro* and *in vivo* studies evaluated clinically, histologically, and biochemically. *Am J Sports Med* 1992;20:104-111.

20. Webber RJ, York JL, Vanderschilden JL, et al: An organ culture model for assaying wound repair of the fibrocartilaginous knee joint meniscus. *Am J Sports Med* 1989;17:393-400.

21. Cox JS, Nye CE, Schaefer WW, et al: The degenerative effects of partial and total resection of the medial meniscus in dogs' knees. *Clin Orthop* 1975;109:178-183.

22. Adams ME, Muir H: The glycosaminoglycans of canine menisci. *Biochem J* 1981;197:385-389.

Future Directions

Determine the effects of altered meniscal function on other knee-joint structures.

Although the importance of the meniscus to normal knee-joint function has become axiomatic, the effects of altered meniscal function on specific joint structures (for example, ligaments, capsule, cartilage, and synovium) are less well understood. This information could help establish a more complete natural history of meniscal insufficiency, which, in turn, could provide sensitive indices for evaluating the efficacy of meniscal repair and replacement.

Define the role of the meniscus in the abnormal joint.

Most studies that have examined meniscal function have done so in the "normal" joint. Essentially no information exists on the function of the meniscus in the abnormal joint, for example, one with varus deformity, valgus deformity, or instability. In these abnormal joint conditions, severely altered stress patterns on the menisci could compromise the architecture and function of the tissue even after restoration of normal joint kinematics. The development of technologies that could be used to examine meniscal function in the dynamic joint, for example, instrumentation that could be used to record hoop stresses and force transmission, would be extremely important in determining the ability to preserve the meniscus at surgery.

Characterize the functional efficacy of meniscal repair and replacement techniques.

The goal of meniscal repair or replacement is to preserve meniscal function. Although many studies have examined meniscal healing or allograft replacement, none have focused on the ability of the repair or replacement to eliminate the degenerative joint changes normally associated with meniscectomy. Such information is of paramount importance if the efficacy of such procedures is to be confirmed.

An appropriate animal model should be used to determine the rate and extent of specific alterations in joint function, composition, and structure that normally accompany partial or total removal of the meniscus. Meniscal function in this animal model must be thoroughly characterized.

Develop finite-element models (FEMs) of the meniscus.

In order to better understand how the meniscus performs its various functions within the knee joint, research efforts should be directed toward the development of a theoretical model of the meniscus. This information would be important in the design and fabrication of stented meniscal replacements. Similar models in articular cartilage research have contributed significantly to the understanding of cartilage mechanics. This FEM development must be coupled with a biomaterial evaluation of meniscal tissue so that the validity of the model could be tested continuously.

Determine the role of specific growth factors in meniscal healing and/or regeneration.

An exogenous fibrin clot (with its inherent cytokines) has been shown in experimental studies to support and stimulate a reparative response in the avascular portion of the meniscus. Identification of the specific cytokines involved and their precise concentration could allow for a clearer understanding of the healing mechanism associated with fibrin clot application. In addition, the ability to incorporate these cytokines in synthetic matrices may allow for enhanced regeneration of meniscal tissue.

Determine the effects of normal aging on the structure, composition, and function of the meniscus.

An understanding of the normal aging process of the meniscus may provide some information as to the susceptibility of the meniscus to injury and degenerative changes as well as providing some insight as to its reparative capabilities. This information may also explain the variations in magnetic resonance imaging signals observed in the meniscus in different age groups.

Determine the architectural remodeling of meniscal allografts and prostheses.

The complex architecture of the normal meniscus is related to its ability to withstand the variety and magnitude of forces experienced in the knee. The extent to which a replacement can duplicate this architecture determines its long-term ability to survive and function within the knee. Factors that affect this remodeling process must be identified.

Identify the origin and phenotypic expression of the cells that repopulate meniscal allografts and prostheses.

The ability of the cells that repopulate a meniscal allograft or prosthesis to synthesize a competent extracellular matrix is a key factor in the ultimate functional survival of the replacement. The factors that affect modulation and meniscofibrochondrocytes must be identified. This information also could be beneficial in determining the ability of a prosthesis to be "seeded" with mesenchymal stem cells.

Characterize the material properties of meniscal repair tissue.

Although significant information exists on the ability of a meniscus to be repaired, comparatively little data exists on the biomaterial character of this repair tissue. Information regarding the strength of this tissue over time is needed to allow the surgeon to formulate a safe, yet expedient rehabilitation program.

Examine the effect of preexisting degenerative joint disease on the remodeling and efficacy of meniscal replacement.

Because the clinical indication for meniscal replacement probably will involve a joint with preexisting degeneration, it is very important to examine the basic science for replacement under similar conditions. As noted in the third recommendation, the comprehensive characterization of the animal model used is mandatory.

Section Four
Ligaments

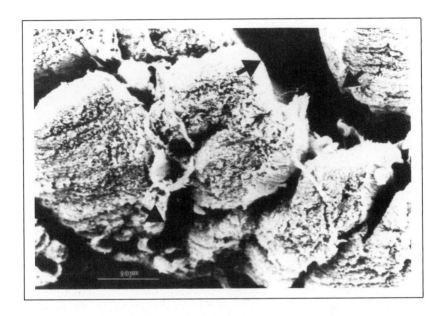

Overview

This section provides a review of the various structures and systems providing stability and dynamic control to the knee joint. Ligaments and their injury and repair mechanisms, the ability of skeletal muscles to produce forces that control motion and stability at the knee and forces that directly strain ligaments, and the nervous system control of muscle forces acting on the knee are discussed. The material presented in this section shows clearly that much more is understood about the biology of ligaments and how they protect the joint than about how muscle forces mediated by the central nervous system control and protect the joint.

Ligaments

Over the past 15 years, significant advances have been made in knowledge of the biology, histology (including ultrastructural analysis), biochemistry, and biomechanics of knee ligaments. Scientific studies continue to provide information that is needed for optimal clinical treatment of ligament injuries. The contribution of ligaments to knee joint stability has been assessed by the study of cadaveric joints with intact ligaments in which stresses and strains are produced in response to joint translations, rotations, and the application of external loads. Isolated bone-ligament-bone preparations also have been studied in detail. Ligaments behave in a viscoelastic manner; that is, their response to stresses and strains is time- and history-dependent. Ligaments demonstrate creep, stress-relaxation, and strain-rate dependent responses to biomechanical testing. Sophisticated, computer-generated models of viscoelastic behavior can demonstrate the biomechanical behavior of ligaments.

The differences between the anterior cruciate ligament (ACL) and the medial collateral ligament (MCL) of the knee have been evaluated using animal models. Results from these studies help explain the outcome of clinical methods of treating injuries of these ligaments. Both ligaments are intra-articular, but MCL fibers are in a nearly parallel arrangement and ACL fibers twist along the long axis of the ligament. The MCL has a higher stiffness and tensile strength than the ACL. In a dog model of MCL injury, the best recovery was obtained in animals in which the ligaments were neither repaired nor immobilized. Biomechanical properties returned towards normal after 48 weeks. However, the recovery of structural properties was much better than that of material properties, partly because of the increased cross-sectional area of the healing ligaments. Results of these studies were confirmed using rabbit models in which the ligaments were ruptured in response to tensile overload rather than from laceration. In both models the healing ligaments can restore joint stability when only the MCL is injured. These data support results of current clinical studies in which excellent outcomes from isolated MCL injuries were obtained without surgical repair or immobilization.

The healing potential for the ACL is much less than for the MCL. Complete tears of the

ACL do not heal, and joint instability usually results. Therefore, experimental studies have focused on surgical techniques for repair or reconstruction of this ligament. The ACL is usually reconstructed using autografts that consist of either a portion of the patellar tendon with bone on either end, the semitendinosus, or the gracilis tendon. The autograft tissue becomes progressively more vascularized over time after implementation and, eventually, is fully vascularized. The biomechanical properties do not recover as well, and partial recovery takes as much as one or two years. Even then most grafts have an ultimate load to failure that is significantly less than that of the normal ACL. Reconstruction with allograft materials also is possible clinically and is receiving attention from basic science investigators. The biologic incorporation and recovery of allografts seems to be relatively similar to that of autografts. Results from animal studies of preservation and sterilization techniques have demonstrated that freezing allograft tissue can reduce its reactivity without being deleterious to mechanical properties. At higher doses, gamma irradiation can lead to a reduction in biomechanical properties.

Muscle

Although normally considered to be the movers of joints, muscles also can be considered to be stabilizers of the joint. Muscles generate forces that result in joint motions and stresses on the ligaments. For example, contraction of the quadriceps muscle produces an anteriorly directed force on the knee that leads to a strain in the ACL. Similarly, activation of the hamstring muscles will produce a posteriorly directed force on the tibia that can reduce or prevent strain in the ACL. In most joint motions, muscles act to decelerate and control forces. Energy is absorbed by the muscular system, rather than totally by the articular surfaces and the ligaments. Muscles often act eccentrically to control these forces, that is, the muscles are activated while being lengthened by external forces; therefore, the muscles are actively resisting lengthening rather than shortening.

Most investigations of the influence of muscles about the knee have centered on the ACL because of its clinical significance. In normal movement, the ACL is strained slightly by quadriceps forces at flexion angles from full extension to 60 degrees of flexion. If there is no ACL, quadriceps activity induces an anterior tibial translation. These data have been used in various rehabilitation protocols to protect an ACL reconstruction. They should also be considered as a factor in the causes of injury to the ACL.

Hamstring activation reduces strain in the ACL at all angles. Gait studies also show hamstring activity as the knee nears extension and the muscles are therefore acting as ACL synergists. The extent to which the muscular activity is protecting or shielding the ACL from stresses and forces in normal and athletic activity is currently unknown, but the effect is probably quite large. The simultaneous activation, or coactivation, of the knee flexors and extensors by the central nervous system (CNS) during joint movement increases joint stiffness and decreases joint displacements. This CNS activity that requires energy to provide opposing movements emphasizes the need for muscles to control forces acting at the joint level.

Following injury to the ACL, distinct changes occur in the CNS control of the knee as evidenced by muscular activity. Quadriceps atrophy and weakness usually accompany ACL injury. There is a decrease in electromyographic (EMG) activity in the quadriceps, with a larger decrement in force production than would be predicted by loss of muscle mass. The hamstring muscles respond very differently after injury of the ACL. The knee flexors maintain their size and strength. In addition, EMG studies show that during gait hamstring activation increases in a manner that would tend to reduce the anterior subluxation made possible by the ACL tear. Surgical reconstruction of the injured ACL allows some return toward normally functioning knee flexors and extensors; however, many patients continue to demonstrate weakness and altered patterns of muscle use. In general, there is a correlation between the clinical success of the procedure and the recovery of more normally functioning muscles.

CNS Control of Joint Function

Discussion of the way muscle action controls joint function predictably leads to consideration of how the CNS controls muscle forces. Both afferent information coming to the CNS from receptors and the mechanisms for motor control should be considered. Results of recent studies have demonstrated the presence of sensory receptors in joint tissues. Afferent nerves are generally classified according to their conduction velocities, which usually correlate with axonal size. Most joint afferent nerve fibers have spot-like receptive fields and are primarily active in response to noxious stimuli, with some small measurable activity during motion. However, these fibers are not very specific in their responses and seem unlikely to be involved with important protective reflexes. The slow conduction velocities of these fibers also mitigate against their involvement with the maintenance of dynamic stability.

The larger nerve fibers innervate large multicellular sensory end organs. Group I fibers terminate on muscle receptors, and group II afferent fibers innervate primarily Ruffinian and Paciniform corpuscles, which respond to tissue stretch and are located throughout the capsule and ligaments. However, there are relatively few of these receptors.

Examination of reflexes mediated by joint afferent fibers raises the concern that these receptors may not be adequate to play a large role in the dynamic stability of the joint. Reflexes evoked by group III and IV afferent fibers were nonspecific and weak. Group II afferent fibers also evoke weak and variable effects in response to electrical stimulation, joint rotation, and joint inflation. It thus appears most likely that ligament afferent fibers do not provide any major reflex effect. However, they still may serve an important protective function. The presence of intact innervation in an unstable joint serves to limit the development of arthrosis. With intact joint afferent fibers, an animal may be able to adopt central nervous system mediated strategies to increase joint stability or minimize any harmful effects. The sensory information is most useful because it can modify the patterns by which the CNS controls movement rather than because it provides instantaneous reflex protection of the joint. The data discussed in the chapter on muscle control of the joint demonstrate that CNS control of joints is quite different in an unstable knee.

The mechanisms by which the nervous system through peripheral receptors, spinal and supraspinal mechanisms, and skeletal muscles provides stability require further study.

Chapter 13

Biology, Healing, and Repair of Ligaments

Savio L-Y. Woo, PhD
Karen J. Ohland, MS
Patrick J. McMahon, MD

Introduction

Ligaments are living, dynamic structures with a very complex role in knee function, capable of hypertrophy, atrophy, and healing responses. Because of the high incidence of ligament injury and the difficulties associated with establishing satisfactory repair techniques, these tissues have been studied intensely. In recent years, it has been recognized that extra-articular ligaments such as the medial collateral ligament (MCL) can heal effectively when injured,[1-4] whereas intra-articular ligaments such as the anterior cruciate ligament (ACL) do not heal effectively.[5-7] Therefore, the choice between nonoperative treatment and surgical repair of knee ligament injuries and the subsequent rehabilitation protocols are controversial. Quantitative information about ligament biology not only will increase knowledge of the behavior of these tissues and their contributions to normal joint function, but also will assist with the management of ligament injury.

This chapter includes discussion of the techniques used for evaluating both normal and healing ligaments. Using a multidisciplinary approach, the normal properties of the MCL and ACL are compared, and the problems and possibilities of restoring function following both MCL and ACL injuries are discussed.

Multidisciplinary Approach for Assessment of Ligament Properties

Ligaments are complex, heterogeneous structures in which the metabolism of the cells within the tissue responds to environmental stimuli and functional needs in a highly regulated fashion. The resulting metabolic changes alter the ultrastructure, chemistry, and physical properties of the ligament. In order to compare the outcomes of different treatment regimens, a multidisciplinary approach, which correlates histologic, biochemical, and biomechanical results, must be used to evaluate both normal and healing ligaments.

Histology

Ultrastructure   Hematoxylin and eosin (H&E) stain is used for routine histological examination of both cells (fibroblasts) and collagen fibers in the healing ligament. The degree of alignment of the collagen fibers, which reflects the organization and, thus, the stiffness and strength of the normal and injured ligaments, can be examined using polarized light microscopy. Polarized light microscopy also is an effective way to visualize the collagen crimp pattern and is helpful in evaluating the architecture of the ligament.[8] Mallory trichrome stain has been used by Goldberg and associates[9] to visualize the interstitial matrix, while Bray and associates[10] have used cationic stains such as ruthenium red and ruthenium hexamine trichloride to enhance the visibility of negatively charged tissue components, particularly glycosaminoglycans. Collagen fibrils are known to vary in size and orientation within ligaments. These variations can be seen using light microscopy, but are best observed using transmission electron microscopy.[11-13]

Cellular   Evaluation of the characteristics of the cells in ligaments is also important because cell characteristics indicate the status of the various metabolic processes. The nuclei of fibroblasts can be seen after H&E staining. Cells can also be examined using immunologic labeling. For example, goat anti-rabbit fibronectin antibodies can be used to label fibronectin-containing cells within the ligament substance.[14] Other immunologic markers may soon help to further characterize ligament cellular elements. Ligament cells also have been examined in culture to evaluate their growth potential[15] as well as their response to such agents as synovial fluid.[16]

Vascular   The blood supply to the ligaments has been documented by several investigators who used vascular injection, microangiographic, and vascular casting techniques.[17-19] Hydrogen washout techniques, which allow assessment of perfusion following sequential manipulations such as application of ligament stress or injury, also have been used to provide information about the vascularity and nutrition of intact ligaments;[20] however, they cannot be used in vivo. Functional blood flow to ligaments in vivo has been measured using laser doppler flowmetry.[21]

Biochemistry

Biochemical analysis of the healing ligament includes measurements of water content, collagen content, collagen type and crosslinks, and total glycosaminoglycans. Water makes up about two thirds of the weight of a normal ligament, and the fibrillar protein collagen makes up 70% to 80% of the remaining dry weight.[22-24]

Collagen is believed to be the principal component that resists tensile stress in a ligament.[25] A normal ligament has 90% type I collagen, less than 10% type III collagen, and smaller quantities of other collagen types. Total collagen is assessed by measuring the hydroxyproline content,[26] while the relative amounts of type I and type III collagen are determined by separation of peptides resulting from cyanogen bromide digestion of the tissue collagen.[27,28] In mature ligament tissues, there is generally a balance between collagen synthesis and degradation, with an estimated collagen half-life between 300 and 500 days.[29] Changes in the ratio of the intermolecular reducible Schiff-base cross-links, as determined by cation-exchange liquid chromatography, are used to evaluate collagen maturation during healing.[30-32] While the presence of proteoglycans may be detected by enzymes such as chondroitinase ABC and chondroitinase AC II, which remove glycosaminoglycan side chains from proteoglycan molecules,[10,33,34] the concentration of glycosaminoglycan can be determined by measuring the hexosamine content.[35]

Biomechanics

Measurement of Knee Joint Stability   Several methods have been developed to assess the roles ligaments play in allowing normal joint motion while maintaining joint stability. Some investigators have measured the force or moment produced by translation or rotation of a joint,[36-38] while others have measured the joint motion produced by application of a known external load.[39-42] However, the findings of these experimental studies have not been in agreement. The discrepancies may result from the different species studied, the variety of testing protocols used, the degrees of constraint to knee motion inherent in the design of the experimental apparatus, or other unknown factors. A normal knee has six degrees of freedom (DOF) of motion: anteroposterior, proximodistal, and mediolateral translations; and varus-valgus, flexion-extension, and internal-external rotations. Therefore, measurement of knee stability with a device that overconstrains coupled motion in several DOF would bias the experimental results.

For example, the influence of the number of DOF on varus-valgus rotation of canine knees was examined using an apparatus designed to apply a varus-valgus bending moment.[39] With the knee flexed at 90 degrees, the varus-valgus knee instability in the five DOF case (all three translations, varus-valgus and internal-external rotations) was much higher (220%) than that for the more constrained three DOF case (anteroposterior translation, varus-valgus and internal-external rotations). This occurred because the tibia was allowed to displace axially and anteroposteriorly in the less constrained case. Thus, five DOF are recommended for examining varus-valgus rotation in the normal knee to avoid artificial constraint of the knee motion. When the contribution of the MCL to valgus knee rotation was measured, the valgus rotation in the three DOF case increased 171% over the intact knee after MCL transection. In the five DOF case, the valgus rotation increased only 21% over the intact knee after MCL transection. Therefore, limiting the knee to three DOF is recommended when assessing the contribution of healing MCL to valgus rotation.

Tensile Testing: Structural Versus Mechanical Properties   Ligament biomechanical properties are generally measured in tension because the main function of ligaments is to resist tensile loading. Tensile testing generally uses the bone-ligament-bone complex as a functional composite (Fig. 1). During testing, elongation of the entire complex and load are obtained. The load-elongation curve represents the structural properties of the composite, which includes the ligament substance and its insertions to bone. These components have different physical properties, and each contributes to the elongation. The stress-strain relationship of the tissue is used to describe the mechanical properties of the ligament substance. If the cross-sectional area is known, the stress can be determined using the load data. For strain, the video dimension analyzer system (described below) is used to measure the change in length/original length. Therefore, the mechanical properties of the ligament substance describe the material characteristics of the ligament alone, without the contribution from other parts of the bone-ligament-bone complex.

Structural Properties of the Bone-Ligament-Bone Complex   A ligament is tested in tension with the the bones affixed to clamps to produce uniform stress distributions across the ligament. The structural properties, as determined from the load-elongation curve recorded during testing, include the linear stiffness (slope of the load-elongation curve), ultimate load, ultimate elongation, and energy absorbed to failure (area under the load-elongation curve) (Fig. 1). If the specimen is properly clamped and tested, elongation between bone and clamps generally has a minimal effect, because the bone and clamps should be much stiffer than the ligament tissue.

Mechanical Properties of Ligament Substance   To determine properties that reflect the behavior of the ligament substance alone, the effects of the insertion sites must be eliminated. This is done by characterizing the ligament substance as a material represented by the stress-strain curves, where stress is defined as the force per unit cross-sectional area. Recently, a laser micrometer system[43,44] has been used to determine the cross-sectional shape and area of the ligament substance. The profile widths of the tissue are measured as the specimen is rotated through 180 degrees in increments of 3 degrees. The data obtained are used to reconstruct the cross-sectional shape and calculate the cross-sectional area.

The strain in a specimen is most commonly calculated using the formula $(l - l_0)/l_0$ where l is the specimen length during a test and l_0 is a reference length, usually the original undeformed length. To

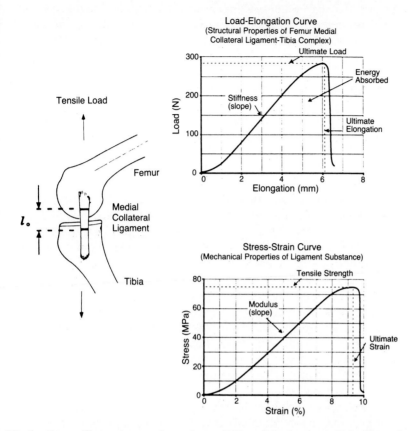

Fig. 1 *Curves illustrating tensile testing to failure of the femur-medial collateral ligament-tibia complex. The structural properties are obtained from the load-elongation curve (**top**), while the mechanical properties of the medial collateral ligament substance are obtained from the stress-strain curve (**bottom**). (Modified with permission from Anderson DR, Weiss JA, Takai S, et al: Healing of the medial collateral ligament following a triad injury. J Orthop Res 1992;10:485-495.)*

avoid direct physical contact with the ligament substance during an experiment, the video dimension analyzer system has been used to measure ligament strain.[45] The video dimension analyzer system tracks the change in distance between two lines stained on the surface of the ligament. The distance between the two lines is converted to an output voltage, which is then calibrated to correspond to a percent strain. Strains of the ligament substance can thus be measured independently of its insertion sites. The mechanical (material) properties of the ligament substance, as determined from the stress-strain curve, include the modulus (slope of the stress-strain curve), tensile strength, and ultimate strain (Fig. 1).

Tensile failure is a result of failure of the weakest link in the complex. It can occur at the insertion sites, within the ligament substance itself, or as a combination of both. Failure at the clamp-bone interface usually indicates improper clamping technique or poor testing procedure. Ultimate load and elongation can be reported whether failure occurs at the insertion site or within the ligament substance, because these parameters represent the ultimate values for the entire structure. Tensile strength (sometimes called ultimate tensile strength or ultimate stress) and ultimate strain are mechanical properties that can be obtained only if failure occurs within the substance of the ligament tissue itself. Failure at the insertion site indicates that the insertion site is the weakest link and, in this case, the highest values obtained from the stress-strain curves will underestimate the true tensile strength of the ligament.

In Situ Versus In Vitro Properties   Although tensile testing of the bone-ligament-bone complex is usually done in vitro, Tipton and associates[46] developed a method for assessing the structural properties of the femur-MCL-tibia complex of rats in situ and compared the results with those obtained in vitro. Anesthetized rats were placed on a loading platform and incisions made to expose the MCL with minimal disruption of the surrounding blood vessels. The popliteal artery was severed just prior to testing and tensile load to failure was applied along the axis of the MCL. Small but significant differences were reported; that is, the linear stiffness and ultimate load obtained for the in situ specimens were 6% and 4% lower, respectively, while the ultimate elongation was 12% higher.

Viscoelasticity   Like other soft connective tissues, ligaments exhibit time- and history-dependent viscoelastic properties that reflect the complex interactions of collagen and the surrounding extracellular matrix. Therefore, the shape of the load-elongation curve for the ligament depends on the previous loading history and the time over which the load is applied. In addition, because of internal energy losses, the loading and unloading curves of a ligament do not follow the same path; instead the curves form a hysteresis loop (Fig. 2). Other important viscoelastic characteristics are creep, an increase in deformation over time under a constant load, and stress relaxation, a decline in stress over time under a constant deformation (Fig. 3).

The viscoelastic behavior of ligaments has important physiological and clinical implications. During walking or jogging, in which the applied strains are repetitive and within a known range,[47,48] cyclic stress relaxation will effectively lower the stress in the ligament substance. This phenomenon may help prevent fatigue failure of ligaments. Similarly, during cyclic loading to a constant load, deformation increases slightly, demonstrating creep behavior.[49] Decreases in joint stiffness and increases in joint laxity (excursion) following exercise have been observed clinically.[50] After a short recovery period there is a return to normal joint stiffness and apparent length as the history-dependent viscoelastic behavior diminishes.

Visualization and analysis of viscoelastic effects are often simplified by considering mechanical or electrical analogues that mimic

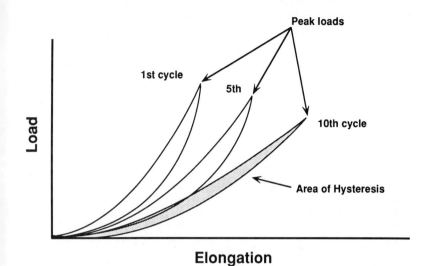

Fig. 2   *Loading (top) and unloading (bottom) curves from cyclic tensile testing of knee ligaments. The two nonlinear curves from any one cycle form a hysteresis loop, with the area between the curves, termed the area of hysteresis, indicative of energy losses within the tissue. (Note: For clarity, the area of hysteresis has been exaggerated.)*

this behavior, such as the Maxwell or Voigt models.[51] Other models have been used to describe and compare the time- and history-dependent viscoelastic properties of ligaments; of these the quasi-linear viscoelastic theory developed by Fung is most notable.[47,48] Although these models do help evaluate and describe the mechanical behavior of ligaments and other soft tissues, "they are no more and no less than models, they demonstrate the behavior but do not necessarily explain it at the molecular level."[51]

Joint Kinematics: Methods for Motion Measurements   Kinematic techniques have provided information about the motion of normal joints and the consequences of ligament injury and/or repair. Different techniques have been used to quantify the amount of motion that occurs in a joint under external loading and with muscle stabilization.[52] Frequently, linear-variable-differential-transducers and rotary-variable-differential-transducers are connected to the two bones of a joint. When the joint moves, the transducers measure the amount of translation or rotation.[53-56] Six-DOF measurements can be made using a magnetic tracking system; the disturbances in the low frequency magnetic field are specific for various joint positions.[57-60] Other investigators have opted to use devices that do not require any mechanical attachments to the femur and tibia, such as acoustic transducers[61] and roentgen-stereophotogrammetric techniques.[62]

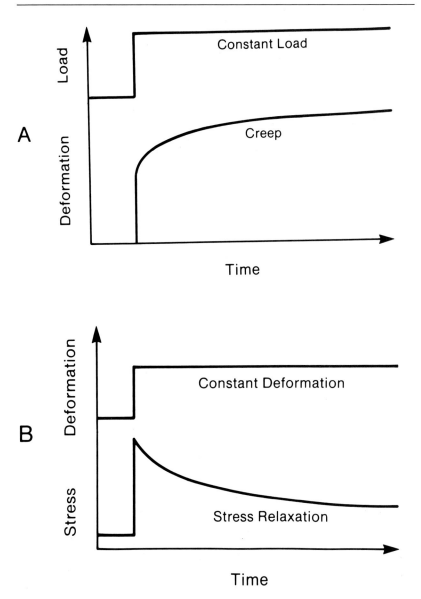

Fig. 3 *Schematic representation of (**top**) creep behavior (increasing deformation over time under a constant load) and (**bottom**) stress relaxation (decreasing stress over time under a constant deformation). (Reproduced with permission from Woo SL-Y, Young EP: Structure and function of tendons and ligaments, in Mow VC, Hayes WC (eds):* Basic Orthopaedic Biomechanics. *New York, Raven Press, 1991, p 203.)*

Joint Kinetics: Methods of Force Measurement   Knowledge of the forces in the ligament of an intact joint (in situ loads) is required to anticipate changes in load distribution that will occur after injury or to reproduce the normal forces during repair. Therefore, different techniques have been developed to determine in situ ligament forces in intact joints. Lewis and associates[63] used buckle transducers to measure ligament forces. Markolf and associates[64] measured the forces in the ACL directly, by drilling a hole approximately in line with the ACL through the tibial plateau and then attaching the bone plug to a load cell. When the knee was subjected to various motions and external loads, the resultant forces were measured. Others have tried to estimate ACL forces by applying strain gauges to the tibial plateau near the ACL insertion site[65] in an attempt to correlate changes in strain of the bone to the forces in the ACL.

Indirect methods have also been used to determine the forces in ligaments. Woo and associates[66] measured the in situ loads in the rabbit MCL by measuring the distance (l) between two dye lines placed on the MCL in the intact knee. All structures of the knee except the MCL were then transected, unloading the MCL, and the new distance (l_0) between the dye lines was measured. After the bone-ligament-bone complex was loaded in a materials testing machine, a load-strain curve was obtained. The load on the curve that corresponded to the level of in-situ strain ($[l - l_0]/l_0$) was the in situ load. Takai and associates[67] determined the loads in the human ACL using a six-DOF kinematic linkage to measure the motion of the knee. The in situ lengths of different portions of the ACL were calculated from the recorded motion. The load-elongation curves were then obtained for the whole ACL as well as for the anterior portion of the ACL alone (that is, with the posterior portion removed). The in situ loads in the whole ACL and in the anterior portion were obtained by combining these load-elongation curves with the in situ length data obtained from the kinematic linkage.

Correlation of Multidisciplinary Results

Analysis of a single tissue or structure will inevitably fail to yield a true understanding of joint function, because the interactions between the various components are critical to joint behavior. The current, though incomplete, understanding of joint kinematics is a result of intense examination of the individual components without regard to the contribution of each to overall joint function.[68] A multidisciplinary approach, which describes the morphological, biochemical, and biomechanical properties, is important for a comprehensive understanding of both normal and healing ligaments. For example, the strength of a ligament cannot be explained solely by quantitative analysis of collagen because the architectural arrangement of the collagen and many other factors also contribute to ligament strength. Additionally, during healing there is a time delay between changes in cellularity and the biochemical detection of the metabolic products of these cells, and there is a further time delay before the cellular and biochemical changes are reflected in the biomechanical properties of the ligament. Therefore, a multidisciplinary approach can be helpful not only for correlating the properties of normal ligaments, but also for understanding the ongoing changes in healing tissues.

Differences Between MCL and ACL

As a result of the frequent involvement of both the MCL and ACL in knee injuries and of differences in their anatomy, environment, and healing response, research has been devoted to contrasting their biomechanical, biochemical, and histological characteristics.

Nutrition and Environment

It has recently been demonstrated that the ACL is capable of deriving nutrition from the synovial fluid;[69-71] however, under certain conditions, the synovial fluid can contain enzymes that are detrimental to ligament metabolic processes. Studies of the ACL in culture have shown that synovial fluid alone does not inhibit collagen synthesis.[16] Yet, results of studies in rabbits have indicated that, after arthrotomy, the synovial sheath appears to protect the ACL against the degradative action of collagenase in the synovial fluid.[72] These and other data[73] suggest that while synovial fluid normally supports ACL metabolism, it may severely limit ligament healing potential after injury or in certain disease states.

Anatomy

Ligaments are dense, collagenous structures attached to bone on either side of a joint. On gross dissection, ligaments are surrounded by loose areolar connective tissue or, if the ligament is intra-articular, synovium. Subdivisions of ligaments have been identified and are known to function in different joint positions.[5,74]

The MCL is an extra-articular ligament that is relatively flat, while the ACL is intra-articular and has fibers that twist along the long axis of the ligament.[75,76] The human MCL does not have an entirely parallel fiber arrangement like that seen in rabbits and other quadrupeds. Poliacu Prosé and associates[77] have examined the collateral ligaments in both humans and felines, and found that the fibers of the MCL are slightly twisted except in the region of the meniscal attachment. Most of the fibers of the MCL were also observed to be taut throughout the range of motion. The ACL's broad attachments to the tibia and femur, however, cause the ligament to twist during knee motion and, as a result, some portions experience tension while other portions are unloaded and buckled.

Histology

Ultrastructural   Ultrastructural studies of ligaments suggest that proteoglycans are nonuniformly distributed and are in close association with cell processes. The extracellular matrix of rabbit MCL has been examined by Bray and associates,[10] who observed an extensive network of thin, electron-dense microfilaments that appeared to irregularly subdivide the extracellular matrix. Small proteoglycan-containing granules were dispersed throughout this network.[10]

The ultrastructure of the ACL was described as fascicular by Kennedy and associates.[78] Regions of endotenon, which appear to bind longitudinal collagen fibers into subfascicles and fascicles, have been found in human, rabbit, and canine ACL.[79,80] Clark and Sidles[81] further described increased interfascicular substance near insertion sites for the ACL in all three species.

Recently, our laboratory and others have used transmission electron microscopy to quantify the distribution of fibril diameters within ligaments.[11-13,82] The fibril diameters are not normally distributed.[13] Both the shape of the ACL distribution and the mean fibril diameter for rabbits are similar to those reported for humans,[12] suggesting analogous collagen fibril populations for the ACL within these species.

The mean fibril diameter is greater for the MCL than for the ACL, and the shapes of their collagen fibril diameter distributions are also significantly different. The ACL is shown to have a predominance of smaller-diameter fibrils. In contrast, the MCL has a more bimodal distribution with both large and small diameter fibrils.[83] It has been suggested that larger-diameter collagen fibrils may provide a greater resistance to tensile loading because of an increase in collagen molecules available to form cross-links.[84] It should be noted, however, that direct evidence is not yet available. Differences in mechanical properties also might arise from differences in the density of collagen fibrils within subfasciculi or from differences in the distributions of fibril diameters.

Cellular   Potential differences between the fibroblasts and pericellular region of the MCL and ACL have been documented using transmission electron microscopy.[14] The cells of the MCL are spindle-shaped, aligned along the long axis of the ligament, and interspersed throughout the fiber bundles. These cells are intimately associated both with collagen fibrils and with neighboring cells. The ACL cells are oval and aligned in columns between the collagen bundles.[23,75,85] They do not appear to be intimately in contact with the collagen matrix, but instead are surrounded by an area of amorphous ground substance. However, more definitive studies of these differences will be needed.

The cells of the ACL and MCL may also exhibit different responses to injury. After rabbit MCLs and ACLs were harvested and placed in cell culture, Nagineni and associates[15] found bigger clusters of cells around the MCL explants. With subculture of these cells, growth rates for the MCL cells were higher than for the ACL cells. These differences may be partially responsible for the differences in the healing capacities of these two ligaments.

Vascular   In rabbits, dogs, and humans, the blood supply to the MCL is provided by the inferior medial geniculate artery while that of the ACL is primarily from the middle geniculate artery.[17,19,86,87] Some differences among species have been observed in the secondary blood supply to these ligaments. However, because many of these vessels have anastomoses throughout the knee joint, variations in experimental procedure may influence the results. The majority of the vessels have been observed on the surface of the ligaments (epiligamentous), with branches connecting to smaller intraligamentous networks.[17,86,87] In addition, fewer intraligamentous vessels are observed in the midsubstance of the ACL in both rabbits[86,88] and dogs.[89] Quantitatively, Dunlap and associates[20] recorded that in dogs the blood flow to the ACL was only 47% of that to the synovium.

Biochemistry

Biochemical differences between the ACL and MCL also have been demonstrated. Compared with the MCL, the rabbit cruciate ligaments contain a similar amount of type I collagen, but a one third higher percentage of type III collagen. In the healing ligament, the percentage of type III collagen is generally higher, reflecting increases in the amount of scar tissue. The cruciate ligaments have twice the amount of glycosaminoglycans, and the reducible collagen cross-link is present in greater amounts.[22]

Elastin is found in small quantities (less than 5%) in most skeletal ligaments. Like other tissue elements, elastin probably has important matrix interactions that influence its mechanical role in ligaments. Although proteoglycans constitute less than 1% of the ligament's dry weight,[90] they may play a key role in ligament function. The association of these molecules with water forms a gel-like extracellular matrix. The absolute amount of glycosaminoglycan may be ligament-specific and may also vary within ligaments. Frank and associates[35] found variable distributions of water, glycosaminoglycan, and collagen along the rabbit MCL. The water content was greatest proximally and decreased toward the tibial insertion. Mean collagen concentration was greatest at the midsubstance and glycosaminoglycan concentration was greatest at the femoral and tibial insertions. Although the nature of proteoglycan-collagen[91] and collagen-collagen[92] interactions is presently not well understood, better characterization of these components may increase understanding of normal ligament biology and of the differential healing responses.

Biomechanical Properties

To reduce the geometric complexity of the ACL and permit more uniform loading, the ACL was divided into medial and lateral portions, and each was tensile tested separately. The mechanical

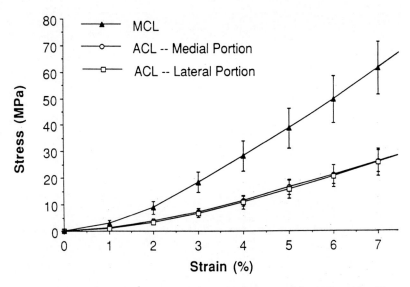

Fig. 4   *The mechanical properties of the mid-substance of the MCL and ACL as represented by the stress-strain curves (Reproduced with permission from Woo SL-Y, Newton PO, MacKenna DA, et al: A comparative evaluation of the mechanical properties of the rabbit medial collateral and anterior cruciate ligaments. J Biomech 1992;25:377-386.)*

properties of the medial and lateral portions of the ACL were found to be similar to each other,[93] but significantly different from those of the MCL (Fig. 4). The modulus (slope of the stress-strain curve) was approximately twice as high for the MCL as for either portion of the ACL. The tensile strength of the MCL was found to be over 70% higher than that of the ACL. Butler and associates,[94] however, demonstrated differences between the portions of human ACL. When loaded to failure in tension, the modulus, tensile strength, and ultimate strain of the anteromedial and anterolateral bundles of the ACL were higher than those of the posterior bundle.[94] The differences in the results of these two studies may be attributable to differences in species, methods for measuring strain, and methods of defining and separating the bundles.

The higher modulus and tensile strength of the MCL as compared with the ACL has been attributed, in part, to differences in their ultrastructural and morphological appearances. Cross-sectional scanning electron micrographs demonstrate this dramatic difference in collagen fiber arrangement (Fig. 5). The subfascicular area fraction of collagen is also significantly greater for the MCL than for the ACL.[13] This indicates that more ground substance, which does not bear tensile load, surrounds the ACL subfascicles. The collagen fibers of the MCL are packed closely together without a prominent interfascicular region of connective tissue. In other words, the MCL has more load-bearing collagen fibers per unit area than the ACL.

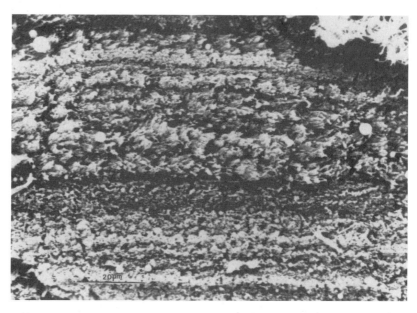

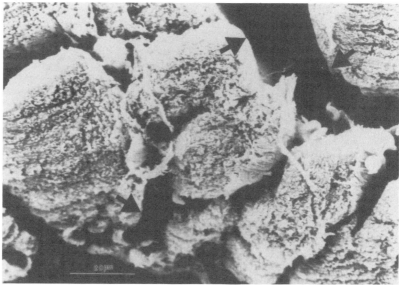

Fig. 5   *Scanning electron photomicrographs (900x) of ligament cross-sections prepared by L. Kitabayashi and A. Sisk.* **Top,** *MCL showing densely packed collagen fibers distributed uniformly.* **Bottom,** *ACL showing collagen fibers arranged in a fascicular pattern, with a large interfascicular region (arrows). (Reproduced with permission from Woo SL-Y, Newton PO, MacKenna DA, et al: A comparative evaluation of the mechanical properties of the rabbit medial collateral and anterior cruciate ligaments. J Biomech 1992;25:377-386.)*

Injury and Repair of Knee Ligaments

Fetto and Marshall[1] reported that the MCL is the most frequently injured ligament of the knee. In a three-year study of a general population of 280,000 people served by the San Diego Kaiser Knee Injury Clinic, 500 severe ligament injuries were diagnosed.[95] Of these, 29% were isolated MCL injuries and an additional 13% were combined MCL and ACL injuries. Others have reported that MCL injury accounts for 55% (450/819) of acute knee injuries.[96] However, the number of ACL injuries is also significant. It has been estimated that in the United States, 100,000 people per year injure an ACL while skiing.[97] Elsewhere, Feagin and associates[97] reported a rate of 72 injuries involving the ACL per 100,000 skier days, and Hewson and associates[98] reported the rate for injuries involving the ACL to be 56 per 100,000 player days in college football. There are 50,000 ligament operations per year in the United States,[99] the majority of which are performed to reconstruct a ruptured ACL.[100] Most isolated ACL (70%), isolated MCL (54%), and combined ACL/MCL (61%) injuries with pathologic motion occurred during sports activities. Football, baseball, soccer, and skiing account for almost equal numbers of acute knee ligament injuries.[96]

Midsubstance injuries or complete tears of the ACL generally do not heal, because the frayed ends do not meet and ligamentous tissue does not fill the gap,[5-7,101,102] even if repair is attempted.[7,103] The sole exception to this poor ACL healing response is seen in avulsion fractures of either the tibial or femoral insertion sites, which heal well as long as the displacement is not large.[104,105] These injuries heal like bony injuries and therefore cannot be classified as ligament healing.[106,107]

Unrepaired midsubstance ACL injuries can lead to secondary damage including MCL injury,[108,109] meniscal tears, and degenerative arthritis of the knee,[96] while untreated MCL injuries appear to heal well with little evidence of subsequent damage to the knee.[2,3] Although it has been suggested that individuals with residual valgus laxity following MCL injury may be at increased risk for ACL injury,[110] clinical studies have demonstrated that the MCL has a reparative capacity that generally results in normal joint function within months of MCL rupture.[1,4] This observation has been substantiated quantitatively in experimental studies using dogs, rabbits, and sheep.[24,111,112] However, while normal ligament has a very orderly organization, the healing tissue is much less organized, with a random pattern of fibers. Orientation of the fibers in the direction of applied physiologic stresses takes a very long time as does the return of stiffness and strength to the healing structures.[113]

Despite extensive clinical and experimental evaluation of MCL injuries and treatment regimens, the preferable treatment method following MCL injury is still debated. It has been suggested that repair may increase the organization of healing MCLs,[114] and result in superior biomechanical properties.[114,115] However, other investigators have found that nonoperative treatment provides as complete a recovery as surgical treatment, with a more rapid return to sports activities. This issue will be discussed in more detail later.

255

MCL Healing: Experimental Studies

Because the ruptured MCL can heal predictably without surgical intervention,[24,111,116] much is known about the quality of healed MCL tissue. MCL healing is a long, complex process involving the same basic phases as wound healing and is apparently subject to the same external influences.[117] Results obtained from in vitro and in vivo animal studies provide significant information regarding both the initial environment to which the ligament is subjected after injury and its healing response with time. Both local and systemic factors can influence the process; this is particularly true of motion or immobilization. A host of other variables (mediators of inflammation and growth factors) offer significant promise for optimizing the healing process.

Effect of Repair and Immobilization Some investigators have postulated that surgical repair of collateral ligaments is required because the torn ends of the ligament are not in close proximity.[114,118] Recently, Grönblad and associates[119] observed that at both 4 and 14 weeks following MCL rupture in the rabbit, more neuropeptide-immunoreactive nerves were present in sutured than in unsutured healing zones. This observation suggests that suturing and the apposition of torn ligament ends have beneficial effects on local nerve regeneration. Korkala and associates[120] histologically examined repaired and nonrepaired ligament injuries in rats at 4 to 5 weeks after surgery. Using scanning electron microscopy, these authors found that the appearance of the nonrepaired ligament was variable, with extensive scarring visible in some cases. Results from biomechanical studies by Clayton and associates[114,121] demonstrated that sutured canine MCLs were stronger than unsutured MCLs at all time periods up to 9 weeks postoperatively. Also, roentgenograms suggested that suturing the ligaments resulted in less valgus joint instability than did not suturing the ligaments.

Although immobilization has often been used in combination with ligament repair to protect the tissue from damage during the early healing phases,[122,123] its detrimental side effects are well known, including increases in joint stiffness, proliferation of fibro-fatty connective tissue, and synovial adhesions.[124] Ligament properties are also compromised by immobilization.

A comparative study of healing following midsubstance transection of canine MCL treated with either no repair and no immobilization or surgical repair and 6 weeks immobilization was performed in our laboratory. Healing in skeletally mature dogs was examined histologically, biomechanically, and biochemically at 6, 12, and 48 weeks postoperatively.[111,125] At 6 weeks, histologic sections of the healing sites in both treatment groups appeared similar. The tissue contained fibroblasts, some of which were aligned along the long axis of the ligament. At 12 weeks, the alignment of the fibroblasts in the longitudinal direction was more pronounced in the surgically repaired ligaments. Similar results were obtained by Korkala and associates[120] and O'Donoghue and associates.[118] By 48 weeks, however, the healing tissues from both the repaired/immobilized and nonrepaired/nonimmobilized groups had microscopic appearances similar to those of normal MCL. Examination with polarized light microscopy, however, revealed that the orientation of the collagen fibers of the MCL remained irregular.

The amount of varus-valgus instability for experimental knees from both groups was significantly higher than for the control knees at 6 weeks, but by 12 weeks the nonrepaired/nonimmobilized group had values similar to normal, whereas the varus-valgus knee instabilities of the repaired/immobilized group were still larger than control. This was also true at 48 weeks (Table 1). The tensile properties of the nonrepaired/nonimmobilized ligaments were superior at all time periods. At 6 weeks, the structural properties of the femur-MCL-tibia complex for both groups were lower than for the controls. By 12 weeks postoperatively, the linear stiffness of the nonrepaired/nonimmobilized femur-MCL-tibia complexes was indistinguishable from that of the contralateral controls. The linear stiffness of the repaired/immobilized femur-MCL-tibia complexes, however, tended to be lower than that of the contralateral controls, suggesting that recovery of the linear stiffness to normal levels is delayed by surgical repair and immobilization. By 48 weeks, the linear stiffness of the experimental femur-MCL-tibia complexes from both groups was not significantly different from that of the contralateral controls. Also, the ultimate load for the nonrepaired/nonimmobilized femur-MCL-tibia complexes remained at about the same level as that of the controls, while the ultimate load for the repaired/immobilized femur-MCL-tibia complexes was only 78% of that of the controls (Table 1).

In both groups, the mechanical properties of the healed MCL substance increased with time, but not as rapidly nor as completely as the structural properties of the femur-MCL-tibia complex. The modulus of the nonrepaired/nonimmobilized MCL was not different from that of the control at 48 weeks, while the modulus of the repaired/immobilized MCL remained significantly lower than that of the control, emphasizing the long-term detrimental effects of repair and immobilization (Table 1). The tensile strength of the MCL in both groups was still lower than that of the control at all times. Tensile strength of the nonrepaired/nonimmobilized MCL reached only two-thirds that of the contralateral control at 48 weeks (Table 1). Biochemical analysis showed that there were no significant differences in collagen content, collagen types, or reducible crosslinks between the groups at any time period.[125]

The effects of different treatment regimens on MCL healing have been examined in clinical studies. O'Donoghue and associates[118] and others[126-128] have recommended surgical repair and subsequent immobilization for MCL injuries. Other investigators have reported that patients respond well to conservative treatment, and immobili-

Table 1 Biomechanical properties of the intact knee and the femur-MCL-tibia complex at 48 weeks postoperatively

Property*	Group I**	Group II+
Intact knee		
V-V knee rotation (E/C)	1.05 ± 0.18	1.58 ± 0.18
Femur-MCL-tibia complex		
Linear stiffness (E/C)	1.03 ± 0.09	0.92 ± 0.12
Ultimate load (E/C)	0.92 ± 0.12	0.81 ± 0.08
MCL substance		
Modulus (MPa) (E)	802 ± 27.0	460 ± 82.6
Modulus (MPa) (C)	912 ± 116	1,110 ± 164
Tensile strength (MPa) (E)	53.8 ± 9.3	41.9 ± 3.3
Tensile strength (MPa) (C)	91.8 ± 7.3	92.1 ± 2.3

(Reproduced with permission from Inoue M, Woo SL-Y, Gomez MA, et al: Effects of surgical treatment and immobilization on the healing of the medial collateral ligament: A long-term multidisciplinary study. *Connect Tiss Res* 1990;25:13-26.)
* E is experimental, C is control
** Nonrepaired/nonimmobilized
+ Repaired/immobilized

zation is not necessary.[1-3,129] However, the severity of injury influences these results. Grade I and II injuries have been shown to heal well.[130,131] Controversy exists regarding the treatment of grade III injuries, in part because isolated grade III injuries are uncommon; many complete MCL tears also involve undiagnosed damage to the ACL or to other joint structures.

Rupture Versus Surgical Transection   Most experimental animal models used to study MCL injury have been created by surgically transecting the ligament in the midsubstance. Surgical transection produces only localized damage to the ligament substance, with no initial damage to the ligament insertions to bone.[132] Thus, this model of injury may not sufficiently represent ligament injuries seen clinically, which frequently involve the entire bone-ligament-bone complex.[2,112,133,134] A new model of ligament injury that includes both a frayed-end tear to the ligament substance and concomitant injury to the insertions to bone has been developed in our laboratory.[135] The rabbit MCL is ruptured by pulling medially on a rod that is passed beneath the ligament. The early healing response after rupture of the MCL (group I) has been compared with that after surgical transection (group II) in skeletally mature rabbits.

Comparison of the varus-valgus knee instabilities and the structural properties of the femur-MCL-tibia complex in groups I and II indicates that the healing response in the two injury models is similar. The varus-valgus instabilities of the experimental knees from both groups are significantly higher than those of the contralateral control knees. The structural properties of the experimental femur-MCL-tibia complexes from both groups are significantly different from those of the controls, but no significant differences are observed between the two groups. Following 6 weeks of healing, however, all group I (ligament rupture) femur-MCL-tibia complexes fail by tibial avulsion, while all group II (surgical transection) femur-MCL-tibia complexes fail in the ligament substance. This difference clearly illustrates that damage occurs at the tibial insertion site when the MCL is ruptured. Histologic examination of the group I specimens confirmed that insertion site damage had occurred. At 10 days postoperatively, the ligament fibers of the insertion are still recoiled, and increased numbers of fibroblasts and blood vessels are evident in the ligament near its insertion to bone. Osteoclastic remodeling is observed at 6 weeks postoperatively.

The longer-term healing responses, up to 52 weeks, following MCL rupture have also been studied.[136] Reossification of the tibial insertion site is observed histologically at 12 weeks, and complete reestablishment of the ligament insertion is achieved by 52 weeks. Varus-valgus instability of the injured knees decreases monotonically with postoperative healing time and is similar to normal at 52 weeks. Over half of the femur-MCL-tibia complexes fail by tibial avulsion at 12 weeks, but at 52 weeks, all specimens fail by midsubstance tears. It should be noted that, in terms of failure modes, the rates of recovery between the ligament substance and insertion sites are asynchronous in the ligament rupture model. The ultimate load of the experimental femur-MCL-tibia complex increases with healing time but remains significantly lower than that of the control, while the mechanical properties of the healing ligament substance are different from those of the control up to 52 weeks. The modulus is less than one third that of the control at 6 weeks and remains unchanged up to 52 weeks postoperatively. The tensile strength of the healing MCL reaches only 25% to 30% of the contralateral control because the cross-sectional area of the healing MCL remains two to three times that of the contralateral control.

The long term results following MCL rupture can be compared with those following surgical transection. Similar results for varus-valgus knee instability have been reported.[125,136] Differences are observed between the ultimate load of the femur-MCL-tibia complex after MCL rupture (~65% of control)[136] and surgical transection (~90% of control).[125] In addition, the tensile strength after MCL rupture (~27% of control) is much lower than that after surgical transection (~60% of control).[125,137]

Effect of Concomitant Injuries   Frequently, more than one ligament is damaged in a traumatized knee. The clinical outcome of combined ACL and MCL injuries is generally worse than that for isolated MCL injuries, regardless of the method of treatment selected.[1,129]

The ability of the MCL to heal under conditions of associated ACL injury has been investigated using a canine knee model that involves either partial or total transection of the ACL.[138] At 6 weeks postoperatively, the varus-valgus instability of the experimental knees from both groups is significantly higher than that of their contralateral controls. At 12 weeks, however, the varus-valgus instability for knees with partial transection of the ACL is similar to that of the controls while varus-valgus instability for knees with total ACL transection is 3.5 times greater than that of the controls. Forbes and associates[139] also found that in rabbit knees with combined ACL and MCL injuries, varus-valgus instability was greater than that of the controls, even after 14 weeks.

The ultimate load for the canine experimental femur-MCL-tibia complex from the partial ACL transected group is similar to that of the control at 12 weeks, while that from the total ACL transected group is only 80% of the control value. However, the mechanical properties of the healed MCL remain significantly different from those of the control ligament. The MCLs from the knees with a totally cut ACL show the least recovery, with the tensile strength reaching only 14% of the control value at 12 weeks (Fig. 6).[138] Because of the marked joint degeneration that develops in the knees with a totally cut ACL, the study was not carried beyond 12 weeks.

The effect of a partial medial meniscectomy and ACL transection on the healing of an MCL rupture was recently studied in our laboratory using skeletally mature rabbits.[140] Campbell[141,142] described this pattern of injury, which was later named the triad injury by O'Donoghue.[122,143] Due to the severity of injury, triad-injured animals experience substantial joint degeneration by 6 weeks postoperatively. Progressive osteophyte formation is observed adjacent to the MCL insertions, and proximal migration of the MCL tibial insertion is observed between 6 and 12 weeks. Histologic examination of the healing MCL substance shows disorganized collagen, inflammation, and fibroblast proliferation that decreases over time. The varus-valgus knee instability is significantly elevated, five times that of the contralateral control following triad injury as compared to twice that of the control following isolated MCL rupture, and it does not decrease with time. Although there is no difference in the linear stiffness of the two injury models at either 6 or 12 weeks, the ultimate load of the triad-injured femur-MCL-tibia complexes is only half that following isolated MCL rupture. The modulus of the healing tissue following triad injury is only 40% of that following isolated MCL rupture and only 5% of contralateral controls.

These experimental results support the clinical observation that the degree of injury has a significant effect on MCL healing and, thus, the selection of an appropriate treatment regimen.[1,129,144] In the laboratory, we have found that ACL reconstruction in this triad injury model can reduce the varus-valgus instability of rabbit knees to levels similar to those following isolated MCL rupture. Such an approach may help improve MCL healing, in part because of the increased valgus stability noted clinically.[1,145] However, the beneficial effect on MCL healing must be determined quantitatively in additional studies.

ACL Healing: Surgical Reconstruction

It is well accepted that a midsubstance ACL tear does not heal intrinsically, and surgical intervention using autografts, allografts,

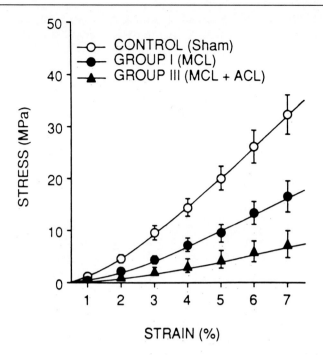

Fig. 6 *Mechanical properties of the femur-MCL-tibia complex at 12 weeks postoperatively. The curve for group II was similar to that for group I. The three groups are as follows: I - isolated MCL transection (intact ACL); II - MCL transection with section of the anteromedial portion of the ACL (partial ACL); and III - both ACL and MCL transection (total ACL). The controls are shown for comparison. (Reproduced with permission from Woo SL-Y, Horibe S, Ohland KJ, et al: The response of ligaments to injury: Healing of the collateral ligaments, in Daniel DM, Akeson WH, O'Connor JJ (eds):* Knee Ligaments: Structure, Function, Injury, and Repair. *New York, Raven Press, 1991, p 361.)*

or synthetic substitutes is often necessary. Intra-articular reconstruction of the ACL using autologous tissue was first reported in 1917 by Hey Groves.[146] Since that time, much has been written on different surgical techniques including the selection and use of various graft materials. At present, the most popular replacements are biologic tissue grafts.

Autografts   The tissues most frequently used as ACL replacements are the central or medial third of the bone-patellar tendon-bone complex,[102,147-153] the semitendinosus tendon,[154-156] and the gracilis tendon.[157] The use of bone-patellar tendon-bone grafts was originally described by Jones[147] and has become the most popular graft because it has available bone blocks for initial fixation.

Experimental animal studies have been performed to evaluate the postimplantation properties of the patellar tendon grafts. Arnoczky and associates[158] found that canine patellar tendon autografts progressed from being initially avascular to being completely ensheathed in a vascular synovial envelope at 6 weeks. Intrinsic revascularization of the graft was complete by 20 weeks, and, at one year, the vascular and histologic appearance of the graft was similar to that of a normal ACL.

The time course of the remodeling process for patellar tendon grafts has also been studied biomechanically in various animal models such as the dog, goat, rabbit, and monkey. Data from dogs reveals that, at the time of transplantation, the femur-patellar tendon-tibia complex has a linear stiffness and ultimate load that are approximately 10% of the control femur-ACL-tibia complex, as a result of fixation site weakness. By 3 months postoperatively, the linear stiffness increases to 20% and ultimate load increases to 30% of control.[152,159] Slightly better biomechanical results for the reconstructed ACL grafts are noted in goats by McPherson and associates[150] and in monkeys by Clancy and associates.[149] Although longer-term studies are necessary to determine whether the properties continue to improve, the general trend for patellar tendon autograft properties has been upward and plateaus at one to two years postoperatively. The ultimate load reaches only 30% to 50% of the control femur-ACL-tibia complex after 2 years, with increases in anteroposterior translation as well as articular degeneration being observed.

It is also noteworthy that the structural properties of the femur-ACL-tibia complex obtained from uniaxial tensile testing depend on the orientation of the ligament and angle of knee flexion.[160] Lower values for the linear stiffness and ultimate load of control or normal femur-ACL-tibia complex, caused by poor specimen orientation as well as misalignment of the ligament with respect to the tensile load, can make the results of a reconstructed femur-ACL-tibia complex seem more favorable. A study of ACL reconstructions in dogs by Nikolaou and associates[161] revealed a very successful outcome using fresh-frozen bone-ACL-bone allografts. They report an ultimate load of the graft complex at 9 months to be 89% of the control femur-ACL-tibia complex, vastly different from the 30% to 40% reported by others. However, their ultimate load values for the control canine femur-ACL-tibia complexes were also much lower than those found by other investigators.[162,163]

Allografts   Allografts, like autografts, can be transplanted as free grafts or with bony insertions. Clinically, the use of autografts has several drawbacks. These problems include increased operative time, size constraints of available tissue, and other complications, which are discussed elsewhere in this book.[164,165] In general, extreme care must be used in the preparation of allografts for transplantation to maintain sterility and to reduce the possibility of disease transmission.

Tissue banks preserve and sterilize allografts by several techniques, including deep freezing, freeze-drying, exposure to ethylene oxide, or cobolt-60 irradiation. These processes could affect the properties of the graft. To assess the effects of freezing on ACL tensile properties, Jackson and associates[166] subjected the ACL substance and insertion sites of the goat to several freeze-thaw cycles in vivo. No significant differences in the linear stiffness, ultimate load, or modulus were noted between the treated ligaments and the contralateral controls at 26 weeks after surgery. Arnoczky and associates[151] compared fresh versus deep-frozen patellar tendon allografts in dogs. The fresh allografts caused a profound inflammatory response. Histologic examination revealed chronic inflammatory cells and evidence of perivascular cuffing. The deep-frozen allografts, in contrast, appeared benign and experienced alterations comparable to those observed in autografts.[158]

Nine months after implantation of a fresh-frozen allograft femur-ACL-tibia complex, ultimate loads were approximately 15% of the normal canine femur-ACL-tibia complex.[163] The linear stiffness and ultimate load values of a freeze-dried ACL allograft-bone complex were 35% and 25% of control, respectively, at one year after implantation. Also, the anteroposterior translation was significantly elevated in the reconstructed knee.[167] At one year, Shino and associates[162] reported that fresh-frozen patellar tendon allografts had ultimate loads that were only 29% of the control femur-ACL-tibia complex. Postoperatively, the transplanted allograft tissue remodels in the same manner as autografts.[162,168,169] By one year after surgery, allograft patellar tendons have been found to be completely revascularized, and to be histologically identical to autografts.[162,170]

In sterile allograft retrieval, the tissue must be removed within 12 hours of cessation of cardiopulmonary function. However, tissue can be removed 24 hours after death if it is secondarily sterilized. The manner in which the allograft is sterilized is important because of the risk for disease transmission. This has raised concern regarding effects of the sterilization process on allograft mechanical properties. Cold ethylene oxide gas is unsuitable because it alters the material properties of the allograft and leads to an increased incidence of joint effusions.[171,172]

The effects of cobolt-60 gamma irradiation on the initial mechanical properties of goat patellar tendon were examined by Gibbons and associates.[173] Fresh-frozen irradiated patellar tendons were compared with fresh-frozen nonirradiated patellar tendons. In their study, 2 Mrad of irradiation did not significantly alter the material properties of the patellar tendon, whereas 3 Mrad significantly reduced the maximum stress, maximum strain, and strain energy to failure. However, Haut and Powlison[174] found that 2 Mrad produced significant decreases in both the ultimate tensile strength (27.5%) and the modulus (43.8%) of human patellar tendons.[174] High-dose irradiation (3 Mrad) creates significant changes in the mechanical properties of allografts, but the effects of low-dose cobolt-60 irradiation (2 Mrad) remain controversial.[173-176] Thus, it appears that before these preparation techniques can be generally accepted, a more complete understanding of their effects on the mechanical behavior of allograft tissues is needed.

Acknowledgments

This work was supported by Department of Veterans Affairs RR&D Grant No. A188-4RA, and National Institutes of Health Grant No. AR39683.

References

1. Fetto JF, Marshall JL: Medial collateral ligament injuries of the knee: A rationale for treatment. *Clin Orthop* 1978;132:206-218.

2. Hastings DE: The non-operative management of collateral ligament injuries of the knee joint. *Clin Orthop* 1980;147:22-28.

3. Indelicato PA: Non-operative treatment of complete tears of the medial collateral ligament of the knee. *J Bone Joint Surg* 1983;65A:323-329.

4. Jones RE, Henley MB, Francis P: Nonoperative management of isolated grade III collateral ligament injury in high school football players. *Clin Orthop* 1986;213:137-140.

5. Girgis FG, Marshall JL, Al Monajem ARS: The cruciate ligaments of the knee joint: Anatomical, functional and experimental analysis. *Clin Orthop* 1975;106:216-231.

6. Hawkins RJ, Misamore GW, Merritt TR: Followup of the acute nonoperated isolated anterior cruciate ligament tear. *Amer J Sports Med* 1986;14:205-210.

7. O'Donoghue DH, Rockwood CA, Frank GR, et al: Repair of the anterior cruciate ligament in dogs. *J Bone Joint Surg* 1966;48A:503-519.

8. Viidik A: Simultaneous mechanical and light microscopic studies of collagen fibers. *Z Anat Entwicklungsgesch* 1972;136:204-212.

9. Goldberg VM, Burstein A, Dawson M: The influence of an experimental immune synovitis on the failure mode and strength of the rabbit anterior cruciate ligament. *J Bone Joint Surg* 1982;64A:900-906.

10. Bray DF, Frank CB, Bray RC: Cytochemical evidence for a proteoglycan-associated filamentous network in ligaments and the extracellular matrix. *J Orthop Res* 1990;8:1-12.

11. Frank C, Bray D, Rademaker A, et al: Electron microscopic quantification of collagen fibril diameters in the rabbit medial collateral ligament: A baseline for comparison. *Connect Tissue Res* 1989;19:11-25.

12. Oakes BW, Leslie J, Jacobsen J et al: Mechanisms of connective tissue rehabilitation, in Howell ML, Parker AW (eds): *Sports Medicine: Medical and Scientific Aspects of Elitism in Sports*. Brisbane, Australian Sports Federation, 1982, vol 8, pp. 39-62.

13. Hart RA, Woo SL-Y, Newton PO: Ultrastructural morphometry of the anterior cruciate and medial collateral ligaments: An experimental study in rabbits. *J Orthop Res* 1992;10:96-103.

14. Lyon RM, Billings E Jr, Woo SL-Y, et al: The ACL: A fibrocartilaginous structure. *Trans Orthop Res Soc* 1989;14:189.

15. Nagineni CN, Amiel D, Green M, et al: Characterization of cell cultures derived from the anterior cruciate and medial collateral ligaments. *Trans Orthop Res Soc* 1991;16:619.

16. Salo P, Frank C, Marchuk L: Synovial fluid does not inhibit collagen synthesis: bovine cruciate ligament studied in vitro. *Acta Orthop Scand* 1990;61:570-574.

17. Arnoczky SP: Blood supply to the anterior cruciate ligament and supporting structures. *Orthop Clin North Am* 1985;16:15-28.

18. Scapinelli R: Studies on the vasculature of the human knee joint. *Acta Anat (Basel)* 1968;70:305-331.

19. Shim S-S, Leung G: Blood supply of the knee joint. A microangiographic study in children and adults. *Clin Orthop* 1986;208:119-125.

20. Dunlap J, McCarthy JA, Joyce ME, et al: Quantification of the perfusion of the anterior cruciate ligament and the effects of stress and injury to the supporting structures. *Am J Sports Med* 1989;17:808-810.

21. Schlehr FJ, Limbird TA, Swiontkowski MF, et al: The use of laser doppler flowmetry to evaluate anterior cruciate blood flow. *J Orthop Res* 1987;5:150-153.

22. Amiel D, Frank C, Harwood F, et al: Tendons and ligaments: A morphological and biochemical comparison. *J Orthop Res* 1984; 1:257-265.

23. Frank C, Amiel D, Akeson WH: Healing of the medial collateral ligament of the knee: A morphological and biochemical assessment in rabbits. *Acta Orthop Scand* 1983;54:917-923.

24. Frank C, Woo SL-Y, Amiel D, et al: Medial collateral ligament healing: A multidisciplinary assessment in rabbits. *Am J Sports Med* 1983;11:379-389.

25. Vogel HG: Correlation between tensile strength and collagen content in rat skin: Effect of age and cortisol treatment. *Connect Tissue Res* 1974;2:177-182.

26. Woessner JF Jr: The determination of hydroxyproline in tissue and protein samples containing small proportions of this amino acid. *Arch Biochem* 1961;93:440-447.

27. Harwood FL, Amiel D: Semiquantitative HPLC analysis of types I and III collagen in soft tissues. *LC-GC Mag Chromatogr Sci* 1986;4:122-126.

28. Miller EJ, Rhodes RK, Furuto DK: Identification of collagen chains as a function of cyanogen bromide peptide patterns using gel permeation high performance liquid chromatography. *Coll Rel Res* 1983;3:79-87.

29. Neuberger A, Slack HGB: The metabolismabolism of collagen from liver, bone, skin and tendon in the normal rat. *Biochem J* 1953;53:47-52.

30. Bailey AJ, Bazin S, Delaunay A: Changes in the nature of the collagen during development and resorption of granulation tissue. *Biochem Biophys Acta* 1973;328:383-390.

31. Akeson WH, Woo SL-Y, Amiel D, et al: The biology of ligaments, in Funk FJ, Hunter LY (eds): *Rehabilitation of the Injured Knee.* St. Louis, CV Mosby, 1984; pp 33-148.

32. Mechanic GL: An automated scintillation counting system with high efficiency for continuous analysis: Cross-links of ^{3}HNaBH$_4$-reduced collagen. *Anal Biochem* 1974;61:354.

33. Hiyama K, Okada S: Crystallization and some properties of chondroitinase from Arthrobacter aurescens. *J Biol Chem* 1975;250:1824-1828.

34. Oike Y, Kimata K, Shinomura T, et al: A mapping technique for probing the structure of proteoglycan core molecules. *J Biol Chem* 1982;257:9751-9758.

35. Frank C, McDonald D, Lieber R, et al: Biochemical heterogeneity within the maturing rabbit medial collateral ligament. *Clin Orthop* 1988;236:279-285.

36. Grood ES, Noyes FR, Butler DL, et al: Ligamentous and capsular restraints preventing straight medial and lateral laxity in intact human cadaver knees. *J Bone Joint Surg* 1981;63A:1257-1269.

37. Piziali RL, Rastegar J, Nagel DA, et al: The contribution of the cruciate ligaments to the load-displacement characteristics of the human knee joint. *J Biomech Eng* 1980;102:277-283.

38. Seering WP, Piziali RL, Nagel DA, et al: The function of the primary ligaments of the knee in varus-valgus and axial rotation. *J Biomech* 1980;13:785-794.

39. Inoue M, McGurk-Burleson E, Hollis JM, et al: Treatment of the medial collateral ligament injury: I. The importance of anterior cruciate ligament on the varus-valgus knee laxity. *Am J Sports Med* 1987; 15:15-21.

40. Nielsen S, Kromann-Andersen C, Rasmussen O, et al: Instability of cadaver knees after transection of capsule and ligaments. *Acta Orthop Scand* 1984;55:30- 34.

41. Nielsen S, Rasmussen O, Ovesen J, et al: Rotatory instability of cadaver knees after transection of collateral ligaments and capsule. *Arch Orthop Trauma Surg* 1984;103:165-169.

42. Woo SL-Y, Gomez MA, Inoue M, et al: New experimental procedures to evaluate the biomechanical properties of healing canine medial collateral ligaments. *J Orthop Res* 1987;5:425-432.

43. Lee TQ, Woo SL-Y: A new method for determining cross-sectional shape and area of soft tissues. *J Biomech Eng* 1988;110:110-114.

44. Woo SL-Y, Danto MI, Ohland KJ, et al: The use of a laser micrometer system to determine the cross-sectional shape and area of ligaments: A comparative study with two existing methods. *J Biomech Eng* 1990;112:426-431.

45. Woo SL-Y, Gomez MA, Seguchi Y, et al: Measurement of mechanical properties of ligament substance from a bone-ligament-bone preparation. *J Orthop Res* 1983;1:22-29.

46. Tipton CM, Matthes RD, Sandage DS: In situ measurement of junction strength and ligament elongation in rats. *J Appl Physiol* 1974;37: 758-761.

47. Woo SL-Y, Gomez MA, Akeson WH: The time and history-dependent viscoelastic properties of the canine medial collateral ligament. *J Biomech Eng* 1981;103:293-298.

48. Woo SL-Y: Mechanical properties of tendons and ligaments: I. Quasistatic and nonlinear viscoelastic properties. *Biorheology* 1982;19:385-396.

49. Weisman G, Pope MH, Johnson RJ: The effect of cyclic loading on knee ligaments. *Trans Orthop Res Soc* 1979;4:24.

50. Skinner HB, Wyatt MP, Stone ML, et al: Exercise-related knee joint laxity. *Am J Sports Med* 1986;14:30-34.

51. Wainwright SA, Biggs WD, Currey JD, et al: *Mechanical Design in Organisms*. Princeton, NJ, Princeton University Press, 1982, pp 6-44.

52. Adams DJ, Shoemaker SC, Harris SL, et al: Effect of initial graft tension and quadriceps force on anterior cruciate ligament (ACL) graft load. *Trans Orthop Res Soc* 1990;15:508.

53. Hefzy MS, Grood ES: Sensitivity of insertion locations on length patterns of anterior cruciate ligament fibers. *J Biomech Eng* 108;73-82:1986.

54. Lewis JL, Lew WD, Schmidt J: Description and error evaluation of an in vitro knee joint testing system. *J Biomech Eng* 1988;110:238-248.

55. Berns GS, Hull ML, Patterson HA: Implementation of a five degree of freedom automated system to determine knee flexibility in vitro. *J Biomech Eng* 1990;112:392-400.

56. Hollis JM, Takai S, Adams DJ, et al: The effects of knee motion and external loading on the length of the anterior cruciate ligament: A kinematic study. *J Biomech Eng* 1991;113:208-214.

57. An K-N, Jacobsen MC, Berglund LJ, et al: Application of a magnetic tracking device to kinesiologic studies. *J Biomech* 1988;21:613-620.

58. Harryman DT II, Sidles JA, Clark JM, et al: Translation of the humeral head on the glenoid with passive glenohumeral motion. *J Bone Joint Surg* 1990;72A:1334-1343.

59. Sidles JA, Harryman DT II, Harris SL, et al: In vivo quantification of glenohumeral stability. *Trans Orthop Res Soc* 1991;16:646.

60. Sidles JA, Harryman DT II, Harris SL, et al: In vivo measurements of glenohumeral and scapulothoracic motion: Implications for fusion position in glenohumeral arthrodesis. *Trans Orthop Res Soc* 1991;16:209.

61. Quinn TP, Mote CD Jr: A six-degree-of-freedom acoustic transducer for rotation and translation measurements across the knee. *J Biomech Eng* 1990;112:371-378.

62. de Lange A, Huiskes R, Kauer JMG: Measurement errors in roentgen-stereophotogrammetric joint-motion analysis. *J Biomech* 1990;23:259-269.

63. Lewis JL, Lew WD, Hill JA, et al: Knee joint motion and ligament forces before and after ACL reconstruction. *J Biomech Eng* 1989;111:97-106.

64. Markolf KL, Gorek JF, Kabo JM, et al: Direct measurement of resultant forces in the anterior cruciate ligament: An *in vitro* study performed with a new experimental technique. *J Bone Joint Surg* 1990;72A:557-567.

65. France EP, Daniels AU, Goble EM, et al: Simultaneous quantitation of knee ligament forces. *J Biomech* 1983;16:553-564.

66. Woo SL-Y, Weiss JA, Gomez MA, et al: Measurement of changes in ligament tension with knee motion and skeletal maturation. *J Biomech Eng* 1990;112:46-51.

67. Takai S, Adams DJ, Livesay GA, et al: Determination of loads in the human anterior cruciate ligament. *Trans Orthop Res Soc* 1991;16:235.

68. Radin EL: The joint as an organ: Physiology and biomechanics, in *Abstracts of the First World Congress of Biomechanics*. La Jolla, CA, University of California, San Diego, 1990. vol II, p 1.

69. Amiel D, Abel MF, Kleiner JB, et al: Synovial fluid nutrient delivery system in the diathrial joint: An analysis of rabbit knee ligaments. *J Orthop Res* 1986;4:90-95.

70. Skyhar MJ, Danzig LA, Hargens AR, et al: Nutrition of the anterior cruciate ligament: Effects of continuous passive motion. *Am J Sports Med* 1985;13:415-418.

71. Whiteside LA, Sweeney RE: Nutrient pathways of the cruciate ligaments: An experimental study using the hydrogen wash-out technique. *J Bone Joint Surg* 1980;62A:1176-1180.

72. Amiel D, Billings E Jr, Lyon R, et al: Collagenase activity in anterior cruciate ligament (ACL): The protective role of the synovial sheath. *Trans Orthop Res Soc* 1990;15:269

73. Olson EJ, Kang JD, Fu FH, et al: The biochemical and histological effects of artificial ligament wear particles: In vitro and in vivo studies. *Am J Sports Med* 1988;16:558-570.

74. Norwood LA, Cross MJ: Anterior cruciate ligament: Functional anatomy of its bundles in rotatory instabilities. *Am J Sports Med* 1979;7:23-26.

75. Lyon RM, Akeson WH, Amiel D, et al: Ultrastructural differences between the cells of the medial collateral and the anterior cruciate ligaments. *Clin Orthop* 1991;272:279-286.

76. Burks RT: Gross anatomy, in Daniel DM, Akeson WH, O'Connor JJ (eds): *Knee Ligaments: Structure, Function, Injury, and Repair*. New York, Raven Press, 1991, pp. 59-76.

77. Poliacu Prosé L, Lohman AH, Huson A: The collateral ligaments of the knee joint in the cat and man: Morphological and functional study of the internal arrangement of fibers. *Acta Anat (Basel)* 1988;133:70-78.

78. Kennedy JC, Weinberg HW, Wilson AS: The anatomy and function of the anterior cruciate ligament: As determined by clinhical and morphological studies. *J Bone Joint Surg* 1974;56A:223-235.

79. Danylchuk KD, Finlay JB, Krcek JP: Microstructural organization of human and bovine cruciate ligaments. *Clin Orthop* 1978;131:294-298.

80. Yahia L-H, Drouin G: Microscopical investigation of canine anterior cruciate ligament and patellar tendon: collagen fascicle morphology and architecture. *J Orthop Res* 1989;7:243-251.

81. Clark JM, Sidles JA: The interrelation of fiber bundles in the anterior cruciate ligament. *J Orthop Res* 1990;8:180-188.

82. Oakes BW, Parker AW, Norman J: Changes in collagen fibre populations in young rat cruciate ligaments in response to an intensive one month's exercise program, in Russo P, Gass G (eds): *Human Adaption.* Williamsburg, KY, Cumberland College of Health Sciences, 1981, pp 223-230.

83. Zar JH: *Biostatistical Analysis.* Englewood Cliffs, Prentice-Hall, 1984, pp 81-82.

84. Parry DA, Barnes GR, Craig AS: A comparison of the size distribution of collagen fibrils in connective tissues as a function of age and a possible relation between fibril size distribution and mechanical properties. *Proc R Soc London (Biol)* 1978;203:305-321.

85. Vasseur PB, Pool RR, Arnoczky SP, et al: Correlative biomechanical and histologic study of the cranial cruciate ligament in dogs. *Am J Vet Res* 1985;46:1842-1854.

86. Bray RC Fisher AWF, Frank CB: Fine vascular anatomy of adult rabbit knee ligaments. *J Anat* 1990;172:69-79.

87. Arnoczky SP, Rubin RM, Marshall JL: Microvasculature of the cruciate ligaments and its response to injury: An experimental study in dogs. *J Bone Joint Surg* 1979;61A:1221-1229.

88. Wallace CD, Amiel D: Vascular assessment of the periarticular ligaments of the rabbit knee. *J Orthop Res* 1991;9:787-791.

89. Alm A, Stromberg B: Vascular anatomy of the patellar and cruciate ligaments: A microangiographic and histologic investigation in the dog. *Acta Chir Scand Suppl* 1974;445:25-35.

90. Pedrini VA, Pedrini-Mille A, Vailas AC: Proteoglycans of ligamentous tissues. *Trans Orthop Res Soc* 1983;8:324.

91. Minns RJ, Soden PD: The role of the fibrous components and ground substance in the mechanical properties of biological tissues: A preliminary investigation. *J Biomech* 1973;6:153-165.

92. Lapiere CM, Nusgens B, Pierard GE: Interaction between collagen type I and type III in conditioning bundles organization. *Connect Tiss Res* 1977;5:21-29.

93. Woo SL-Y, Newton PO, MacKenna DA, et al: A comparative evaluation of the mechanical properties of the rabbit medial collateral and anterior cruciate ligaments. *J Biomech* 1992;25:377-386.

94. Butler DL, Guan Y, Kay MD, et al: Location-dependent variations in the material properties of anterior cruciate ligament subunits. *Trans Orthop Res Soc* 1991;16:234.

95. Miyasaka KC, Daniel DM, Stone ML et al: The incidence of knee ligament injuries in the general population. *Am J Knee Surg* 1991;4:3-8.

96. Hirshman HP, Daniel DM, Miyasaka K: The fate of unoperated knee ligament injuries, in Daniel DM, Akeson WH, O'Connor JJ (eds): *Knee Ligaments: Structure, Function, Injury, and Repair*. New York, Raven Press, 1991, pp 481-503.

97. Feagin JA Jr, Lambert KL, Cunningham RR, et al: Consideration of the anterior cruciate ligament injury in skiing. *Clin Orthop* 1987;216:13-18.

98. Hewson GF, Mendini RA, Wang JB: Prophylactic knee bracing in college football. *Am J Sports Med* 1986;14:262-266.

99. Jensen JE, Conn RR, Hazelrigg G, et al: Systematic evaluation of acute knee injuries. *Clin Sports Med* 1985;4:295-312.

100. Daniel DM, Teiege RA, Grana WA, et al: Knee and leg: Soft-tissue trauma, in *Orthopaedic Knowledge Update 3*. Park Ridge, IL, American Academy of Orthopaedic Surgeons 1990, pp 557-573.

101. Noyes FR, Mooar PA, Matthews DS, et al: The symptomatic anterior cruciate-deficient knee: Part I: The long-term functional disability in athletically active individuals. *J Bone Joint Surg* 1983;65A:154-162.

102. Ballock RT, Woo SL-Y, Lyon RM, et al: Use of patellar tendon autograft for anterior cruciate ligament reconstruction in the rabbit: A long-term histologic and biomechanical study. *J Orthop Res* 1989;7:474-485.

103. O'Donoghue DH, Frank GR, Jeter GL, et al: Repair and reconstruction of the anterior cruciate ligament in dogs: Factors influencing long term results. *J Bone Joint Surg* 1971;53A:710-718.

104. Robinson SC, Driscoll SE: Simultaneous osteochondral avulsion of the femoral and tibial insertions of the anterior cruciate ligament. *J Bone Joint Surg* 1981;63A:1342-1343.

105. Eady JL, Cardenas CD, Sopa D: Avulsion of the femoral attachment of the anterior cruciate ligament in a seven-year-old child: A case report. *J Bone Joint Surg* 1982;64A:1376-1378.

106. Zaricznyj B: Avulsion fracture of the tibial eminence: Treatment by open reduction and pinning. *J Bone Joint Surg* 1977;59A:1111-1114.

107. Meyers MH, McKeever FM: Fracture of the intercondylar eminence of the tibia. *J Bone Joint Surg* 1959;41A:209-222.

108. Finsterbush A, Frankl U, Matan Y, et al: Secondary damage to the knee after isolated injury of the anterior cruciate ligament. *Am J Sports Med* 1990;18:475-479.

109. Bonamo JJ, Fay C, Firestone T: The conservative treatment of the anterior cruciate deficient knee. *Am J Sports Med* 1990;18:618-623.

110. Shapiro MS, Markolf KL, Finerman GAM, et al: The effect of section of the medial collateral ligament on force generated in the anterior cruciate ligament. *J Bone Joint Surg* 1991;73A:248-256.

111. Woo SL-Y, Inoue M, McGurk-Burleson E, et al: Treatment of the medial collateral ligament injury: II. Structure and function of canine knees in response to differing treatment regimens. *Am J Sports Med* 1987;15:22-29.

112. Laws G, Walton M: Fibroblastic healing of grade II ligament injuries: Histological and mechanical studies in the sheep. *J Bone Joint Surg* 1988;70B:390- 396.

113. Viidik A: Structure and function of normal and healing tendons and ligaments, in *Abstracts of the First World Congress of Biomechanics*. La Jolla, CA, University of California, San Diego, 1990, vol II. p 1.

114. Clayton ML, Weir GJ Jr: Experimental investigations of ligamentous healing. *Am J Surg* 1959;98:373-378.

115. Vailas AC, Tipton CM, Matthes RD, et al: Physical activity and its influence on the repair process of medial collateral ligaments. *Connect Tiss Res* 1981;9:25-31.

116. Gomez MA, Woo SL-Y, Inoue M, et al: Medial collateral ligament healing subsequent to different treatment regimens. *J App Physiol* 1988;66:245-252.

117. Andriacchi T, Sabiston P, DeHaven K, et al: Ligament: Injury and repair, in Woo SL-Y, Buckwalter JA (eds): *Injury and Repair of the Musculoskeletal Soft Tissues*. Park Ridge, IL, American Academy of Orthopaedic Surgeons, 1988, pp 103-128.

118. O'Donoghue DH, Rockwood CA Jr, Zaricznyj B, et al: Repair of knee ligaments in dogs: I. The lateral collateral ligament. *J Bone Joint Surg* 1961;43A:1167-1178.

119. Grönblad M, Korkala O, Konttinen Y, et al: Immunoreactive neuropeptides in nerves in ligamentous tissue: An experimental neuroimmunohistochemical study. *Clin Orthop* 1991;265:291-296.

120. Korkala O, Rusanen M, Gronblad M: Healing of experimental ligament rupture: findings by scanning electron microscopy. *Arch Orthop Traumat Surg* 1984;102:179-182.

121. Clayton ML, Miles JS, Abdulla M: Experimental investigations of ligamentous healing. *Clin Orthop* 1968;61:146-153.

122. O'Donoghue DH: Surgical treatment of fresh injuries to the major ligaments of the knee. *J Bone Joint Surg* 1950;32A:721-738.

123. Starke W: Fibullar ligament rupture during growth. *Unfallchirurg* 1989;92:6-10.

124. Woo SL-Y, Matthews JV, Akeson WH, et al: Connective tissue response to immobility: A correlative study of biomechanical and biochemical measurements of normal and immobilized rabbit knees. *Arth Rheum* 1975;18:257-264.

125. Inoue M, Woo SL-Y, Gomez MA, et al: Effects of surgical treatment and immobilization on the healing of the medial collateral ligament: A long-term multidisciplinary study. *Connect Tiss Res* 1990;25:13-26.

126. Ginsburg JH, Ellsasser JC: Problem areas in the diagnosis and treatment of ligament injuries of the knee. *Clin Orthop* 1978;132:201-205.

127. Price CT, Allen WC: Ligament repair in the knee with preservation of the meniscus. *J Bone Joint Surg* 1978;60A:61-65.

128. Weaver JK, Derkash RS, Freeman JR, et al: Primary knee ligament repair: Revisited. *Clin Orthop* 1985;199:185-191.

129. Warren RF, Marshall JL: Injuries of the anterior cruciate and medial collateral ligaments of the knee: A long-term follow-up of 86 cases: Part II. *Clin Orthop* 1978;136:198-211.

130. Ellsasser JC, Reynolds FC, Omohundro JR: The non-operative treatment of collateral ligament injuries of the knee in professional football players: An analysis of seventy-four injuries treated non-operatively and twenty-four injuries treated surgically. *J Bone Joint Surg* 1974;56A:1185-1190.

131. Kannus P: Long-term results of conservatively treated medial collateral ligament injuries of the knee joint. *Clin Orthop* 1988;226:103-112.

132. Walsh S, Frank C: Two methods of ligament injury: A morphological comparison in a rabbit model. *J Surg Res* 1988;45:159-166.

133. Horwitz MT: Injuries of the ligaments of the knee joint: An experimental study. *Arch Surg* 1939;38:946-954.

134. Palmer I: On the injuries to the ligaments of the knee joint. *Acta Chir Scand Suppl* 1938;53:1-282.

135. Weiss JA, Woo SL-Y, Ohland KJ, et al: Evaluation of a new injury model to study medial collateral ligament healing: Primary repair varus nonoperative treatment. *J Orthop Res* 1991;9:516-528.

136. Ohland KJ, Weiss JA, Anderson DR, et al: Long-term healing of the medial collateral ligament (MCL) and its insertion sites. *Trans Orthop Res Soc* 1991;16:158.

137. Chimich D, Frank C, Shrive N, et al: The effects of initial end contact on medial collateral ligament healing: A morphological and biomechanical study in a rabbit model. *J Orthop Res* 1991;9:37-47.

138. Woo SL-Y, Young EP, Ohland KJ, et al: The effects of transection of the anterior cruciate ligament on healing of the medial collateral ligament: A biomechanical study of the knee in dogs. *J Bone Joint Surg* 1990;72A:382-392.

139. Forbes I, Frank C, Lam T, et al: The biomechanical effects of combined ligament injuries on the medial collateral ligament. *Trans Orthop Res Soc* 1988;13:186.

140. Anderson DR, Weiss JA, Takai S, et al: Healing of the medial collateral ligament following a triad injury. *J Orthop Res* 1992;10:485-495.

141. Campbell WC: Reconstruction of the ligaments of the knee. *Am J Surg* 1939;43:473-480.

142. Campbell WC: Repair of the ligaments of the knee: Report of a new operation for repair of the anterior crucial ligament. *Surg Gynecol Obstet* 1936;62:964-968.

143. O'Donoghue DH: An analysis of end results of surgical treatment of major injuries to the ligaments of the knee. *J Bone Joint Surg* 1955;37A:1-13,124.

144. Sandberg R, Balkfors B, Nilsson B, et al: Operative versus non-operative treatment of recent injuries to the ligaments of the knee: A prospective randomized study. *J Bone Joint Surg* 1987;69A:1120-1126.

145. Andersson C, Odensten M, Good L, et al: Surgical or non-surgical treatment of acute rupture of the anterior cruciate ligament. *J Bone Joint Surg* 1989;71A:965-974.

146. Hey Groves EW: Operation for the repair of the crucial ligaments. *Lancet* 1917;2:674.

147. Jones KG: Reconstruction of the anterior cruciate ligament: A technique using the central one-third of the patellar ligament. *J Bone Joint Surg* 1963;45A:925-932.

148. Ryan JR, Drompp BW: Evaluation of tensile strength of reconstructions of the anterior cruciate ligament using the patellar tendon in dogs: A preliminary report. *South Med J* 1966;59:129-134.

149. Clancy WG Jr, Narechania RG, Rosenberg TD, et al: Anterior and posterior cruciate ligament reconstruction in rhesus monkeys: A histological, microangiographic, and biomechanical analysis. *J Bone Joint Surg* 1981;63A:1270-1284.

150. McPherson GK, Mendenhall HV, Gibbons DF, et al: Experimental mechanical and histologic evaluation of the Kennedy ligament augmentation device. *Clin Orthop* 1985;196:186-195.

151. Arnoczky SP, Warren RF, Ashlock MA: Replacement of the anterior cruciate ligament using a patellar tendon allograft. *J Bone Joint Surg* 1986;68A:376-385.

152. Yoshiya S, Andrish JT, Manley MT, et al: Augmentation of anterior cruciate ligament reconstruction in dogs with prostheses of different stiffnesses. *J Orthop Res* 1986;4:475-485.

153. Hurley PB, Andrish JT, Yoshiya S, et al: Tensile strength of the reconstructed canine anterior cruciate ligament: A long-term evaluation of the modified Jones technique. *Am J Sports Med* 1987;15:393.

154. Cho KO: Reconstruction of the anterior cruciate ligament by semitendinosus tenodesis. *J Bone Joint Surg* 1975;57A:608-612.

155. Lipscomb AB, Johnston RK, Synder RB, et al: Secondary reconstruction of anterior cruciate ligament in athletes by using the semitendinosus tendon: Preliminary report of 78 cases. *Am J Sports Med* 1979;7:81-84.

156. Mott HW: Semitendinosus anatomic reconstruction for cruciate ligament insufficiency. *Clin Orthop* 1983;172:90-92.

157. Noyes FR, Butler DL, Grood ES, et al: Biomechanical analysis of human ligament grafts used in knee-ligament repairs and reconstructions. *J Bone Joint Surg* 1984;66A:344-352.

158. Arnoczky SP, Tarvin GB, Marshall JL: Anterior cruciate ligament replacement using patellar tendon: An evaluation of graft revascularization in the dog. *J Bone Joint Surg* 1982;64A:217-224.

159. Yoshiya S, Andrish JT, Manley MT, et al: Graft tension in anterior cruciate ligament reconstruction: An in vivo study in dogs. *Am J Sports Med* 1987;15:464-470.

160. Woo SL-Y, Hollis JM, Adams DJ, et al: Tensile properties of the human femur-anterior cruciate ligament-tibia complex: The effects of specimen age and orientation. *Am J Sports Med* 1991;19:217-225.

161. Nikolaou PK, Seaber AV, Glisson RR, et al: Anterior cruciate ligament allograft transplantation: Long-term function, histology, revascularization, and operative technique. *Am J Sports Med* 1986;14:348-360.

162. Shino K, Kawasaki T, Hirose H, et al: Replacement of the anterior cruciate ligament by allogeneic tendon graft: An experimental study in the dog. *J Bone Joint Surg* 1984;66B:672-681.

163. Vasseur PB, Rodrigo JJ, Stevenson S, et al: Replacement of the anterior cruciate ligament with a bone-ligament-bone anterior cruciate ligament allograft in dogs. *Clin Orthop* 1987;219:268-277.

164. Roberts TS, Drez D Jr, Banta CJ III: Complications of anterior cruciate ligament reconstruction, in Sprague NF III (ed): *Complications in Arthroscopy*. New York, Raven Press, 1989, pp 169-177.

165. Webster DA, Werner FW: Freeze-dried flexor tendons in anterior cruciate ligament reconstruction. *Clin Orthop* 1983;181:238-243.

166. Jackson DW, Grood ES, Cohn BT, et al: The effects of *in situ* freezing on the anterior cruciate ligament. *J Bone Joint Surg* 1991;73A:201-213.

167. Jackson DW, Grood ES, Arnoczky SP, et al: Freeze dried anterior cruciate ligament allografts: Preliminary studies in a goat model. *Am J Sports Med* 1987;15:295-303.

168. Shino K, Inoue M, Horibe S, et al: Reconstruction of the anterior cruciate ligament using allogenic tendon: Long-term followup. *Am J Sports Med* 1990;18:457-465.

169. Gibbons MJ, Butler DL, Grood ES, et al: Effects of gamma irradiation on the initial mechanical and material properties of goat bone-patellar tendon-bone allografts. *J Orthop Res* 1991;9:209-218.

170. Shino K, Inoue M, Horibe S, et al: Maturation of allograft tendons transplanted into the knee: an arthroscopic and histological study. *J Bone Joint Surg* 1988;70B:556-560.

171. Roberts TS, Drez D, McCarthy W, et al: Anterior cruciate ligament reconstruction using freeze-dried, ethylene oxide-sterilized, bone-patellar tendon-bone allografts: Two year results in thirty-six patients. *Am J Sports Med* 1991;19:35-41.

172. Silvaggio VJ, Fu FH, Georgescu HI, et al: The induction of IL-1 by freeze dried ethylene oxide treated bone-patellar tendon-bone allograft wear particles: An in vitro study. *Trans Orthop Res Soc* 1991;16:207.

173. Gibbons MJ, Butler DL, Grood ES, et al: Effects of gamma irradiation on the initial mechanical and material properties of goat bone-patellar tendon-bone allografts. *J Orthop Res* 1991;9:209-218.

174. Haut RC, Powlison AC: Order of irradiation and lyophilization on the strength of patellar tendon allografts. *Trans Orthop Res Soc* 1989;14:514.
175. Butler DL, Noyes FR, Walz KA, et al: Biomechanics of human knee ligament allograft treatment. *Trans Orthop Res Soc* 1987;12:128.
176. Paulos LE, France EP, Rosenberg TD, et al: Comparative material properties of allograft tissues for ligament replacement: Effects of type, age, sterilization and preservation. *Trans Orthop Res Soc* 1987;12:129.

Chapter 14

Nervous System Control of Joint Function

Peter Grigg, PhD

Introduction

From the viewpoint of a neurophysiologist, the nervous system does not control joint function in a strict sense. Our limbs are articulated, and the nervous system controls limb movement. Thus, a discussion on control of joint function essentially covers the field of movement control, a topic that is far too broad to cover in the allotted time and space. Several excellent reviews discuss in detail the control of limb movements,[1] and the role of proprioceptive mechanisms in movement control.[2]

Because this symposium deals with ligament injury, I have chosen to discuss whether some specific aspect of joint function, such as protection from potentially injurious stimuli, might be mediated by the nervous system. Johansson and associates[3] and Sjölander[4] discuss whether sensory mechanisms in ligaments have a role in stabilizing joints; these authors are in favor of joint protection by such mechanisms. Because of the study by Johansson and associates,[3] it is not necessary to review all of the relevant literature. I will discuss only the key components of the literature that I believe support my hypothesis that while articular sensory neurons may protect a joint by allowing an animal to adopt movement strategies that minimize damage from a chronic injury, they do not regulate or protect joints through reflex mechanisms.

It is well known that rotation of freely-moving joints is restricted by the passive stretching of ligaments, joint capsule, and muscles and tendons that span the joint. This chapter addresses the question of whether there are active, neuromuscular mechanisms that regulate joint position or that protect the joint from overrotation. The conceptual basis for such mechanisms comes from familiar mechanisms in the nervous system. For example, negative feedback systems regulate several variables, such as blood pressure and blood PCO_2, keeping some of them within a desired range. Also, there are neural mechanisms for protection against noxious stimuli that result in such movement as eye blinking or withdrawal of a limb from noxious stimuli.

In considering whether similar neural mechanisms operate around joints, first I will briefly describe what sensors are present in and around joints, and the types of stimuli to which they are sensitive. Second, I will review the evidence that these sensors, when activated, can initiate or regulate neural mechanisms that significantly alter the status of the joint. I will describe primarily the cat knee, because it appears to be a typical joint and has been widely used in studies of joint innervation.

Neural Sensors in Joint Tissues

The soft-tissue components of all joints have a sensory innervation. Some tissues, such as menisci, are poorly innervated, while others, such as the capsule, are richly innervated. The many types of sensory endings have different functions, are distributed unevenly throughout the joint, and are innervated by axons of different sizes. Because axons of different diameters conduct action potentials with different velocities, a useful starting point is to classify axons according to their conduction velocities. Table 1 shows the relative numbers of afferent axons of different diameters in the posterior and medial articular nerves of cat knees.

Table 1 shows that fine afferent nerve fibers (groups 3 and 4), which are believed to terminate in noncorpuscular sensory endings, make up the overwhelming majority of sensory neurons innervating joints.[5,6] Also, there is a difference in the fraction of axons of various types that arise from different parts of the joint, as shown by the differences between medial and posterior articular nerves. There are few group 2 and no group 1 fibers in the medial articular nerves.

Properties of Afferent Nerve Fibers

Fine Afferent Nerve Fibers

Fine afferent nerve fibers, those with group 3 and 4 axons, have spot-like receptive fields when studied with a fine indenting probe.[7] Many have multiple receptive fields. When the joint is rotated, the majority of group 3 and about half of group 4 afferent nerve fibers respond to joint rotations. A small fraction of them, a few from group 4 and more from group 3, respond to gentle rotations that are limited in movement. Most fine afferent nerve fibers, however, respond optimally only when the joint is subjected to a forceful, noxious rotation that goes beyond an innocuous movement. A noxious rotation, as defined by Schaible and Schmidt,[8] is one against tissue resistance, strong enough to cause abrupt limb withdrawal in conscious cats and a rise in blood pressure in anesthetized cats. Thus, the majority of group 3 and 4 fibers in joints appear to be consistent

Table 1 Approximate numbers of afferent fibers of different sizes in the medial and posterior articular nerves of cat knees

	Medial Articular Nerves*	Posterior Articular Nerves*
Group 1	0	27
Group 2	57	150
Group 3	132	85
Group 4	441	408
Total number of afferent fibers	630	680
Percent that are group 3 or 4 (fine) afferent fibers	91	74

*The actual number of nerve fibers in each nerve varies between nerves. The numbers above are based on the average number of fibers in the nerve and the relative proportions of fibers of different types. (Data from Heppelmann et al[5] and Langford et al.[6])

with those in other systems, where they have very high mechanical thresholds, and function as nociceptor neurons.

The types of rotational stimuli that activate group 3 and 4 afferent nerve fibers are complex. A given afferent nerve fiber may respond to a variety of rotations, in different directions. For example, an individual fine afferent nerve fiber might be sensitive to both flexion and extension, or to both external and internal rotation, or to other combinations of the rotations. There is no consistent pattern of excitatory stimuli for those neurons, except that it can be stated that stimuli are effective only when they rotate the joint to its limit. Noxious external rotation is the single excitatory stimulus for most group 3 and 4 afferent nerve fibers in the knee. Phasic components of movement are not effective stimuli.

Therefore, some transducer mechanism must account for the punctate and complex rotational sensitivity of these afferent nerve fibers. However, it is not clear what that mechanism might be. The fact that receptive fields are spot-like implies that the endings do not sense tension, because indentations adjacent to a spot would cause tensile loading at that spot. True stretch-sensitive neurons, when studied with punctate stimuli, have receptive fields that extend beyond the morphologic limits of the receptor organ itself. Understanding the mechanism underlying group 3 and 4 receptor activation would be valuable in understanding their complex responses to joint rotations.

Another important feature of the fine afferent nerves is that their sensitivity is increased by experimentally-induced inflammation of the joint. Following inflammation of the knee, all fine afferent nerves are more responsive to mechanical stimuli.[9,10] Afferent nerves that formerly required noxious stimuli respond to (previously ineffective) gentle rotations; those that had been silent at midrange joint positions discharge spontaneously. For example, in a knee held statically at midrange, inflammation caused an eightfold increase in the afferent inflow from the knee.[9] In the posterior articular nerves, inflammation caused the group 4 afferent nerves that are mechanically sensitive to increase from 7% to 45%. The percentage of nerves that responded to joint movements increased from 0% to 54%.[10] These findings, and the observations of high thresholds in normal joints, indicate that a primary role for these neurons is as nociceptors.

The afferent neurons of the group 3 and 4 populations, then, have attributes that would serve well in a joint protection mechanism. First, they are activated when the joint is rotated into extreme positions, being otherwise silent. They are optimally activated by stimuli that appear to be potentially damaging to the joint. Their responsiveness is markedly enhanced by joint inflammation. Importantly, there is a very large number of neurons (over 1,300 in the cat's knee) that would serve as suitable sensors for such a mechanism. On the other hand, their relative lack of specificity is a problem. This population of neurons does not encode the directions of movements, because direction is confounded in the discharge of each neuron. Most fine afferent nerve fibers respond to external rotations, but they also respond to rotations in a number of other directions. Because of this fact, it is difficult to determine how activation of this population of afferent neurons could evoke an appropriate reflex motor response. It is possible that the fine afferent nerve fiber population might signal that some extreme rotation had occurred, and another mechanism might be used to determine the direction of the movement. It appears that when activated, these neurons evoke a single common protection response—joint flexion. An additional problem for a protection mechanism lies in the very slow conduction velocities of the fine afferent nervous system. It could take as long as 1,000 milliseconds for action potentials in group 4 axons to reach the human spinal cord. This is hardly suitable for any mechanism designed to provide dynamic stability.

Group 1 and Group 2 Afferent Nerve Fibers

Group 1 and 2 nerve fibers innervate large, multicellular sensory end-organs. Group 1 fibers terminate strictly in muscle receptors (muscle spindles and Golgi tendon organs). Their presence in articular nerves reflects the fact that articular nerves contain afferents from other sources, such as the popliteus muscle.

Group 2 nerve fibers are easy to study because of their large size, and they have, therefore, attracted a lot of experimental attention. Group 2 afferent nerve fibers innervate two types of sensory end-organs: ruffinian corpuscles, and small lamellated (paciniform) corpuscles.

The ruffinian endings are found on the flexion side of the joint (that is, the side of the joint facing the direction of joint flexion) and are activated when the joint is extended. The ruffinian corpuscles are sensitive to tissue stretch.[11,12] However, the adequate stimulus is the resulting tissue load, not capsule deformation.[13] No response is observed until the joint approaches the limit of extension. Their response is then proportional to joint extensional moment. Ruffinian endings have very low thresholds for activation. In cat knees, the modal extension moment at threshold was about 250 g/cm.[14]

Unlike the ruffinian endings, the pacinian or lamellated endings have not been unequivocally isolated and their properties characterized. Group 2 endings in the medial region of the knee capsule, where there are few if any ruffinian corpuscles, are compression sensitive when studied in isolated tissue,[15] and have phasic responses when studied using rotational stimuli.[16] The location of phasic endings in Clark's study[16] of the cat knee corresponds roughly with the distribution of the lamellated endings seen in histologic studies; they are distributed throughout the entire joint capsule as well as in muscles around the joint.[17] Regardless of the type of ending, the group 2 phasic endings in medial articular nerves are activated by joint rotation into extreme angles and have a response that adapts to zero within approximately 10 seconds.[16]

Thus, group 2 afferent nerve fibers also provide a signal that could be used as a potential input signal for a mechanism that would protect joints. Some group 2 afferent nerve fibers are activated by joint rotations that approach limits of movement, and are quite specific for direction of rotation. Phasic receptors likewise signal that the joint is at a limit of rotation. With regard to a major role in dynamic joint stabilization, it is a concern that there are relatively few of these afferent nerve fibers. Group 2 fibers make up a small fraction of the afferent inflow from the knee joint, and not all group 2 fibers are limit sensors. Eighty-three percent of the group 2 fibers in the posterior articular nerves are extension sensors[14] and about 55% of the group 2 fibers in the medial articular nerves are either slowly adapting or phasic limit detectors. Therefore, it can be estimated that a cat's knee would be innervated by only approximately 150 limit-sensing group 2 afferent nerve fibers. Also, any dynamic stabilizing mechanism would have to operate despite a significant conduction delay for afferent action potentials—about 20 msec from the knee to the spinal cord.

Reflexes Mediated by Activation of Joint Afferent Nerve Fibers

Because afferent signals coming from joints appear more or less appropriate to serve in a joint protection mechanism, the question of whether or not they serve such a function has attracted considerable experimental attention.

Fine Afferent Nerve Fibers

When activated, group 3 and 4 afferent fibers appear to serve as the afferent limb of a flexion reflex, a standard role for nociceptors. Very intense stimuli, which would excite fine afferent fibers, evoke knee flexion.[18,19] He and associates[20] recorded from single flexor motoneurons, and observed their response to gentle rotations into flexion and extension. The knee was then inflamed with an injection of kaolin and carrageenan, which sensitized fine afferent fibers but did not affect group 2 afferent fibers. Subsequent flexion and extension rotations, which now would activate some fine afferent fibers excited flexor motoneurons. Thus, activation of the fine afferent fibers had a flexion effect. Note also that fine afferent fibers, at least in this circumstance, do not evoke selective responses depending on the direction of the stimulus. Both extension and flexion evoke a common response, excitation of knee flexor motoneurons.

Ferrell and associates[21] also used inflammation to show that fine afferent fibers mediate flexion responses. They produced a knee inflammation, causing activation of fine afferent fibers, and observed an increase in the magnitude of the flexion reflex.

Group 2 Afferent Nerve Fibers

Several experimental methods have been devised to test for reflex effects that are mediated by group 2 afferent fibers. Because some experimental designs are flawed, and others are limited in scope, I shall critically examine several different experimental methods.

Electrical Stimulation   Electrical stimulation of articular nerves causes excitability changes in motoneurons, observed either directly from motoneurons, or indirectly using electromyographic (EMG) recordings. These observations support the basic concept that some reflex connection is made between joint afferent fibers and motor units. Electrical stimulation at intensities sufficient to maximally excite group 2 afferent fibers evokes weak and variable effects.[18,19] However, because electrical stimuli would excite axons in unnatural combinations, it is not possible to interpret these results beyond the fact that some connections are made in the spinal cord.

Natural Stimulation of the Joint   Natural (mechanical) stimulation of joints overcomes the problem associated with electrical stimuli. In various studies, different natural stimuli have been used, and several different means have been used to measure the resulting effects.

Inflation of the joint capsule.   Afferent nerve fibers in the joint are known to be activated by fluid injection into the joint space.[22] Several investigators have documented, in humans, a decrease in the H reflex or a decrease in the maximal force that the quadriceps muscles can generate following knee joint inflation.[23,24] While experiments of this sort show convincingly that some reflex mechanism is present, little can be said about what subpopulation of afferent fibers cause the effect. It might, for example, be a flexion response mediated by low-threshold fine afferent fibers.

Rotation of the knee, in animal experiments.   The electrical stimulation experiments imply that when joint afferent fibers are activated, direct synaptic effects are generated in motoneurons. Several experiments have been devised to test for resulting excitability changes in motoneurons. Direct recordings from motoneurons, EMG changes, changes in motor unit force output, and changes in the magnitude of the monosynaptic reflex have all been used to test for reflex effects from joint afferents. A striking finding in reviewing this literature is that the results are quite inconsistent. For example, extending the knee has been shown in various studies to generate either positive or negative feedback in motoneurons acting about the knee.[25] This is an important issue to resolve, because this type of experiment directly addresses the question at hand: When a joint is rotated in a way that is known to excite joint afferent fibers, are any reflex actions observed in the musculature that crosses the knee?

The principal factor underlying the inconsistency of the previous studies appears to be the fact that reflex effects evoked in such an experimental design are very weak. This is a problem for two reasons. First, if the stimulus that rotates the leg causes any movement of any other part (muscle or skin) of the experimental animal, reflex effects caused by afferent fibers in those structures could overshadow the weak effects mediated by joint afferent fibers. Second, in order to avoid effects of anesthetic agents on reflex mechanisms, it is necessary to perform these experiments in unanesthetized, spinal or decerebrate animal models. In such models, the excitability of motoneurons is depressed and inherently variable. To eliminate the effect of this variability, one experimental design[25] presented large numbers of trials at random, over a long period of time, and then averaged the resulting data. That design measured the excitability of particular motoneuron populations, using the electrically-evoked monosynaptic reflex. Motoneuron excitability was measured while the knee was rotated to the limit of extension, using stimuli that were shown to excite the group 2 capsular stretch sensors. Knee extensions were presented and data were collected automatically, using a computer, so that there was no experimenter bias. The hind limbs, hips, and lumbar spinal muscles of the test animal were extensively denervated, and the animal was held in a very rigid fixation device. Effects resulting from knee extensions were evaluated with the medial and posterior articular nerves intact and after they were cut. If residual effects remained after the articular nerves were cut, indicating that afferent fibers other than joint afferent fibers contributed to the effects seen, the data were not used.

With all of these components of the experimental design in place, it was possible to show that knee joint extensions evoked a positive feedback mechanism in motoneurons acting about the knee. The key feature of this feedback was that it was very weak. When muscle afferent fibers were excited by the same knee extension stimuli, they were much larger than the joint-mediated reflex. A more recent experiment by Ferrell and associates[26] has confirmed this general finding. They used local, discrete indentation of the posterior capsule as stimuli. Thus, their design was very unlikely to be subject to mechanical artifacts. They recorded changes in the responses of tonically active motoneurons, and found that quadriceps motor units are excited by activity in afferent fibers from the posterior capsule. Thus, when appropriate methodology is used to test for reflex effects caused by group 2 afferent fibers in the posterior articular nerves, weak positive feedback is observed.

In subsequent experiments, Baxendale and Ferrell[27] extended the basic concept of how joint reflexes might work. They found that activity in joint afferent fibers could modulate transmission in the flexion and crossed extension reflex pathway. They evoked the flexion reflex in the cat hindlimb, by electrically stimulating the peroneal nerve. They observed the resulting flexion and crossed extension reflexes by recording EMG responses in hindlimb muscles. The thresholds for evoking these reflexes changed when the knee joint angle was changed. For example, when the knee was extended, the threshold for knee flexion was lowered, indicating that some component of the flexion reflex system was excited, lowering the threshold for the reflex. The effect was lost when the joint was injected with local anesthetic, blocking joint afferent activity. Although this result is compelling, it is unclear how it is mediated by joint afferent fibers.

The effects were observed when the knee was within the range of angles (60 to 180 degrees) in which it is freely moving. It has been shown that very few joint afferent neurons are active at joint angles less than 160 degrees.[14,28,29] Thus, it would be of great interest if these experiments could be extended, using extension stimuli that optimally excite the group 2 afferent fibers, and perhaps also using noxious rotations. When, in a similar experimental design, the excitability of the group 3 and group 4 afferent fibers was recruited into activity by inflammation of the knee, there was a marked increase in the excitability of the flexion reflex, and a loss of the joint angle effect.[21] Clearly, this phenomenon needs to be studied more thoroughly. It is a concern that the effects only have been studied using stimuli that are not optimal, that is, stimuli that activate few if any joint afferent fibers.

Natural Stimulation of Single Ligaments   A third experimental design that tests for joint reflexes has looked specifically for reflexes evoked by mechanical stimulation of single ligaments. In these experiments, single ligaments have been stimulated by stretching. Measures of reflex effects have been quite limited: (1) gamma (fusimotor) neurons have been recorded from, and (2) motor unit output has been recorded, either as force or EMG recordings. An important limitation in these experiments is that the optimal stimulus for ligament afferent fibers is not known. Without knowing what types of and how many nerve endings are present in the ligaments, and to what stimuli they are sensitive, it is difficult to appropriately design the experiments and interpret the results of those that have been done.

Ligament Innervation

The Medial Collateral Ligament (MCL)

In their studies of the medial articular nerves, Schmidt and associates did not report any differences in the properties of fine afferent nerve fibers that had endings in the capsule, the patellar tendon, or the MCL.[7-9] Thus, the properties of fine afferent fibers in the MCL would be similar to the properties of other medial articular nerve fine afferent fibers. They have spot-like receptive fields, and respond primarily to intense, noxious rotations. A small number of stretch-sensitive group 2 afferent fibers have also been described in the MCL.[30,31] These afferent fibers are excited by tensile loading of the ligament and have relatively low thresholds, as low as 5 g of tensile load.

The Cruciate Ligaments

The innervation of the cruciate ligaments appears to be generally similar to that of the MCL. However, very little data is available. Several investigators have described ruffinian endings in the cruciate ligaments.[32] It would be expected, on the basis of the many other studies that show that ruffinian endings are stretch-sensitive, that the afferent neurons from these endings would be sensitive to axial stretching. According to Pope and associates,[33] there are ligament afferent fibers that respond to axial loading. They also reported other ligament afferent fibers that were compression but not tension sensitive. However, because of the relative paucity of cruciate afferent fibers, it is not clear how many fibers are compression rather than tension sensitive. Further, it is not known how sensitive the stretch-sensitive fibers are to axial stress. While capsule afferent fibers are readily obtained and recorded from, the yield of afferent neurons identified as being from the cruciate ligament is very small indeed.

Their paucity notwithstanding, some sensors in the ligaments appear to have attributes that would be appropriate in a joint-protection mechanism. Some MCL afferent fibers are excited by axial loading, and by intense rotations. Some afferent fibers in the cruciate ligaments are excited by axial loading. In both cases, this is a stimulus for which an appropriate response would be to unload the joint.

Reflex effects caused by ligament stimulation have been tested using two basic methods: (1) To determine the effects on gamma motoneurons, a muscle is stretched sinusoidally, activating muscle spindle receptors. A ligament is then loaded by pulling a loop of thread tied around it. This pulling activates ligament afferent fibers, which reflexly affect gamma motoneurons, causing observable changes in the discharge rate of the muscle receptor. Control observations are made with the posterior articular nerve cut. Johansson and associates[3] have shown effects on both dynamic and static gamma motoneurons caused by pulling a loop of thread that is tied around the ligament. They hypothesize that the effect of this action is to modify muscle stiffness, thus stabilizing the joint. (2) The effects on alpha motoneurons were tested by seeking reflex effects mediated by ligament afferent fibers. Ekholm and associates[34] recorded flexor monosynaptic reflexes while pulling the MCL with a loop of thread. Flexor facilitation was observed.

In both of these studies, it is not clear what afferent fibers would be activated by the stimulus. Pulling the loop of thread will create axial loads along the ligament, but also will produce compression loads under the thread. Given the rather large loads applied to the thread (up to 40 N), it seems likely that fine afferent fibers under the thread would be activated, thereby evoking a flexion reflex response. In the case of the MCL, it is also a concern that the thread would have to pass through local wounds, which might result in local fine afferent fiber activation when the thread was pulled.

In another experimental design,[35] loads simply have been applied to a ligament, and evoked EMG signals are sought in muscles around the joint. Petersen and Stener[36] used a somewhat similar design, in which they forcibly abducted the tibia in humans in order to load the MCL; EMG responses were sought. They observed that no muscular responses were evoked by the stimuli. It should be stressed that experiments like this have several potential problems. The EMG is a relatively insensitive measure of motoneuron excitability, because active fibers may be distant from the recording electrodes, and because quiescent motoneurons would not show inhibition and extremely intense stimuli would be needed to show excitation. Thus, dual dangers exist: (1) applied stimuli can spread to structures other than the intended ligament; and (2) nociceptors may be activated by the intense stimuli. Thus, it is not clear how any outcome can be interpreted.

Summary

In summary, the mechanism of the reflex connections made by joint afferent fibers is not completely understood. A strong case can be made that fine afferent fibers in the knee evoke a flexion reflex at the knee joint. Fine afferent fibers are numerous, and are best activated by extreme and potentially damaging rotations and by inflammations of the joint. However, the reflex effects of fine afferent fibers have been incompletely studied.

Group 2 afferent fibers also weakly mediate reflexes. Two well-controlled studies show that those connections mediate a positive feedback system that would reinforce movements into extension.

Some group 2 afferent fibers also appear to have another effect, modifying transmission through the flexor reflex system. Whatever neurons mediate this effect, they are a very small fraction of the total population of afferent fibers available. More work needs to be done to explore the neural systems that mediate this effect and its significance.

Very little can be said about reflexes mediated by ligament afferent fibers. The strongest argument to support my contention that they are insignificant is that in the studies where reflexes were evoked using joint rotations,[25] the joint nerves were intact. Thus, ligament as well as capsule afferent fibers were present in the nerves mediating the effect. The weakness of the observed effects is in contrast with the hypothesis that a powerful role is played by ligament afferent fibers. Thus, it is unlikely that the same ligament endings, studied alone using similar stimuli, would have any major reflex effect. In some experiments, ligaments were pulled with thread. These results cannot be interpreted until it can be shown whether or not the stimulus is activating fine afferent fibers.

Some experiments showed reflex effects on gamma motoneurons; it remains to be seen whether any resulting changes in muscle stiffness are great enough to provide a significant change in joint stiffness.

Some experiments showed a reflex effect mediated through the flexion reflex; it is unknown whether these effects have any significance in movement control. Even if joint afferent fibers were to mediate reflexes with an appropriate organization, there is the possibility that the loop times (time for conduction in afferent and efferent axons, synaptic delays, and time for muscle to develop force) would be too long to permit a role in protecting against anything except very slow joint rotation.[37]

Despite the fact that joint afferent neurons do not appear to elicit reflexes that serve as a dynamic stabilizing mechanism, there is strong evidence that joint afferent fibers do serve a protective function. The protection is observed, however, only if the joint is made mechanically unstable. O'Connor and associates,[38] in experiments with dog knees, have shown that cutting the joint nerves and then cutting the anterior cruciate ligament (ACL) results in an unstable joint that develops symptoms of osteoarthritis, including degeneration of articular cartilage. However, the articular nerves have an important role in limiting the extent of the disease. If the articular nerves are intact when the ACL is cut, the resulting disease is significantly diminished. Joint denervation alone has no effect. Thus, in the absence of joint nerves, an unstable joint is much more subject to injury. This suggests that joint afferent fibers can function in an unstable joint so as to allow the animal to adopt movement strategies that would stabilize it and/or avoid excess loadings. Presumably, this would be by signaling extreme and/or potentially damaging joint positions to the dog's central nervous system.

References

1. Soechting JF, Flanders M: Arm movements in three-dimensional space: Computation, theory, and observation. *Exerc Sport Sci Rev* 1991;19:389-418.

2. Hasan Z, Stuart DG: Animal solutions to problems of movement control: The role of proprioceptors. *Ann Rev Neurosci* 1988;11:199-223.

3. Johansson H, Sjölander P, Sojka P: Receptors in the knee joint ligaments and their role in the biomechanics of the joint. *Crit Rev Biomed Eng* 1991;18:341-368.

4. Sjölander P: A sensory role for the cruciate ligaments. *Umea University Medical Dissertations* 1989, series 245.

5. Heppelmann B, Heuss C, Schmidt RF: Fiber size distribution of myelinated and unmyelinated axons in the medial and posterior articular nerves of the cat's knee joint. *Somatosens Res* 1988;5:273-281.

6. Langford LA, Schmidt RF: Afferent and efferent axons in the medial and posterior articular nerves of the cat. *Anat Record* 1983;206:71-78.

7. Schaible H-G, Schmidt RF: Activation of groups III and IV sensory units in medial articular nerve by local mechanical stimulation of knee joint. *J Neurophysiol* 1983;49: 35-44.

8. Schaible H-G, Schmidt RF: Responses of fine medial articular nerve afferents to passive movements of knee joints. *J Neurophysiol* 1983;49:1118-1126.

9. Coggeshall RE, Hong KA, Langford LA, et al: Discharge characteristics of fine medial articular afferents at rest and during passive movements of inflamed knee joints. *Brain Res* 1983;272:185-188.

10. Grigg P, Schaible H-G, Schmidt RF: Mechanical sensitivity of group III and IV afferents from posterior articular nerve in normal and inflamed cat knee. *J Neurophysiol* 1986;55:635-643.

11. Boyd IA: The histological structure of the receptors in the knee-joint of the cat correlated with their physiological response. *J Physiol* 1954;124:476-488.

12. Grigg P, Hoffman AH: Properties of Ruffini afferents revealed by stress analysis of isolated sections of cat knee capsule. *J Neurophysiol* 1982;47:41-54.

13. Fuller MS, Grigg P, Hoffman AH: Response of joint capsule neurons to axial stress and strain during dynamic loading in cat. *J Neurophysiol* 1991;65:1321-1328.

14. Grigg P: Mechanical factors influencing response of joint afferent neurons from cat knee. *J Neurophysiol* 1975;38:1473-1484.

15. Grigg A, Hoffman AH, Fogarty KE: Properties of Golgi-Mazzoni afferents in cat knee joint capsule, as revealed by mechanical studies of isolated joint capsule. *J Neurophysiol* 1982;47:31-40.

16. Clark FJ: Information signaled by sensory fibers in medial articular nerve. *J Neurophysiol* 1975;38:1464-1472.

17. Strasmann T, Halata Z: Applications for 3-D image processing in functional anatomy: Reconstruction of the cubital joint region and spatial distribution of mechanoreceptors surrounding this joint in Monodelphis domestica, a laboratory marsupial. *Eur J Cell Biol* 1989;48(suppl 25):107-110.

18. Gardner E: Reflex muscular responses to stimulation of articular nerves in the cat. *Am J Physiol* 1950;161:133-141.

19. Skoglund S: Anatomical and physiological studies of knee joint innervation in the cat. *Acta Physiol Scand* 1956;36(suppl 124):1-101.

20. He X, Proske U, Schaible H-G, et al: Acute inflammation of the knee joint in the cat alters responses of flexor motoneurons to leg movements. *J Neurophysiol* 1988;59: 326-340.

21. Ferrell WR, Wood L, Baxendale RH: The effect of acute joint inflammation on flexion reflex excitability in the decerebrate, low-spinal cast. *Q J Exp Physiol* 1988;73:95-102.

22. Ferrell WR: The effect of acute joint distension on mechanoreceptor discharge in the knee of the cat. *Q J Exp Physiol* 1987;72:493-499.

23. DeAndrade JR, Grant C, Dixon AStJ: Joint distension and reflex muscle inhibition in the knee. *J Bone Joint Surg* 1965;47A:313-322.

24. Fahrer H, Rentsch HU, Gerber NJ, et al: Knee effusion and reflex inhibition of the quadriceps: A bar to effective retraining. *J Bone Joint Surg* 1988;70B:635-638.

25. Grigg P, Harrigan EP, Fogarty KE: Segmental reflexes mediated by joint afferent neurons in cast knee. *J Neurophysiol* 1978;41:9-14.

26. Ferrell WR, Rosenberg JR, Baxendale RH, et al: Fourier analysis of the relation between the discharge of quadriceps motor units and periodic mechanical stimulation of cat knee joint receptors. *Exp Physiol* 1990;75:739-750.

27. Baxendale RH, Ferrell WR: The effect of knee joint afferent discharge on transmission in flexion reflex pathways in decerebrate cats. *J Physiol* 1981;315:231-242.

28. Clark FJ, Burgess PR: Slowly adapting receptors in cat knee joint: Can they signal joint angle? *J Neurophysiol* 1975;38:1448-1463.

29. Ferrell WR: The adequacy of stretch receptors in the cat knee joint for signalling joint angle throughout a full range of movement. *J Physiol* 1980;299:85-99.

30. Andrew BL: The sensory innervation of the medial ligament of the knee joint. *J Physiol* 1954;123:241-250.

31. Stener B: Experimental evaluation of the hypothesis of ligamento-muscular protective reflexes: I. A method for adequate stimulation of tension receptors in the medial collateral ligament of the knee joint of the cat, and studies of the innervation of the ligament. *Acta Physiol Scand* 1959;48(suppl 166):5-26.

32. Halata Z, Haus J: The ultrastructure of sensory nerve endings in human anterior cruciate ligament. *Anat Embryol (Berl)* 1989;179:415-421.

33. Pope DF, Cole KJ, Brand RA: Properties of ACL mechanoreceptive afferents. *J Biomech* 1990;23:717.

34. Ekholm J, Eklund G, Soglund S: On the reflex effects from the knee joint of the cat. *Acta Physiol Scand* 1960;50:167-174.

35. Solomonow M, Baratta R, Zhou BH, et al: The synergistic action of the anterior cruciate ligament and thigh muscles in maintaining joint stability. *Am J Sports Med* 1987;15: 207-213.

36. Petersen I, Stener B: Experimental evaluation of the hypothesis of ligamento-muscular protective reflexes: III. A study in man using the medial collateral ligament of the knee joint. *Acta Physiol Scand* 1959;48(suppl 166):51-61.

37. Pope MH, Johnson RJ, Brown DW, et al: The role of the musculature in injuries to the medial collateral ligament. *J Bone Joint Surg* 1979;61A:398-402.

38. O'Connor BL, Visco DM, Brandt KD, et al: Neurogenic acceleration of osteoarthritis: The effects of prior articular neurectomy on the development of osteoarthritis after anterior cruciate ligament transection in the dog. *J Bone Joint Surg* 1992;74A:367-376.

Chapter 15

Skeletal Muscle and the Knee Joint

William E. Garrett, Jr, MD, PhD
David J. Kuester, MD
Thomas M. Best, MD

Introduction

This chapter will review the effects of muscle activity on the knee joint. The function of muscle is to create and control joint motion. Therefore, it is important to know the complete relationship of muscle to joints. However, this review will be more specific regarding muscle as it might relate to injury of the knee joint. Muscle activity that might cause injury or protect from injury will be discussed along with the changes that occur in muscle following injury.

Muscle Forces That Act on Joints

When muscles act on the knee joint, the primary focus is usually on the muscle groups responsible for flexion and extension of the knee. This is because the knee joint works principally as a hinge joint, with one degree of freedom. It is true that some degree of tibial rotation on the femur is also possible as a second degree of freedom, but this is of less importance to this discussion. The knee extensor muscle is the quadriceps femoris. The flexor muscles are primarily the hamstring muscles, including the biceps femoris, semitendinosus, and semimembranosus, although other muscles also function as knee flexors. The sartorius, gracilis, gastrocnemius, and popliteus also cause knee flexion.

Joint motion can be caused by mechanical factors as well as muscle action. For instance, the gravitational effects of hip flexion will cause knee flexion in the standing position. Similarly, deceleration of hip flexion will cause knee extension during gait, at the end of the swing phase. As hip flexion is decelerated, inertial forces cause the knee to extend. It is not always obvious when motion is caused by muscle action across the knee, or by mechanical factors that might be generated by muscles acting primarily on other joints.

Striated (skeletal) muscles stop or limit motion as well as create it. During gait, the knee flexor muscles act more as a decelerator of knee extension than as the primary cause of knee flexion (for example, during normal walking). Knee flexion that begins in late stance and continues into the swing phase is not associated with significant hamstring activation. However, as the knee approaches extension prior to heel strike, the hamstrings act to decelerate the extending knee. To a large extent, then, the knee flexors act as antiextensors rather than as flexors. This is also true for the quadriceps muscles, which act as antiflexors as well as extensors.

Muscles function somewhat differently when they are acting to decelerate or control motion. Muscles that are activated during elongation are described as undergoing eccentric action. This is in contrast to the concept of muscle that is being shortened while activated (concentric action) or muscle that is activated while its length is kept constant (isometric action). Eccentric action allows absorption of energy, or negative work. In contrast to concentric action, muscle is more efficient during eccentric action. It can produce significantly more force, and the same force can be produced with less energy consumption. In addition, muscle understretch can produce force because of the passive properties of the connective tissue. These viscoelastic effects are thought to be entirely passive and do not require active metabolism and contractile protein activity.

It is important to consider how muscles assist in controlling forces within joints. It is surprising how much the musculoskeletal system is at risk of injury when muscles do not assist in the control of these joint forces. Many orthopaedic surgeons have treated a tibial plateau fracture or a ruptured lumbar disc in a patient who stepped off a curb or from a relatively small height. In these patients, it is clear that there is enough energy to fracture the knee joint when unexpected forces are delivered directly to the articular surface. A consideration of Newton's second Law of Motion explains how this occurs.

Force (F) = Mass (M) x Acceleration (A) or F = M x A.

Acceleration is a measure of how fast the velocity changes.

$$\text{Acceleration} = \frac{\text{Change in Velocity } (\delta v)}{\text{Change in Time } (\delta t)}$$

further,

$$\text{Velocity} = \frac{\text{Change in Distance } (\delta x)}{\text{Change in Time } (\delta t)}$$

Therefore,

$$F = M \times \delta v/\delta t$$
$$= M \times \delta^2 x/\delta t^2$$

Therefore, force is related to the distance and time over which the change in velocity (acceleration/deceleration) occurs. The stopping distance is an equivalent indicator of force magnification due to impact. In walking and running, the body's center of mass changes through cyclic motions that are accentuated by athletic activities, such as jumping. If the body were to instantly decelerate its center of mass, the time over which the change in velocity occurred would approach zero. It is not the velocity that causes injury, but how quickly it changes. Therefore, the quantity $\delta v/\delta t$ would approach infinity, along with the resultant force transmitted to the joint. Muscle contraction allows a more gradual change in velocity and increases the stopping distance.

For example, studies of gait show that as the foot approaches heel strike, the knee extensors and hip flexors become active. They are very active during foot strike and their function is to slow the decrease in the body's center of mass, with the deceleration occurring gradually. One very important function of muscle is to protect the joint by controlling the high forces of physical activity. Clinically, it is interesting to recall how little trauma can cause injury when the muscles are not aligned to protect the joint and, conversely, how much force can be withstood if the muscles function properly.

Control of Muscles That Act on Joints

The knee joint and essentially every other moving joint in the body are influenced by muscles that can generate opposite joint motions (such as flexion and extension). One muscle group, the agonist, acts to achieve a certain motion, while the opposing muscle group is called the antagonist. Frequently, muscles are simultaneously active and the net effect of combined muscular activity, or coactivation, on the joint must be considered. Muscles that produce the same effect on a joint are called synergists. In the knee, the four quadriceps muscles are synergistic during extension of the knee. The knee flexors, the hamstrings, act as antagonists.

The control of the muscle groups affecting the knee is very complex and not completely understood by neurophysiologists. Presently, the continued impetus to understand the basics of motor control is augmented by the field of robotics, in which even relatively simple motions seem slow and jerky compared with the fluid, coordinated motion produced by the limbs of animals. The control of muscle movement is far too complex to discuss in detail in this chapter. Fuchs and associates[1] and Hasan and Stuart[2] present more complete discussions on motor control.

The central nervous system controls a broad spectrum of movement and motor activity. The least complex level involves movements that require no thought processes by the brain. Withdrawal from painful stimuli and the familiar tendon jerk reflex are examples of reflex movements mediated directly through the spinal cord. A much more complex level of movement consists of learned patterns voluntarily controlled by the brain and modified by a variety of sensory information. An example of complex movement might be ballet dancing. A third level of motor control that falls between simple reflexes and complex, voluntary motion consists of a variety of repetitive motions. Examples include walking, running, and chewing. These movements can be initiated by the brain and require little thought or control.

It was previously thought that various reflexes such as the muscle stretch reflex might allow these repetitive motions, and that afferent signals from the periphery might cause an appropriate motor signal without much processing at the level of the central nervous system. However, it is now clear that these repetitive movements are under the control of networks in the spinal cord and the brain stem called central pattern generators. These networks intricately link the motor nerves controlling the various phases of repetitive motions. For example, the hip, knee, and ankle muscles are properly activated to allow walking. The appropriate agonists and antagonists of the separate joints are active at the appropriate time to allow the rhythmic motor activity. Further, it is clear that the rudimentary control of gait is possible even without afferent input into the spinal cord.[1]

These pattern generators are present in the spinal cord and brain stem and are capable of commanding repetitive motor functions even in the absence of information from peripheral afferent nerves or descending signals from the brain. However, afferent and supraspinal information into these spinal levels allows for the huge amount of control and interaction with the environment that characterizes motor control in animals. Afferent information from the periphery includes signals from muscles and tendons, skin, and joints. These afferent signals interact at the spinal cord level and also are transmitted to the brain. The brain modifies its motor signal based on peripheral afferent information as well as other sensory information coming from visual, vestibular, and other systems.

All of these levels are highly integrated, acting together. Consideration of the number of cells involved helps to illustrate this point. In the cat spinal cord, for example, a dorsal root entering a segment of the spinal cord contains approximately 15,000 fibers. These fibers carry afferent information from the periphery. In contrast, there are only half as many efferent motor fibers in the ventral root. Between the afferent dorsal root fibers and the efferent ventral root fibers, there are an estimated 300,000 to 400,000 spinal interneurons to integrate peripheral input with descending tracts from the brain to control the motoneurons. Thus, there is tremendous opportunity for modulation of the stimulus from the brain to the motoneurons.

The preceding discussion of motor control points to several pertinent facts regarding muscle control of joints. First, much of the control originates from spinal cord centers that are intrinsically capable of exerting gross motor control. Second, rather complex patterns of motor control can be learned and retained by the central nervous system as stored motor programs. And third, there is tremendous opportunity for fine control of the pattern generators and motor control based on interaction with peripheral afferent information and with sensory and cognitive information from the central nervous system.

It may be helpful to consider applying these principles to a common problem, the anterior cruciate ligament (ACL)-deficient knee, during walking. Sensory information from the knee and the ligament specifically are not necessary to generate knee flexor and extensor muscle function because pattern generators and learned motor programs exert this control. However, the absence of the ACL may deprive the spinal cord of some helpful afferent information. In addition, abnormal motion caused by instability can provide other sensory information from joint receptors and muscle-tendon receptors that can influence central control. New sensory information induced by mechanical changes in the ACL-deficient knee can lead to alterations in the central pattern generators and motor programs to exert a modified level of control of muscle forces about the knee.

Afferent Nerves From Muscle and Tendon

Having considered the interaction of peripheral afferent nerves in motor control, it is important to note the types of afferent nerves coming from muscle and tendon. Muscle contributes all types of afferent fibers to the spinal cord. In fact, more than two thirds of the nerve fibers in a nerve leading directly to a muscle are afferent. Group I fibers are large, myelinated fibers originating from muscle spindles (Ia) and Golgi tendon organs (Ib). Muscle spindles are specialized receptors in muscle that are sensitive to both static and changing muscle length. Along with afferent nerves, they are also supplied by efferent fibers, the (gamma) motoneurons, which can actively control the receptor characteristics of the spindles. The Golgi tendon organs are usually situated near muscle-tendon junctions and are sensitive to force in the tendon and muscle.

The type II fibers in muscle come from the neuromuscular spindles and other muscle receptors, including Ruffini receptors (force-sensitive), paciniform receptors (stretch- and pressure-sensitive), pacinian corpuscles (pressure- and vibration-sensitive), and free nerve endings (pressure- and contraction-sensitive). Group III fibers innervate free nerve endings and blood vessels. Group IV fibers are small, unmyelinated fibers that compose almost half of all the afferent fibers. These fibers innervate free nerve endings, most of which respond to noxious stimuli and are often termed nociceptors.

Muscle afferent neurons are involved with several well-known reflex movements. The tendon jerk reflex involves the sudden stretching of the patellar tendon. The muscle spindles sense the sudden stretch and the afferent neurons directly excite the efferent alpha motoneurons to contract and resist the stretch, leading to the characteristic muscle contraction that causes the quadriceps to shorten briefly. This is effected by direct afferent to efferent neuron contact without the necessity of internuncial neuronal activation. This, then, is a monosynaptic reflex. There are also pathways that tend to activate the synergists of the muscle and those that inhibit contraction of the antagonists; these pathways involve internuncial neurons.

Another muscle reflex is the stretch reflex, which is based directly on peripheral afferent neuron input. It occurs in response to a more sustained stretch on the muscle and lasts longer than the tendon jerk reflex. A stretched muscle responds by generating muscle excitation to resist the stretch. This is accomplished with group Ia and group II afferent neurons from the muscle spindles.

In both of these reflexes, afferent pathways exist within muscles, which lead to mechanisms to resist muscle length change caused either by quick or sustained stretch. Thus, not only is muscle the dynamic force to control joint forces, it is also a very powerful sensor that provides information to the central nervous system, provides fine control of movement, and protects joints.

Ligament and Muscle Interactions

Aside from the question of how joints are influenced by muscles as both initiators and controllers of motion, there is growing interest in the possible role of muscles as agonists or antagonists to certain ligaments. The most studied interaction is the relationship of the ACL to the musculature surrounding the knee. The hamstrings have the ability to pull the tibia posteriorly on the femur and can therefore have a synergistic relationship with the ACL in preventing anterior subluxation of the tibia. Similarly, the quadriceps muscles tend to pull the tibia anteriorly and thereby act as an antagonist to the ACL. The muscle pairs interact oppositely with the posterior cruciate ligament; the quadriceps act as an agonist and the hamstrings as an antagonist.

The relationship of these interactions has been evaluated in several mechanisms. The ACL will be discussed primarily because most of the current interest and information is obtained from clinical studies of muscle forces in anterior cruciate ligament injury and reconstruction. The interaction has been investigated from several approaches. Can the antagonist quadriceps be all or part of the cause for rupture of the ACL? Can the agonistic hamstrings prevent rupture of the ACL? These questions concern muscle interactions with a normal cruciate. Another line of questioning concerns muscle changes after ACL tear. Can muscle action help to substitute for the function of an absent ACL? Does muscle deteriorate after an ACL tear? Finally, questions are being asked about the fate of muscles after successful ACL reconstruction. Do muscles regain their normal function and properties when the ACL is surgically reconstructed?

Quadriceps as an ACL Antagonist

Clinical investigations reported in the literature support the fact that ACL injuries often occur during noncontact sports; perhaps the majority of ACL injuries do not involve contact. The athletic maneuvers responsible often involve sudden deceleration or sudden change in direction. Because there is often no contact to impart energy, the mechanical energy to decelerate or change direction is derived in large part from muscle, especially the quadriceps muscle. Several investigations have shown that the ACL is strained by activation of the quadriceps muscle.[3,4] Passive knee extension also causes a strain in the ACL.[5] The combination of knee extension and quadriceps activation causes even more strain in the ACL. Arms and associates[5] showed that the strain in the human knee ACL depends on several factors. During passive motion, the flexion angle affects ACL strain. Strain is at a minimum at 30 to 35 degrees and increases as the angle moves to full extension and to flexion. Maximum strain occurs at 120 degrees. In addition to flexion angle, muscle activation affects strain in the ligament. Simulated isometric quadriceps contraction induced a strain in the ACL from full extension to 60 degrees of flexion. However, isometric quadriceps contraction at flexion angles greater than 60 degrees did not induce a strain on the ACL. These results have been confirmed by Renström and associates[6] and Yasuda and Sasaki.[3] Further, the latter authors estimate that the anterior shear force that must be resisted by the ACL is 14% of the force in the quadriceps.

Without a functioning ACL, quadriceps muscle forces induce an anterior subluxation of the tibia on the femur. This is consistent with studies that demonstrate the resistance of the ACL to anterior tibial motion. Grood and associates[7] found that the quadriceps force increased rapidly as terminal extension was reached and that sectioning of the ACL did not affect the force, but did result in anterior tibial displacement between 0 and 30 degrees. Franklin and associates[8] demonstrated a radiographic assessment of anterior tibial subluxation in ACL-deficient knees. Quadriceps contractions were performed in full extension with an ankle weight of 15 lbs causing a subluxation of 5 mm more than on the normal side.

These investigations have been directed primarily toward the effect of quadriceps contraction as it relates to rehabilitation after ACL surgery. Studies to date have not looked at the very high loads that might be involved with an injury to the ACL. However, clinical experience has shown that ACL tears may result from athletic activities involving sudden deceleration or rotation of the body. In these activities, muscular power is used to resist or alter kinetic energy of the body. Much of the force is transmitted through the knee joint and these forces are generated by the quadriceps. It is quite possible that the force generated by an activated quadriceps muscle is part of the force causing an injury to the ligament. It is also helpful to consider the physical principles discussed earlier.

Hamstrings as ACL Agonists

Given the forces acting to displace the tibia anteriorly, action of the hamstring muscles might help absorb energy and prevent injury to the ACL. Several of the studies previously noted also investigated the effect of hamstring activation on ACL strain. Renström and associates[6] found that hamstring activity reduced strain in the ACL at all angles tested. During simultaneous quadriceps and hamstring activation, the hamstrings reduced the strain produced by quadriceps at all angles and reduced ACL strain to less than that seen in passive motion from full extension to 30 degrees of flexion. Similar results were obtained by Yasuda and Sasaki.[3] Iverson and associates[9] examined the effects of hamstring contraction in subjects undergoing knee ligament laxity testing at 15 degrees and 90 degrees of knee flexion. With the knee in 90 degrees of flexion, the anterior drawer sign was easily eliminated by tensing the hamstrings. At 15 degrees of knee flexion, a reduction of up to 31% resulted from hamstring contraction.

Gait studies show that the hamstrings are very active near terminal swing and early stance phases of all speeds of gait. These are the times when the ACL may be strained because of maximum knee extension and contraction of the quadriceps muscle. Therefore, even in normal knee motion during gait, the hamstrings may function as agonists or synergists of the ACL.

Using a feline model, Solomonow and associates[10] proposed a ligament-hamstring reflex arc that would serve to improve dynamic stability in normal knees. When ligament loads became sufficiently high, the hamstrings were synergistically excited, resulting in reduced ligament strain. However, Grabiner and associates[11] tested nine males with intact ACLs and concluded that no hamstring excitation was used to reduce ACL strain during nonweightbearing isometric knee extension in healthy knees.

The proposal of a reflex arc that might protect the ACL is quite intriguing.[10] Certainly static strain of the ACL influences quadriceps and hamstring muscles. However, there is no clear consensus and little data to determine whether hamstring activation in normal and running gait is generated in response to reflex action, spinal cord pattern generators, or supraspinal drive. Reflex activation may occur from afferent signals in the joint structures or muscle-tendon units. In another chapter of this book, Dr. Peter Grigg discusses the possibilities for interactions from the ligaments. Pope and associates[12] provided earlier data that ligament strain was very unlikely to result in significant protection from a reflex because of the obligate time delays from nerve conduction, synaptic transmission, and muscle force generation after activation.

Coactivation and Effects on Ligaments

Thus far, the separate effects of quadriceps and hamstring forces acting at the knee have been discussed. The nervous system often employs simultaneous activation, or coactivation, of both muscle groups. As expected, this significantly changes the stiffness of the joint. Markolf and associates[13] used a clinical laxity tester to evaluate in vivo knee stability. Active tensing of the knee muscles increased knee stiffness by two to four times and reduced laxity by 25% to 50% of the control side.

Isolated knee extension exercises have been shown to result in coactivation of the quadriceps and hamstring muscles. The quadriceps initiate the extension but the hamstrings become coactive near terminal extension. Draganich and associates[14] showed that all hamstring muscles were active from nine degrees of flexion to full extension with generally increasing activity. Faster speeds of extension were associated with higher bursts of hamstring activity. These data from studies of ballistic extension are very similar to the results mentioned earlier from studies of gait. The hamstrings are activated just prior to heel strike to decelerate the hip and knee, while the quadriceps become active to halt the fall of the body's center of gravity after heel strike. In the ballistic movements and during gait, the coactivation of the hamstrings will increase joint stiffness and act synergistically with the ACL to control anterior tibial subluxation. Several investigators have shown that coactivation has a role in maintaining knee joint stability. Baratta and associates[15] showed that the level of activation would lead to a constant opposing torque in the hamstring muscles near full extension. Renström and associates[6] and Draganich and Vahey[4] demonstrated that hamstring coactivation could reduce strain in the ACL produced by quadriceps forces alone. However, the coactivation of the hamstrings was not sufficient to reduce the strain in the ACL to the level of strain in passive knee motion at angles from more than 45 degrees of flexion to full extension.

The occurrence of coactivation raises the possibility that the relative torques produced by the hamstrings and quadriceps might be important factors in the causation or prevention of knee injuries.[16] Without coactivation only the absolute torques produced by the muscles rather than the ratio may be of interest. Prietto and Caiozzo[17] have shown that the hamstring-quadriceps ratio is a function of the speed of isokinetic testing at specific angles. When appropriate corrections for gravity and angle specificity are applied, the hamstring-quadriceps ratio ranges from 33% to 38%. Although the literature has placed some emphasis on this ratio, it may not be as important as once anticipated. For instance, it does not seem to be related to the likelihood of injury in high school football players.[18] In addition, it seems to be highly variable from one individual to another, especially if angle-specific torques are not measured and gravitational effects are not corrected. It is also probably true that the balance or coordination among muscle groups is more related to the degree of activation of the muscle by the central nervous system than relative maxima of each muscle group.

Effects of ACL Injury on Quadriceps Muscles

Several studies have characterized the changes in the quadriceps muscles following ACL injury. Most of these studies show that quadriceps mass and the maximum force generated by the quadriceps are diminished. Several authors have evaluated torque output for knee extensors in the chronically injured ACL-deficient knee. These studies all show a significant decrease in torque that can be generated by the knee extensors.[19-22] The significant decreases in torque were accompanied by atrophy of the quadriceps muscle. This has been determined by measurement of thigh circumference and by quantitative computed tomography or magnetic resonance imaging.[21,23] Imaging studies have been a more precise measure of atrophy because of the changes in subcutaneous fat and because of the differential atrophy among the different muscle groups.

Imaging studies show a discrepancy between muscle atrophy and strength deficits. Although there is significant quadriceps atrophy, the magnitude of the atrophy is smaller than the magnitude of the strength deficit.[20,23] Muscle atrophy is caused primarily by a decrease in fiber cross-sectional area. (Strength is usually proportional to cross-sectional area if the muscle is fully or equally activated.) A decrement of only 5% in cross-sectional area led to a decrement in torque output of nearly 25% when testing isokinetically at 30 degrees/sec.[21,24] These findings have led to the proposal that a torn ACL leads to a diminished central nervous system drive to the quadriceps muscle. This decreased drive has been observed with electromyography.[24] Differences in torque production were more pronounced at lower isokinetic testing velocities in which maximum torques are higher. Therefore, the decrement in central drive may be higher as maximum torque values increase.

Effects of ACL Injury on the Hamstring Muscles

Chronic injury to the ACL does not lead to the same changes in the hamstrings as in the quadriceps. Recent studies have demonstrated little atrophy or even slight hypertrophy of the hamstrings in patients with chronic ACL tears.[21,23] Just as imaging studies failed to show atrophy, isokinetic dynamometry showed no strength deficits in hamstrings, compared with the contralateral normal knee.[25] However, previous studies have shown mild deficits in hamstring strength.[26]

Walla and associates[27] studied a group of patients with ACL injuries that were treated nonsurgically. They attributed improved function to increased control of the hamstrings in the injured knee. It was believed that muscular coordination was a much more important predictor of success than laxity or pivot shift instability tests. Although the control was attributed to voluntary or reflex mechanisms, determination of the level of central nervous system control was not possible. A similar study has also emphasized the importance of hamstring function in patients with chronic ACL deficiency. Giove and associates[16] found higher levels of sports participation in patients whose hamstring strength equalled or exceeded their quadriceps strength.

Dynamic studies of muscle activity during gait have provided some insight into the different reactions of knee flexors and extensors to chronic ACL injury. Several studies now show that the electromyographic profiles of muscle activity respond differently in the two muscle groups after ACL injury. Limbird and associates[28] studied the electromyographic profiles of the lower extremity muscles to demonstrate adaptations following ACL rupture. There were significant differences during two periods in the gait cycle, the swing to stance transition and the early swing phase. During loading, muscle activity was decreased in the quadriceps and increased in the hamstrings. During early swing, muscle activity increased in the quadriceps and decreased in the hamstrings. Branch and associates[29] also found similar changes. Recently, Shiavi and associates[30] confirmed and extended these studies. They demonstrated that these changes in muscle activity result in a greater posteriorly directed force and a greater flexor moment. These changes could help to avoid any anterior subluxation made possible by the lack of an ACL.

Effects of ACL Reconstruction on Muscles

Improvements in reconstructive procedures over the years have led to a relatively high probability of restoration of knee stability. Surgery and a subsequent rehabilitation program might restore the deficits in the quadriceps. However, even at five years following reconstruction, significant strength deficits persisted in reconstructed knees.[31] Elmqvist and associates[22] investigated recovery of contractile ability of the quadriceps muscle following ACL reconstruction. Even after one year, quadriceps peak torque averaged only approximately 80% of that of the uninjured limb. The inability of the quadriceps to regain normal strength has been a consistent focus of several studies following ACL reconstructions.[32] It is possible that prolonged immobilization or restriction of normal function may be a contributing factor. Accelerated rehabilitation programs are more common now. However, even the accelerated program has allowed recovery to approximately 90% of normal and not to a normal range.[33]

Several studies have attempted to correlate the objective and functional results of surgery with the function of the quadriceps and hamstrings. Of course, it is impossible to determine whether a good result allowed normal strength recovery or whether the muscle recovery allowed a good functional result, but certainly the factors are related. Arvidson and associates[34] found the maximum torque produced by the quadriceps after reconstruction was significantly less in the involved leg than in the uninvolved leg for the fair and poor functional groups. However, in the good and excellent outcomes, the maximum quadriceps torque was equal to that of the normal leg. Odensten and associates[35] also found that return to preinjury functional status was correlated with increased quadriceps strength. Seto and associates[31] examined individuals five years after ACL reconstruction and assessed strength, stability, function, and activity of muscle. For intra-articular reconstructions, a significant correlation was observed between quadriceps and hamstring strength and the functional activity scores. Interestingly, the muscle performance scores correlated better with the activity level than did the tests for stability.

Summary

It is quite clear that the muscles about the knee strongly influence the function of the ligaments; conversely, the state of the knee ligaments influences muscle function. Muscle activity can affect the stresses and strains on the knee ligaments, which in turn enables it to cause or prevent injury. Injury to ligaments leads to adaptations in the muscles moving the knee. As yet, the treatment regimens have not been able to restore consistently normal or predictable ligament and muscle function. Further study into muscle and ligament interactions should prove interesting and helpful.

References

1. Fuchs AF, Anderson ME, Binder MD, et al: The neural control of movement, in Patton HD, Fuchs AF, Hille B, et al (eds): *Textbook of Physiology: Excitable Cells and Neurophysiology*, ed 21. Philadelphia, Saunders, 1989, vol 1, pp 503-509.
2. Hasan Z, Stuart DG: Animal solutions to problems of movement control: The role of proprioceptors. *Ann Rev Neurosc* 1988;11:199-223.
3. Yasuda K, Sasaki T: Exercise after anterior cruciate ligament reconstruction: The force exerted on the tibia by the separate isometric contractions of the quadriceps or the hamstrings. *Clin Orthop* 1987;220:275-283.
4. Draganich LF, Vahey JW: An in vitro study of anterior cruciate ligament strain induced by quadriceps and hamstrings forces. *J Orthop Res* 1990;8:57-63.
5. Arms SW, Pope MH, Johnson RJ, et al: The biomechanics of anterior cruciate ligament rehabilitation and reconstruction. *Am J Sports Med* 1984;12:8-18.
6. Renström P, Arms SW, Stanwyck TS, et al: Strain within the anterior cruciate ligament during hamstring and quadriceps activity. *Am J Sports Med* 1986;14:83-87.
7. Grood ES, Suntay WJ, Noyes FR, et al: Biomechanics of the knee-extension exercise: Effect of cutting the anterior cruciate ligament. *J Bone Joint Surg* 1984;66A:725-733.
8. Franklin JL, Rosenberg TD, Paulos LE, et al: Radiographic assessment of instability of the knee due to rupture of the anterior cruciate ligament. *J Bone Joint Surg* 1991;73A:365-372.
9. Iverson BF, Stürup J, Jacobsen K, et al: Implications of muscular defense in testing for the anterior drawer sign in the knee: A stress radiographic investigation. *Am J Sports Med* 1989;17:409-413.
10. Solomonow M, Baratta R, Zhou BH, et al: The synergistic action of the anterior cruciate ligament and thigh muscles in maintaining joint stability. *Am J Sports Med* 1987;15:207-213.

11. Grabiner MD, Campbell KR, Hawthorne DL, et al: Electromyographic study of the anterior cruciate ligament-hamstrings synergy during isometric knee extension. *J Orthop Res* 1989;7:152-155.
12. Pope MH, Johnson RJ, Brown DW, et al: The role of the musculature in injuries to the medial collateral ligament. *J Bone Joint Surg* 1979;61A:398-402.
13. Markolf KL, Graff-Radford A, Amstutz HC: In vivo knee stability: A quantitative assessment using an instrumented clinical testing apparatus. *J Bone Joint Surg* 1978;60A:664-674.
14. Draganich LF, Jaeger RJ, Kralj AR: Coactivation of the hamstrings and quadriceps during extension of the knee. *J Bone Joint Surg* 1989;71A:1075-1081.
15. Baratta R, Solomonow M, Zhou BH, et al: Muscular coactivation: The role of the antagonist musculature in maintaining knee stability. *Am J Sports Med* 1988;16:113-122.
16. Giove TP, Miller SJ III, Kent BE, et al: Non-operative treatment of the torn anterior cruciate ligament. *J Bone Joint Surg* 1983;65A:184-192.
17. Prietto CA, Caiozzo VJ: The in vivo force-velocity relationship of the knee flexors and extensors. *Am J Sports Med* 1989;17:607-611.
18. Grace TG, Sweetser ER, Nelson MA, et al: Isokinetic muscle imbalance and knee-joint injuries: A prospective blind study. *J Bone Joint Surg* 1984;66A:734-740.
19. Noyes FR, Mangine RE, Barber S: Early knee motion after open and arthroscopic anterior cruciate ligament reconstruction. *Am J Sports Med* 1987;15:149-160.
20. LoPresti C, Kirkendall DT, Streete GM, et al: Quadriceps insufficiency following repair of the anterior cruciate ligament. *J Orthop Sports Phys Ther* 1988;9:245-249.
21. Lorentzon R, Elmqvist LG, Sjöström M, et al: Thigh musculature in relation to chronic anterior cruciate ligament tear: Muscle size, morphology, and mechanical output before reconstruction. *Am J Sports Med* 1989;17:423-429.
22. Elmqvist LG, Lorentzon R, Johansson C, et al: Knee extensor muscle function before and after reconstruction of anterior cruciate ligament tear. *Scand J Rehab Med* 1989;21:131-139.
23. Karlya Y, Itoh M, Nakamura T, et al: Magnetic resonance imaging and spectroscopy of thigh muscles in cruciate ligament insufficiency. *Acta Orthop Scand* 1989;60:322-325.
24. Elmqvist LG, Lorentzon R, Langstrom M, et al: Reconstruction of the anterior cruciate ligament: Long-term effects of different knee angles at primary immobilization and different modes of early training. *Am J Sports Med* 1988;16:455-462.
25. Fridén T, Zätterström R, Lindstrand A, et al: Disabilty in anterior cruciate ligament insufficiency: An analysis of 19 untreated patients. *Acta Orthop Scand* 1990;61:131-135.
26. Murray SM, Warren RF, Otis JC, et al: Torque-velocity relationships of the knee extensor and flexor muscles in individuals sustaining injuries of the anterior cruciate ligament. *Am J Sports Med* 1984;12:436-440.
27. Walla DJ, Albright JP, McAuley E, et al: Hamstring control and the unstable anterior cruciate ligament-deficient knee. *Am J Sports Med* 1985;13:34-39.
28. Limbird TJ, Shiavi R, Frazer M, et al: EMG profiles of knee joint musculature during walking: Changes induced by anterior cruciate ligament deficiency. *J Orthop Res* 1988;6:630-638.
29. Branch TP, Hunter R, Donath M: Dynamic EMG analysis of anterior cruciate deficient legs with and without bracing during cutting. *Am J Sports Med* 1989;17:35-41.

30. Shiavi R, Limbird T, Borra H, et al: Electromyography profiles of knee joint musculature during pivoting: Changes induced by anterior cruciate ligament deficiency. *J Electromyograph Kinesiol* 1991;1:49-57.

31. Seto JL, Orofino AS, Morrissey MC, et al: Assessment of quadriceps/ hamstring strength, knee ligament stability, functional and sports activity levels five years after anterior cruciate ligament reconstruction. *Am J Sports Med* 1988;16:170-180.

32. Snyder-Mackler L, Ladin Z, Schepsis AA, et al: Electrical stimulation of the thigh muscles after reconstruction of the anterior cruciate ligament. *J Bone Joint Surg* 1991;73A:1025-1036.

33. Shelbourne KD, Nitz P: Accelerated rehabilitation after anterior cruciate ligament reconstruction. *Am J Sports Med* 1990;18:292-299.

34. Arvidsson I, Eriksson E, Knutsson E, et al: Reduction of pain inhibition on voluntary muscle activation by epidural analgesia. *Orthopedics* 1986;9:1415-1419.

35. Odensten M, Lysholm J, Gillquist J: Long-term follow-up study of a distal iliotibial band transfer (DIT) for anterolateral knee instability. *Clin Orthop* 1983;176:129-135.

Future Directions

Ligament Biology and Healing

In the past decade a number of cellular and mechanical properties of ligaments and ligament healing have been described. In the next decade emphasis should be placed on cells and factors involved in healing and on more sensitive mechanical probes.

Ligament injury and healing can be understood only by understanding the basic molecular biology of ligaments. The embryology and biology of ligaments must be advanced. We need to understand the complex relationship among their cell types, extracellular matrix, and biomechanical properties. The cellular nature of the sheath, the midsubstance, and the insertions require more detailed understanding.

The following specific goals are suggested:

Develop new methods of examining ligament composition, structure, and function.

Fundamental information on structure and function could be simultaneously derived from rigorous comparative studies. Collagen, proteoglycan, elastin, fibronectin, and cytoskeletal interactions and function may be quantifiable in whole-tissue models. The functional role of crimp should be determined. In vitro organ-culture and cell-culture models of ligaments need to be developed to study the fundamental nature of ligament cells and their interactions with their mechanical and chemical environment. Studies of normal ligament composition, structure, and function will establish the standard against which rehabilitation/reconstruction must be measured.

It is important to develop biochemical, biomechanical, and morphologic correlative studies to evaluate how the normal ligament and its insertion sites respond to the mechanical and chemical environment. Similar approaches also should be used to study homeostasis and remodeling after the healing has taken place. The data obtained can be applied to the principles of rehabilitation.

Obtain detailed analyses of the composition, structure, and function of the healing ligament.

These analyses are needed to provide a more rational approach to the clinical management of ligament pathologies. The factors that affect the outcome of the healing process are just beginning to be understood. Experimental studies in which a realistic model is used to investigate the healing process of the ligament structure from insertion site to insertion site will provide important information. For instance, do ligament injuries that include the insertion sites require specific treatments to restore normal blood supply, ligament continuity, and, thus, joint function? Additionally, the effect of drugs, particularly growth factors, and the response of ligaments to other potentially useful extrinsic manipulations must be determined.

Conduct studies to obtain information about in vivo ligament mechanics, kinematics, and forces.

The complex nature of the forces and strains in different parts of ligaments under various static and dynamic loading conditions must be established if we are to understand more about normal ligament function. Similarly, forces and strains in the ligament and the healing (repair) site must be quantified if we are to develop a better understanding of the relationship between tissue-loading and tissue-remodeling. Although we know that ligaments and ligament scars do respond to their stress environment, it is not clear how to optimize these effects from a functional point of view (that is, length and other viscoelastic behaviors).

Learn more about the healing process in ACL reconstruction.

The identity of the cells involved in the healing process is not understood. Because the cellular composition of the ligaments is not understood, the access of reparative cells to injury needs to be investigated. The intrinsic cellular difference between the anterior cruciate ligament and the medial collateral ligament must be understood. Once these cells are identified, the bioactive factors that modify their activities can be determined and explored to optimize clinical outcomes.

Neuromuscular Control of Joint Stability

The forces applied to joints and ligaments during daily activities and especially during athletic activities are more than adequate to rupture ligaments and to create osteochondral injury. Protection of the joint is greatly facilitated by muscles that can control and absorb forces, control or alter articulation patterns, and potentially relieve other joint structures from injurious stresses. Very little is known about the forces produced in muscles about joints and how these forces add or relieve stress on ligaments and joint surfaces. Even less is known about the nervous system control of these muscle forces. Control can be medi-

ated at supraspinal, spinal, and peripheral mechanisms. A better understanding of the interaction of joint forces and neuromuscular control is likely to provide effective strategies for injury prevention and for rehabilitation following surgical and nonsurgical treatment.

The following specific directions are suggested:

Improve understanding of the relationship between muscle forces and stresses on ligaments and joint surfaces.

Information is needed regarding activation levels and forces produced by muscles during normal and athletic activities. These forces can produce or reduce stress in ligaments and joint surfaces, and, therefore, can cause or prevent injury depending on the circumstances. Cadaveric and animal studies should be undertaken to evaluate relationships between muscle and ligament loads and deformations. In vivo biomechanical studies are needed to evaluate muscle activation and coordination and the interaction of joint and muscle forces. Modeling studies also should be helpful.

Investigate nervous system coordination of muscles around joints.

Because muscles can exert forces in excess of those required to injure ligaments, it is necessary to understand how the movement of limbs is controlled and coordinated. The role of afferent sensory mechanisms and central motor programs needs to be better understood. Studies are needed of the coordination of normal limb movements in human subjects and of how the central nervous system and muscles might be coordinated and retrained following injury.

Determine the number and location of neural receptor structures in ligaments and capsules.

Information is needed on what local mechanical states cause sensory neuron activation. Proper understanding of mechanotransduction by neurons would make it possible to use mechanoreceptors as noninvasive probes for local ligament loading.

Section Five

Instability and Force Measurement

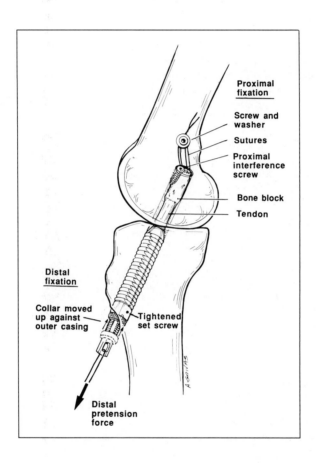

Proximal
fixation

Screw and
washer

Sutures

Proximal
interference
screw

Bone block

Tendon

Distal
fixation

Collar moved
up against
outer casing

Tightened
set screw

Distal
pretension
force

Overview

The force applied to a ligament and its resulting elongation determine the function of the ligament and its ability to resist abnormal displacements without injury. The restraining function of ligaments is exemplified by the complex interaction between the external forces and moments about the knee joint and the anatomic structures that resist these forces. Both static and dynamic anatomic restraints provide knee joint stability, and an interruption in their interaction may lead to ligament rupture or osteocartilaginous injury. Static restraints to external forces are represented mainly by anatomic joint congruity and weightbearing, compressive joint loadings, and the ligamentous structures. Dynamic restraints are by means of muscle forces that act directly through muscle insertions such as the semimembranous and popliteus muscle insertions and also include semimembranous and popliteus muscle insertions into capsular structures.

Analysis of complicated motion patterns and the resultant joint positions describes the highly complex interplay between static and dynamic structures that provide joint stability. Three-dimensional (3-D), computer-simulated knee models permit study and analysis of the relationship between various static and dynamic variables. Direct clinical application of these concepts to anterior cruciate ligament (ACL) replacements helps determine the ideal anatomic insertion regions. Computer-simulated conditions provide clinically relevant data that often cannot be obtained using other methods. Replacements for the ACL were believed to be too weak or not to heal in situations

in which it had been found that the correct anatomic location had not been duplicated, and graft failure resulted from excessive forces and elongations. Early work on posterior cruciate ligament (PCL) attachment sites is currently in progress.

Mathematic models can be applied to a host of clinically relevant problems dealing with restoration of joint stability after ligament injuries. However, model projections and model findings must be validated by experimental data. The inherent weaknesses of models, as well as their strengths, are discussed in this section.

Variables that affect graft tension, remodeling, and ultimately the ability to surgically restore joint stability include the anatomic placement of the ligament graft, its pre-tensioning, the method of internal graft fixation, and the material and structural properties of the particular graft selected.

The actual force levels in ligament grafts and the change in forces as a result of placement and tensioning variables have been inferred because accurate measurement of ligament forces in vivo has not been possible. New, miniature force measurement devices are now available, and investigators are pursuing this research. Data obtained from experimental studies in which the actual forces in the ligaments are measured will affect our entire understanding of ligament function and surgical reconstruction. In this section, data derived from the use of instruments that measure ligament elongation, as opposed to ligament force, are summarized. The studies covered herein provide information on the elongation that the ACL and ligament replacement grafts may undergo under a variety of loading conditions.

One approach the surgeon uses to adjust the tension in the ligament replacement is to control the resting length of the graft by the amount of tension applied on the graft construct. The actual resultant forces in the ligament fibers or fiber bundles can only be approximated. It is, in fact, somewhat unsettling that the actual level of forces in a ligament replacement are unknown, because this level is believed to greatly influence graft remodeling. The ability to more precisely duplicate normal ligament forces within ligament replacements will affect profoundly the replacement's postoperative remodeling and return in strength.

It has been hypothesized that the marked postoperative weakening of ligament replacements is caused partly by inability to reproduce in the graft the forces and the elongations of the collagen fibers found in the original ligament. Moreover, ligament replacements may not achieve normal strength and normal morphology, including collagen fiber diameters, because of the abnormal loading states in those replacements.

Existing clinical studies indicate that a variety of postoperative rehabilitation programs are used, often on an empirical basis, after reconstruction of the ACL, PCL, or other ligament structures. Most surgeons and therapists have adopted immediate postoperative motion programs. However, the types of activities that can be allowed and the timing of these activities after surgery are unknown. For example, when is it safe to allow turning or twisting activities after ACL replacement? What levels of force are caused by specific activities? Which activities are safe and which activities will result in deleterious forces and elongations that stretch out the graft? Research, summarized in part in this section, has been carried out on modifications of traditional postoperative rehabilitation programs and on identification of activities that may unduly load ligament replacements in the early postoperative period.

Clinicians advocating aggressive early return to physical activities after major ligament surgery should be cautious because the true levels of force placed on the ligament graft and articular cartilage are not known. If it were possible to identify those knees in which healing and remodeling events are delayed and the ligament

graft is less than ideal strength, further time and protective measures could be instituted.

The levels of force and the strains on ligaments in vivo depend partly on the restraining function of the other ligament structures about the knee. For example, injury to the medial ligaments results in increased forces on the ACL during valgus knee rotations. In chronic injuries in which medial joint opening is excessive, an ACL replacement would be subjected to higher levels of force than in situations in which the medial ligaments are intact. This is relevant clinically because of the need to recognize when medial or lateral ligament reconstructions must accompany ACL or PCL reconstruction. The clinical data and guidelines in this area are still somewhat controversial.

A reasonable amount of knowledge exists on the interrelationship of primary and secondary ligamentous restraints to specific joint replacements. For example, clinical diagnosis of lateral and posterolateral ligament injuries requires knowledge of the restraining functions of the various individual structures that compose the arcuate ligament complex. In addition, the restraint provided by the PCL at different flexion angles is known. Having the ability to measure more precisely the magnitude of subluxations of the medial and lateral tibial plateaus will allow the clinician to diagnose all ligament injuries in a knee with abnormal rotatory subluxations of the medial and lateral tibiofemoral joints. At present, the ligament-sectioning studies performed in the laboratory provide data on the types of joint subluxations that result from combined ligament injuries. However, the means to measure these subluxations in clinical cases is not well defined.

In summary, this section focuses on the force levels and strains in ligaments: first, in the normal state to examine their interaction; and second, in injury states to determine how one ligament injury affects other ligament structures. In addition, the ways are considered in which the complex interactions among external loading, joint positions, and dynamic muscle forces affect ligament force levels and elongations. The effects of these factors on ligament replacements provide potential strategies for increasing success rates after ligament reconstruction procedures.

Chapter 16

Ligamentous Restraints to Posterior Subluxation of the Lateral Tibial Plateau

J. David Grauer, MD

Introduction

Posterior subluxation of the lateral tibial plateau is one of the least understood abnormal knee motions. It is relatively uncommon and may occur as an isolated entity, but more often occurs simultaneously with anterior cruciate insufficiency, or most frequently with posterior cruciate insufficiency.

The functional impairment resulting from isolated posterior subluxation of the lateral tibial plateau is not well documented. There is no accurate information related to the natural history of these injuries because isolated posterolateral injuries are uncommon, and many may go undiagnosed or are not seen by the physician. Nevertheless, functional impairment secondary to this injury may include giving way of the limb, difficulty ascending or descending stairs or slopes, difficulty with twisting or pivoting, and medial joint line pain.[1,2] When combined with posterior cruciate ligament (PCL) disruption, posterolateral instability is more likely to cause functional impairment.[3-9]

Early analysis of posterior subluxation of the lateral tibial plateau included an attempt to correlate the physical examination with intraoperative findings.[1,2,10-13] The specific pathology included a variety of lesions, including injury to the popliteus tendon, arcuate ligament, fibular collateral ligament, lateral gastrocnemius, and biceps femoris with or without injury to the PCL. More recently, cadaveric ligament sectioning studies have been used to define more accurately the direction and degree of abnormal joint motion produced by injury.[14-20] These studies have improved the ability to diagnose and understand the pathomechanics of posterior subluxation of the lateral tibial plateau. However, the role of surgical intervention (the optimal form of reconstruction for chronic instabilities) and its long-term results remain unstudied.

Anatomy

The anatomy of the posterolateral knee has been accurately described by Kaplan,[21] and more recently by Seebacher and associates.[22] Confusion regarding terminology (short lateral ligament, arcuate ligament versus complex) has existed.[11,21] In addition, the anatomy in this region is much more variable than that of the medial side.[22] Seebacher and associates[22] have divided the posterolateral structures into three layers. Layer I, which is most superficial, is formed by the iliotibial tract anteriorly and the superficial portion of the biceps femoris posteriorly. Layer II is formed anteriorly by the quadriceps retinaculum and posteriorly by the patellofemoral ligaments and their insertions on the terminal fibers of the lateral intermuscular septum proximally, and the fabella or posterolateral capsule and lateral gastrocnemius attachment to the lateral femoral condyle. Layer II also includes the patellomeniscal ligament. Layers I and II adhere to the lateral margin of the patella. The deepest layer, layer III, is the lateral joint capsule, which forms two laminae posteriorly. The superficial lamina encompasses the lateral collateral ligament (LCL), while the deep lamina contains the popliteal hiatus and terminates posteriorly with the fabellofibular and/or arcuate ligament.

The popliteal musculotendinous junction is a very important stabilizing element of the posterolateral corner.[23] The popliteus muscle arises from the posteromedial aspect of the proximal tibia, its tendon coursing proximally and laterally through a hiatus in the coronary ligament posterior to the lateral meniscus. It passes between the lateral femoral condyle and the fibular collateral ligament to insert immediately anterior to the femoral attachment of the fibular collateral ligament. The course of the popliteus tendon is roughly parallel to that of the PCL and it, thus, is placed kinematically to act as a synergist with the PCL to resist posterior tibial displacement.[23] The popliteus tendon also may aid in statically resisting varus and external rotation of the tibia on the femur.[21,24] The dynamic role of the popliteus muscle and tendon is one of tibial internal rotation and prevention of tibial external rotation.[24] The concept of the popliteus muscle and tendon functioning as a dynamic stabilizer and posterior retractor of the posterior horn of the lateral meniscus[23,25,26] has not been supported by a recent study demonstrating an infrequent direct attachment of the popliteus tendon to the posterior horn of the lateral meniscus.[27]

The arcuate ligament is a Y-shaped structure arising from the apex of the fibular styloid process, passing posterior to the popliteal musculotendinous junction.[22] Its vertical limb attaches firmly to the "condylar plate," a condensation of tissues on the posterior femur.[22] The more horizontal limb fans out over the popliteus muscle to insert into the fibers of the oblique popliteal ligament.[22] The arcuate ligament is firmly attached to the underlying popliteal musculotendinous junction, and often reinforces the underlying posterolateral capsule.[22] The arcuate ligament may or may not be present, a factor that seems to depend on the degree of development of the fabella and fabellofibular ligament. In specimens with a large fabella and fabellofibular ligament, the arcuate ligament may be absent.[20]

The fabella is present in approximately 20% of knee specimens.[23] The fabellofibular ligament is a variable structure that attaches along with the arcuate ligament on the fibular styloid process, passing along the posterolateral capsule to the fabella in the lateral head of the gastrocnemius. According to Seebacher and associates,[22] in most specimens the fabellofibular and arcuate ligaments are both present. When the fabella is absent or poorly developed, the fabellofibular ligament is absent and only the arcuate ligament is present.[22] In contrast to the arcuate ligament, the arcuate complex refers to the arcuate, popliteus, and lateral collateral ligaments and the lateral head of the gastrocnemius, as defined by Hughston.[1,24]

The anatomy of the posterolateral knee represents a complex relationship between both static and dynamic structures. These structures are represented in a variable pattern. The popliteal musculotendinous junction can provide dynamic stability by resisting external rotation of the tibia. The posterolateral capsule is statically reinforced by either the fabellofibular or arcuate ligament, or, in 67% of cases, by both ligaments.

Functional Biomechanics

Recent laboratory studies have greatly contributed to the understanding of the pathologic motion present with disruption of the posterolateral structures.[19,20] In vitro laxity studies using the selected ligament sectioning method have helped to define the role of these structures in preventing posterior translation as well as varus and external tibial rotation.[19,20,28]

Gollehon and associates[19] evaluated 17 cadaver knees before and after sequential sectioning of the "deep lateral ligaments" (popliteus and arcuate ligaments), LCL, and PCL. A servocontrolled hydraulic materials testing system machine was used to measure (1) anterior and posterior translation and coupled internal and external tibial rotation with application of a 125-N anterior and posterior force; (2) varus and valgus rotation with application of 15 N·m varus and valgus torque; and (3) internal and external tibial rotation with coupled anterior and posterior translation, coupled varus and valgus rotation, and coupled medial and lateral translation with application of 6 N.m internal and external tibial torque.

Preliminary testing of two specimens showed no difference in tibial translation between isolated division of the popliteus ligament and combined division of the popliteus and arcuate ligaments, so these were divided together as the deep ligament.

Grood and associates[20] evaluated 15 cadaver knees before and after sectioning of the PCL (including meniscofemoral ligaments, if present), posterolateral structures (including the posterolateral capsule, arcuate ligament, popliteus tendon, and fabellofibular ligament), and the LCL. A specially designed apparatus that allowed the limb to hang freely under its own weight was used to measure (1) anterior and posterior translation and coupled internal and external rotation with application of a 100-N anterior and posterior force; (2) varus and valgus rotation with application of a 20-N·m varus and valgus torque; and (3) internal and external tibial rotation and coupled anterior and posterior tibial translation with application of a 5-N·m internal and external tibial torque.

Wascher and associates[28] evaluated five cadaver knees before and after sectioning the LCL and posterolateral structures (including the posterolateral capsule, arcuate ligament, popliteus tendon, and fabellofibular ligament) prior to an in vitro evaluation of the biceps femoris tenodesis procedure. A previously described knee testing apparatus developed by Markolf and associates[29] was used to measure varus and valgus rotation with applied 10-N·m varus and valgus torque and internal and external tibial rotation with applied 10-N·m internal and external tibial torque. The knees were tested in the intact state at 0, 30, 60, and 90 degrees of flexion. The arcuate ligament complex (including the fabellofibular ligament, if present) and the popliteus tendon were sectioned at the level of the joint line and testing was repeated. The LCL was then sectioned at the level of the joint line and testing repeated.

Anterior-Posterior Translation With Anterior-Posterior Force

Gollehon and associates[19] demonstrated that isolated sectioning of the PCL produced posterior tibial translation at all flexion angles, increasing progressively (3 to 13 mm) from 0 to 90 degrees of flexion. Isolated sectioning of either the LCL or the deep ligament failed to produce posterior translation, whereas combined LCL and deep ligament sectioning produced small increases (3 mm) in posterior translation at all flexion angles. Combined sectioning of the PCL, LCL, and deep ligaments produced a marked increase in posterior translation (20 to 25 mm) at all flexion angles. No combination of sectioning of the PCL, LCL, or deep ligaments produced anterior translation with applied anterior force.

Grood and associates[20] reported increased posterior tibial translation (1 to 11 mm) at all flexion angles, increasing progressively from 0 to 90 degrees of flexion, following isolated sectioning of the PCL. Sectioning of any single posterolateral structure did not produce an increase in posterior translation; however, when at least two of the three structures were sectioned, a small increase (1.5 to 3 mm) in posterior translation was seen at 0 to 45 degrees of flexion only. Combined sectioning of the PCL and posterolateral structures produced larger increases in posterior translation (7 to 22 mm) at all flexion angles, with the greatest increase at 90 degrees. No combination of sectioning of the PCL, LCL, or posterolateral structures produced anterior translation with applied anterior force.

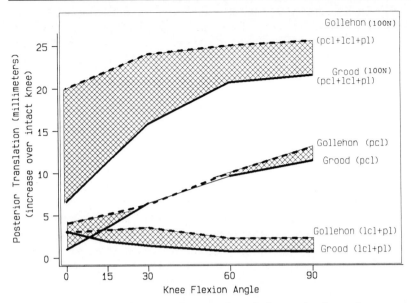

Fig. 1 *Increase in posterior translation with applied posterior force after sectioning of the lateral collateral ligament(LCL), posterolateral structures (PL), and/or posterior cruciate ligament (PCL). Gollehon and associates[19] applied 125 N and measured at 100 N; Grood and associates[20] measured at 100 N.*

The posterior translation that resulted with applied posterior force after sectioning of the PCL and posterolateral structures was similar in these two studies (Fig. 1).[19,20] Although small increases in posterior tibial translation are seen with combined sectioning of the LCL and posterolateral structures, a much more significant increase occurs after sectioning of the PCL.

Varus-Valgus Rotation With Varus-Valgus Torque

Gollehon and associates[19] found no increase in varus or valgus rotation after isolated sectioning of the anterior cruciate ligament or PCL. A small increase (1 to 4 degrees) in varus rotation was noted at all flexion angles after isolated sectioning of the LCL, and only at 90 degrees of knee flexion following isolated sectioning of the deep structures. Progressively greater increases in varus rotation were noted at all flexion angles with combined sectioning of the LCL and deep structures (5 to 9 degrees) and sectioning of the PCL, LCL, and deep structures (14 to 19 degrees). After sectioning of the LCL and deep structures, this increase was greatest at 30 degrees; with sectioning of the PCL, LCL, and deep structures, the increase was greatest at 60 degrees. No increase in valgus rotation was seen after any combination of sectioning.

Grood and associates[20] reported very small increases (less than 1 degree) in varus and valgus rotation following isolated sectioning of the PCL. By comparing the results of isolated sectioning of the posterolateral structures, they found that sectioning of the LCL alone produced significant increases in varus rotation. Isolated sectioning of the LCL produced an increase of 2.5 to 5.7 degrees of varus rotation at all flexion angles, with the greatest increase at 30 degrees. A further increase (8 to 21 degrees) at all flexion angles was seen with added sectioning of the PCL, with the greatest increase at 90 degrees.

Wascher and associates[28] also saw no increase in varus rotation at any flexion angle with isolated sectioning of the posterolateral structures. Sectioning of the LCL and posterolateral structures produced an increase in varus rotation of 4 to 9 degrees at all flexion angles, with the greatest increase at 30 degrees.

These three studies are in agreement regarding the contribution of the PCL, LCL, and posterolateral ligaments to varus rotational stability in the knee (Fig. 2).[19,20,28] Isolated sectioning of the posterolateral structures exclusive of the LCL appears to have no effect as increases in varus rotation occur only after sectioning of the LCL. This increase is seen at all flexion angles, and is greatest at 30 degrees. The posterolateral structures and PCL are important secondary restraints to varus rotation, because further increases in varus are seen following sectioning of these structures.

Internal and External Tibial Rotation With Internal and External Torque

Gollehon and associates[19] reported no increase in internal rotation following any combination of sectioning of the PCL, LCL, or deep structures. Isolated sectioning of the deep structures produced an increase (6 degrees) in external rotation only at 90 degrees of flexion. Isolated sectioning of the LCL caused increased external rotation (2 to 3 degrees) at 0, 30, and 90 degrees of flexion. Combined sectioning of the LCL and deep structures produced larger increases in external rotation (6 to 13 degrees) at all flexion angles, with the greatest increase at 30 degrees. Isolated sectioning of the PCL resulted in no change in external rotation, but when the PCL was sectioned after the LCL and deep structures, further increases in external rotation occurred at 60 and 90 degrees of flexion.

Grood and associates[20] found a slight (2.6 degree) increase in internal rotation following isolated sectioning of the PCL at 90 degrees only. No change in external rotation was noted following isolated sectioning of the PCL. Sectioning only two of the three posterolateral structures produced an increase (3.6 to 6 degrees) of external rotation at all flexion angles, which was greatest at 30 degrees. The specific structures sectioned were not reported, although the trend correlates with the combined LCL and deep structure sectioning results presented by Gollehon and associates.[19] When the PCL and posterolateral structures were sectioned, there was a further increase in external rotation at 30, 60, and 90 degrees, with the great-

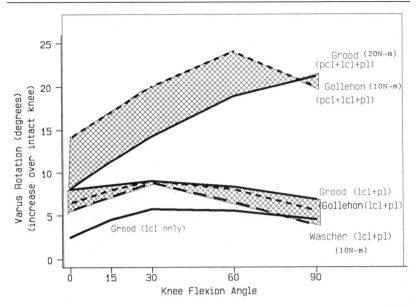

Fig. 2   *Increase in varus rotation with applied varus force after sectioning of the lateral collateral ligament (LCL), posterolateral structures (PL), and/or posterior cruciate ligament (PCL). Gollehon and associates[19] applied 15 N·m and measured at 10 N·m; Grood and associates[20] measured at 20 N·m.*

est increase at 90 degrees. Presumably, no increase in internal rotation was seen, although this was not specifically reported.

Wascher and associates[28] noted small increases (1.5 to 2.5 degrees) in external rotation at 30, 60, and 90 degrees of flexion following isolated sectioning of the posterolateral structures. Combined sectioning of the LCL and posterolateral structures produced greater increases (8 to 14 degrees) in external rotation at all flexion angles; it was greatest at 30 and 60 degrees. Isolated sectioning of the posterolateral structures did not produce an increase in internal rotation. An unexpected finding in this study was the small but significant increases (1.5 to 3.5 degrees) in internal rotation that were seen following combined sectioning of the LCL and posterolateral structures. This was observed at all flexion angles, was greatest at 90 degrees, and was a smaller increase than that observed in external rotation.

These three studies provide similar conclusions regarding the role of the PCL, LCL, and posterolateral ligaments in resisting external rotation of the tibia (Fig. 3).[19,20,28] Together the LCL and the posterolateral structures prevent external rotation of the tibia, particularly from 15 to 60 degrees of flexion. Both Gollehon and associates[19] and Wascher and associates[28] demonstrated small increases in external rotation following posterolateral sectioning exclusive of the LCL. This occurred only at 90 degrees in Gollehon and associates' study,[19] and occurred at 30, 60, and 90 degrees in the study done by

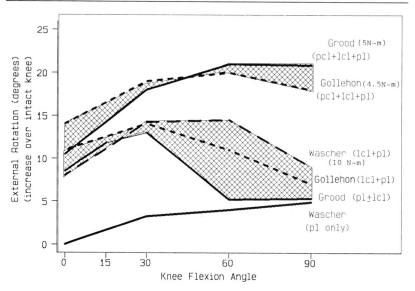

Fig. 3 *Increase in external tibial rotation with applied external torque after sectioning of the lateral collateral ligament (LCL), posterolateral structures (PL), and/or posterior cruciate ligament (PCL). Gollehon and associates[19] applied 6 N·m and measured at 4.5 N·m; Grood and associates[20] measured at 5 N·m; and Wascher and associates[28] measured at 10 N·m.*

Wascher and associates.[28] This may be attributed to the greater torque (10 versus 6 N·m) used in the latter study.

The discrepancy between results of the three studies regarding tibial rotation with applied internal tibial torque following sectioning of the LCL and posterolateral capsule is uncertain. Only Wascher and associates[28] reported a small increase in internal tibial rotation. However, increased internal tibial rotation has been reported by Nielson and associates,[14] who noted small increases from 30 to 130 degrees of knee flexion. The increases in internal rotation are much less than those seen in external rotation; the significance of this is unknown. Thus, it appears that the posterolateral capsule, and arcuate, fabellofibular, and popliteus ligaments exclusive of the LCL do contribute to prevention of external tibial rotation; however, as long as the LCL is intact, this contribution is minor. Once the LCL is sectioned, much larger increases in external rotation laxity occur, particularly at the intermediate flexion angles (15 to 60 degrees). Additional sectioning of the PCL causes a further increase in external rotation, most pronounced at 90 degrees.

Gollehon and associates[19] and Cooper and associates[24] also reported on the effect of ligament sectioning on coupled rotations and translations. The intact knee exhibits obligatory tibial internal rotation with application of an anterior force, and tibial external rotation with application of a posterior force. No combination of sectioning of the LCL, posterolateral structures, and PCL produced an increase in coupled internal rotation with applied anterior force. Isolated sectioning of the PCL eliminated coupled external rotation with posterior force, but did not affect coupled internal rotation with anterior force. Combined sectioning of the LCL and posterolateral structures produced an increase in coupled external rotation with posterior force at all flexion angles; it was greatest (20-degree increase) at 30 degrees. Further sectioning of the PCL failed to produce a significant further increase in coupled external rotation, but it remained greater than in the intact knee. Coupled posterior translation with applied external tibial rotation was also affected by ligament sectioning.[19,24] Combined sectioning of the LCL and posterolateral structures caused a significant increase of coupled posterior translation with applied external tibial torque at all flexion angles. Additional sectioning of the PCL caused a further increase in coupled posterior translation at 60 and 90 degrees. Isolated sectioning of the PCL did not alter coupled posterior translation.

Grood and associates[20] also evaluated coupled motions before and after ligament sectioning. Coupled external tibial rotation with applied posterior force decreased at 30 and 90 degrees after isolated PCL sectioning. A marked increase in coupled external rotation occurred at 30 and 90 degrees (greatest at 30 degrees) after sectioning of all posterolateral structures. This was slightly increased even further at 90 degrees with additional sectioning of the PCL. Coupled posterior translation with applied external tibial torque increased only at 90 degrees after isolated PCL sectioning. Sectioning of all posterolateral structures resulted in an increase in posterior translation at 30 degrees with applied external rotation. Combined PCL, LCL, and posterolateral sectioning caused large increases (8.5 to 11.9 mm) in coupled posterior translation at all flexion angles.

Both Gollehon and associates'[19] and Grood and associates'[20] studies essentially support the same conclusions regarding coupled motion. Sectioning of the posterolateral structures, including the LCL, produces an increase in external rotation coupled with applied posterior force at all flexion angles, which is greatest at 30 degrees. Additional PCL sectioning produces very small, but probably insignificant, further increases in coupled external rotation. Isolated sectioning of the PCL results in a decrease in coupled external rotation, but if the LCL and posterolateral structures are also divided, a larger increase in coupled external rotation occurs than when all structures are intact. Coupled posterior translation with applied tibial external rotation increases after sectioning of the LCL and posterolateral structures and is greatest at 30 degrees. Additional PCL sectioning causes a further increase in coupled posterior translation, particularly at 60 and 90 degrees of flexion.

Clinical Relevance

Knowledge of the individual role of the PCL, LCL, and posterolateral structures in prevention of posterior translation as well as varus and external rotation is necessary during clinical evaluation of a patient with injury to these structures. An injury confined to the posterolateral capsule, arcuate and/or fabellofibular ligaments, and popliteal ligament may produce small increases in external rotation at 30, 60, and 90 degrees, but this is probably not detectable clinically. Additional injury to the LCL will produce larger increases in external rotation that are detectable clinically, particularly at 30 degrees. A large increase in external rotation at 90 degrees also indicates injury to the PCL.

In order to produce a significant increase in varus rotation, the LCL must be injured. Varus rotation will increase even more, particularly at 30 degrees, with additional injury to the posterolateral structures. Isolated PCL injury will produce significant posterior translation, especially at 90 degrees, while additional injury to the LCL and posterolateral structures will produce an even greater increase in posterior translation at all flexion angles, but will nearly equalize the posterior translation present at 30 and 90 degrees.

Thus, in a patient with suspected injury to the LCL, posterolateral structures, and/or PCL, careful attention should be paid to posterior translation at 30 and 90 degrees flexion, to varus rotation at 0 and 30 degrees, and to external tibial rotation at 30 and 90 degrees. An increase in posterior translation that is greater at 90 than 30 degrees suggests an isolated injury to the PCL, while a marked increase in posterior translation, which is nearly equal at 30 and 90 degrees, suggests a combined PCL, LCL, and posterolateral injury. An increase in varus rotation at 30 degrees suggests injury to the LCL, but if varus is also increased at full extension or is markedly increased, an additional injury to the PCL and/or posterolateral structures may be present. Finally, if external tibial rotation is significantly increased and the maximum is 30 degrees, then a combined injury to the LCL and posterolateral structures is likely. If a large increase in external rotation is present at 90 degrees, then additional injury to the PCL should be suspected.

Summary

Although posterolateral knee injuries are uncommon and have been recognized only relatively recently, excellent in vitro data have greatly contributed to better understanding of this problem.[14-20] Before diagnosis and treatment of knee ligament injuries can be successful, a thorough understanding of the anatomy and biomechanics is necessary. Early recognition and diagnosis of this problem should result in improved opportunities for acute repair of injured structures, but the natural history of posterolateral knee injuries is still unclear.

Several methods of surgical treatment have been proposed for chronic posterolateral knee injuries.[2,10-13,24,30,31] However, before definitive recommendations for treatment can be made, extensive study of these procedures and their long-term follow-up results is necessary.

References

1. Hughston JC, Andrews JR, Cross MJ, et al: Classification of knee ligament instabilities: Part II. The lateral compartment. *J Bone Joint Surg* 1976;58A:173-179.

2. Hughston JC, Jacobson KE: Chronic posterolateral rotatory instability of the knee. *J Bone Joint Surg* 1985;67A:351-359.

3. Cain TE, Schwab GH: Performance of an athlete with straight posterior knee instability. *Am J Sports Med* 1981;9:203-208.

4. Cross MJ, Powell JF: Long-term followup of posterior cruciate ligament rupture: A study of 116 cases. *Am J Sports Med* 1984;12:292-297.

5. Dandy DJ, Pusey RJ: The long-term results of unrepaired tears of the posterior cruciate ligament. *J Bone Joint Surg* 1982;64B:92-94.

6. Fowler PJ, Messieh SS: Isolated posterior cruciate ligament injuries in athletes. *Am J Sports Med* 1987;15:553-557.

7. Parolie JM, Bergfeld JA: Long-term results of nonoperative treatment of isolated posterior cruciate ligament injuries in the athlete. *Am J Sports Med* 1986;14:35-38.

8. Satku K, Chew CN, Seow H: Posterior cruciate ligament injuries. *Acta Orthop Scand* 1984;55:26-29.

9. Torg JS, Barton TM, Pavlov H, et al: Natural history of the posterior cruciate ligament-deficient knee. *Clin Orthop* 1989;246:208-216.

10. Hughston JC, Norwood LA Jr: The posterolateral drawer test and external rotational recurvatum test for posterolateral rotatory instability of the knee. *Clin Orthop* 1980;147:82-87.

11. Baker CL Jr, Norwood LA, Hughston JC: Acute posterolateral rotatory instability of the knee. *J Bone Joint Surg* 1983;65A:614-618.

12. Baker CL Jr, Norwood LA, Hughston JC: Acute combined posterior cruciate and posterolateral instability of the knee. *Am J Sports Med* 1984;12:204-208.

13. Fleming RE, Blatz DJ, McCarroll JR: Posterior problems in the knee: Posterior cruciate insufficiency and posterolateral rotatory insufficiency. *Am J Sports Med* 1981;9:107-113.

14. Nielsen S, Rasmussen O, Ovesen J, et al: Rotatory instability of cadaver knees after transection of collateral ligaments and capsule. *Arch Orthop Trauma Surg* 1984;103:165-169.

15. Nielsen S, Ovesen J, Rasmussen O: The posterior cruciate ligament and rotatory knee instability: An experimental study. *Arch Orthop Trauma Surg* 1985;104:53-56.

16. Nielsen S, Helmig P: The static stabilizing function of the popliteal tendon in the knee. *Arch Orthop Trauma Surg* 1986;104:357-362.

17. Markolf KL, Mensch JS, Amstutz HC: Stiffness and laxity of the knee—The contributions of the supporting structures: A quantitative *in vitro* study. *J Bone Joint Surg* 1976;58A:583-594.

18. Jakob RP, Hassler H, Stapubli H-U: Observations on rotatory instability of the lateral compartment of the knee. *Acta Orthop Scand Suppl* 1981;52:1-32.

19. Gollehon DL, Torzilli PA, Warren RF: The role of the posterolateral and cruciate ligaments in the stability of the human knee. *J Bone Joint Surg* 1987;69A:233-242.

20. Grood ES, Stowers SF, Noyes FR: Limits of movement in the human knee: Effect of sectioning the posterior cruciate ligament and posterolateral structures. *J Bone Joint Surg* 1988;70A:88-97.

21. Kaplan EB: Some aspects of functional anatomy of the human knee joint. *Clin Orthop* 1962;23:18-29.

22. Seebacher JR, Inglis AE, Marshall JL, et al: The structure of the posterolateral aspect of the knee. *J Bone Joint Surg* 1982;64A:536-541.

23. Muller W: Kinematics and rotation, in *The Knee: Form, Function, and Ligament Reconstruction*. New York, Springer-Verlag, 1983, pp 39-99.

24. Cooper DE, Warren RF, Warner JJP: The posterior cruciate ligament and posterolateral structures of the knee: Anatomy, function, and patterns of injury, in Tullos HS (ed): American Academy of Orthopaedic Surgeons *Instructional Course Lectures, XL*. Park Ridge, IL, American Academy of Orthopaedic Surgeons, 1991, pp 249-270.

25. Last RJ: Some anatomical details of the knee joint. *J Bone Joint Surg* 1948;30B:683-688.

26. Last RJ: The popliteus muscle and the lateral meniscus: With a note on the attachment of the medial meniscus. *J Bone Joint Surg* 1950;32B: 93-99.

27. Tria AJ Jr, Johnson CD, Zawadsky JP: The popliteus tendon. *J Bone Joint Surg* 1989;71A:714-716.

28. Wascher DC, Grauer JD, Markolf KL: Biceps tendon tenodesis for posterolateral instability of the knee: An in vitro laxity study. Presented at the Combined Congress of the International Arthroscopy Association and the International Society of the Knee, Toronto, Ontario, Canada, May 13-17, 1991.

29. Markolf KL, Gorek JM, Kabo JM: New insights into load bearing functions of the anterior cruciate ligament, in Mow V, Ratcliffe A, Woo SL-Y (eds): *Biomechanics of Diarthrodial Joints*. New York, Springer-Verlag, 1990, vol 1, pp 155-175.

30. DeLee JC, Riley MB, Rockwood CA Jr: Acute posterolateral rotatory instability of the knee. *Am J Sports Med* 1983;11:199-207.

31. Clancy WG Jr: Repair and reconstruction of the posterior cruciate ligament, in Chapman MW (ed): *Operative Orthopaedics*. Philadelphia, JB Lippincott, 1988, vol 3, pp 1651-1665.

Chapter 17

Measurement of Force in the Anterior Cruciate Ligament

Keith L. Markolf, PhD

Introduction

The anterior cruciate ligament (ACL) has long been recognized as a key structure in providing knee stability. Its biomechanical control of tibiofemoral motions has been studied extensively, as evidenced by numerous cruciate sectioning studies available in the literature. Less well understood are the forces developed in the ligament when external loads are applied to normal knees, and to knees with ligamentous deficits.

This chapter summarizes the results of two studies performed at UCLA in which in vitro forces in the ACL were measured in intact knees before and after sectioning of the medial collateral ligaments (MCL).

Prior Studies of ACL Force

The most widely used method for indirect study of ligament forces has been the selected sectioning technique. With this technique, a prescribed displacement (or rotation) is imparted to the knee specimen, a ligament is cut, and the reduction of force (or moment) is taken to reflect the portion of the applied force originally carried by the sectioned structure. With this method, the force in the ligament is not directly measured, but is inferred from the changes in the response curves. Such ligament sectioning studies on unloaded knee specimens are found rather frequently in the literature,[1-4] more recently reported studies have centered on knee specimens with tibiofemoral contact force applied.[5-7]

Buckle transducers have been used to measure forces in selected fiber bundles of the natural ACL,[8-10] and more recently on the entire ACL in conjunction with measurements of forces in autogenous graft substitutes augmented with the ligament augmentation device (LAD) synthetic ligament.[11] The forces recorded reflect only that portion carried by the instrumented fibers; foreshortening and distortion of the instrumented cruciate fibers may introduce artifacts in the reported measurements.

Direct measurements of ligament strain have been reported that used mercury-filled strain gauges that were sutured to selected ligament fibers.[12,13] Fiber strain measurements also have been recorded by attaching miniature Hall effect transducers to the ACL with sharp barbs that penetrate the ligament surface.[14] Unfortunately, these localized measurements of ligament strain have not been correlated directly with total ligament force. A complicating factor common to all of these techniques is that specific bands of the ligament are tensioned at different portions of the loading cycle.

Strain gauges have been applied to the tibial plateau near the ACL insertion site to measure changes in bone strain caused by ligament loading.[15] Again, these measurements cannot be related directly to ligament force; the recorded bone strain is also sensitive to compressive forces applied across the joint. In other attempts to estimate the forces developed in the natural ACL, load transducers have been used to measure the forces in steel cables that have been passed through the anatomic pathway of the excised ACL.[16] Although these cable force measurements may be used to estimate ACL forces, the stiffness of the cable and its anatomic placement within the broad attachment sites of the ACL could present substantial sources of error.

In Vitro ACL Force Studies at UCLA

Studies of forces developed in the cruciate ligaments in vitro have been hampered by the lack of suitable experimental techniques for directly measuring ligament force. A new technique recently developed at UCLA makes direct measurement of total ACL resultant force possible without foreshortening or distorting the ligament's normal anatomy.[17] The technique involves attachment of a specially designed load cell to a mechanically isolated cylinder of cancellous bone containing the tibial attachment of the base of the ACL. The transducer measures the resultant force generated in the ligament as controlled loads are applied to the specimen (Fig. 1). The major advantage of this method is that the ligament fibers are not mechanically altered and remain in their anatomic position. All three components of the resultant force are recorded and the direction of pull can be calculated if desired. A disadvantage of the method is movement of the base plug as cruciate loads are applied; this produces an error in the force measurement that tends to underestimate the true load on the ligament. Another disadvantage is the limited level of cruciate ligament force that can be tolerated before the bone cap pulls off its attachment to the load cell; with poor quality cancellous bone, the interface strength can be relatively low (100 N or less).

This technique has been used to record ACL forces during a series of controlled loading experiments; studies with intact cadaveric

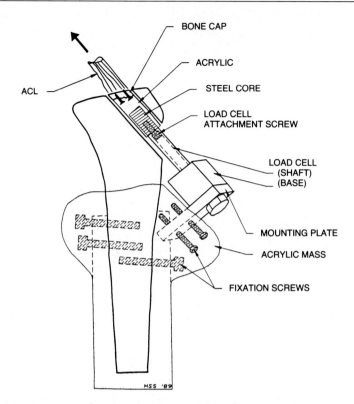

Fig. 1 *Schematic diagram of the load cell-bone plug construct used in these studies. Because the bone plug containing the tibial insertion of the ACL is mechanically isolated from the tibia, all forces generated in the ligament pass directly through the load cell. (Reproduced with permission from Markolf KL, Gorek JF, Kabo JM, et al: Direct measurement of resultant forces in the anterior cruciate ligament: An* in vitro *study performed with a new experimental technique.* J Bone Joint Surg *1990;72A:557-567.)*

specimens[17] and after sectioning of the medial collateral ligament[18] will be summarized here.

The Intact Knee

Rationale for the Loading Tests   Knee hyperextension has been cited as a mechanism for isolated rupture of the ACL;[19] this often occurs when the foot and tibia are fixed and the forward momentum of the upper body produces a forced extension moment at the knee. This loading condition is simulated by fixing the femur, attaching a goniometer linkage, and applying a manual, anteriorly-directed force to the distal tibia, thereby producing an extension moment.

The classic football "clipping" injury involves application of a medially directed force to a planted or fixed lower extremity. This generates a valgus moment that causes medial joint space opening; this mechanism often produces combined ACL-MCL injuries. In bench tests, varus-valgus moment is produced by fixing the femur and applying a measured mediolateral force to the distal tibia at a known distance from the joint line. Knowledge of cruciate forces during this loading condition can provide guidelines for prophylactic knee bracing.

Tibial torque is a recognized loading made for injury to the ACL. In skiing, crossing the tips or catching an edge involves application of tibial torque, frequently to an extended or hyperextended knee. Tibial torque generated by twisting or changing direction while running has also been implicated in ACL injuries. In both instances, the tibia and foot are fixed, and angular momentum of the upper body transmits a torque to the knee joint. With the torsional bench test, the femur is fixed and a manual torque is applied to the distal tibia through an instrumented torque cell.

In addition to providing better understanding of knee injury mechanisms, the bench tests also provide information important for patient care. Passive manual knee extension is routinely performed during physical examinations and rehabilitation. Active quadriceps extension against a fixed resistance is a common rehabilitation exercise to restore muscle strength. This loading condition is simulated by applying a constant quadriceps tendon force through a pulley system while allowing the knee to extend against manual resistance. Knowledge of cruciate forces produced during these loading experiments is important for determining range of motion and extension exercises to be allowed after cruciate reconstruction procedures.

Summary of ACL Force Magnitudes in Intact Knees   Passive extension of the knee generated ligament force only during the last 10 degrees of extension; the ligament force at 5 degrees of hyperextension ranged from 50 N to 240 N (mean 118 N). When a 200-N quadriceps tendon pull was applied to a knee extending slowly against tibial resistance, the ACL force increased at all knee flexion angles (Fig. 2).

Internal tibial torque always generated greater ligament force than external tibial torque; higher ligament forces were recorded as the knee was extended (Fig. 3). The greatest ligament forces in this study (133 N to 370 N) were generated when 10 N·m of internal tibial torque was applied to a hyperextended knee.

Ligament forces generated by 15 N·m of applied varus moment ranged from 94 N to 177 N at full extension; 15 N·m of applied valgus moment generated a mean ligament force of 56 N, which remained unchanged with knee flexion (Fig. 4). The force in the ACL during straight anterior tibial translation was approximately equal to the applied anterior tibial force.

Clinical Implications   The high ligament forces recorded beyond full extension suggest that hyperextension can contribute to ACL rupture. The absence of ligament force beyond 10 degrees of flexion suggests that passive range of motion beyond this point would be

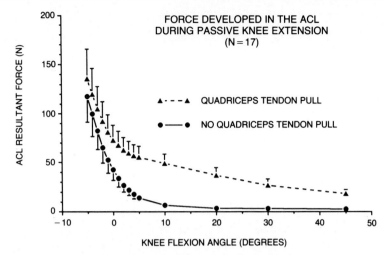

Fig. 2   *Mean force generated in the ACL during passive knee extension without and with 200 N quadriceps tendon pull. Error bars indicate the 95% confidence interval for the mean. (Reproduced with permission from Markolf KL, Gorek JF, Kabo JM, et al: Direct measurement of resultant forces in the anterior cruciate ligament: An* in vitro *study performed with a new experimental technique.* J Bone Joint Surg *1990;72A:557-567.)*

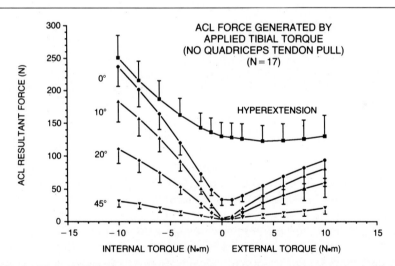

Fig. 3   *Mean ACL force generated by application of internal and external tibial torque. Error bars indicate the 95% confidence interval for the mean. The curve labeled hyperextension represents specimens sustaining a 10 N·m extension moment. (Reproduced with permission from Markolf KL, Gorek JF, Kabo JM, et al: Direct measurement of resultant forces in the anterior cruciate ligament: An* in vitro *study performed with a new experimental technique.* J Bone Joint Surg *1990;72A:557-567.)*

safe for a knee undergoing rehabilitation following ligament injury or reconstruction. The increases in ligament force observed during application of quadriceps tendon pull would suggest that active quadriceps extension against resistance in the flexion range of 0 to

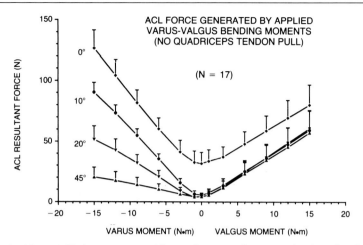

Fig. 4 *Mean ACL force generated by application of varus and valgus bending moment. Error bars indicate the 95% confidence interval for the mean. (Reproduced with permission from Markolf KL, Gorek JF, Kabo JM, et al: Direct measurement of resultant forces in the anterior cruciate ligament: An in vitro study performed with a new experimental technique. J Bone Joint Surg 1990;72A:557-567.)*

45 degrees would not be advisable if one desired to limit forces in the ACL or a ligament substitute.

The change in ligament force caused by an applied valgus moment was surprisingly constant, ranging from 0 to 45 degrees of knee flexion. This implies that the restraining moments generated by other medial structures (primarily the MCL) were also constant over this flexion range. In contrast, the ligament force generated from an applied varus moment decreased with increasing knee flexion, indicating possible recruitment of additional lateral structures. Thus, for applied varus moment, the ACL is markedly more susceptible to high ligament forces when the knee is extended, an observation that is consistent with a type of ACL injury that involves cutting inside and away from a planted foot, with the knee near extension.

The patterns of ligament force generation from tibial torsion also aids in understanding commonly observed ACL injury mechanisms. The ligament force generated by both internal and external tibial torque decreases as the knee is flexed from 0 to 45 degrees, indicating that a flexed knee may be less vulnerable to ACL injury from twisting. Hypertension of an externally rotated tibia markedly increases ACL force. This is consistent with a mechanism for ACL rupture during skiing, whereby a skier catches a tip and applies high external tibial torque to a hyperextended knee (often with associated valgus stress). Near extension, the ligament force generated by internal torque is more than double that generated by external torque. Internal tibial torque near extension can be produced when a skier crosses the tips and the upper body is thrust forward over an extended knee.

If a surgically implanted ligament substitute is overtensioned at 20 or 30 degrees of knee flexion, forcing the knee to full extension can generate high forces in the graft and possibly compromise graft fixation in the tunnel holes. If a goal of rehabilitation is to limit graft forces in the early recuperative period, passive and active motion to full extension should be avoided. Selection of an appropriate brace should be considered for control of tibial torsion and varus-valgus angulation near extension.

The MCL-Deficient Knee

The MCL is the most frequently injured knee ligament; injuries are common at all levels of sports activity.[19] The vast majority of athletes with isolated injury of the MCL return to their previous level of sports participation, yet most have some element of residual abnormal medial joint opening regardless of the type of treatment.[20-23] Experiments using animal models also support this finding. In two separate reports, Woo and associates[24,25] noted that surgically transected MCLs healed with some element of residual valgus laxity in both dogs and rabbits.

Injuries to the ACL are frequently associated with MCL sprains. In a study of 265 patients with injury to the MCL, 20% of patients with grade I MCL injuries also ruptured the ACL; this incidence rises to 53% with grade II injuries, and to 78% with grade III injuries.[19] These associations suggest that load sharing occurs between these two important structures, particularly during injury situations.

The functions of the ACL and MCL in limiting knee motions have been documented in prior ligament sectioning studies.[2,4,7,20,26] In vitro measurements of forces in these ligaments using buckle transducers have identified tibial torque and varus-valgus moment as knee loading states that load these structures.[7,20,27] However, no studies have documented the effects of MCL sectioning on force generated in the ACL.

Summary of ACL Force Magnitudes in MCL Deficient Knees

Sectioning of the MCL did not change the ACL force generated by applied varus moment. When valgus moment was applied to the knees, ligament force increased dramatically after MCL sectioning; the increases were greatest at 45 degrees of flexion (Fig. 5).

Sectioning of the MCL had variable effects on ACL force during internal rotation, but dramatically increased force in the ACL during external rotation; these increases were greatest at 45 degrees (Fig. 6). Sectioning of the MCL increased mean total internal-external tibial rotation produced by 10 N·m of tibial torque; increases averaged 12.6 degrees (0 degrees of flexion) to 19.6 degrees (20 degrees of flexion).

Application of anterior tibial force to an intact knee increased ACL force; this force increase was maximum near the midrange of tibial rotation, and minimum with external tibial rotation. Section-

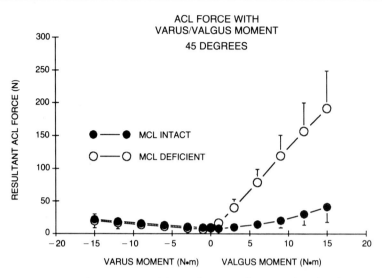

Fig. 5 *Mean ACL force generated by application of varus-valgus bending moment before and after sectioning of the MCL at 45 degrees of knee flexion. Error bars indicate the 95% confidence interval for the mean. (Reproduced with permission from Shapiro MS, Markolf KL, Finerman GAM, et al: The effect of section of the medial collateral ligament on force generated in the anterior cruciate ligament. J Bone Joint Surg 1991;73A:248-256.)*

ing of the MCL did not change the ACL force generated by straight anterior tibial pull near the midrange of tibial rotation. With the tibia in an externally rotated position, ACL force increased after MCL sectioning; the force increases were greater for flexed knee positions (Fig. 7).

Clinical Implications   In the intact knee, ACL force generated by applied external torque progressively diminishes as the knee is flexed.[12] In an MCL-deficient knee, this pattern is reversed; ACL force is markedly greater, and increases as the knee is flexed. This indicates that the MCL is more active in resisting external torque as the knee is progressively flexed. This conclusion is further substantiated by the observation that increases in torsional laxity after sectioning of the MCL are greater for flexed knees.

Similar observations during varus-valgus testing have led to the conclusion that the MCL is more active in resisting a valgus moment as knee flexion increases. The loss of restraining force caused by sectioning of the MCL is compensated for by increased tension developed in the ACL and perhaps other structures such as the posterior capsule.

Results of tibial torque tests performed with superimposed anterior tibial force further illustrate concepts of load sharing between the ACL and MCL. In neutral rotation, the ACL carries virtually all the applied anterior tibial force. When the tibia of an intact knee is externally rotated and anterior tibial force is applied, the MCL

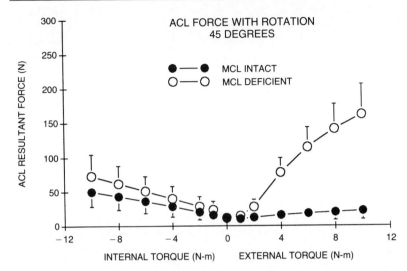

Fig. 6   *Mean ACL force generated by application of internal-external tibial torque before and after sectioning of the MCL at 45 degrees of knee flexion. Error bars indicate the 95% confidence interval for the mean. (Reproduced with permission from Shapiro MS, Markolf KL, Finerman GAM, et al: The effect of section of the medial collateral ligament on force generated in the anterior cruciate ligament.* J Bone Joint Surg *1991;73A:248-256.)*

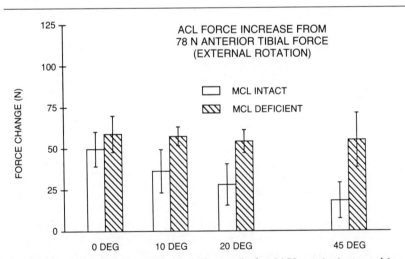

Fig. 7   *Mean increase in ACL force (before and after MCL sectioning) resulting from application of 78 N anterior tibial force to a tibia externally rotated by 10 N·m of external tibial torque. Error bars indicate the 95% confidence interval for the mean. (Reproduced with permission from Shapiro MS, Markolf KL, Finerman GAM, et al: The effect of section of the medial collateral ligament on force generated in the anterior cruciate ligament.* J Bone Joint Surg *1991;73A:248-256.)*

is strained, thereby reducing the force generated in the ACL. When the MCL is sectioned and the knee is locked into a new externally rotated position, the ACL force generated by the same anterior tibial force increases markedly. This indicates that the MCL had been actively resisting the applied force prior to its being sectioned. As noted in the varus-valgus and torsional tests, this ability of the MCL to resist applied anterior tibial force is greater as the knee is flexed.

Valgus moment and external torque are loading modes that could be responsible for combined injuries to the ACL and MCL. The MCL is a primary restraint to these loading states, and thereby effectively shields the ACL from load. Once the MCL has ruptured, the ACL will experience a sudden increase in tension, possibly at a level that can cause rupture. An MCL-deficient knee will experience the greatest ACL force from these loading modes when it is flexed.

The magnitudes of the force increases after MCL sectioning were quite striking. These increases are interesting because many athletes with residual abnormal medial joint opening from a prior MCL injury continue to participate in sports. As noted previously,[19] even athletes with third-degree MCL injuries typically return to play after a period of recuperation, but it is probable that abnormal medial joint opening always remains to some extent. It might be expected that for the loading conditions tested in this study, increased medial joint opening would result in an increase in ACL force. Athletes with residual medial joint opening might therefore be at high risk for subsequent ACL injury. Although this clinical finding has not been reported, studies I have performed offer an additional rationale for the common practice of protecting MCL-insufficient knees with mediolateral knee braces. The brace may act not only to protect the MCL, but also to limit forces in the ACL.

Clinical experience has shown that patients with combined injuries to the ACL and MCL do quite poorly with nonoperative treatment.[19] When the ACL is intact, nonoperative treatment with controlled early motion frequently results in functional regeneration of the MCL, although in a slightly lengthened condition.[22,25] The present study indicates that the ACL is significantly loaded when the MCL is nonfunctional. Perhaps as suggested by Inoue and associates,[28] the ACL generates sufficient restraining force to prevent medial joint opening at low levels of activity, thereby facilitating MCL healing.

Finally, it should be noted that ACL reconstruction is frequently performed on knees that have concurrent MCL injury, or residual medial joint opening from an old injury with stretched-out secondary restraints. My belief is that high graft tensions would be generated in such knees during the healing period if the knee is unprotected. Limitation of medial joint opening might be a justification for the use of a knee brace in such patients.

Summary

The absence of ligament force beyond 10 degrees of flexion suggests that passive flexion-extension motions ranging from 10 degrees to full flexion would be safe for a knee undergoing rehabilitation after repair or reconstruction of the ACL. The increases in ACL force caused by quadriceps tendon pull indicate that active quadriceps extension against resistance in the flexion range of 0 to 45 degrees would not be advisable if one desired to limit forces in the ACL or a ligament substitute. For applied varus moment, the ACL is markedly more susceptible to elevated ligament forces when the knee is near full extension. My data indicate that a flexed knee should be less vulnerable to ACL injury from applied tibial torque. Joint load acts to protect the knee from high ACL forces generated by applied straight anterior tibial force; no such protective mechanism was demonstrated for applied internal or external tibial torque.

The MCL normally acts to resist external torque, valgus moment, and anterior tibial force (when the tibia is externally rotated). In doing so, it effectively helps prevent the ACL from experiencing high forces; this protection is greatest when the knee is flexed. In an MCL-deficient knee, increased force is borne by the ACL, especially when the knee is flexed. My data suggest that an individual with residual valgus laxity as a result of a previous injury to the MCL may be at increased risk for potentially injurious ACL forces generated by these loading modes.

References

1. Butler DL, Noyes FR, Grood ES: Ligamentous restraints to anterior-posterior drawer in the human knee: A biomechanical study. *J Bone Joint Surg* 1980;62A:259-270.

2. Grood ES, Noyes FR, Butler DL, et al: Passive restraints in the human knee: Varus-valgus rotations. *Trans Orthop Res Soc* 1978;3:22.

3. Piziali RL, Seering WP, Nagel DA, et al: The function of the primary ligaments of the knee in anterior-posterior and medial-lateral motions. *J Biomech* 1980;13:777-784.

4. Seering WP, Piziali RL, Nagel DA, et al: The function of the primary ligaments of the knee in varus-valgus and axial rotation. *J Biomech* 1980;13:785-794.

5. Fukubayashi T, Torzilli PA, Sherman MF, et al: An *in vitro* biomechanical evaluation of anterior-posterior motion of the knee: Tibial displacement, rotation, and torque. *J Bone Joint Surg* 1982;64A:258-264.

6. Markolf KL, Bargar WL, Shoemaker SC, et al: The role of joint load in knee stability. *J Bone Joint Surg* 1981;63A:570-585.

7. Shoemaker SC, Markolf KL: Effects of joint load on the stiffness and laxity of ligament-deficient knees: An *in vitro* study of the anterior cruciate and medial collateral ligaments. *J Bone Joint Surg* 1985;67A:136-146.

8. Ahmed AM, Burke DL, Hyder A: Effect of tibial prerotation on the ligamentous response of the flexed knee to passive anterior shear. *Trans Orthop Res Soc* 1986;11:127.

9. Barry D, Ahmed AM: Design and performance of a modified buckle transducer for the measurement of ligament tension. *J Biomech Eng* 1986;108:149-152.

10. Lewis JL, Lew WD, Schmidt J: A note on the application and evaluation of the buckle transducer for the knee ligament force measurement. *J Biomech Eng* 1982;104:125-128.

11. Lew WD, Engebretsen L, Lewis JL, et al: Method for setting total graft force and load sharing in augmented ACL grafts. *J Orthop Res* 1990;8:702-711.

12. Edwards RG, Lafferty JF, Lange KO: Ligament strain in the human knee. *J Basic Eng* 1980;92:131-136.

13. Kennedy JC, Hawkins RJ, Willis RB: Strain gauge analysis of knee ligaments. *Clin Orthop* 1977;129:225-229.

14. Arms SW, Pope MH, Johnson RJ, et al: The biomechanics of anterior cruciate ligament rehabilitation and reconstruction. *Am J Sports Med* 1984;12:8-18.

15. France EP, Daniels AU, Goble EM, et al: Simultaneous quantitation of knee ligament forces. *J Biomech* 1983;16:553-564.

16. Grood ES, Hefzy DL, Butler DL, et al: On the placement and the initial tension of anterior cruciate ligament substitutes. *Trans Orthop Res Soc* 1983;8:92.

17. Markolf KL, Gorek JF, Kabo JM, et al: Direct measurement of resultant forces in the anterior cruciate ligament: An *in vitro* study performed with a new experimental technique. *J Bone Joint Surg* 1990;72A:557-567.

18. Shapiro MS, Markolf KL, Finerman GAM, et al: The effect of section of the medial collateral ligament on force generated in the anterior cruciate ligament. *J Bone Joint Surg* 1991;73A:248-256.

19. Fetto JF, Marshall JL: Medial collateral ligament injuries of the knee: A rationale for treatment. *Clin Orthop* 1978;132:206-218.

20. Derscheid GL, Garrick JG: Medial collateral ligament injuries in football: Nonoperative management of grade I and grade II sprains. *Am J Sports Med* 1981;9:365-368.

21. Holden DL, Eggert AW, Butler JE: The nonoperative treatment of Grade I and II medial collateral ligament injuries to the knee. *Am J Sports Med* 1983;11:340-344.

22. Indelicato PA: Non-operative treatment of complete tears of the medial collateral ligament of the knee. *J Bone Joint Surg* 1983;65A:323-329.

23. Kannus P: Long-term results of conservatively treated medial collateral ligament injuries of the knee joint. *Clin Orthop* 1988;226:103-112.

24. Frank C, Woo SL, Amiel D, et al: Medial collateral ligament healing: A multidisciplinary assessment in rabbits. *Am J Sports Med* 1983;11:379-389.

25. Woo SL, Inoue M, McGurk-Burleson E, et al: Treatment of the medial collateral ligament injury: II. Structure and function of canine knees in response to differing treatment regimens. *Am J Sports Med* 1987;15:22-29.

26. Markolf KL, Mensch JS, Amstutz HC: Stiffness and laxity of the knee: The contributions of the supporting structures: A quantitative *in vitro* study. *J Bone Joint Surg* 1976;58A:583-594.

27. Ahmed AM, Hyder A, Burke DL, et al: In-vitro ligament tension pattern in the flexed knee in passive loading. *Orthop Res* 1987;5:217-230.

28. Inoue M, McGurk-Burleson E, Hollis JM, et al: Treatment of the medial collateral ligament injury: I. The importance of anterior cruciate ligament on the varus-valgus knee laxity. *Am J Sports Med* 1987;15:15-21.

Chapter 18

Measurement of Force in Cruciate Ligament Reconstructions

Jack L. Lewis, PhD
William D. Lew, MS

Introduction

Appropriate force levels in graft tissues used to reconstruct the cruciate ligaments of the knee are thought to be important for long-term success of the reconstruction. Several investigators have reported that during the early phase of tissue remodeling and revascularization there is a decrease in the strength and stiffness of grafts used to reconstruct the anterior cruciate ligament (ACL).[1-3] After this initial decline, the mechanical properties of the graft tissues were found to increase gradually without reaching normal levels. This early graft weakening probably occurs because the graft has not yet been adequately incorporated into the joint, as well as because there is degradation of the graft tissue as it remodels and revascularizes. This decrease in graft strength often results in protection of reconstructions during the initial postoperative period, to avoid subjecting the graft tissue to high loads.[4] However, more aggressive rehabilitation, with an increased likelihood that high graft loads will occur, has been advocated recently to prevent loss of joint motion and muscle strength.[5] The benefits of mobilization and the deleterious effects of immobilization on the mechanical properties of normal and repaired ligaments have been investigated.[6,7]

Forces, or loads, that are too high or too low can be damaging to the successful remodeling of a graft. Surgical reconstruction and rehabilitation procedures are tailored to avoid these extremes, thereby implying that certain midrange levels of graft force may be beneficial, with some load levels possibly better than others. This implication leads to the following questions: Is there an optimal load history for a particular graft-fixation system that will enhance the graft's remodeling into a normal functioning ligament? Is the decline in a graft's mechanical properties a result of not knowing this optimal load history? Is there an optimal load range that will satisfy the need for graft protection, yet allow aggressive rehabilitation to regain motion and strength? Answering these questions requires understanding the factors that determine graft forces.

The purpose of this chapter is (1) to identify and examine factors thought to influence graft forces, particularly mechanical surgical factors; (2) to review current and proposed methods or mechanical conditions under which grafts are installed and summarize the in vitro graft forces resulting from these methods; and (3) to describe ongoing research into measurement of in vivo graft forces. These measurements are the initial steps in establishing an optimal load history for graft remodeling, and for developing methods for achieving these forces in humans.

Factors That Affect Graft Force

This discussion will emphasize the ACL, because its reconstruction has been the subject of a great deal of research effort, and has been the focus of the authors' work.

Interaction With Other Joint Structures

When a load is applied to the knee, from muscle activity and/or from external forces, the stabilizing joint load will be shared by the ACL and the other passive joint structures. This is demonstrated symbolically by the spring model in Figure 1. ACL or graft forces will depend not only on their own mechanical state, but also on the mechanical state of the other passive joint structures. It is the nature of the ACL or graft to share load.

External Joint Loads

A second important point is that forces generated in the ACL or graft will depend on the loads applied to the knee. Several investigators have documented the load states that create forces in the intact ACL.[8-10] The results of these studies indicate that the ACL is loaded primarily near extension, during anterior tibial load, varus moment (more than valgus), internal tibial rotation (more than external rotation), and hyperextension. No significant forces occur in the ACL during passive flexion-extension. Forces in the normal ACL will be discussed in more detail in another chapter. Joint loads that generate forces in the intact ACL will not necessarily load a graft in an identical manner; however, the general principle remains the same. The forces in the ACL or the graft will depend on the joint loads applied.

We can use the above two points as a basis for identification and examination of factors believed to affect forces in a graft used to reconstruct the ACL. The mechanical surgical variables that influence graft force will be considered, then factors that cause graft creep after fixation will be examined.

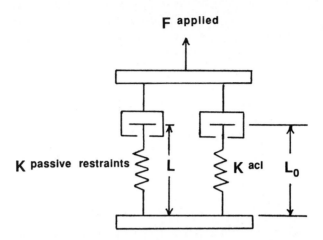

Fig. 1 *Spring model representing the interaction between the ACL or graft (with stiffness, K^{ACL}, and maximum unloaded length, L_0) and the remaining passive restraints (soft tissue and articular contact), as they stabilize an applied load to the knee, $F_{APPLIED}$, from an external force and/or muscular activity.*

Mechanical Surgical Variables

Mechanical surgical variables are those variables that are under the influence, if not control, of the surgeon at the time of surgery. Mechanical surgical variables identified at this time include the graft tunnel or fixation location, maximum unloaded graft length, pre-tension magnitude, pre-tension direction, flexion angle at which the pre-tension is applied, presence of an extra-articular procedure, augmentation of a biologic graft, and distribution of graft segment attachment sites in a composite graft. The two most important variables appear to be graft tunnel or fixation location and the maximum unloaded graft length, L_0, which is the distance between the origin and insertion of the graft when it just begins to carry load. Although L_0 is an independent variable, it can be influenced by pre-tension magnitude and direction, and the flexion angle at which the pre-tension is applied. After fixing the graft to one side of the joint, pre-tension is defined as the load applied to a graft while attaching it to the other side.

Graft Pre-tension   Early use of pre-tension was empirical; pre-tension was applied to restore normal anteroposterior laxity to the joint, although specific levels of pre-tension required to achieve this condition were not specified.[11,12] Some have advocated applying pre-tension to a graft with the joint near 30 degrees of flexion; others have advocated applying pre-tension at extension.[13-15] Various magnitudes of graft pre-tension have been suggested.[16,17] Although the patellar tendon has become the most frequently used graft tissue, other tissues such as the semitendinosus and gracilis tendons are also used,[18,19] resulting in the need to apply pre-tension from either the proximal or the distal directions. Bylski-Austrow and associates[13] reported an in vitro study in which they simulated an ACL graft with an instrumented, flexible wire cable that approximated the stiffness of the normal ACL, and studied the effect of pre-tension magnitude and flexion angle on graft force with the joint under load. Pre-tension magnitude had a small effect on graft force; however, the flexion angle at which the pre-tension was applied was found to be more important, with pre-tension applied at 30 degrees of flexion producing greater forces than that applied at extension.

In an in vitro study, the authors determined the effect on ACL graft force and knee motion, of the direction of the pre-tension application (distal, distal with posterotibial force, proximal), the magnitude of the pre-tension force (5 lbs, 15 lbs), and the flexion angle at which the pre-tension was applied (extension, 30 degrees of flexion).[20] Ten fresh cadaveric knees were tested using an experiment setup that included buckle transducers for the measurement of ACL and graft forces and an instrumented spatial linkage for the measurement of three-dimensional knee motion, as 100-N anterotibial loads were applied with a pneumatic load apparatus at 0, 30, 60, and 90 degrees of flexion. Measurements were also made during an unloaded state before the anterior load was applied at each flexion angle. After measuring ACL force and motion data in a knee that had an intact ACL, the ACL was resected and a 10 mm bone-patellar tendon-bone graft was harvested from that knee. Fixation tunnels were drilled through the anteromedial ACL tibial attachment and the posterosuperior portion of the ACL femoral attachment. Distal fixation of the graft was achieved using a cylindrical fixture consisting of a threaded outer casing that lined an enlarged distal fixation hole, and an inner cylinder that freely moved with the outer casing, and within which the distal bone block was fixed with bone cement (Fig. 2).

The graft was initially secured proximally using increasing sizes of interference screws. With the graft fixed proximally, distal fixation was achieved by adjusting a moveable collar on the threaded outer surface of the inner cylinder, up against the end of the outer casing, while eight possible combinations of 5 and 15 lbs of distal pre-tension were applied through the inner cylinder with a spring scale, at extension and 30 degrees of flexion, with and without addition of a manual posterotibial force (Fig. 3). After each pre-tension setting, graft forces and joint motion were recorded under the anterior loads at the test flexion angles. The graft was then fixed distally in the cylindrical fixture, and the test procedure was repeated under the four magnitude (5 and 15 lbs) and flexion angle (0 and 30 degrees) combinations for proximal pre-tension. A factorial analysis was used to determine the significance of the effect of the pre-tension variables on the force and motion data, with an alpha level of 0.05 considered significant.

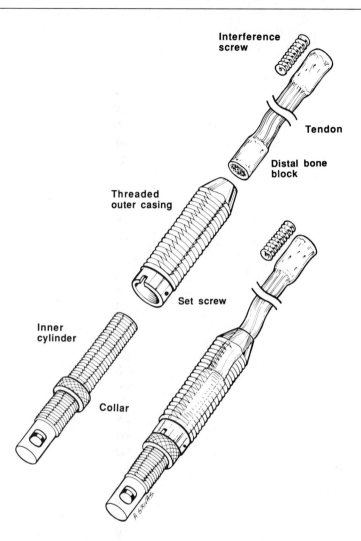

Fig. 2 *Cylindrical fixture for distal fixation. The distal bone block was fixed with bone cement within the inner cylinder, which had a threaded outer surface to allow movement of a collar. The threaded outer casing was inserted through an enlarged tibial fixation hole. With the inner graft cylinder capable of sliding freely within the outer casing, distal fixation was achieved by advancing the collar on the inner cylinder up against the end of the outer casing, and tightening a set screw.*

The factorial analysis indicated that the graft force was affected significantly by the flexion angle at which the pre-tension was applied and by the direction of application of the pre-tension force, but not by the pre-tension magnitude. Figure 4 presents the means of the forces in the intact ACL and graft, with the joint under anterior load, when the three pre-tension directions (distal, distal with postero-tibial force, proximal) were applied at extension and at 30 degrees of

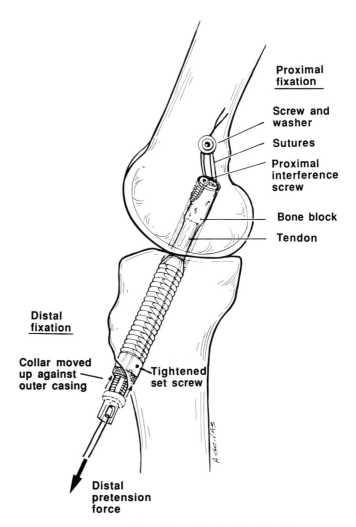

Fig. 3 *Distal pre-tension test. The graft was fixed with an interference screw proximally, and was reinforced by tying sutures through the bone block to a screw and washer. Distal pre-tension was applied with the weight of the distal lower limb simulated and the limb supported as it would be in surgery, and distal fixation was achieved by rotating the collar of the inner cylinder up against the end of the outer casing.*

flexion. Because pre-tension magnitude was not a significant variable, results for 5 and 15 lbs of pre-tension graft force were averaged for each pre-tension direction-flexion angle combination. Proximal pre-tension resulted in the largest graft forces with the knee under anterotibial load at extension, followed by distal pre-tension with posterotibial force, and then distal pre-tension alone. As the anterior loads were applied from 30 to 90 degrees of flexion, however, the graft forces with proximal pre-tension became lower than with

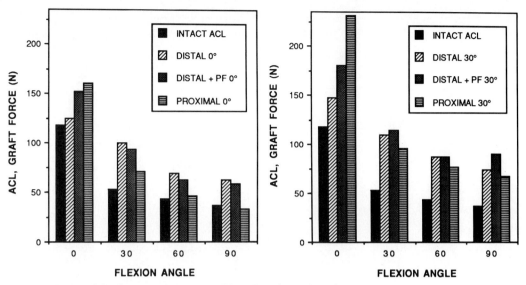

Fig. 4 *Means of the forces in the intact ACL and graft resulting from the anterotibial loads at the four test flexion angles, when the three pre-tension directions (distal, distal with posterotibial force (PF), proximal) were applied at extension (**left**) and at 30 degrees of flexion (**right**).*

distal pre-tension with and without posterior force. The graft forces with distal pre-tension were the most isotonic over the flexion range, while the graft forces with proximal pre-tension were the least isotonic. The graft forces were greater when the pre-tension was applied at 30 degrees of flexion than at extension, and this difference was greatest for proximal and least for distal pre-tension (Fig. 4). Figure 4 also demonstrates that graft forces for all combinations of pre-tension variables were always greater in the intact ACL. Substantial forces also occurred in the graft during the unloaded states.

When the graft was fixed under any of the pre-tension directions at either extension or 30 degrees of flexion, the joint was overcorrected; that is, the tibia in the unloaded state was positioned posteriorly and rotated externally, compared with its configuration in the normal knee with an intact ACL (Fig. 5). This abnormal configuration was more pronounced for distal pre-tension with and without posterior force than for proximal pre-tension. When the anterotibial loads were applied, the joints displaced anteriorly, but were still in a configuration posterior to the normal anterior-loaded joint.

This study demonstrates that the flexion angle at which pre-tension is applied influences graft force, but the pre-tension magnitude has little effect, which is in agreement with Bylski-Austrow and associates.[13] Our results also showed that the direction in which a given level of pre-tension is applied affects graft force.

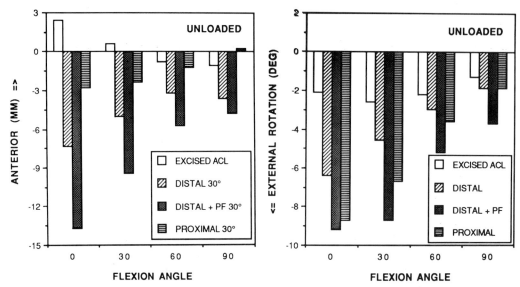

Fig. 5   *Left, Means of the anteroposterior joint configurations during the unloaded state at the four text flexion angles for the excised ACL state, and for the three pre-tension directions (distal, distal with posterotibial force (PF), proximal) applied at 30 degrees of flexion. Because factorial analysis indicated that pre-tension magnitude was not a significant variable affecting anteroposterior displacement, the 5- and 15-lb displacement results were averaged for each pre-tension direction-flexion angle combination. The joint configuration (tibial position relative to the fixed femur) in all test states was defined relative to the tibial position in the normal unloaded knee with an intact ACL. Right, Means of the transverse rotational (internal-external) joint configurations during the unloaded state at the four test flexion angles for the excised ACL state, and for the three pre-tension directions (distal, distal with posterotibial force (PF), proximal). Because the factorial analysis indicated that pre-tension magnitude and flexion angle were not significant variables affecting transverse rotation, the configurations for the 5- and 15-lb pre-tension magnitudes, and the 0 and 30 degree pre-tension flexion angles, were averaged for each pre-tension direction.*

Maximum Unloaded Graft Length or L_0   Although the pre-tension variables can directly affect graft force, these variables are dependent in the sense that they all influence one fundamental mechanical variable, L_0. The three pre-tension variables establish the relative configuration of tibia and femur at the time of fixation, which, in turn, determines the condition when graft force is just increasing from zero, or L_0. To show how L_0 works, the effect of L_0 of a composite graft on the mechanics of the reconstructed joint was assessed in an in vitro study.[21] ACL forces were measured with a buckle transducer during the application of 90-N anterotibial loads at 0, 30, 60, and 90 degrees of flexion in five normal knee specimens. The ACL was then excised, and a three-segment composite graft was prepared, consisting of the semitendinosus and gracilis tendons left distally based, and augmented with a synthetic augmentation

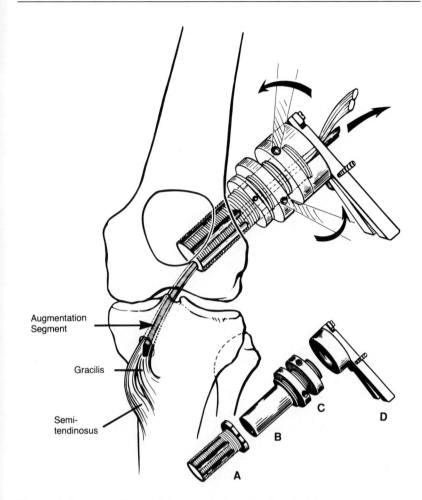

Fig. 6   *Schematic of femoral fixation device with threaded outer casing (A), moveable inner cylinder with tunnel for graft (B), threaded collars (C), and tissue clamp (D). (Reproduced with permission from Lewis JL, Lew WD, Engebretsen L, et al: Factors affecting graft force in surgical reconstruction of the anterior cruciate ligament.* J Orthop Res *1990;8:514-521.)*

device. Fixation tunnels were drilled through the anteromedial ACL tibial attachment and the center of the ACL femoral attachment. The proximal tunnel was enlarged to accommodate the threaded outer casing of a fixation device (Fig. 6). This device consisted of the outer casing, a moveable inner cylinder with a tunnel to accommodate passage of the graft, a pair of threaded collars on the inner cylinder, and a clamp for graft fixation. It was possible to continuously adjust the L_0 of a graft secured in the clamp by varying the double collar assembly of the fixation device.

Two inner cylinders were available for testing. The graft tunnel was located centrally in one cylinder, so that the graft could be fixed at the center of the anatomic ACL attachment. The tunnel in the second cylinder was offset from the center by 5 mm (Fig. 6). Rotation of this offset cylinder within the outer casing allowed continuous variation of the femoral fixation site about the central anatomic site. A buckle transducer was installed around the entire composite graft and was calibrated at 30 degrees of flexion. With the graft passing through the inner cylinder with the central tunnel and fixed proximally in the tissue clamp, a 90-N anterior load was applied to the tibia at 30 degrees of flexion. With the external load applied, the collars of the fixation jig were adjusted until the total force in the graft, as indicated by the calibrated buckle transducer, was equal to the force in the intact ACL that had been measured under that same joint load. This procedure was used to provide a standardized starting condition from which to examine changes in L_0. Because of the geometric complexities of the graft attachment sites, L_0 was not measured directly. Instead, the resultant graft force with the knee under load, which depends on L_0, was measured and controlled. After matching the total graft force to the intact ACL force at 30 degrees, the external load was released and the graft buckle transducer readings were recorded during the application of the antero-tibial loads at 0, 30, 60, and 90 degrees of flexion.

L_0 was then varied at 30 degrees of flexion by an amount expected to cause a significant change in graft force (usually 1 to 3 mm), and the graft forces were recorded during the anterior load sequence. L_0 was then changed by another amount in the same direction, and by one or more increments in the opposite direction, with the anterior load sequence repeated after each change.

The effect of the variation in L_0 on the total graft force for the anatomic femoral hole location at extension and 90 degrees of flexion for the five specimens is presented in Figure 7, *top* and *bottom*, respectively. A straight line was fit to the data to show the approximate level of change in graft force with variation in L_0. Variation in L_0 changed the total graft force at all flexion angles. The ratio of percent change in total graft force to change in L_0, averaged over all specimens and flexion angles, was 22% per mm. L_0 was considered to have a significant effect on total graft force because a 3-mm change in L_0 could produce an over 50% change in graft force at all four flexion angles tested.

Femoral Attachment Site   The locations of the graft attachment sites on the tibia and femur determine graft force as well as L_0. Numerous locations for ACL graft attachment sites have been recommended. Although the rationale for many of these is empirical, the current mechanical criterion for locating grafts is isometry; that is, the graft is positioned in such a way that the separation distance between the sites remains relatively constant over the range of passive flexion-extension. This criterion is used because an improperly-placed graft might become overloaded in flexion or extension, resulting in fixation or graft substance failure as well as restricted range of motion during function. Regions for potential ACL graft

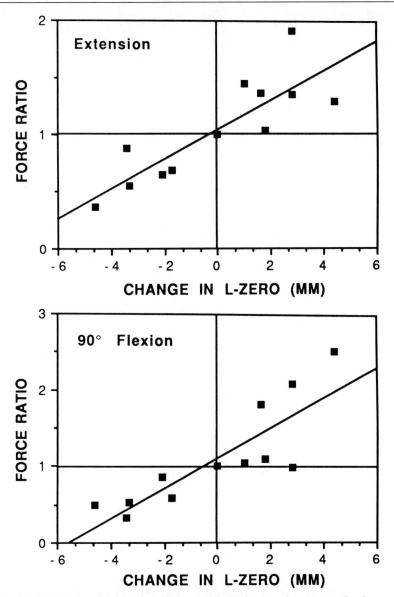

Fig. 7 *Top, Ratio of the total graft force with the knee under anterior load at extension after a change in L$_0$, to the graft force under anterior load at extension with the initial L$_0$ determined by standardizing the graft force to the intact ACL force at 30 degrees of flexion, versus the change in L$_0$ for the five specimens with the graft located in the central anatomic site.* **Bottom,** *Ratio of the total graft force with/without a change in L$_0$, versus the change in L$_0$ at 90 degrees of flexion. (Reproduced with permission from Lewis JL, Lew WD, Engebretsen L, et al: Factors affecting graft force in surgical reconstruction of the anterior cruciate ligament. J Orthop Res 1990;8:514-521.)*

attachments most likely to provide isometric behavior have been described in several studies.[22,23] Briefly, results of these studies showed that the separation distance is affected more by the femoral attachment site than by the tibial site, and that the separation distance is more sensitive to the position of the femoral site in the anteroposterior direction than in the proximodistal direction. Isometry will be further discussed in another chapter.

Bylski-Austrow and associates[13] reconstructed the ACL with an instrumented, flexible wire cable and measured graft force as a function of femoral attachment position. Graft forces with the joint under anterior load increased with flexion when the graft was fixed at a site on the anterior margin of the femoral anatomic ACL attachment region. Graft forces were greater in extension than flexion when the femoral site was either over-the-top or on the posterior margin of the anatomic ACL attachment region. Of all the sites tested, a point on the distal margin of the anatomic region provided the most isotonic force pattern over the range of flexion.

We generated similar force data in an experiment in which we used a semitendinosus-gracilis-augmentation segment composite graft, as described in the L_0 section of this chapter.[21] The inner cylinder with the central tunnel of the femoral fixation fixture (Fig. 6) was capable of placing the composite graft in the center of the anatomic ACL attachment site. When the inner cylinder with the central tunnel was replaced by the inner cylinder with the offset tunnel, the femoral attachment was varied 5 mm anterior, posterior, distal, and proximal to the central anatomic site. At each site, the graft force was standardized to the force in the intact ACL at 30 degrees of flexion under a 90-N anterotibial load. Figure 8, *top* and *bottom* present the total graft force in the anterior and posterior sites, respectively, normalized to the graft force in the central anatomic location, for the five specimens under anterotibial load. Variation in tunnel location produced minimal changes in total graft force near extension, but had a greater effect on graft force in flexion. The graft forces in the anterior and distal tunnel locations were greater than those in the anatomic site in flexion, while forces in the posterior site were less than those in the anatomic location. These results seem to indicate that the femoral tunnel location is important to prevention of large graft forces in flexion, and that tunnel placement has little influence on graft forces near extension, at least for the tunnel locations tested and for fixation at 30 degrees of flexion.

Graft Augmentation   Other factors that can influence graft force are augmentation and the distribution of the attachment sites of the biologic and augmentation segments of a composite graft. Augmentation refers to the addition of either a biologic or synthetic segment, which is placed in parallel with biologic graft material, to share load with the biologic graft. The goal of augmentation may be either to share the load permanently with the graft material, or to share the load temporarily when the biologic material weakens during graft remodeling and revascularization. We have studied load sharing between a bone-patellar tendon-bone graft and a commercially-available, polypropylene augmentation device.[18] The graft was located

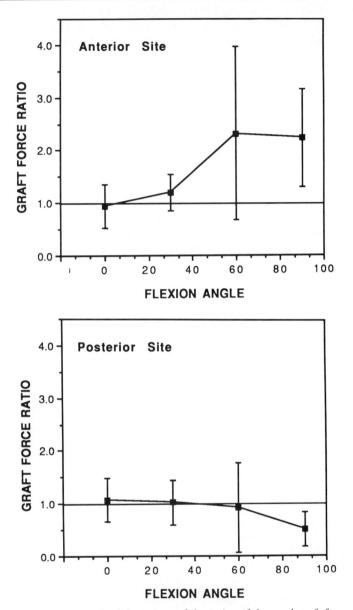

Fig. 8   *Means and standard deviations of the ratios of the total graft force with the graft placed 5 mm anterior (**top**) or posterior (**bottom**) to the anatomic site, to the graft force with an anatomic placement, for the five specimens under anterior load at each of the four flexion angles. (Reproduced with permission from Lewis JL, Lew WD, Engebretsen L, et al: Factors affecting graft force in surgical reconstruction of the anterior cruciate ligament. J Orthop Res 1990;8:514-521.)*

isometrically, and was fixed at 30 degrees of flexion under distal pre-tension. Total graft force and load sharing were measured by buckle transducers under anterotibial loads at several flexion angles. Results from this study showed that load sharing did occur between the segments, reducing the load in the tendon portion of the graft. However, the level of load sharing between the graft segments was not controllable when using the pre-tension method at the time of graft fixation.

Composite Graft With Distributed Femoral Attachment Sites   Use of augmentation raises the possibility of more closely simulating the natural ACL by distributing the graft segments' attachment sites.[24-27] However, this also increases the number of mechanical surgical variables involved, because L_0 and the location of the attachment site for each band can be varied. We performed a systematic in vitro study of these variables with a patellar tendon graft and augmentation segment.[28] The study was undertaken to assess the biomechanical effect of the distribution of the femoral attachment sites of the segments of the composite graft, as well as the prescribed level of load sharing between these segments, as reflected by the control of L_0 of each segment. A cylindrical fixture that allowed variation of the distribution of the femoral attachments of the graft segments was used for proximal fixation. Distal fixation was obtained using a force-setting device (Fig. 9). Total graft force and load sharing between the graft segments were measured using buckle transducers, and total anteroposterior joint laxity was measured using an instrumented spatial linkage, as anterotibial loads were applied at various test flexion angles. Forces and laxity were recorded both for various combinations of load sharing established with the force-setting device at extension, and for distributions of femoral attachments of the graft segments, which spanned the area of the normal ACL attachment region.

Total graft force and anteroposterior laxity were not affected by either the set level of load sharing at extension or the location of femoral attachment sites. Relative load sharing over the flexion range was not affected by the particular level of load sharing set at extension, but femoral hole location significantly influenced the way load sharing changed over the flexion range. This implies that as long as a desired level of load sharing can be established at a particular flexion angle, the manner in which load sharing changes over the flexion range can be controlled by a suitable choice of femoral attachment sites for the individual bands of a composite graft.

Lateral Extra-articular Procedures   Lateral extra-articular procedures have been used as a backup for an intra-articular ACL reconstruction, in order to reinforce the lateral secondary restraints and augment the intra-articular graft during tissue remodeling.[14,29] In light of recent improvements in intra-articular ACL reconstruction, this concept has been challenged by some who have concluded that patients who undergo an extra-articular procedure in conjunction with an intra-articular reconstruction have no better outcome than those who undergo an intra-articular procedure alone.[30,31] Others

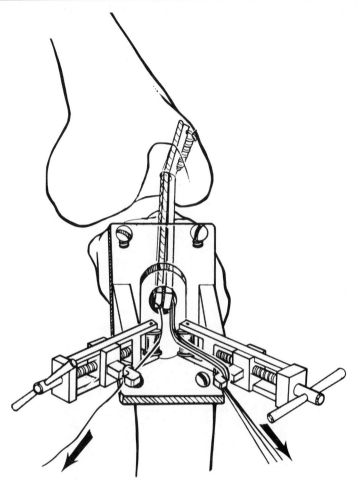

Fig. 9 *Schematic of the force-setting device. The sutures from the tendon and augmentation segments are fixed to the screw mechanisms on the device. With the knee under a standardized external load at a particular flexion angle, the maximum unloaded lengths of the segments (L_0) were independently varied using the screw mechanisms, so that each segment carried a prescribed portion of the total graft force. Graft forces could be monitored by buckle transducers installed on the graft segments within the joint for in vitro testing, or by load cells mounted externally on the screw mechanisms for in vivo testing. (Reproduced with permission from Lew WD, Engebretsen L, Lewis JL, et al: Method for setting total graft force and load sharing in augmented ACL grafts. J Orthop Res 1990;8:702-711.)*

have concluded that addition of an extra-articular procedure to an intra-articular reconstruction improves the outcome of patients in special situations, such as young, large, athletically-active individuals with severe instability due to a lack of lateral secondary restraints.[32] In addition to increasing the degree of morbidity, extra-articular procedures frequently stretch out over time and overconstrain the joint by placing the tibia in an abnormal amount of fixed external rotation.[23,33-35] Some have found that pre-tensing the extra-articular tissue at the time of its fixation contributes to this excessive externally-rotated configuration; however, it is possible to pre-tense the extra-articular tissue just enough to take up the slack without abnormally rotating the tibia externally.[33] Others have addressed the stretching-out and constraint issues by measuring the distances between potential extra-articular attachments on the tibia and femur, in an attempt to locate sites that will result in near isometric behavior and, thereby, reduce the risk of tissue overload in the range of motion.[23,35] Actual load sharing between extra-articular and intra-articular reconstruction segments was never directly measured, but was inferred from strain measurements in one study.[33] Load sharing occurs between intra-articular and extra-articular graft tissues; however, the interaction between them is poorly understood.

Engebretsen and associates[34] began to study this interaction by measuring joint motion and forces in a composite intra-articular graft (bone-patellar tendon-bone graft augmented with a commercially-available synthetic device) with and without an iliotibial tenodesis. Intra-articular fixation holes were drilled through the anteromedial portion of the ACL tibial attachment and the postero-superior portion of the femoral attachment. The intra-articular graft segments were fixed proximally with an interference screw. Buckle transducers were installed on both graft segments and were calibrated at 30 degrees of flexion. Distal fixation was achieved by attaching the segments to a force-setting jig (Fig. 9) mounted on the medial tibial surface over the opening of the distal fixation hole of the intra-articular graft. With the joint under an anterotibial load at 30 degrees of flexion, the total graft force of the intra-articular reconstruction was standardized to match the force in the intact ACL under the same anterior load, so that the total force was shared equally among the graft segments. Forces and motions were measured during an unloaded state and a 90-N anterotibial load at 0, 30, 60, and 90 degrees of flexion with the standardized intra-articular reconstruction alone. The reconstruction was removed at the distal end, and a tenodesis was prepared using a 20-mm portion of the posterior iliotibial band. A buckle transducer was installed on the iliotibial band. The standardized intra-articular reconstruction was fixed as described above, then the tenodesis was secured with a soft-tissue screw and washer at Krackow's F-9 site on the lateral femoral condyle, while under 27-N pre-tension at 30 degrees of flexion. The test sequence was repeated, and both the tenodesis and intra-articular graft were taken down. The tenodesis was then fixed first, followed by the addition of the standardized intra-articular reconstruction, and the test sequence was repeated.

Forces in the intra-articular graft were significantly reduced when the tenodesis was added to the intra-articular reconstruction (Fig. 10, *left*). Addition of the tenodesis seemed to disrupt the mechanical state established by the standardized intra-articular reconstruction. When the tenodesis was performed first, followed by the intra-articular reconstruction, total graft force was not statistically signifi-

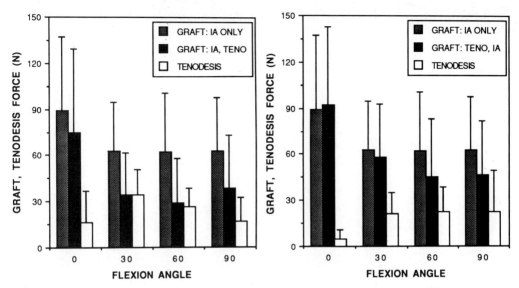

Fig. 10   *Left, Means and standard deviations of the total force in the intra-articular graft when the standardized intra-articular reconstruction was performed alone (GRAFT:IA ONLY) and when the tenodesis was added to the intra-articular reconstruction (GRAFT: IA, TENO), and of the force in the tenodesis (TENODESIS) when it was added to the intra-articular reconstruction, for the seven specimens under anterior load at the four flexion angles.*
Right, *Means and standard deviations of the total force in the intra-articular graft when the intra-articular reconstruction was performed alone (GRAFT: IA ONLY) and when the intra-articular reconstruction was added to the tenodesis (GRAFT: TENO, IA), and of the force in the tenodesis (TENODESIS) when the intra-articular reconstruction was added. (Reproduced with permission from Engebretsen L, Lew WD, Lewis JL, et al: The effect of an iliotibial tenodesis on intra-articular graft forces and knee joint motion. Am J Sports Med 1990;18:169-176.)*

cantly different from that for intra-articular reconstruction alone (Fig. 10, *right*). The tenodesis in both conditions was more highly loaded from 30 to 90 degrees of flexion than in extension. The total graft force was significantly greater than the tenodesis force at extension, but they were not significantly different from 30 to 90 degrees of flexion. Load sharing between the tenodesis and intra-articular graft was indicated by the equivalence of the reduction in the total graft force to that carried in the tenodesis, whether the tenodesis was added before or after the intra-articular graft. When the tenodesis was added, the configuration of the knee in the anteroposterior direction was returned to within normal limits. However, the knee was significantly externally rotated in both the unloaded and anterior loaded conditions, relative to its state with an unloaded intact ACL.

Factors Causing Graft Creep After Fixation

The question of whether the mechanical conditions established at surgery remain after fixation and early use of the joint has been addressed by several investigators. King and associates[36] performed static load relaxation tests on isolated femur-MCL-tibia complexes, as a function of differing peak loads, and of whether or not the specimens had a prior load history. They found that the peak loads initially decreased, then stabilized to a relatively constant residual load after a period of time. The peak loads and residual loads were related linearly, and a prior load history resulted in less relaxation with a higher residual load for a given peak load. These data suggest that if the recent load history of a graft is known, and if the force in the graft can be controlled at the time of fixation, the peak graft load required at fixation to provide a desired residual load after fixation could be predicted.

More and Markolf[37] performed an in vitro study where they reconstructed the ACL with a commercially-available synthetic ligament. After repeated anteroposterior tibial loading, the anteroposterior laxity of the joints increased from the level immediately after fixation. This creep effect was reduced to within acceptable limits by preconditioning the graft while one end was fixed in the joint. This study points out that in situ preconditioning allows the fibers in either a biologic or synthetic graft to reorient themselves, and allows any soft tissues trapped between the graft and bone to become stabilized.

We performed an in vitro study using five goat knees, with the goal of setting the force in the segments of a composite graft with the joint under load, and then quantifying the effect of repeated exercise or loading of the graft segments and of fixation of the graft segments on the resulting level of graft force. The ACLs were reconstructed using a bone-patellar tendon-bone graft, along with a synthetic augmentation segment. Before implantation, the graft segments were preconditioned by stretching on a suture table. The segments were fixed proximally with an interference screw and were attached to a force-setting device mounted distally on the anterior tibia (Fig. 9). Rather than using a tibial tunnel, the segments were directed over the anteromedial edge of the tibia in two separate troughs. Buckle transducers were installed on the segments external to the joint but proximal to the force-setting device. Just before attaching them to the force-setting device, the segments were preconditioned in situ by applying loads to them while exercising the joint.

After preconditioning the segments and attaching them to the force-setting device, a prescribed level of total force and load sharing were set in the segments with the joint under a standardized anterotibial load. Then, the standardized external load was removed, and the joint was exercised by flexing and extending multiple times, and by repeatedly applying anterior loads. The standardized load was then reapplied, and the forces in the graft segments were recorded. If the forces in the segments decreased from their set levels as a result of creep in the graft segments themselves, or as a result of compression of other joint structures in contact with the loaded graft, the graft segments would be reset to the initial desired

Table 1 Ability to achieve desired graft force under load

Specimen	Intended Set Force (N)*		Check Force Level (N)*		Final Force Level (N)*	
	PT	AUG	PT	AUG	PT	AUG
1	30	30	24	14	31	31
2	30	23	27	19	28	22
3	22	22	17	17	26	24
4	22	22	17	16	23	20
5	22	22	19	21	25	28

*After setting forces in the tendon (PT) and augmentation (AUG) segments under a standardized anterior load (Intended Set Force), the joint is exercised by flexion-extension and application of 15 lbs (67 N) of anterotibial loads ten times each. The standardized load was reapplied to see if the set forces had changed (Check Force Level). If the graft forces decreased, the graft was reset or overset, exercised, checked, and, if necessary, reset. This was repeated until exercise did not affect the set forces (Final Force Level).

levels, or sometimes overset to account for the reduction in graft force. The exercise sequence would be repeated, followed by measurement of the segment forces under the standardized external load until the level of set force was not affected by the exercise sequence (Table 1).

From these tests, we concluded that a desired level of total graft force and load sharing could be chosen and set with the joint under a prescribed external load, and could be maintained within an average of 27% of the desired level after repeating the exercise resetting sequence from two to five times. These results made us confident that a particular graft state, set both in total force and load sharing, would remain after later reloading of the joint. The tests also demonstrated a drop of over 50% in set values with joint reloading if the exercise-resetting sequence was not performed. This work was a preliminary study to develop methodology for an in vivo study, and numbers sufficient for statistical significance were not generated. Although the study provided evidence to support the ability to set load and load sharing, and maintain them in the immediate postoperative period, it did not address the changes that undoubtedly occur in the subsequent healing phase in vivo.

Methods for Installing ACL Grafts

Up to this point, this chapter has identified and quantified the effect of factors believed to influence graft force. We will now examine surgical methods used to install an ACL graft, and discuss how these methods might influence the mechanical variables that were identified.

Pre-tension and Isometry Approach

The pre-tension and isometry approach, which occurs in a multitude of variations, is used in essentially all ACL reconstructions. As described on page 336, the graft is initially fixed at one end, and then it is secured at the other end while tension is being applied to it.

Some clinicians measure the pre-tension magnitude, while others do not. Some clinicians apply minimal pre-tension or no pre-tension at all. The fixation sites on the tibia and femur are chosen so that the graft is isometric during flexion and extension of the joint. The criterion for adequate graft placement is a predetermined level of joint laxity, which is considered adequate for normal joint function. Isometry is established either by eye or by the use of such devices as an isometer, which quantifies the change in separation distance over the flexion range between candidate bone fixation sites or tunnels. Isometry will be discussed in another chapter. The question of interest here is "What forces in the graft result from using the pre-tension method?"

To address this question, we studied the effect of the pre-tension variables (direction, magnitude, flexion angle) on graft force and joint motion, as previously described in this chapter. An earlier in vitro study was also performed in which graft forces were measured in five specimens under anterotibial loads, and the ACL was reconstructed first using a distally-based gracilis-semitendinosus-augmentation segment composite graft, and then reconstructed using a free bone-patellar tendon-bone graft with an augmentation segment.[18] Fixation tunnels were located for isometric behavior using an isometer. Buckle transducers were installed on each graft segment for the measurement of total graft force and load sharing. The three-segment graft was fixed under 15 lbs proximal pre-tension, and the two-segment graft was fixed under 15 lbs distal pre-tension, both at 30 degrees of flexion. As shown in Figure 11, the graft forces under the anterotibial loads were found to be relatively reproducible over the five knees tested, although the graft forces were not reproducible compared to normal, because they were significantly higher than the forces in the natural ACL under similar conditions in flexion. This suggested to us that pre-tension overloads the graft, yet produces a relatively constant state for variable knees.

Our interpretation of the results from both pre-tension studies, in terms of the variables previously discussed, is that variation in L_0 was the cause of the lack of control over the mechanical state of the reconstructed joint. For a given set of pre-tension variables, the displacements of the tibia relative to the femur under anterior load typically differed for each knee tested. The joint was often overconstrained in a posterior and externally rotated configuration. Although proximal pre-tension generated higher graft forces compared to distal pre-tension (Fig. 4), the joint configuration more closely approximated normal under proximal pre-tension than under distal pre-tension (Fig. 5). This demonstrates that there is a weak correlation between joint laxity and graft force. A satisfactory laxity range can have a wide range of graft forces.

This lack of a strong link between graft force and joint laxity reflects the sensitivity of graft force to L_0. The graft shares load with other passive joint structures, and varying L_0 of the graft will change the state of load sharing. The pre-tension method of fixation essen-

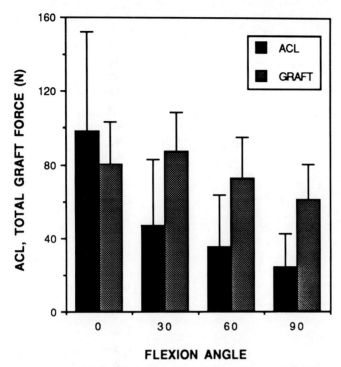

Fig. 11 *Means and standard deviations of the force in the intact ACL and the total force in the composite graft for the five specimens under 90-N anterotibial loads at 0, 30, 60, and 90 degrees of flexion, where the two-segment composite graft was fixed under 15 lbs of distal pre-tension at 30 degrees of flexion.*

tially alters L_0, depending on the pre-tension variables used; however, neither L_0 nor graft force or load sharing are ever measured directly. Joint displacement or laxity is considered to be the outcome variable by which the success of the reconstruction is evaluated. It is not surprising that there is considerable variability in joint forces when using this approach.

Force-setting Approach

In light of the deficiencies inherent in the pre-tension approach, we have developed and explored an alternative method in which the mechanical criterion for graft installation is graft force. We call this the force-setting approach. In this method, the graft is fixed in such a way as to achieve a prescribed graft force with the joint under some standardized external load. The advantage of this approach is that the graft force can be set to a constant level among specimens, for a particular joint load. Because forces rather than displacements are set, a potential disadvantage of this method is that joint displacements under load might not fall within an acceptable range, depending on the mechanical state of the graft and joint. However, this problem has not occurred in our in vitro use of the technique. We have restricted our use of this method to cadaver and animal testing, and do not recommend its use in humans until the safety and efficacy of the approach have been established.

This approach involves temporarily mounting a force-setting device near the external opening of the fixation tunnel on one side of the joint. This device consists of one or more advancing screw mechanisms, with an attached load cell mounted in line with each screw. Figure 9 shows the force-setting device we use for in vitro knee testing. The single-band graft, or individual segments of a composite graft, are initially fixed on one side of the joint, with the other ends of the graft segments temporarily attached to the force-setting device on the other side of the joint. With a standardized external load applied to the joint, the screw mechanisms are used to adjust the L_0s of the graft segments until a desired level of total force and load sharing are achieved. We have demonstrated this technique in an in vitro study involving eight specimens.[38] Intact ACL forces and joint motion were first measured during 90-N anterotibial loads applied at 0, 30, 60, and 90 degrees of flexion. A composite graft was then prepared, which consisted of a bone-patellar tendon-bone graft, augmented with a synthetic device.

The force-setting device was installed on the anteromedial tibia, over the opening of the distal fixation tunnel (Fig. 9). After fixing the composite graft proximally with an interference screw in the posterosuperior region of the anatomic ACL attachment, a 90-N anterotibial load was applied to the joint at 30 degrees of flexion, and the screw mechanisms were adjusted until a desired level of graft force and load sharing was achieved. The force in the intact ACL under the same anterior load at 30 degrees of flexion was used as the target graft force. This was typically near 40 N. After the segment forces were set, the anterior load was released, and the total graft force and load sharing were recorded during the anterior load sequence at the four test flexion angles. Figure 12 compares the total graft forces, which were set at 30 degrees of flexion to match normal, and the respective intact ACL forces. Figure 13 shows the load sharing between the graft segments at the four test flexion angles, when the load sharing was set at 30 degrees of flexion so that each segment carried one half of the total force. It is evident from the data that the total graft force was controlled so that it more closely reproduced the force in the intact ACL, compared with the pre-tension graft forces in Figure 10. The load sharing throughout the flexion range remained close to the level set at 30 degrees of flexion.

The force-setting method is essentially a way to adjust L_0 in a continuous manner so that the total graft force can be set to achieve some prescribed mechanical goal. This concept can be extended to setting the level of load sharing by controlling L_0 of each segment of a composite graft independently. Although the chosen criteria in the demonstration study were to match the intact ACL force at 30

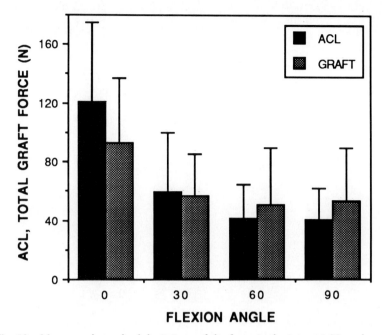

Fig. 12 *Means and standard deviations of the force in the intact ACL and total force in the composite graft for the eight specimens under 90-N anterotibial loads at 0, 30, 60, and 90 degrees of flexion. The force in the composite graft was set to match the force in the intact ACL at 30 degrees of flexion with the knee under a 90-N anterotibial load, so that each graft segment carried 50% of the total force.*

degrees of flexion and to have equal load sharing between the two segments, force levels satisfying other criteria could also be prescribed and set. Graft pre-tension, with its variables of direction, flexion angle, and magnitude, seems to provide inadequate control over L_0 and the immediate postoperative state of the joint. The force-setting technique uses L_0 as the primary variable to dictate forces in the graft segments with the joint under a standardized external load, and allows increased control over the immediate postoperative mechanical state of the joint. Even though force is the variable being monitored, L_0, which is not being measured directly, is the parameter being controlled and set. The force-setting approach is useful in cadaver testing to reduce variability between specimens. Researchers are continuing to assess its utility in animal and human surgery.

In Vivo Measurement of Graft Forces

Graft force is suspected to be important for graft remodeling and function. Up to this point, we have reviewed in vitro studies of mechanical surgical variables affecting graft force. The real question

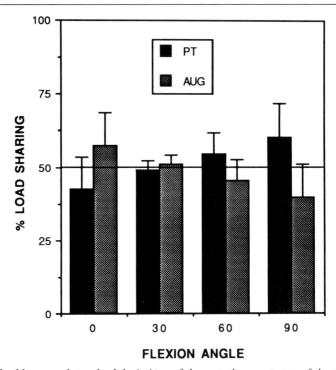

Fig. 13 *Means and standard deviations of the actual percentages of the total graft force carried by the patellar tendon (PT) and augmentation (AUG) segments when the graft was set at 30 degrees of flexion to have 50% load sharing in the two graft segments, for the eight specimens under anterotibial load at each of the four flexion angles. (Reproduced with permission from Lew WD, Engebretsen L, Lewis JL, et al: Method for setting total graft force and load sharing in augmented ACL grafts. J Orthop Res 1990;8:702-711.)*

of interest, however, is how do these variables affect in vivo performance of a graft? How relevant are the in vitro studies of graft force to the in vivo situation? To answer these questions, several investigators have begun to study graft forces in vivo. Direct measurement of graft forces in living subjects is a challenging task, and minimal work has been done. Pope and associates[39] have arthroscopically installed their Hall Effect Strain Transducers in humans. This work will be discussed in detail in another chapter. Cummings and associates[40] used a curved beam implantable force transducer to measure load in the patellar tendon of a goat during function. Lewis and associates[9] used buckle transducers to measure the force in the medial collateral ligaments of dogs. We have been developing a method for using buckle transducers to measure forces in the segments of a composite ACL graft in a goat model. The test method and some early results will be discussed below.

The in vivo graft force measurements were based on the force-setting method, using a patellar tendon graft, augmented with a polypropylene augmentation device. The tendon and augmentation segments were secured with interference screw fixation proximally,

Table 2 In vivo forces (Newtons) in the augmentation device at two weeks after surgery in two goats

Load State	Animal No. 1*	Animal No. 2**
Straight walking	23	27
15-lb (67-N) anterotibial force at 60 degrees flexion, anesthesia	15	15
Manual anterior drawer at 60 degrees flexion, anesthesia	32	40

*Femoral fixation of the patellar tendon failed within two weeks
**Patellar tendon graft partially ruptured, and stretched out

and were directed over two separate troughs on the anteromedial tibia for temporary fixation to a force-setting device mounted distally on the tibia. Buckle transducers were installed on the tendon and augmentation segments as they passed over the anteromedial tibia, external to the joint and proximal to the force-setting device. This configuration prevented impingement of the transducers with the femur in the intercondylar region, and also kept the transducers from being displaced as a result of repeated motion of the joint, which can lead to fatigue failure of the lead wires. This test setup was used to measure graft forces in the functioning goat, to assess the ability to set graft forces under anterotibial load in vivo, and to establish the relation between the set force and the functional forces. Three goats have been instrumented to date. A summary of the results is shown in Tables 2 and 3.

There have been considerable technical difficulties, and all three tests failed for various reasons. However, several useful conclusions can be drawn from the preliminary data. First, the graft did carry load, even in the early healing period at two weeks after surgery. A total graft force of nearly 30 N was measured during level walking at two weeks, even though the patellar tendon had failed in animals 1 and 2 (Table 2). The animals had a considerable limp, but were bearing weight on the limb. This force was the same order of magnitude as the forces occurring during clinical laxity testing, which indicates that there were significant forces in the ACL graft during normal function. This is contrary to earlier findings in the normal canine MCL, which showed significantly less force during function than with clinical laxity testing.[9] The present results pertain to the early healing period and, no doubt, are influenced by surgical artifact. A second result is that the prescribed force magnitude and load sharing could be reasonably maintained after fixation and closure in vivo (Table 3). However, the results also demonstrated that application of other load states to the joint generated different graft forces and load sharing, as would be expected.

The graft force and load sharing can probably be set; however, the joint load states to be applied while the forces are being set, must still be established. An important point regarding the surgical technique was evident in that two of the three tests failed because of overloading of the patellar tendon graft, with subsequent failure of

Table 3 In vivo forces in anesthetized animals immediately after surgery

| Load State | Animal No. 1* | | Animal No. 2* | | Animal No. 3* | |
	PT	AUG	PT	AUG	PT	AUG
Intended set force (N)	35	8	28	7	7	28
Force (N) after fixation, closure, multiple cycles of flexion/extension	25	13	28	11	18	42

*Forces in the tendon (PT) and augmentation (AUG) segments with a 15-lb (67 N) anterotibial load applied at 60 degrees of flexion

tissue or fixation. The tendon fixation in Goat No. 1 failed on the femoral side, where two K-wires were used for fixation of the tendon-bone block. The tendon segment of Goat No. 2 stretched out, probably because of failure near the buckle transducer. In both cases, it appeared as if the cause of the overload was improper placement of the femoral tunnel. Large loads in the tendon graft were recorded in both cases during hyperflexion. The animals were not immobilized postoperatively. Although this represents a technical problem in this study, it probably illustrates a real problem in surgery on human beings.

Our results to date represent a learning curve to a certain extent, but they also demonstrate the possible fate of grafts implanted in human beings, and the complex interaction of graft force and mechanical surgical variables. The in vivo measurements generally support the validity of the in vitro tests, but they also show that greater care must be taken in in vivo surgery. In addition, the in vivo measurements raise the question of the mechanical goal of surgery. Our understanding of the factors affecting graft force has been improved, and we are having some success in controlling graft force. However, there remains the question of what level of graft force is desirable for optimal tissue remodeling. The quantitative relation between load history and graft remodeling is unknown. This remains a promising avenue for research.

Summary

Several mechanical surgical variables affecting graft force, which are under the control of the surgeon, have been identified, including the maximum unloaded graft length (L_0), fixation or tunnel location, extra-articular procedures, augmentation, and distribution of attachment sites in a composite graft. L_0 is, in turn, influenced by the pre-tension variables of the flexion angle at which the pre-tension is applied and the direction of the pre-tension force. Pre-tension magnitude was found to have less effect. All of the studies of these variables have been in cadavers, and work is just underway to confirm these findings in living animals and human beings. Early in vivo work supports the in vitro findings, but studies of the long-term consequences of particular chosen surgical variables are just beginning. It is not known what graft force occurs in human beings or what optimum graft force is required for the maturation of a graft into a functioning ligament. Early results are encouraging. Understanding of the process is improving, and there is hope that better control can be gained over the starting and end points of ligament reconstruction.

Acknowledgments

The authors gratefully acknowledge the financial support provided by NIH grants AR38398 and AR39255, and a gift from the Mahadh Foundation.

References

1. Butler DL, Hulse DA, Kay MD, et al: Biomechanics of cranial cruciate ligament reconstruction in the dog: II. Mechanical properties. *Vet Surg* 1983;12:113-118.

2. Clancy WG, Narechania RG, Rosenberg TD, et al: Anterior and posterior cruciate ligament reconstruction in Rhesus monkeys: A histological, microangiographic, and biomechanical analysis. *J Bone Joint Surg* 1981;63A:1270-1284.

3. Drez DJ Jr, DeLee J, Holden JP, et al: Anterior cruciate ligament reconstruction using bone-patellar tendon-bone allografts: A biological and biomechanical evaluation in goats. *Am J Sports Med* 1991;19: 256-263.

4. Grood ES, Suntay WJ, Noyes FR, et al: Biomechanics of the knee extension exercise: Effect of cutting the anterior cruciate ligament. *J Bone Joint Surg* 1984;66A:725-734.

5. Shelbourne KD: Accelerated rehabilitation after anterior cruciate ligament reconstruction. *Am J Sports Med* 1990;18:292-299.

6. Woo SL-Y, Gomez MA, Sites TJ, et al: The biomechanical and morphological changes in the medial collateral ligament of the rabbit after immobilization and remobilization. *J Bone Joint Surg* 1987;69A:1200-1211.

7. Woo SL-Y, Inoue M, McGurk-Burleson E, et al: Treatment of the medial collateral ligament injury: II. Structure and function of canine knees in response to differing treatment regimens. *Am J Sports Med* 1987;15:22-29.

8. Ahmed AM, Hyder A, Burke DL, et al: In-vivo ligament tension pattern in the flexed knee in passive loading. *J Orthop Res* 1987;5: 217-230.

9. Lewis JL, Lew WD, Shybut GT, et al: Biomechanical function of knee ligaments, in Finerman G (ed): *Symposium on Sports Medicine: The Knee.* St. Louis, CV Mosby, 1985, pp 152-168.

10. Markolf KL, Gorek JF, Kabo JM, et al: Direct measurement of resultant forces in the anterior cruciate ligament: An in vitro study performed with a new experimental technique. *J Bone Joint Surg* 1990;72A:557-567.

11. Jones KG: Reconstruction of the anterior cruciate ligament: A technique using the central one-third of the patellar ligament. *J Bone Joint Surg* 1963;45A:925-932.

12. Noyes FR, Butler DL, Paulos LE, et al: Intra-articular cruciate reconstruction: I. Perspectives on graft strength, vascularization, and immediate motion after replacement. *Clin Orthop* 1983;172:71-77.

359

13. Bylski-Austrow DI, Grood ES, Hefzy MS, et al: Anterior cruciate ligament replacements: A mechanical study of femoral attachment location, flexion angle at tensioning, and initial tension. *J Orthop Res* 1990;8:522-531.

14. Clancy WG Jr, Nelson DA, Reider B, et al: Anterior cruciate ligament reconstruction using one-third of the patellar ligament, augmented by extra-articular tendon transfers. *J Bone Joint Surg* 1982;64A:352-359.

15. Jackson DW, Windler GE, Simon TM: Intraarticular reaction associated with the use of freeze-dried, ethylene oxide-sterilized bone-patella tendon-bone allografts in the reconstruction of the anterior cruciate ligament. *Am J Sports Med* 1990;18:1-11.

16. Burks RT, Leland R: Determination of graft tension before fixation in anterior cruciate ligament reconstruction. *Arthroscopy* 1988;4:260-266.

17. Yoshiya S, Andrish JT, Maley MT, et al: Graft tension in anterior cruciate ligament reconstruction: An in vivo study in dogs. *Am J Sports Med* 1987;15:464-470.

18. Hanley P, Lew WD, Lewis JL, et al: Load sharing and graft forces in anterior cruciate ligament reconstructions with the Ligament Augmentation Device. *Am J Sports Med* 1989;17:414-422.

19. Zaricznyj B: Reconstruction of the anterior cruciate ligament using free tendon graft. *Am J Sports Med* 1983;11:164-176.

20. Gertel TH, Lew WD, Lewis JL, et al: Effect of ACL graft pretension direction, magnitude and flexion angle of knee biomechanics. Presented at the Program-Combined Congress of the International Arthroscopy Association and the International Society of the Knee, Toronto, May 1991.

21. Lewis JL, Lew WD, Engebretsen L, et al: Factors affecting graft force in surgical reconstruction of the anterior cruciate ligament. *J Orthop Res* 1990;8:514-521.

22. Hefzy MS, Grood ES, Noyes FR: Factors affecting the region of most isometric femoral attachments: Part II. The anterior cruciate ligament. *Am J Sports Med* 1989;17:208-216.

23. Sidles JA, Larson RV, Garbini JL, et al: Ligament length relationships in the moving knee. *J Orthop Res* 1988;6:593-610.

24. Roberts TS, Drez D Jr, McCarthy W, et al: Anterior cruciate ligament reconstruction using freeze-dried, ethylene oxide-sterilized, bone-patellar tendon-bone allografts: Two year results in thirty-six patients. *Am J Sports Med* 1991;19:35-41.

25. Engebretsen L, Lew WD, Lewis JL, et al: Knee mechanics after repair of the anterior cruciate ligament: A cadaver study of ligament augmentation. *Acta Orthop Scand* 1989;60:703-709.

26. McCarthy JA, Steadman JR, Dunlap J, et al: A nonparallel, nonisometric synthetic graft augmentation of a patellar tendon anterior cruciate ligament reconstruction: A model for assessment of stress shielding. *Am J Sports Med* 1990;18:43-49.

27. Veltri DM, Fulkerson JP: Isometricity of y-graft replacement of the anterior cruciate ligament. *Trans Orthop Res Soc* 1990;15:55.

28. Chao TTH, Lew WD, Hong B, et al: Biomechanical effect of distributed femoral attachment site of augmented ACL graft. *Trans Orthop Res Soc* 1991;16:204.

29. Zarins B, Rowe CR: Combined anterior cruciate-ligament reconstruction using semitendinosus tendon and iliotibial tract. *J Bone Joint Surg* 1986;68A:160-177.

30. O'Brien SJ, Warren RF, Wickiewicz TL, et al: The iliotibial band lateral sling procedure and its effect on the results of anterior cruciate ligament reconstruction. *Am J Sports Med* 1991;19:21-25.

31. Strum GM, Fox JM, Ferkel RD, et al: Intraarticular *versus* intra-articular and extraarticular reconstruction for chronic anterior cruciate ligament instability. *Clin Orthop* 1989;245:188-198.

32. Noyes FR, Barber SD: The effect of an extraarticular procedure on allograft reconstructions for chronic ruptures of the anterior cruciate ligament. Presented at the Program-Combined Congress of the International Arthroscopy Association and the International Society of the Knee, Toronto, May 1991.

33. Draganich LF, Reider B, Ling M, et al: A in vitro study of an intra-articular and extraarticular reconstruction in the anterior cruciate ligament deficient knee. *Am J Sports Med* 1990;18:262-266.

34. Engebretsen L, Lew WD, Lewis JL, et al: The effect of an iliotibial tenodesis on intraarticular graft forces and knee joint motion. *Am J Sports Med* 1990;18:169-176.

35. Krackow KA, Brooks RL: Optimization of knee ligament position for lateral extraarticular reconstruction. *Am J Sports Med* 1983;11:293-302.

36. King G, McPherson R, Shrive N, et al: Rabbit medial collateral ligament tension is dependent on time and loading history. *Trans Orthop Res Soc* 1991;16:157.

37. More RC, Markolf KL: Measurement of stability of the knee and ligament force after implantation of a synthetic anterior cruciate ligament. *J Bone Joint Surg* 1988;70A:1020-1031.

38. Lew WD, Engebretsen L, Lewis JL, et al: Method for setting total graft force and load sharing in augmented ACL grafts. *J Orthop Res* 1990;8:702-711.

39. Pope MH, Beynnon BD, Howe JG, et al: In vivo study of the anterior cruciate ligament strain biomechanics in the normal knee. *Abstracts of the First World Congress of Biomechanics* 1990;2:320.

40. Cummings JF, Holden JP, Grood ES, et al: In vivo measurement of patellar tendon forces and joint position in the goat model. *Trans Orthop Res Soc* 1991;16:601.

Chapter 19

The Measurements of the Anterior Cruciate Ligament Strain In Vivo

Bruce D. Beynnon, PhD
Malcolm H. Pope, DMSc, PhD
Robert J. Johnson, MD
James G. Howe, MD
Braden C. Fleming, MS

Introduction

The anterior cruciate ligament (ACL) is the most frequently totally disrupted knee ligament.[1-4] A loss of the ACL eventually results in changes of the tibiofemoral joint, because one of the primary functions of this ligament is to prevent anterior subluxation of the tibia in relation to the femur. Knee ligament injuries in the United States occur at an estimated rate of 1.5 million per year.[5] Liljedahl and Nordstrand[6] and Dye and associates[7] demonstrated that rupture of the ACL may lead to knee instability, abnormal knee kinematics, increased erosion of joint cartilage, and production of abnormal osseous metabolic activity. Palmer[8] found that arthrosis can occur with repeated episodes of instability following ACL injury. Results of these and many other studies have led to recommendations to consider surgical reconstruction of disrupted ACLs in active individuals. Unfortunately, the management of ACL injuries has remained inconsistent because of the lack of objective clinical and biomechanical data.

Specific treatment procedures often are based on a surgeon's clinical experience rather than on objective biomechanical or prospective data. Therefore, further research is needed to define the characteristics and behavior of the normal ACL, so that injuries to this structure can be diagnosed consistently and treated effectively. Our research in this area has included in vivo studies preceded by extensive in vitro investigations. We have studied normal ACL strain during activities common to diagnostic procedures and ACL rehabilitation protocols, investigated the effect of functional knee bracing on the ACL, and measured ACL reconstruction strain biomechanics at the time of implantation.

Experimental Background

The clinical diagnosis of an ACL injury is not straightforward because several structures interact with each other to provide stability to the knee joint. Clinical tests for knee laxity[9-17] as well as instrumented knee arthrometers have been developed in an attempt to provide an accurate and easy means of diagnosing instabilities in the knee. Large interobserver and intraobserver errors have indicated that these clinical examinations[18-20] and commercial machines[18,21-25] do not reproducibly diagnose knee injuries. Most clinicians still use their hands to evaluate the integrity of the ACL. Their patients, therefore, depend on the experience of the clinician rather than on a universally accepted objective test.

After a knee injury has been diagnosed, the challenge remains as to the treatment procedure to follow and the type of rehabilitation protocol to use. Traditionally, the rehabilitation protocol following ACL reconstruction has been conservative, requiring joint immobilization for up to six weeks to allow tissues to heal and joint inflammation to decrease. However, innumerable investigators have reported the deleterious effects of knee immobilization on leg muscles, articular cartilage, periarticular bone, ligaments, and capsular structures.[26-31] Noyes and associates[32] have shown that continuous passive motion (CPM) after open or arthroscopic ACL reconstruction does not permanently elongate the ligamentous reconstruction; they recommend early protected joint mobilization with CPM to decrease the morbidity associated with reconstruction procedures. Because early unprotected motion of the knee joint could permanently elongate the newly reconstructed ACL and fixation system, many advocate controlled CPM immediately following ACL reconstruction, whereas others believe that early aggressive mobilization of such reconstructions avoids many of the disadvantages while not significantly endangering the healing tissues.[33] Knowledge of safe and effective activities that would not excessively strain the ACL or its replacement are vital in developing objective rehabilitation protocols. Although rehabilitation activities have been evaluated in in vitro studies,[34-41] evidence suggests that in vivo muscle tone and muscle contraction patterns alter the strain behavior of the ACL observed in the in vitro environment.[42-46] Our investigation is the first to characterize comprehensively the effects of different rehabilitation activities on the normal human ACL in vivo.

Functional knee braces, which often are prescribed for patients to augment the later phases of their rehabilitation program, have been defined as those designed to provide stability for unstable knees.[47] Variable results have been reported for studies on the effectiveness of braces and on patient satisfaction with the stability provided by the braces.[48,49] Data from recent biomechanical studies show that application of a functional knee brace effectively controls excessive tibiofemoral knee motion during low anterior shear loading, but does not do so at the high loads that occur during sports events.[48-51] Unfortunately, the ability of different functional braces to shield the ACL from strain in vivo was not directly measured in these studies.

Data from prospective, long-term follow-up studies of ACL injuries, when combined with in vivo ACL strain data, may reveal an optimal treatment program for ACL injuries. Such variables as the type of replacement graft, the position of the tunnels, and the amount of initial tension required to secure the graft contribute to the technical difficulty of ACL reconstruction and result in a variety of outcomes. Yoshiya and associates[52] recognize that the initial tension at the time of its fixation can affect the vascularity of an autogenous tissue replacement. In addition, graft tension at the time of implantation and fixation of an ACL replacement directly affects knee laxity and the success of an ACL reconstruction procedure.[52-56] Too much initial tension may constrain the knee, while insufficient initial tension may produce a lax knee joint. Results of studies performed on human cadaveric specimens indicate that different graft positions create markedly different strain patterns during passive range of motion testing.[34,54,57-68] For example, if the femoral tunnel is in an anterior position relative to the anatomic ACL insertion, the graft will tighten excessively during knee flexion, and if the femoral tunnel is more posterior, the graft will tighten as the knee is extended.[34,63] The goal of an ACL reconstruction is to restore the normal knee joint kinematics. Therefore, our work has included an in vivo study in which we compared the strain biomechanics of the normal ACL with those of the replacement graft at the time of surgical reconstruction.

Materials and Methods

Normal ACL Study

ACL strain was measured in ten healthy male subjects from 18 to 40 years of age (a mean of 25 years).[45] The patients were all candidates for exploratory arthroscopy or arthroscopic meniscectomy and had normal ACLs. Patients suspected of having an ACL injury were excluded from the study. Local anesthesia was used for both the surgical and experimental procedures so that the study subjects retained full control of their lower extremity musculature. This study was approved by the institutional review board, an informed consent was obtained from each patient, and no monetary compensation was given.

After the routine surgical procedure was complete, the Hall Effect Strain Transducer (HEST), a highly compliant displacement transducer developed at our research institute, was prepared for insertion (Fig. 1). The sterile HEST was arthroscopically inserted through a 9-mm lateral portal sleeve on to the anteromedial band of the ACL. The 9-mm sleeve was removed, allowing the output wires and removal sutures attached to the HEST to exit through the lateral portal so that the HEST could be connected to the data acquisition computer. Portal wounds were stapled closed and covered with a sterile dressing. Each patient was positioned so that he was sitting

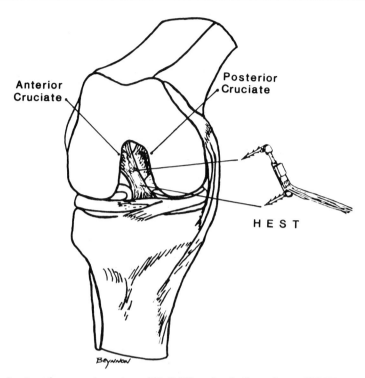

Fig. 1 *Attachment orientation of Hall Effect Strain Transducer (HEST) on anteromedial bundle of ACL. (Reproduced with permission from Beynnon BD, Pope MH, Wertheimer CM, et al: The effect of functional knee braces on anterior cruciate ligament strain* in vivo. *J Bone Joint Surg, in press.)*

on the end of an operating table modified so that a t-bar could be attached to the end of the table, allowing knee flexion angles to be controlled during the various tests.

The HEST measures the ACL displacement pattern without loading or stretching the ligamentous tissue. However, under some knee loading conditions, the ACL may exhibit marked laxity and be described as unstrained. For example, when a posterior shear force is applied across the knee joint during the Lachman's test, the ACL is palpably slack and, as the posterior shear load is released and an anterior load is applied, the ACL becomes taut, and is a load-bearing structure. Because the HEST will measure displacement when the ACL is either slack or taut, we have chosen to calculate strain with a reference length based on this slack-taut transition state of the ACL to differentiate between slack and taut states. This reference length was evaluated in two study patients. A procedure was designed that used simultaneous arthroscopic visualization and palpation of the anteromedial band with a barbed probe embedded next to the HEST, while a custom-designed load cell was used to apply anteroposterior shear loading to the tibia at 30 degrees of knee flexion.[45] The investigator palpated the anteromedial band by gently pulling on the probe, while arthroscopically observing this portion of the ligament tent and simultaneously applying shear load across the tibiofemoral joint in a continuous fashion. As the shear load was applied in an anterior direction the investigator was able to detect and arthroscopically visualize a transition in the anteromedial band. This transition was defined as the palpated slack-taut transition. The investigator documented it by closing a switch, located at the load cell grip, at the instant the transition was palpated. This enabled correlation of applied shear load to the HEST length, defined as reference length L_0, at which the transition occurred. This reference length was used in the calculation of strain. When the ligament elongates beyond L_0, it is considered strained (or is in a load-bearing state), and when the ligament contracts and becomes smaller in length, it is considered unstrained (or is in an unloaded, slack state). Strain (e) is calculated, using an engineering strain formulation, as a change in length from a reference length (L_0) divided by that reference length, and is expressed as a percentage:

$$e = \frac{L - L_0}{L_0} \times 100$$

An electrogoniometer was then attached to the leg of each patient to allow continuous measurement of the knee flexion-extension and internal-external rotation angles. A custom anteroposterior load cell was developed to apply a cyclic anteroposterior shear load to the knee joint at the level of the proximal tibia. A second load cell (isoquad load cell) was attached to the horizontal arm of the t-bar, such that the distal portion of each patient's anterior tibia could be strapped to it and could record the level of knee extension force during isometric quadriceps activities. The output from the HEST, electrogoniometer, anteroposterior load cell, and isoquad load cell were recorded at 10 Hz intraoperatively through a computerized data acquisition system. Each transducer was independently calibrated before its use on a study patient.

The experimental protocol consisted of activities that often are encountered in post ACL reconstruction rehabilitation programs. Each test represented a different knee motion that challenged the ACL and caused strain to occur. The tests consisted of anteroposterior shear testing of the tibia relative to the femur at 30 and 90 degrees of knee flexion (The Lachman and Drawer tests, respectively), active and passive range of knee motion, an isometric quadriceps contraction at 30 and 90 degrees of knee flexion, and squatting with and without external resistance. For the Lachman and Drawer tests, each patient was seated on the end of the operating table and the distal tibia of his instrumented leg was strapped to the horizontal portion of the t-bar (Fig. 2). The t-bar angle was set so that the leg remained at 30 degrees of knee flexion. The anteroposterior load cell was then positioned in a transverse plane, directed through the mid-tibial tuberosity. Four cycles of continuous anterior and posterior shear loads to limits of ± 150 N were applied by

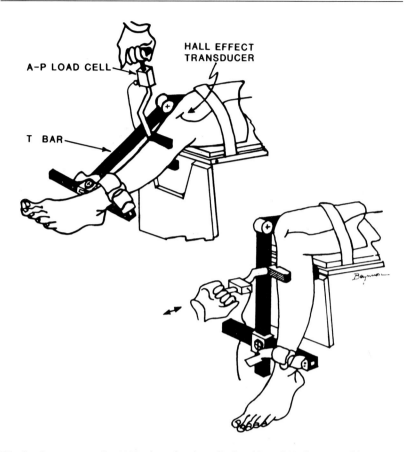

Fig. 2 *Anteroposterior (AP) shear load applied at 90 and 30 degrees of knee flexion. (Reproduced with permission from Beynnon BD, Howe JG, Pope MH, et al: The measurement of anterior cruciate ligament strain* in vivo. Int Orthop *(SICOT) 1992;16:1-12.)*

the investigator. The leg was repositioned at 90 degrees of knee flexion (Drawer test) and the four loading cycles were repeated. The anteroposterior load cell was then removed, and the patient's leg was unstrapped from the t-bar allowing it to swing freely.

The t-bar was secured so it would not interfere with the patient's leg during the active and passive range of motion tests. For the passive range of motion test (PROM), the investigator held the patient's heel and guided the tibia from 5 to 110 degrees of knee flexion in a continuous manner. For the active range of motion test (AROM), each patient was instructed to extend and flex his knee in a cyclic pattern between 5 and 110 degrees of knee flexion. Eight of the ten patients also underwent an AROM with a 10-lb weight boot. For each activity, four continuous cycles of data were collected. While this was being done an attached electrogoniometer measured the knee flexion-extension and the internal-external rotation of the tibia relative to the femur.

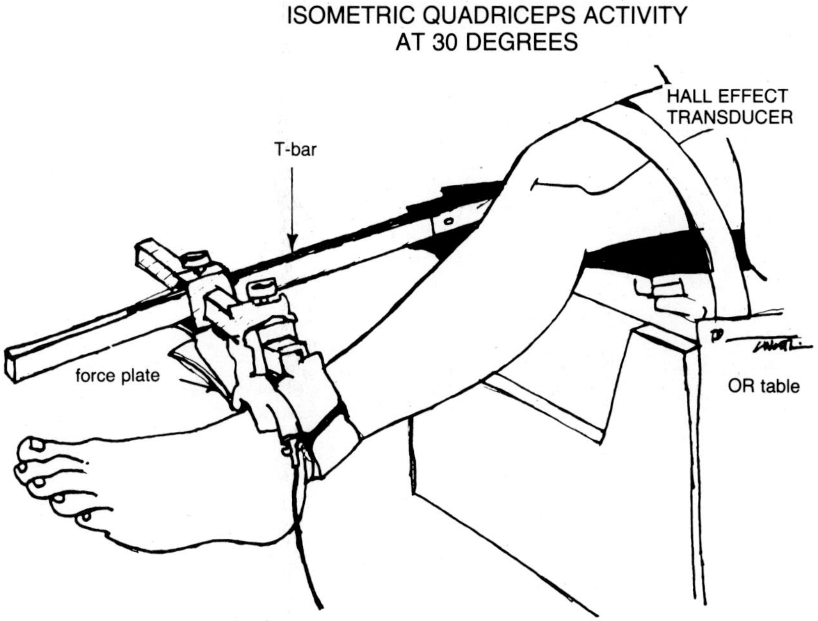

ISOMETRIC QUADRICEPS ACTIVITY
AT 30 DEGREES

Fig. 3   *Isometric quadriceps extension activity at 30 degrees of knee flexion.*
(Reproduced with permission from Beynnon BD, Howe JG, Pope MH, et al: The
measurement of anterior cruciate ligament strain in vivo. Int Orthop *(SICOT)*
1992;16:1-12.)

The distal tibia of the instrumented leg was strapped to the isoquad load cell located on the horizontal portion of the t-bar (Fig. 3)
while the patient remained in the seated position on the operating
table. The moment arm from the knee joint to the isoquad load cell
was measured with a hand-held tape and recorded for the extension
torque calculation. The patient was instructed to contract his quadriceps muscle by extending his leg against the stationary isoquad
load cell four times to approximately 80% of his maximal effort. This
was performed at both 30 and 90 degrees of knee flexion.

Six subjects performed a squatting activity with and without the
resistance of a rehabilitative Sport Cord. For these tests, the patient
was assisted off the operating table and onto a six degree of freedom
(three forces and three moments) force plate. The foot of the instrumented leg was placed on the plate, and the uninjured leg was put on
a footstool of equal height located next to the plate. Each patient
was fitted with a three degree of freedom electrogoniometer for the
ankle in addition to the two degree of freedom electrogoniometer
already attached to the knee. A tension load cell was placed in series
with the handle of the Sport Cord to record the level of force created
by the Sport Cord during a squatting exercise (Fig. 4). Force outputs

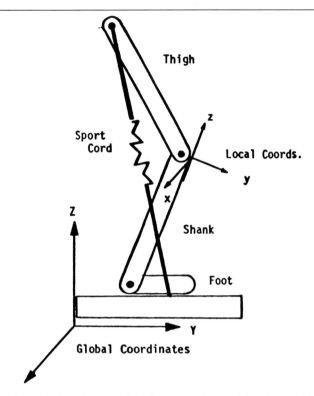

Fig. 4 *Sagittal plane knee model of the squatting activity. (Reproduced with permission from Pope MH, Stankewich CJ, Beynnon BD, et al: The effect of knee musculature on ACL strain in-vivo. J Electromyography Kinesiol 1991;1:191-198.)*

from the plate and Sport Cord load cell, combined with the kinematic data from the electrogoniometers, were then input into a four-bar linkage model we developed to predict knee joint moments and forces.[69] A description of the free body diagram is presented in Figure 4. Once positioned on the force plate, each patient was instructed to perform four continuous squatting exercises. The Sport Cord was then placed under both feet of the subject and stretched so that the patient could hold the handles stationary at the hip while performing four continuous squats against its resistance. For these tests, the data were collected intraoperatively at 20 Hz and then input into a postprocessing computer-based linkage model.[69] After the experimental protocol was complete, the HEST was removed from the joint and the remaining wounds were closed and dressed.

Functional Brace Study

This study was undertaken to quantify whether functional bracing can alter normal ACL strain, either detrimentally or beneficially. ACL strain measurements were conducted on otherwise healthy male subjects ranging from 18 to 35 years of age who were candidates for diagnostic arthroscopy or arthroscopic meniscectomy, and were found to have normal ACLs on arthroscopic examination. Local anesthesia was used for both the surgical and experimental procedures. ACL displacement was measured with the arthroscopically implanted HEST, using the techniques described above for the normal ACL study by Beynnon and associates.[70]

Seven different functional braces were tested within this portion of the study. The braces tested included three custom fit designs and four off-the-shelf designs. The three custom fit braces were: The C.Ti Standard with the ACL cable system (Innovation Sport, Irvine, CA), The Lenox Hill Derotation Brace (Lenox Hill Brace Shop, Long Island, NY), and The Townsend Knee Brace (Townsend Industries, Inc., Bakersfield, CA). The four off-the-shelf braces included: The Donjoy 4-point Sport ACL Brace with ACL accessory strap (Donjoy, Inc., Carlsbad, CA), The 3D Dynamic Functional Knee Brace (3-D Orthopaedic, Inc., Dallas, TX), The Lerman Multi-Lig II Brace (United States Manufacturing Co., Pasadena, CA), and the Bledsoe Sports Rehab Brace (Medical Technology, Grand Prairie, TX). Each of the custom braces was sized and attached to the patient's leg by a licensed orthotist according to the manufacturer's specifications. The off-the-shelf braces were sized and attached by the investigator as instructed by a representative of each brace manufacturer. Because of the operating room time limitations placed on our experiments, a maximum of three braces could be tested on each subject.

Strain was measured during activities commonly encountered in rehabilitation programs after ACL reconstruction. Clinical implications of this study rest on the hypothesis that if a functional brace can provide some protection to the normal ACL, it also will protect athletes with an injured or reconstructed ACL. The four activities tested were anteroposterior shear loading of the tibia at 30 degrees of flexion (Fig. 5), isometric quadriceps contraction at 30 degrees of knee flexion (Fig. 6), AROM, and internal-external torque applied to the tibia with the knee flexed to 30 degrees (Fig. 7).

The first three activities were evaluated as described in the normal ACL study.[45] For the fourth activity, an instrumented torque-boot was attached to the patient's leg, allowing the investigator to apply internal and external torque alternately to a minimum of ± 5 N·m. Four continuous cycles of internal-external torque were recorded while the electrogoniometer attached to the knee recorded internal-external tibiofemoral rotation (Fig. 7).

For the experimental protocol, the unbraced leg was tested for each of the four activities, then a knee brace was applied and the four activities were repeated. The Lachman and AROM tests were repeated on the unbraced knee between each brace test. This study design allowed three comparisons of ACL strain values to be made for each activity: between the unbraced and repeated unbraced tests; between each brace and the unbraced condition; and among the braces.

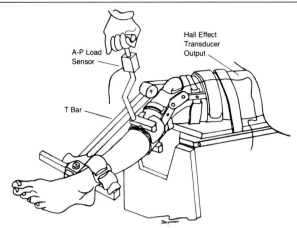

Fig. 5   *Anteroposterior (AP) shear load at 30 degrees of flexion with U.S. Manufacturing functional knee brace applied to patient. (Reproduced with permission from Beynnon BD, Pope MH, Wertheimer CM, et al: The effect of functional knee braces on anterior cruciate ligament strain* in vivo. J Bone Joint Surg, *in press.)*

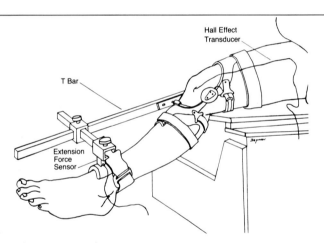

Fig. 6   *Isometric quadriceps extension activity with C.Ti. functional knee brace applied to patient. (Reproduced with permission from Beynnon BD, Pope MH, Wertheimer CM, et al: The effect of functional knee braces on anterior cruciate ligament strain* in vivo. J Bone Joint Surg, *in press.)*

Reconstructed ACL Study

This work involved measuring the displacement of an ACL replacement graft at the time of surgical reconstruction.[70,71] The HEST allows us to measure the displacement pattern of the replacement graft immediately after fixation, so that we can compare it with the normal ACL data. Graft elongation patterns, as recorded with the HEST, can be used to document restoration of normal ACL biomechanics (an indirect indicator of normal knee kinematics). Ten patients undergoing acute arthroscopic reconstruction of their ACLs

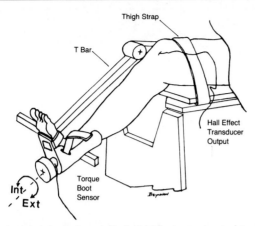

Fig. 7 *Internal-external torque applied with the instrumented torque boot sensor at 30 degrees of knee flexion. (Reproduced with permission from Beynnon BD, Pope MH, Wertheimer CM, et al: The effect of functional knee braces on anterior cruciate ligament strain* in vivo. *J Bone Joint Surg, in press.)*

with bone-patella tendon-bone grafts participated in this portion of the study. Interference screws were used for graft fixation in all patients. After the graft was fixed and the wounds closed, the HEST was inserted through the lateral portal onto the anteromedial aspect of the replacement graft as described above. A sterile electrogoniometer was attached to the leg to measure knee motion angles. The reconstruction joint was then subjected to 20 continuous cycles of PROM while the electrogoniometer and HEST outputs were recorded as described previously. Because the grafts are fixed in place with an initial tension, they do not undergo the slack-taut transition during the Lachman or PROM test that was described for the normal ACL. Therefore, the elongation reference was chosen as the HEST length with the joint in an extended position (10 degrees). After the experimental protocol was complete, the HEST was removed from the joint and the remaining wounds were closed and dressed.

Statistical Analysis

For the normal ACL study, each subject served as his own control with statistical comparison of strain values made within patients using the student's *t* test. Statistical analysis was based only on the load-bearing strain values. For each of the three activities (anteroposterior shear loading, isometric quadriceps contraction, and range of motion) a comparison was made between flexion angles (30 and 90 degrees of knee flexion) at specific load levels or between active and passive range of motion (at 10-degree increments). For the AROM with a weight boot and for squatting with and without a Sport Cord, only descriptive analysis was performed.

The functional brace study was structured as a balanced incomplete block design (Table 1). Two comparisons were of interest: the

Table 1 Incomplete block experimental design for the functional knee brace study

Subject*	Brace Type**										
	3D	US	TN	DJ	CT	BL	LH	N	R1	R2	R3
1	X		X					X	X	X	
2			X		X			X	X	X	
3			X			X		X	X	X	
4						X	X	X	X	X	
5		X	X				X	X	X	X	X
6		X			X	X		X	X	X	X
7		X	X	X				X	X	X	X
8	X	X						X	X	X	
9	X				X		X	X	X	X	X
10	X			X			X	X	X	X	X
11	X					X		X	X	X	
12				X		X	X	X	X	X	X
13				X	X			X	X	X	
Total	5	4	5	4	4	5	5	13	13	13	6

*Out of the 27 subjects tested, 13 were used in the data analysis. Seven study patients were omitted because of technical failures, while another seven were not used because of inconsistent repeated measures (caused by impingement of the HEST as the knee was brought into full extension at 0 degrees).
**3D = 3-D Orthopaedic Brace
  US = United States Manufacturing, Lerman Multi-Lig II Brace
  TN = Townsend Brace
  DJ = DonJoy 4-point Sport ACL Brace
  CT = C.Ti. Brace with ACL Cable System
  BL = Bledsoe Sports Rehab Brace
  LH = Lenox Hill Derotation Brace
  N = Normal Unbraced Test
  R1 = Repeat Unbraced Test #1
  R2 = Repeat Unbraced Test #2
  R3 = Repeat Unbraced Test #3
  (Reproduced with permission from Beynnon BD, Pope MH, Wertheimer CM, et al: The effect of functional knee braces on anterior cruciate ligament strain *in vivo. J Bone Joint Surg*, in press.)

first between the different braces, and the second between the unbraced and repeated unbraced test conditions. For each loading activity, differences in strain values were calculated between the braced and unbraced conditions, and between the unbraced and repeated unbraced conditions. The comparisons were performed at 40, 100, and 180 N for anterior shear loading; at 5 and -5 N·m for corresponding internal and external torques; at 30 N·m of extension torque for isometric quadriceps contraction; and at 20 degrees of knee extension for AROM (the knee flexion angle where maximum ACL strain occurred). Within the structure of this model, we also were able to determine if there was a significant difference between all the braces as a group and the unbraced condition. For this analysis, the mean difference of braced to unbraced conditions for each study patient, calculated across all braces, was tested for significant differences in comparison to the null or zero value (indicating no difference). This portion of the analysis was performed using the student's t test. Tests were made for all four loading activities at each of the previously described load intervals. An identical procedure was used to determine if there were differences between braced and repeated unbraced conditions.

An investigation of each brace's performance was also conducted. For this analysis, differences in strain values were calcu-

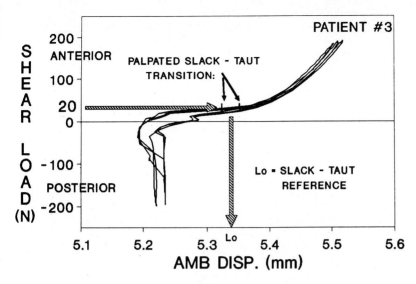

Fig. 8 *Anteroposterior (AP) shear loading at 30 degrees of knee flexion (Lachman test). Shear load (N) versus ACL anteromedial bundle (AMB) displacement (mm). (Reproduced with permission from Beynnon BD, Howe JG, Pope MH, et al: The measurement of anterior cruciate ligament strain* in vivo. Int Orthop *(SICOT) 1992;16:1-12.)*

lated between the braced and unbraced conditions, averaged across patients, and then used in calculation of the paired t statistic. To evaluate the effect of bracing, the difference between the braced and unbraced conditions was calculated at common load intervals and then averaged across patients. This convention was used to determine if brace application could strain shield the ACL (or produce negative difference values), cause a prestraining effect on the ACL (evidenced by positive difference values), or produce no effect at all (a zero difference value).

Results

Normal ACL Study

The L_0 strain reference for these studies was calculated by means of a graph of anteroposterior load, measured by the instrumented load cell and plotted against HEST displacement at a flexion angle of 30 degrees. The palpated slack-taut transition is clearly shown in Figure 8. The two arrows on the graph labeled palpated slack-taut transition indicate the positions on the graph where the investigator was able to arthroscopically observe and palpate the transition between the slack and taut states for two cycles. The difference in displacement between these two points indicates the reference may be defined within the resolution of the measurement technique (0.3% strain). Similar results were found for the second patient.

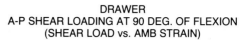

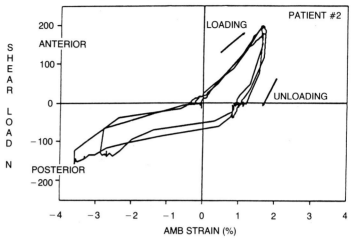

DRAWER
A-P SHEAR LOADING AT 90 DEG. OF FLEXION
(SHEAR LOAD vs. AMB STRAIN)

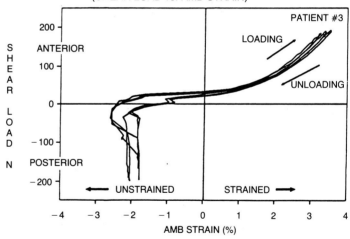

LACHMAN
A-P SHEAR LOADING AT 30 DEG. OF FLEXION
(SHEAR LOAD vs. AMB STRAIN)

Fig. 9 *In vivo ACL anteromedial bundle (AMB) strain pattern for anteroposterior shear loading at 90 degrees (Drawer test) and 30 degrees (Lachman test) of knee flexion. These data are for a typical study subject. (Reproduced with permission from Beynnon BD, Howe JG, Pope MH, et al: The measurement of anterior cruciate ligament strain in vivo. Int Orthop (SICOT) 1992;16:1-12.)*

Because this was observed to occur consistently at 20 N of anterior shear and the inflection point of the anteroposterior load versus HEST displacement relation, the analysis of data for the next eight study patients used the HEST length at the inflection point as a

Table 2 Lachman and Drawer AMB strain values at 150-N anterior shear force

Subject #	Lachman % Strain	Drawer % Strain	Difference Between Drawer and Lachman % Strain
1	4.7	2.0	2.7
2	4.4	3.6	0.8
3	3.7	2.7	1.0
4	4.6	1.8	2.8
5	2.8	1.6	1.2
6	3.3	2.4	0.9
7	3.0	0.3	2.7
8	3.9	0.6	3.3
9	2.4	1.3	1.1
10	4.2	1.4	2.8
Average	3.7	1.8	1.9
SD	0.8	0.9	1.06
			$(t = 5.6, p < 0.01)$

(Reproduced with permission from Beynnon BD, Howe JG, Pope MH, et al: The measurement of anterior cruciate ligament strain *in vivo*. *Int Orthop* (SICOT) 1992;16:1-12.)

strain reference. Figure 9 describes the load versus strain behavior of the ACL anteromedial band during the Lachman and Drawer tests for a typical patient.

Anterior shear loading to 150 N at 30 degrees of knee flexion (Lachman test) produced a mean strain value of 3.7%, while corresponding shear loading at 90 degrees of knee flexion (Drawer test) produced a mean strain of 1.8%. Across all patients the strain developed in the anteromedial band during the Lachman testing was consistently greater than during the Drawer test with an anterior applied load ($p \leq 0.01$). The data are presented in Table 2.

Figure 10 shows the extension torque versus strain relation for a typical patient during an isometric quadriceps contraction at 30 and 90 degrees of knee flexion. Isometric quadriceps contraction at the level of 27 N·m produced a mean unstrained anteromedial band value of −2.5% at 90 degrees of knee flexion, and a mean strain of 3.2% at 30 degrees of flexion. At 90 degrees of flexion no significant change in strain occurred during isometric quadriceps contraction ($p \leq 0.01$). However, at 30 degrees of flexion, the strain increased significantly during muscle contraction ($p \leq 0.01$). The strain pattern at 30 degrees of flexion was significantly greater in comparison to that measured at 90 degrees of flexion during isometric contraction (Table 3).

During PROM (Fig. 11), the mean unstrained minimum value was −4.1% (range −2.6% to −8.2%) at 50 degrees of knee flexion. At this minimum, the anteromedial band was always unstrained across all patients, indicating it was slack or unloaded. At 10 degrees of knee flexion the mean peak was 0.1% (range 0.4% to −1.0%). The transition of the mean curve between the strained and unstrained anteromedial band occurred at 11.5 degrees of flexion.

AROM (Fig. 11) produced a peak ACL strain value of 3.1% (range 4.1% to 1.5%) at 20 degrees of flexion, while the minimum ACL strain of −3.5% (range 0.5% to −5.7%) occurred at 110 degrees of

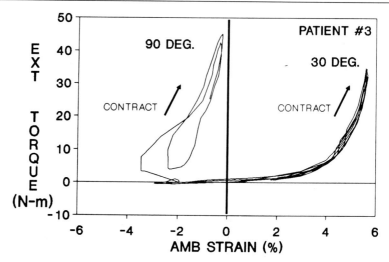

Fig. 10 *In vivo ACL anteromedial bundle (AMB) strain pattern for isometric quadriceps contraction at 30 and 90 degrees of knee flexion. Quadriceps induced extension torque (N·m) versus AMB strain (%), for a typical study subject. (Reproduced with permission from Beynnon BD, Howe JG, Pope MH, et al: The measurement of anterior cruciate ligament strain* in vivo. Int Orthop *(SICOT) 1992;16:1-12.)*

Table 3 Isometric quadriceps contraction, raw data

Subject	% Strain at 90 Degrees Flexion		% Strain at 30 Degrees Flexion	
	Rest: (0 N·m)	Contraction: (27 N·m)	Rest: (0 N·m)	Contraction: (27 N·m)
1	−1.5	−0.55	−1.5	2.2
2	2.5	−0.1	0.3	2.6
3	−9.0	−8.5	−2.0	3.0
4	−3.8	−4.1	0.2	1.8
5	1.6	1.6	2.5	3.4
6	−8.0	−4.5	0.0	4.5
7	−2.2	−2.0	1.5	2.5
8	−5.0	−5.0	1.0	2.9
9	0.1	0.2	3.3	6.0
Mean	−3.4	−2.5	0.6	3.2
SD	3.5	3.2	1.7	1.3
	No significant difference between rest and contracton at 90 degrees		Significant difference (p<0.01) between rest and contraction at 30 degrees (t = 5.7)	

(Reproduced with permission from Beynnon BD, Howe JG, Pope MH, et al: The measurement of anterior cruciate ligament strain *in vivo*. *Int Orthop* (SICOT) 1992;16:1-12.)

flexion. For AROM, the transition of the mean curve between the strained and unstrained anteromedial band occurred at 48 degrees of flexion. The addition of a 10-lb weight boot did not cause the strain values at each flexion increment to increase in comparison to the same activity without the weight boot, although the strain values were elevated (Fig. 12). There was no significant difference between the strain values for AROM and PROM between 50 and 110 degrees of flexion. However, the AROM strain values were significantly

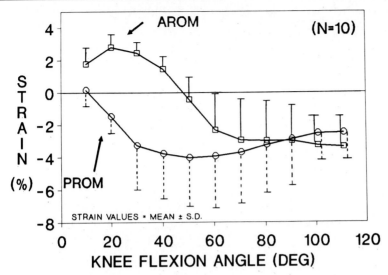

Fig. 11 *In vivo ACL anteromedial bundle (AMB) strain pattern for active range of motion (AROM) and passive range of motion (PROM). Average strain values measured from ten study subjects. (Reproduced with permission from Beynnon BD, Howe JG, Pope MH, et al: The measurement of anterior cruciate ligament strain in vivo. Int Orthop (SICOT) 1992;16:1-12.)*

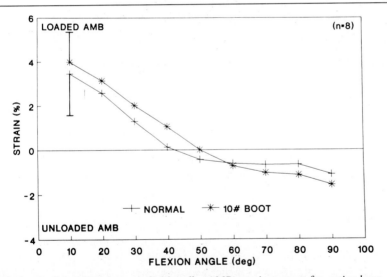

Fig. 12 *In vivo ACL anteromedial bundle (AMB) strain pattern for active knee flexion with and without a 10-lb weight boot attached to the distal aspect of a patient's leg. Mean values are shown for eight study subjects.*

greater at the 40, 30, 20, and 10 degree increments of extension (p≤0.01) (Fig. 11).

For the squatting activity, the additional resistance of a rehabilitative Sport Cord did not significantly change the ACL strain values a all knee flexion angles between 110 and 15 degrees of flexion

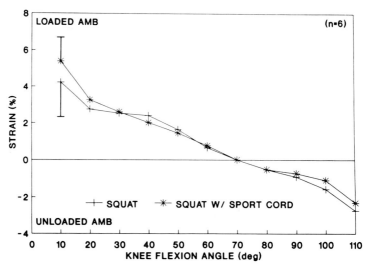

Fig. 13 *In vivo ACL anteromedial bundle (AMB) strain pattern for the squatting activity with and without a resistive Sport Cord. Included are the mean strain values measured from six study subjects.*

(Fig. 13). Maximum strain for both the squat and the squat with the Sport Cord was measured at 10 degrees of flexion. The mean peak ACL strain was 4.2% during the free squat and 5.4% with the Sport Cord. For the free squat, the transition between strained and unstrained ligaments occurred at 70 degrees during the flexion phase and at 42 degrees during extension. In all patients, there was a greater strain during the flexion phase of squatting than during the extension phase. As predicted by the four-bar-linkage model, the patellar tendon forces reached a peak in the deepest part of the free squat. The calculated shear force across the tibiofemoral joint was directed anteriorly throughout most of the free squat and became posteriorly directed at approximately 75 degrees of knee flexion.

Functional Knee Brace Study

For anterior shear loading, no significant differences in strain values were found between the braces at each of the load intervals tested (40, 100, 180 N). This was also the case for the repeated unbraced comparisons at each load interval. For the braces as a group compared with the unbraced condition, no significant difference was found at the 40- or 180-N load level, but a significant difference was found at the 100-N load level ($p \leq 0.05$). Comparison of the individual braces to the unbraced condition revealed a similar trend (Fig. 14). None of the braces was able to reduce the ACL anteromedial band strain at the 40- and 180-N levels. Only the Donjoy and Townsend braces were able to reduce significantly the anteromedial band strain at the 100-N load level (Table 4). Compari-

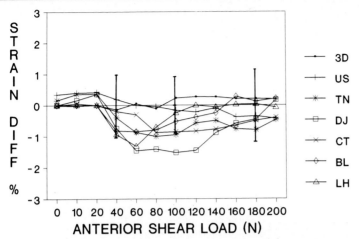

Fig. 14 *Functional knee brace study results for anterior shear loading applied to the tibia relative to femur at 30 degrees of flexion. Mean difference plots (using the convention of braced minus unbraced ACL strain value) at selected shear loads for all seven braces (N=5). The differences were used to provide controlled comparisons of strain values within each patient. A zero difference indicates no effect by the brace, while negative differences show a protective strain shielding by the brace, and positive differences show a deleterious increase in ACL strain. An identical method was used for data presentations in Figures 15, 16, and 17. The 95% significance levels for means of braced to unbraced differences are displayed centered at zero strain value for 40-, 100-, and 180-N load levels. (Reproduced with permission from Beynnon BD, Pope MH, Wertheimer CM, et al: The effect of functional knee braces on anterior cruciate ligament strain in vivo. J Bone Joint Surg, in press.)*

Table 4 Functional knee brace study results

	Anterior Shear at 100 N*	AROM at 20 degrees	Internal Torque (5 N·m)	Isometric Quads (30 N·m)
Donjoy	p≤0.05	N.S.	p≤0.05	N.S.
Townsend	p≤0.05	N.S.	p≤0.05	N.S.
C.Ti.	N.S.	N.S.	p≤0.05	N.S.
Lenox Hill	N.S.	N.S.	p≤0.05	N.S.
Bledsoe	N.S.	N.S.	N.S.	N.S:
U.S. Manuf.	N.S.	N.S.	N.S.	N.S.
3-D Orthop	N.S	N.S.	N.S.	N.S.

*Anterior shear loading at 40 and 180 N produced nonsignificant (N.S.) differences in strain values across all braces.
(Reproduced with permission from Beynnon BD, Pope MH, Wertheimer CM, et al: The effect of functional knee braces on anterior cruciate ligament strain *in vivo. J Bone Joint Surg*, in press.)

son of each individual repeated unbraced test with the original unbraced test revealed no significant differences in ACL strain values.

There were no significant differences in anteromedial band strain values for the braces at the isometric extension torque of 30 N·m. There also were no significant differences in anteromedial band strain values between braces as a group and the unbraced test condition. Analysis of each brace individually also revealed no significant difference in anteromedial band strain values between the braced

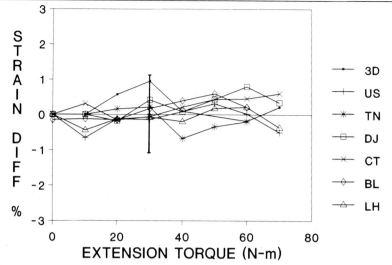

Fig. 15 *Functional knee brace study results from isometric quadriceps contraction at 30 degrees of knee flexion. Mean difference plots (braced minus unbraced ACL strain value) at selected quadriceps extension torques for all seven braces. Included are the 95% significance limits for the means of the braced to unbraced differences, displayed centered at the zero strain value for isometric quadriceps extension torque to the level of 30 N·m. (Reproduced with permission from Beynnon BD, Pope MH, Wertheimer CM, et al: The effect of functional knee braces on anterior cruciate ligament strain* in vivo. *J Bone Joint Surg,* in press.)*

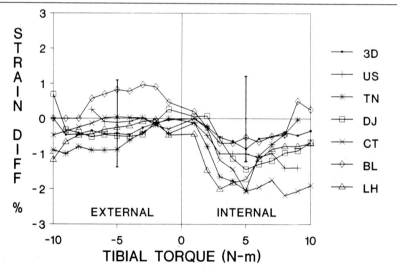

Fig. 16 *Functional knee brace study results for internal-external torque applied to the tibia at 30 degrees of knee flexion. Mean difference plots (braced minus unbraced strain value) at selected torque levels for all seven braces. Included are the 95% significance limits for the means of the braced to unbraced differences, displayed centered at the zero strain value, for internal (+ values) and external (−values) of tibial torque. (Reproduced with permission from Beynnon BD, Pope MH, Wertheimer CM, et al: The effect of functional knee braces on anterior cruciate ligament strain* in vivo. *J Bone Joint Surg,* in press.)*

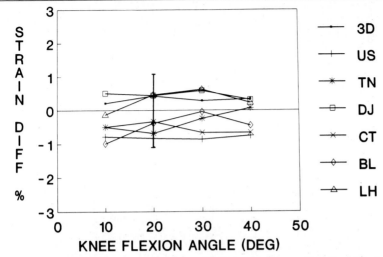

Fig. 17 *Functional knee brace study results for active range of motion. Mean difference plots (braced minus unbraced strain value) at selected knee flexion angles for all seven braces. Included are the 95% significance limits for the means of braced to unbraced differences, displayed centered at the zero strain value, for active range of knee motion at 20 degrees of flexion. (Reproduced with permission from Beynnon BD, Pope MH, Wertheimer CM, et al: The effect of functional knee braces on anterior cruciate ligament strain* in vivo. *J Bone Joint Surg, in press.)*

and the unbraced condition at 30 N·m of extension torque (Fig. 15, Table 4).

For both internal and external torques applied at 5 N·m, no significant differences were found between the braces. Comparison of the braces as a group to the unbraced condition revealed no significant differences for external torque. However, for applied internal torque the anteromedial band strain values were significantly less in comparison with the unbraced conditions. At 5 N·m of internal torque, the mean anteromedial band strain value with the braces applied was 1.3% less than the normal unbraced value (p = 0.01). Comparison of each individual brace with the unbraced conditions produced a similar trend. The Donjoy, Townsend, C.Ti., and Lenox Hill braces significantly reduced anteromedial band strain values in comparison to the unbraced conditions at an applied internal torque of 5 N·m. The ability of each brace to provide protective anteromedial band strain-shielding was dependent on the magnitude of applied torque (Fig. 16).

For AROM, no significant differences in strain values were found between the braces at the knee position of 20 degrees. This was also the case for the repeated unbraced comparisons. No significant differences were found between the braces as a group and the unbraced condition. Analysis of each brace individually also revealed no significant difference in the ACL anteromedial band strain values at all flexion angles during AROM when compared with the unbraced condition (Fig. 17).

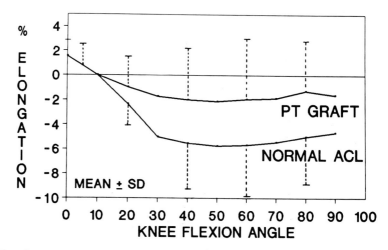

Fig. 18   *In vivo bone-patella tendon-bone graft mean elongation values for passive range of motion of the knee (N = 10), and normal ACL anteromedial bundle data (N = 10).*

Reconstructed ACL Study

Results for the PROM test are reported as a percent elongation rather than a percent strain because the graft remains taut throughout the range of knee motion. An absolute strain reference cannot be obtained using the procedure outlined for the normal ACL study. The mean bone-patella tendon-bone graft elongation pattern for all study subjects is presented in Figure 18. The graph pattern demonstrates a relative increase in strain as the knee is extended and as the knee is flexed beyond 50 degrees. This relationship is similar to the normal ACL data presented in Figure 11.

Discussion

Although others have used in-vitro techniques to infer in vivo biomechanics,[9,13,37-41,61-63,66,72-74] this study presents the first objective in vivo data on the strain patterns of the normal and reconstructed ACL during various activities common to rehabilitation and daily living events. The ability to differentiate between the slack-taut transition that the ACL experiences, and then use this transition displacement as a reference length in the calculation of strain has allowed assessment of various exercises. The choice of a load bearing strain reference is based on the following three observations: (1) The applied anteroposterior shear load versus HEST displacement relationship (Fig. 8) produced a hysteresis loop pattern with two characteristic regions. The region of the curve to the right of the inflection point is a repeatable, closed hysteresis loop indicating a taut anteromedial band, while the region to the left of

Table 5 Rank comparison of activities based on peak strain measurements during activity

Activity	Peak in-vivo ACL Strain	Test Subjects (n)
Squatting with Sport Cord	5.4%	6
Squatting without Sport Cord	4.2%	6
AROM with 10-lb weight boot	4.0%	8
Lachman at 150 N	3.7%	10
AROM	3.1%	15
Isometric Quadriceps Contraction at 30 degrees to 27 N·m Ext Torque	3.0%	14
Anterior drawer at 150 N	1.8%	10
PROM	0.1% at 0 degree flexion	10
Isometric Quadriceps Contraction at 90 degrees to 27 N·m Ext Torque	0.0%	10

AROM = Active flexion-extension of the knee
PROM = Passive flexion-extension of the knee

the inflection point consists of a repeatable, open hysteresis loop and is characteristic of a slack structure. (2) The applied anterior shear load at the inflection point of this curve consistently measured 20 N of force across all patients (who were similar in size, weight, and gender). This force corresponds to the force that must be applied to offset the gravity load on the tibia as it is held over the edge of the operating table. Static equilibrium of forces in the sagittal plane would predict that an anterior shear force equal in magnitude but opposite in direction must be applied to overcome the posterior shear force resulting from the weight of the tibia, just before the ACL becomes a restraint to an increased magnitude of anterior shear load. (3) Simultaneous anteroposterior shear loading and palpation of the anteromedial band found the slack-taut transition occurred at the inflection point of the applied anteroposterior load versus HEST displacement relation. Based on these observations, we used the HEST displacement value at the inflection point of the applied anteroposterior shear versus HEST displacement relation, performed at 30 degrees of flexion, as a reference length for the calculation of strain.

Through the use of local anesthesia, we were able to include the effects of active muscle tone and contraction while measuring ACL strain and directly evaluating brace performance. Rehabilitation activities may now be ranked according to the amount of strain that each produces on the ACL (Table 5).

This work has revealed that for a similar load magnitude of 150 N, anterior shear testing of the knee with a normal ACL at 30 degrees of flexion (the Lachman test) produced more strain than anterior shear testing at 90 degrees of flexion (the Anterior Drawer test). This finding is in contrast to earlier in vitro work,[34] and the difference may exist because the in vitro studies chose an arbitrary reference length for the calculation of strain, or because there are differences in muscle tone between in vitro and in vivo subjects. Our in vivo results are in agreement with those of previously published studies that used either instrumented knee laxity testing or clinical impressions to assess the behavior of the ACL under clinical examination conditions.[3,12,75-79] Our findings confirm that clinical evaluation of the ACL might best be performed at a knee flexion angle between 20 and 30 degrees, where an appreciation of the largest magnitude of anteroposterior laxity may be gained.

ACL strain was not significantly increased during isometric quadriceps contraction when the knee was maintained at 90 degrees of flexion. Isometric quadriceps strengthening should, therefore, be safe in the ACL-injured or reconstructed knee if the flexion angle is maintained at 90 degrees. At 30 degrees of knee flexion, isometric quadriceps activity produced a large increase in ACL strain, and should be carefully controlled, especially during the early stages of rehabilitation where reconstruction fixation may be tenuous.

For PROM using distal thigh and heel support loading, the ACL remained at or below the zero strain level until the joint was brought beyond 11.5 degrees extension. Therefore, continuous passive motion of the knee between the limits of extension and 110 degrees of knee flexion should be safe for the reconstructed ACL immediately following surgery, when the leg is supported near the ankle throughout flexion-extension motion without applied varus-valgus loading, internal-external torques, or anterior shear forces.

AROM of the knee consistently produced strain between 10 degrees and 48 degrees of knee flexion, and no strain between 48 and 110 degrees of flexion. AROM rehabilitation programs may now be prescribed with the two flexion angle regions adapted to the clinician's requirements. The addition of a 10-lb weight boot to a subject's foot during the AROM activity increased but did not significantly change the ACL strain values at all flexion angles in comparison to the same activity without a weight boot.

Investigation of ACL strain during squatting, both with and without a Sport Cord, revealed positive strain values between 70 degrees and full extension. Only slightly elevated strain values were found during squatting activities with application of the Sport Cord. A ranked maximum strain value comparison between the different rehabilitation activities is presented in Table 5. These data may be used as an objective basis for prescribing rehabilitation activities after surgical reconstruction of the ACL.

The functional knee brace study demonstrated that brace performance depends on both the magnitude of anterior shear load and internal torque applied across the tibiofemoral joint. Functional knee braces offered no significant strain shielding effect when an anterior shear load of 180 N was applied to the knee joint. It appears that some of the knee braces can protect the ACL only during applied anterior shear loads less than 100 N. These load magnitudes are small in comparison to those produced during activities of daily living.[80-83]

Only four of the seven braces tested (Donjoy, Lenox Hill, Townsend, and C.Ti.) had a strain shielding effect on the ACL when the knee was subjected to an internal torque. Actual joint mechanics may play a large role in this finding. Because the joint is more compliant in the transverse plane during internal-external tibial torque, the brace-soft-tissue interface may perform rigidly and resist applied internal torque before the ligaments restrain that applied internal torque.

Finally we found that there is no apparent advantage of the custom brace design in comparison to the off-the-shelf braces. Romash and Henningsen[84] revealed similar findings in tests performed with the KT-1000 on five custom and five off-the-shelf brace designs.

For the PROM activity, there were similarities between the in vivo normal ACL anteromedial band data and the reconstructed bone-patella tendon-bone graft data immediately after fixation. This suggests restoration of normal joint kinematics for this group of subjects.

Acknowledgments

The Department of Orthopaedics and Rehabilitation gratefully acknowledges the assistance provided by grants #R01-AR39213 and R01-AR40174 from the National Institutes of Health.

References

1. Eriksson E: Reconstruction of the anterior cruciate ligament. *Orthop Clin North Am* 1976;7:167-179.

2. Feagin JA Jr, Curl WW: Isolated tear of the anterior cruciate ligament: 5-year follow-up study. *Am J Sports Med* 1976;4:95-100.

3. Johnson RJ: The anterior cruciate: A dilemma in sports medicine. *Int J Sports Med* 1982;3:71-79.

4. Marshall JL, Rubin RM: Knee ligament injuries: A diagnostic and therapeutic approach. *Orthop Clin North Am* 1977;8:641-668.

5. Grazier KL, Holbrook TL, Kelsey JL, et al: *The Frequency of Occurrence, Impact, and Cost of Musculoskeletal Conditions in the United States.* Chicago, American Academy of Orthopaedic Surgeons, 1984.

6. Liljedahl S-O, Nordstrand A: Injuries to the ligaments of the knee: Diagnosis and results of operation. *Injury* 1969;1:17-24.

7. Dye SF, Anderson CT, Stowell MT: Unrecognized abnormal osseous metabolic activity about the knee of patients with symptomatic ACL deficiency. Presented at the ACL Study Group, Snowmass, CO, March 1988.

8. Palmer I: On the injuries to the ligaments of the knee joint. *Acta Chir Scand Suppl* 1938;81:1-282.

9. Galway RD, Beaupré A, MacIntosh DL: Pivot shift: A clinical sign of symptomatic anterior cruciate insufficiency. *J Bone Joint Surg* 1972;54B:763-764.

10. Hughston JC, Andrews JR, Cross MJ, et al: Classification of knee ligament instabilities: Part I. The medial compartment and cruciate ligaments. *J Bone Joint Surg* 1976;58A:159-172.

11. Hughston JC, Andrews JR, Cross MJ, et al: Classification of knee ligament instabilities: Part II. The lateral compartment. *J Bone Joint Surg* 1976;58A:173-179.

12. Jakob RP, Hassler H, Staeubli H-U: Observations on rotatory instability of the lateral compartment of the knee: Experimental studies on the functional anatomy and the pathomechanism of the true and the reversed pivot shift sign. *Acta Orthop Scand Suppl* 1981;191:1-32.

13. Langrana NA, Bronfeld J: Computer-assisted analysis of ligament constraints in the knee. *Clin Orthop* 1985;196:42-50.

14. Losee RE, Johnson TR, Southwick WO: Anterior subluxation of the lateral tibial plateau: A diagnostic test and operative repair. *J Bone Joint Surg* 1978;60A:1015-1030.

15. MacIntosh DL, Galway HR: The lateral pivot shift: A symptomatic and clinical sign of anterior cruciate insufficiency. Presented at the Annual Meeting of the American Orthopaedic Association, Tucker's Town, Bermuda, June 1972.

16. Markolf KL, Mensch JS, Amstutz HC: Stiffness and laxity of the knee: The contributions of the supporting structures: A quantitative *in vitro* study. *J Bone Joint Surg* 1976;58A:583-594.

17. Noyes FR, Grood ES, Butler DL, et al: Clinical laxity tests and functional stability of the knee: Biomechanical concepts. *Clin Orthop* 1980;146:84-89.

18. Fleming BC, Johnson RJ, Shapiro E, et al: Clinical versus instrumental knee testing. *Clin Orthop*, in press.

19. Marks JS, Palmer MK, Burke MJ, et al: Observer variation in the examination of knee joints. *Ann Rheum Dis* 1978;37:376-377.

20. Pope MH, Johnson R, Kristiansen T, et al: Variations in the examinations of the medial collateral ligament. *J Clin Biomech* 1987;2:71-73.

21. Emery M, Moffroid M, Boerman J, et al: Reliability of force/displacement measures in a clinical device designed to measure ligamentous laxity at the knee. *J Orthop Sports Phys Ther* 1989;10:441-447.

22. Forster IW, Warren-Smith CD, Tew M: Is the KT1000 knee ligament arthrometer reliable? *J Bone Joint Surg* 1989;71B:843-847.

23. Highgenboten CL, Jackson A, Meske NB: Genucom, KT-1000, and Stryker knee laxity measuring device comparisons. *Am J Sports Med* 1989;17:743-746.

24. King JB, Kumar SJ: The Stryker knee arthrometer in clinical practice. *Am J Sports Med* 1989;17:649-650.

25. Sherman O, Markolf K, Weibel W, et al: Instrumented testing of normal and ACL deficient knees: A comparison of two devices. *Trans Orthop Res Soc* 1985;10:275.

26. Häggmark T, Eriksson E: Cylinder or mobile cast brace after knee ligament surgery: A clinical analysis and morphologic and enzymatic studies of changes in the quadriceps muscle. *Am J Sports Med* 1979;7:48-56.

27. Józsa L, Järvinen M, Kannus P, et al: Fine structural changes in the articular cartilage of the rat's knee following short-term immobilisation in various positions: A scanning electron microscopical study. *Int Orthop* 1987;11:129-133.

28. Józsa L, Réffy A, Järvinen M, et al: Cortical and trabecular osteopenia after immobilization: A quantitative histological study of the rat knee. *Int Orthop* 1988;12:169-172.

29. Józsa L, Thöring J, Järvinen M, et al: Quantitative alterations in intramuscular connective tissue following immobilization: An experimental study in the rat calf muscles. *Exp Mol Pathol* 1988;49: 267-278.

30. Kennedy JC: Symposium: Current concepts in the management of knee instability. *Contemp Orthop* 1982;5:59-78.

31. Noyes FR: Functional properties of knee ligaments and alterations induced by immobilization. *Clin Orthop* 1977;123:210-242.

32. Noyes FR, Mangine RE, Barber S: Early knee motion after open and arthroscopic anterior cruciate ligament reconstruction. *Am J Sports Med* 1987;15:149-160.

33. Shelbourne KD, Nitz P: Accelerated rehabilitation after anterior cruciate ligament reconstruction. *Am J Sports Med* 1990;18:292-299.

34. Arms SW, Pope MH, Johnson RJ, et al: The biomechanics of anterior cruciate ligament rehabilitation and reconstruction. *Am J Sports Med* 1984;12:8-18.

35. Arms S, Donnermeyer D, Renstrom P, et al: The effect of knee braces on anterior cruciate ligament strain. *Trans Orthop Res Soc* 1987;12:245.

36. Baker BE, VanHanswyk E, Bogosian S IV, et al: A biomechanical study of the static stabilizing effect of knee braces on medial stability. *Am J Sports Med* 1987;15:566-570.

37. Kennedy JC, Hawkins RJ, Willis RB: Strain gauge analysis of knee ligaments. *Clin Orthop* 1977;129:225-229.

38. Renström P, Arms SW, Stanwyck TS, et al: Strain within the anterior cruciate ligament during hamstring and quadriceps activity. *Am J Sports Med* 1986;14:83-87.

39. Sapega AA, Moyer RA, Schneck C, et al: Testing for isometry during reconstruction of the anterior cruciate ligament: Anatomical and biomechanical considerations. *J Bone Joint Surg* 1990;72A:259-267.

40. Trent PS, Walker PS, Wolf B: Ligament length patterns, strength, and rotational axes of the knee joint. *Clin Orthop* 1976;117:263-270.

41. Wang CJ, Walker PS: The effects of flexion and rotation on the length patterns of the ligaments of the knee. *J Biomech* 1973;6:587-596.

42. Beynnon BD, Fleming BC, Erickson AR, et al: Characterization of the anterior cruciate ligament strain pattern in vivo. Presented at the Annual Meeting of the American Society of Biomechanics, Champaign, IL, September 1988.

43. Beynnon BD, Pope MH, Fleming BC, et al: An in-vivo study of the ACL strain biomechanics in the normal knee. *Trans Orthop Res Soc* 1989;14:324.

44. Beynnon BD, Pope MH, Wertheimer CM, et al: The effect of functional knee braces on anterior cruciate ligament strain *in vivo*. *J Bone Joint Surg*, in press.

45. Beynnon BD, Howe JG, Pope MH, et al: The measurement of anterior cruciate ligament strain *in vivo*. *Int Orthop* (SICOT) 1992;16:1-12.

46. Kain CC, McCarthy JJ, Arms S, et al: An *in-vivo* study of the effect of transcutaneous electrical muscle stimulation on ACL deformation. *Trans Orthop Res Soc* 1987;12:106.

47. American Academy of Orthopaedic Surgeons: *Knee Braces: Seminar Report*. Chicago, American Academy of Orthopaedic Surgeons, 1985.

48. Colville MR, Lee CL, Ciullo JV: The Lenox Hill brace: An evaluation of effectiveness in treating knee instability. *Am J Sports Med* 1986;14:257-261.

49. Cook FF, Tibone JE, Redfern FC: A dynamic analysis of a functional brace for anterior cruciate ligament insufficiency. *Am J Sports Med* 1989;17:519-524.

50. Branch T, Hunter R, Reynolds P: Controlling anterior tibial displacement under static load: A comparison of two braces. *Orthopedics* 1988;11:1249-1252.

51. Wojtys EM, Goldstein SA, Redfern M, et al: A biomechanical evaluation of the Lenox Hill knee brace. *Clin Orthop* 1987;220:179-183.

52. Yoshiya S, Andrish JT, Manley MT, et al: Graft tension in anterior cruciate ligament reconstruction: An in vivo study in dogs. *Am J Sports Med* 1987;15:464-470.

53. Burks RT, Leland R: Determination of graft tension before fixation in anterior cruciate ligament reconstruction. *Arthroscopy* 1988;4:260-266.

54. Grood ES, Hefzy MS, Butler DL, et al: On the placement and the initial tension of anterior cruciate ligament substitutes. *Trans Orthop Res Soc* 1983;8:92.

55. Kurosaka M, Yoshiya S, Andrish JT: A biomechanical comparison of different surgical techniques of graft fixation in anterior cruciate ligament reconstruction. *Am J Sports Med* 1987;15:225-229.

56. Robertson DB, Daniel DM, Biden E: Soft tissue fixation to bone. *Am J Sports Med* 1986;14:398-403.

57. Arnoczky SP, Tarvin GB, Marshall JL: Anterior cruciate ligament replacement using patellar tendon: An evaluation of graft revascularization in the dog. *J Bone Joint Surg* 1982;64A:217-224.

58. Butler DL, Noyes FR, Grood ES, et al: Mechanical properties of transplants for the anterior cruciate ligament. *Trans Orthop Res Soc* 1979;4:81.

59. Butler DL, Noyes FR, Grood ES, et al: The effects of vascularity on the mechanical properties of primate anterior cruciate ligament replacements. *Trans Orthop Res Soc* 1983;8:93.

60. Graf B: Isometric placement of substitutes for the anterior cruciate ligament, in Jackson DW, Drez D Jr (eds): *The Anterior Cruciate Deficient Knee: New Concepts in Ligament Repair.* St. Louis, CV Mosby, 1987, pp 102-113.

61. Grood ES, Hefzy MS, Lindenfield TN: Factors affecting the region of most isometric femoral attachments: Part I. The posterior cruciate ligament. *Am J Sports Med* 1989;17:197-207.

62. Hefzy MS, Grood ES: Sensitivity of insertion locations on length patterns of anterior cruciate ligament fibers. *J Biomech Eng* 1986;108:73-82.

63. Hefzy MS, Grood ES, Noyes FR: Factors affecting the region of most isometric femoral attachments: Part II. The anterior cruciate ligament. *Am J Sports Med* 1989;17:208-216.

64. Melhorn JM, Henning CE: The relationship of the femoral attachment site to the isometric tracking of the anterior cruciate ligament graft. *Am J Sports Med* 1987;15:539-542.

65. Penner DA, Daniel DM, Wood P, et al: An in vitro study of anterior cruciate ligament graft placement and isometry. *Am J Sports Med* 1988;16:238-243.

66. Sidles JA, Larson RV, Garbini JL, et al: Ligament length relationships in the moving knee. *J Orthop Res* 1988;6:593-610.

67. Siegel MG, Grood E, Hefzy S: Analysis and placement of the anterior cruciate ligament substitute. *Orthop Trans* 1984;8:69.

68. Wilcox PG, Jackson DW: Arthroscopic anterior cruciate ligament reconstruction. *Clin Sports Med* 1987;6:513-524.

69. Pope MH, Stankewich CJ, Beynnon BD, et al: The effect of knee musculature on ACL strain *in-vivo. J Electromyography Kinesiol* 1991;1:191-198.

70. Beynnon BD: The in vivo biomechanics of the anterior cruciate ligament, reconstruction, and application of a mathematical model to the knee joint, thesis. Burlington, University of Vermont, 1991.

71. Fleming BC, Beynnon BD, Erickson AR, et al: An *in-vivo* study of the reconstructed anterior cruciate ligament at the time of implantation. *Trans Orthop Res Soc* 1990;15:84.

72. Kurosawa H, Yamakoshi K-I, Yasuda K, et al: Simultaneous measurement of changes in length of the cruciate ligaments during knee motion. *Clin Orthop* 1991;265:233-240.

73. Torzilli PA, Greenberg RL, Insall J: An *in vivo* biomechanical evaluation of anterior-posterior motion of the knee. *J Bone Joint Surg* 1981;63A:960-968

74. Martin MS: The effect of flexion, tibial rotation and depth on the 3-D orientation length and straightness of the human cruciate ligaments, thesis. Cincinnati, University of Cincinnati, 1987.

75. Daniel DM, Malcom LL, Losse G, et al: Instrumented measurement of anterior laxity of the knee. *J Bone Joint Surg* 1985;67A:720-726.

76. Henning CE, Lynch MA, Glick JR Jr: An in vivo strain gage study of elongation of the anterior cruciate ligament. *Am J Sports Med* 1985;13:22-26.

77. Markolf KL, Graff-Radford A, Amstutz HC: In vivo knee stability: A quantitative assessment using an instrumented clinical testing apparatus. *J Bone Joint Surg* 1978;60A:664-674.

78. Torg JS, Conrad W, Kalen V: Clinical diagnosis of anterior cruciate ligament instability in the athlete. *Am J Sports Med* 1976;4:84-93.

79. Torzilli PA, Greenberg RL, Hood RW, et al: Measurement of anterior-posterior motion of the knee in injured patients using a biomechanical stress technique. *J Bone Jont Surg* 1984;66A;1438-1442.

80. Morrison JB: Bioengineering analysis of force actions transmitted by the knee joint. *J Biomed Eng* 1968;3:164-170.

81. Morrison JB: Function of the knee joint in various activities. *J Biomed Eng* 1969;4:573-580.

82. Morrison JB: The mechanics of the knee joint in relation to normal walking. *J Biomech* 1970;3:51-61.

83. Noyes FR, Butler DL, Grood ES, et al: Biomechanical analysis of human ligament grafts used in knee-ligament repairs and reconstructions. *J Bone Joint Surg* 1984;66A:344-352.

84. Romash MM, Henningsen HJ: Comparative functional testing of knee braces. Presented at the Fifty-Sixth Annual Meeting of the American Academy of Orthopaedic Surgeons, Las Vegas, NV, Feb 1989.

Chapter 20

Placement of Knee Ligament Grafts

Edward S. Grood, PhD

Introduction

The knee is a complex mechanism in which the ligaments, capsular structures, menisci, joint cartilage, and bones all interact to provide normal motion and function. When knee ligaments are injured, it is impossible to restore the normal anatomy and mechanical properties of the injured structure or the joint as a whole. Thus, some deficit always remains after surgery. As a result, controversy exists regarding the optimum surgical technique to stabilize the knee following ligament injuries.

The outcome of knee ligament reconstruction is influenced by numerous factors. Not all of the factors are well understood and some of them are not readily controllable. One factor that is under direct control of the surgeon is placement of the ligament graft. In this paper, the term graft is used to refer to all types of ligament replacements, and the term placement is used to mean all the geometric variables that describe how the graft is implanted within the knee. The geometric variables include the route used in passing the graft from tibia to femur (for example, over the top versus through bone tunnels), the location of the intra-articular entrance of any bone tunnels or troughs (also called the attachment location), the orientation of the tunnels within the bones, any twists placed in the graft, and the site of its fixation to bone. Related factors, which cannot be considered independent of placement, are the amount of pre-tension applied before fixation and the position of the knee at the time of pre-tensioning.

Improper placement and tensioning are known to result in a number of postsurgical complications. These include a reduced range of motion immediately after surgery, failure of the graft's attachment to bone, and incomplete removal of pathologic laxity.[1] Other complications, such as the return of laxity over time, might also result, in part, from improper placement.

Placement Goals

A major goal of recent surgical placement techniques has been to locate attachments that yield an isometric graft.[2-10] The concept of isometry is a misnomer because not all graft fibers are expected to remain isometric as the knee is flexed. The primary objective of isometric placement is to prevent excessive elongation or slackening of the graft as the knee is flexed or extended from the angle where the graft is pre-tensioned and fixed to bone. Excessive elongation produces large graft forces that can limit the full range of motion, fail attachments to bone, or cause permanent stretching over time. Excessive slacking results in pathologic laxity.

Other goals in the selection of appropriate graft placement include avoiding deleterious bone impingement, restoring the normal relationship between physiologic laxity and flexion angle, and restoring normal load sharing among the ligaments.

It has not yet been established that locating isometric attachments is the proper or most important goal of placement. Two possibilities need to be considered in this regard. First, intraoperative determination of isometric attachments might yield locations that are not isometric in the intact or reconstructed knee. A number of factors already have been identified that affect the accuracy of intraoperative determination of isometric attachments. Second, because the majority of fibers in normal ligaments are not isometric, an isometric graft might not restore normal knee mechanics. In fact, a recent study by Galloway and associates[11,12] suggests a nonisometric intraoperative posterior cruciate graft is better in this regard than an isometric one.

Important variables, other than attachment location, are the amount of pre-tension applied and the flexion angle where the graft is fixed (tensioning angle)[13,14] because they establish the initial mechanical state of the graft and of the knee. Lewis and associates[15-17] have demonstrated abnormal load sharing among the ligaments following reconstruction and have developed improved methods for tensioning that might allow the surgeon to restore more completely normal knee mechanics. Clearly, the goals of placement should not be limited to obtaining isometric placement at the time of surgery.

This chapter is divided into three major sections. The first section covers some of the properties of ligaments and ligament length patterns that underlie the concept of isometric placement. The second section reviews studies on the isometry of both medial and lateral capsular and collateral ligament reconstructions. This section also includes a discussion of Burmester Curves, which have been used to explain the attachments of the collateral ligaments and capsular structures as well as to predict appropriate bone attachments for extra-articular reconstructions. The third section considers the cruciate ligaments. Emphasis is placed on the anterior cruciate ligament (ACL) because it is more frequently injured and reconstructed than the posterior cruciate ligament (PCL). As a result, the majority of published studies also focus on the ACL.

Basic Concepts

As early as 1911, Fick[18] recognized that ligaments do not act as a single uniform structure. Rather, ligaments are composed of fibers, often described as being grouped into two or three bands, that are not all tense at the same time. Fick noted that knee flexion angle was an important variable that determined which bands are tense and which are slack.[18]

In the period since Fick's work, it has been demonstrated that the location of ligament fibers' attachment to bone plays an important role in the way knee flexion affects fiber tension. Fiber tension is important because it is an indicator that the fiber has been recruited to resist joint motions. The relationship between fiber tension, flexion angle, and attachment location is mediated by three separate relationships: (1) how the tension in a fiber depends on its length, (2) how the length of a fiber varies with knee flexion angle, and (3) how the relationship between length and flexion angle depends on the fiber's attachment location.

Length-Tension Relationship

The elastic properties of ligaments allow them to stretch and develop the tension needed to resist further tibiofemoral displacements or to become slack and nonfunctional. However, ligament fibers develop tension only within a small range of lengths. This is illustrated in Figure 1, which shows a length-tension curve reconstructed from tensile failure test data on young human ACL fiber bundles.[19] When the distance between bone attachments is less than L_0, the fiber bundle is slack and nonfunctional. If the distance between attachments is more than 1.12 to 1.16 L_0, the fiber bundle fails and becomes nonfunctional. Thus, the fiber bundle can function only when its length is within the small range of lengths beginning at L_0 and ending with failure at lengths 12% to 16% greater than L_0. Because failure begins in the upper region of this range, normal function probably uses only the lower region of the range, the shaded region in Figure 1. The size of this region has been estimated to include strains of 5% and less.[20] This estimate is supported by recent in vivo measurements of strain in the ACL anterior medial band. A strain of 4.0% ± 0.8% was measured when a 150-N anterior shear force was applied to the knee at 30 degrees of flexion.[21] It is not yet known what strains and tensions are developed by locomotor and other activities of daily living.

Length-Flexion Angle Relationship

Because ligament fibers function only within a small range of lengths and because the fiber's length varies with the flexion angle, most fibers function only over a limited range of flexion angles. A curve that shows how fiber length depends on flexion angle is called a length pattern.

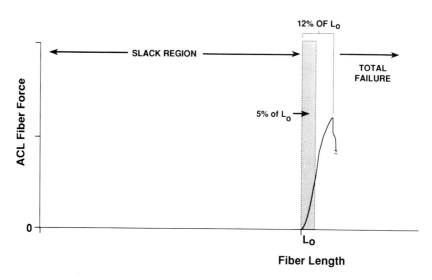

Fig. 1   *Force-length curve for human ACL fibers. Fiber force is shown as a function of the distance between attachments (length). In-vivo functional activities are thought to occur within the shaded region, which corresponds to fiber strain of only 5%.*

Length patterns of ligament fiber bundles and bands have been studied by numerous investigators. Because the actual length of a fiber bundle is hard to measure directly, investigators often have used the distance between attachments in place of length. The distance between attachments and fiber length is the same only when the fiber follows a straight line path between its attachments.

Figure 2 shows three different fiber length patterns described by Krackow and Brooks,[22] based on studies of extra-articular reconstructions. Other length patterns are also possible. The shaded regions show the range of flexion angles within which the fiber is expected to develop a tension and be functional. The size of the region is estimated by assuming the longest length on a curve corresponds to a fiber strain of 5%. When the length falls to a strain of zero, the fiber becomes slack and nonfunctional. Some fibers will function in extension (type II), others primarily in flexion (type III), and others within an intermediate range of angles (type I).

Dependence of Length Pattern on Femoral Attachment Location

While a fiber's length pattern is affected by many factors, it is particularly sensitive to the location of the fiber's femoral attachment and much less sensitive to that of the fiber's tibial attachment. Bartel and associates,[23] studying medial reconstructions, were probably the first to note this observation. Similar results have also

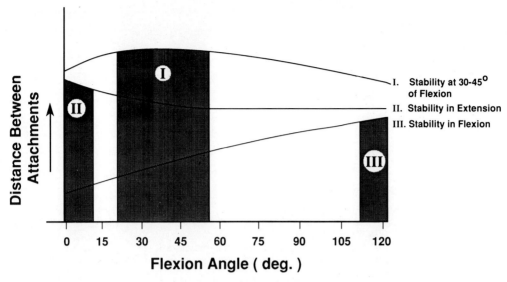

Fig. 2 *Three types of length patterns. Type I is appropriate for combating instability between 30 and 45 degrees of flexion because this is the region in which the ligament, so positioned, would be tightest. Type II would be appropriate for a situation where stability was sought in full extension, and type III would be appropriate for achieving stability in flexion. Other patterns are also possible. (Adapted with permission from Krackow KA, Brooks RL: Optimization of knee ligament position for lateral extraarticular reconstruction.* Am J Sports Med *1983;11:293-302.)*

been reported for the cruciate ligaments[24] and lateral extra-articular reconstructions.[22]

A simple model that explains these experimental findings and also shows how the length pattern is altered by a change in femoral attachment location was described by Grood and associates[3] (Fig. 3). The tibia and tibial attachment (T) of a fiber are stationary in the model. It is assumed, for the sake of simplicity, that flexion of the femur occurs about a fixed center of rotation (CR). This fixed center is considered to be located at the average center of rotation for real knee flexion. With this simplification, all femoral attachments will follow circular paths about the center of rotation. The radius of the circle is determined by the distance from the femoral attachment to the center of rotation. The circular path followed by the femoral attachments makes it easier to visualize how the length of any fiber changes with knee flexion.

Consider the fiber shown, which attaches anterior to the CR at location F_a. This fiber will lengthen during the first 90 degrees of flexion as its femoral attachment rises up the circle until it is directly above the center of rotation. Further flexion causes the fiber to shorten as its femoral attachment follows the descending portion of the circle. The length pattern for this fiber is shown in the graph.

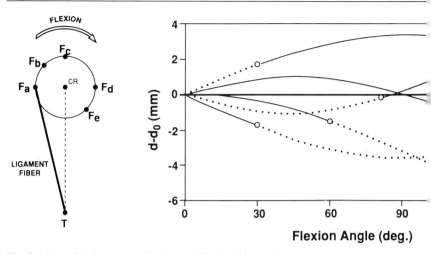

Fig. 3 *Length patterns are determined by the femoral attachment location. A ligament fiber is shown with tibial attachment, T, and femoral attachment F_a. Other femoral attachments are represented by points F_b through F_e. The femur is assumed to flex about a fixed center of rotation, CR. The graph shows how the distance between attachments (d) referenced to the distance between attachments at 0 degrees (d_o) varies with flexion to 120 degrees. The curves are solid in the region over which the ligament fiber is tense and dotted in the region over which it is slack. The functional region is obtained by assuming the fiber is strained 5% at its maximum length.*

The curve is drawn as a solid line when the fiber length is within 5% of its maximum length (and assumed to be tense) and as a fine dotted line when it is shorter (and assumed to be slack).

Length patterns, drawn in a similar fashion for the four other femoral attachments, show wide diversity for small changes of the femoral attachment location. A fiber attached at site F_b lengthens during the first 45 degrees of flexion and shortens during the last 90 degrees. The opposite occurs with a fiber attached at site F_e.

The model shows that the overall shape of a fiber's length pattern depends on where, around the circle, the fiber attaches. Further, it is easy to verify that the shape of the length pattern is not affected by the circle's radius. However, the magnitude of the change in length will be in direct proportion to the distance between the femoral attachment and the CR.

The effect of changing the tibial attachment also can be studied with this model. Moving the attachment directly toward or away from the CR will change neither the basic shape of the length pattern nor the flexion angle where the fiber is longest and shortest. Moving the tibial attachment perpendicular to the line connecting it to the CR also will have only a small effect. This effect is primarily caused by how the change in tibial attachment location alters the relative position of the femoral attachment around the circle. The relative position is measured from the bottom of the circle, defined by the intersection of the circle with the line connecting the CR to the tibial attachment. If the tibial attachment of the fiber shown in Figure 3 is moved to the left, the bottom of the circle also shifts to the left causing the femoral attachment side F_a to be located at a lower point on the rising side of the circle. This causes a small change in the flexion angles where the fiber is longest and shortest without changing the basic shape of the length pattern.

The model presented above is only approximate because the knee does not have a fixed center of rotation. Nevertheless, the basic features described can be seen in length patterns measured on human knees in vitro.

Contour Plots

The finite size of a ligament's femoral attachment makes it impossible for all fibers within a ligament to have the same length pattern. To map out the behavior of the fibers requires a large number of length pattern curves. An even greater number of curves are required if one is interested in studying potential graft attachments that lie outside the anatomical insertion of the injured ligament. Sidles and associates[10] and others[3,4] have avoided this problem by using contour plots to illustrate the effect of femoral attachment location. A typical contour plot (Fig. 4) is composed of a series of contour lines. A single contour line contains all attachments that produce the same maximum fiber strain. The region bounded by the contour line with the smallest maximum strain contains the most isometric attachments. Thus, contour plots show both the shape and size of the region of most isometric attachments.

The contour plots also show the directions along which a change in attachment location has the smallest and largest effect on maximum strain. These directions correspond to the direction along and perpendicular to the contour lines, respectively. In addition, the spacing between lines provides a visual clue as to how rapidly the changes occur. A disadvantage of contour plots is that they do not show the shape of the underlying length pattern curve. Thus, the flexion angles at which fibers are tense or slack is not presented. Moreover, each contour plot assumes a single tibial attachment.

Extra-articular Reconstructions

Medial Reconstructions

The earliest studies of placement[22,23,25,26] focused on extra-articular repairs and reconstructions. Bartel and associates[23] were probably the first to recognize that length patterns were more sensitive to the femoral attachment site than to the tibial attachment site. They found that advancing the medial collateral ligament's (MCL) femoral origin produced large ligament strains, while advancing its tibial attachment produced only small strains. Because tibial advance-

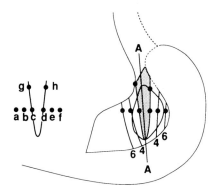

LATERAL CONDYLE

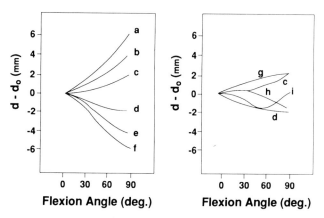

Fig. 4 *Typical contour plot for the anterior cruciate ligament. This figure was determined for knee flexion from 0 to 90 degrees while an anterior force of 100 N was applied to the tibia. The tibial attachment site used in the analysis was located in the geometric center of the ACL's tibial insertion. (Reproduced with permission from Hefzy MS, Grood ES, Noyes FR: Factors affecting the region of most isometric femoral attachments: Part II. The anterior cruciate ligament. Am J Sports Med 1989;17:208-216.)*

ments are more difficult to perform, some surgeons now choose to recess the MCL's femoral attachment into the medial condyle, thereby removing the slack in the ligament without changing its attachment location.

Although most studies on placement have been based on the measurement or computation of length patterns, Menschik[25,26] has developed an alternate approach for determining acceptable attachments. This approach is based on both the four-bar mechanism model of the knee first proposed by Strasser,[27] (Fig. 5) and on a mathematical theory for analyzing mechanism motion developed by Burmester.[28] In simple terms, Burmester's theory allows the determination of all pairs of femoral and tibial attachments that remain

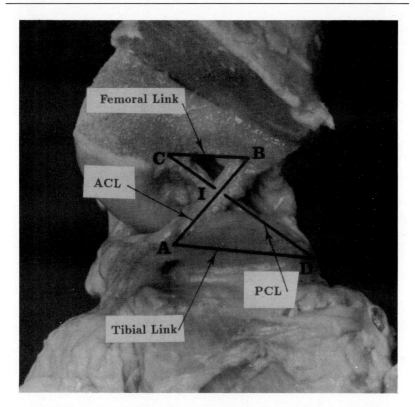

Fig. 5 *A human knee with the lateral femoral condyle removed, exposing the cruciate ligaments. Superimposed is a diagram of a four-bar linkage comprising the anterior cruciate ligament AB, the posterior cruciate ligament CD, the femoral link CB joining the ligament attachment points on the femur, and the tibial link AD joining their attachment points on the tibia. (Reproduced with permission from O'Connor J, Shercliff T, FitzPatrick D, et al: Geometry of the knee, in Daniel DM, Akeson WH, O'Connor JJ (eds):* Knee Ligaments: Structure, Function, Injury, and Repair. *New York, Raven Press, 1990, pp 163-199.)*

the same distance apart (that is, attachments that are isometric) as the mechanism is moved through small (infinitesimal) motions. Collectively, the pairs of attachment points make two curves (Fig. 6). These curves are called cubics because of their mathematical form. One cubic contains all possible femoral attachments, the other all possible tibial attachments. A single pair of attachments is obtained by drawing a straight line through the instant center for knee flexion that, in the four-bar mechanism model of the knee, is located at the point where the cruciate links cross each other. The tibial and femoral attachments are the points where this line crosses the tibial and femoral cubics. All other pairs can be obtained by rotating the line about the center of rotation.

Mueller[29] has used Burmester curves to explain the attachment locations of the collateral ligaments and capsular structures. This use appears to be supported by the good agreement between attach-

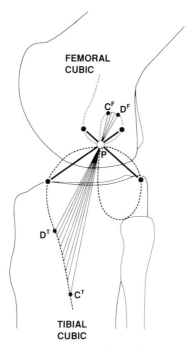

Fig. 6 *Burmester curves for the four-bar mechanism. There are two separate curves, a femoral cubic and a tibial cubic. Pairs of nearly isometric attachments can be obtained by passing a line through instant center, P, and extending the line until it crosses both cubics. The points C^F and C^T where the line crosses the cubics are nearly isometric. Other pairs of nearly isometric attachments can be found by rotating the line about the instant center. The lines shown here represent theoretical fibers of the medial collateral ligament. (Reproduced with permission from Mueller W:* The Knee: Structure, Function, Injury, and Repair. *Berlin, Springer-Verlag, 1983.)*

ment locations found in Mueller's dissections and the shape of the Burmester curves. However, there are several reasons for believing Burmester curves cannot be used to explain ligament attachments.

First, Mueller[29] recognized that Burmester theory is based on small motions. This led him to question whether the distance between pairs of Burmester attachments remains isometric over a full range of knee flexion. Sidles (personal communication, 1986) found that while Burmester attachments were not isometric, the change in length was indeed small. However, Sidles also found tibial attachments, not on the Burmester curve, that were as and more isometric than those on the Burmester curve. Although the region that contained these attachments was only a few millimeters wide in the proximodistal direction, it covered nearly the entire width of the tibia in the anteroposterior direction. Thus, the tibial Burmester attachments are not more isometric than other tibial attachments when a large range of knee motion is considered.

There is a second, and perhaps more significant, problem in the clinical application of Burmester curves. Their shape is not unique

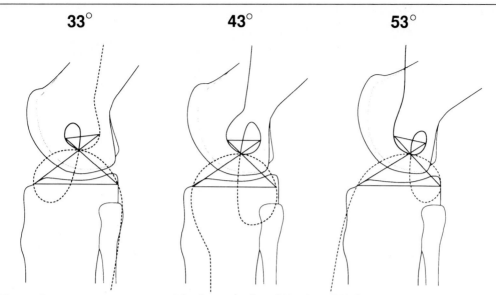

Fig. 7   *Burmester curves computed for flexion angles of 33, 43, and 53 degrees. The curves for 43 degrees of flexion are nearly identical to the curves published by Menschik[25,26] and Mueller.[29] Note that most of the tibial cubics for 33 and 53 degrees of flexion are not on the tibia, and, thus, they are not possible ligament attachments.*

and it depends strongly on the flexion angle assumed when they are computed. Menschik[25,26] only published the curve for 43 degrees of flexion. Figure 7 shows curves computed for three flexion angles. The one for 43 degrees agrees well with Menschik's curves; the others demonstrate the widely varying shapes that are possible with only small changes in flexion angles. None of the others show any similarity to the attachments of the normal collateral ligaments. Further, there is no criterion for why the curve for 43 degrees of flexion should be used over the other curves.

Lateral Reconstructions

Krackow and Brooks[22] measured the length patterns of a large number of tibial and femoral attachments for lateral extra-articular reconstructions and found that no pair of attachments was isometric. In order to eliminate a positive pivot shift sign, they recommended a pair of attachments whose length pattern was longest near 20 to 30 degrees of flexion. This ensures the reconstruction will be under tension and able to resist tibial subluxation near these angles. The recommended femoral attachment was located at the junction of the lateral femoral condyle and the femoral shaft at site F_9 in Figure 8, *left*. The tibial attachment was located at Gerdy's tubercle, T_3 site. A length pattern for this pair of attachments is shown in Figure 9, along with patterns for several other femoral attachments

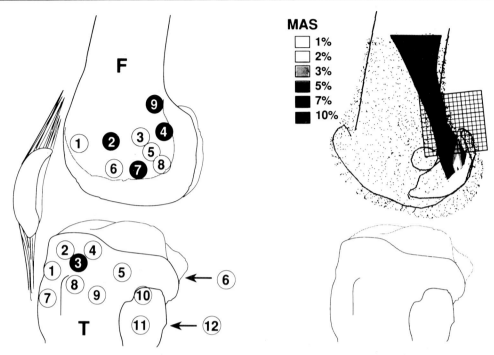

Fig. 8 *Left, Extra-articular attachments studied by Krackow and Brooks.[22] F = femur, T = tibia. Point F-5 is the origin of lateral collateral ligament at lateral epicondyle, T-10 is the insertion of the lateral collateral ligament, and T-3 is Gerdy's tubercle. (Reproduced with permission from Krackow KA, Brooks RL: Optimization of knee ligament position for lateral extraarticular reconstruction. Am J Sports Med 1983;11:293-302.)* **Right,** *Extra-articular isometry map of Sidles and associates[10] for 0 to 110 degrees of flexion. Tibial load is anterior during flexion. The articular surface and lateral aspect of the knee are shown as scattered points. The lateral articular margin, lateral collateral ligament attachment, notch roof, lateral notch margin, and posterior femoral midline are continuous lines. The squares in the grid are 2 mm on a side. (Reproduced with permission from Sidles JA, Larson RV, Garbini JL, et al: Ligament length relationships in the moving knee. J Orthop Res 1988;6:593-610.)*

paired with the same tibial attachment. The closest other femoral attachment studied, F_4, had a length pattern that was longest near 60 degrees of flexion.

Krackow's results are consistent with contour plots of maximum absolute strain for lateral extra-articular reconstructions determined by Sidles and associates.[10] These contour plots were determined from measurement of three-dimensional motion and bone anatomy of human cadaveric specimens. The resulting contour plots are shown in Figure 8, *right*, rotated and scaled to the same size as the adjacent figure from Krackow and Brooks.[22] As noted above, the most isometric region is the one with the smallest maximum absolute strain. This region is close to Krackow and Brooks' site F_4 and is directly posterior to the femoral attachment of the lateral collateral ligament, about 6 mm from the cartilage margin (Fig. 8, *right*).

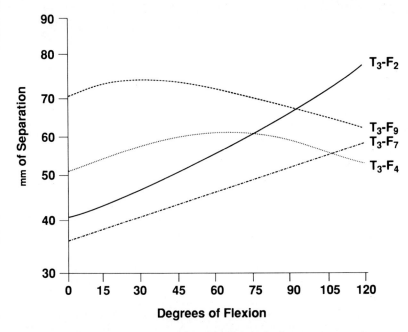

Fig. 9 *Each curve shown has been averaged over the five specimens after normalizing to a common mean. The widely differing contours of these four curves show the influence of changing the femoral attachment while the tibial connection, T_3, remains the same. (Reproduced with permission from Krackow KA, Brooks RL: Optimization of knee ligament position for lateral extraarticular reconstruction. Am J Sports Med 1983;11:293-302.)*

However, the position of the region of smallest maximum absolute strain varied greatly between knees. Sidles and associates[10] speculated this variation was caused by an observed sensitivity of extra-articular length patterns to axial tibial rotation.

Engebretsen and associates[30] studied the effect on knee mechanics of an iliotibial band tenodesis, fixed at Krackow's F_9 site. The tenodesis was performed before and after an intra-articular reconstruction with a patellar tendon graft. The tenodesis held the tibia in an abnormal externally rotated position whether performed before or after the intra-articular reconstruction. In contrast, the intra-articular reconstruction did not alter tibial rotation. The tenodesis also unloaded the patellar tendon graft. The ability to unload the patellar tendon graft was greater when the tenodesis was performed after the intra-articular reconstruction.

Intra-articular Reconstructions

Normal Anatomy and Length Patterns

Knowledge of fiber function in a normal cruciate ligament is a prerequisite to the development of ligament substitutes or reconstructive procedures that mimic their function. Even after numerous studies,[6,18,31-38] there is no consensus on the anatomy of either cruciate ligament. In the ACL, some investigators identify two[18,31,33] or three[34,38] primary bands, while others maintain the ACL comprises a continuum of fibers.[6,35-37] It is not surprising, therefore, that there is also disagreement on the flexion angles where fibers are tense and functional.

There is general agreement that the most isometric ACL fibers originate anteroproximally on the femur and insert anteromedially on the tibia.[4,18,36,38] However, disagreement still exists over the remainder of the ligament's anatomy and function. Fuss[36] has proposed that only the most anteromedial fibers are tight in full flexion, with the remaining fibers progressively recruited as the knee is extended. Amis and Dawkins,[38] however, report that some posterior fibers are also tense in full flexion. Kurosawa and associates[39] describe the anteromedial band as being longest between 60 and 70 degrees of flexion, with it becoming shorter as the knee is brought to full flexion or full extension. A recent study by Blankevoort and associates[40] shows the anterior portion of the ACL to have a variable length pattern. In three knees, it was slack in extension and in one knee, it was only tense in extension.

Some of the disagreement in the literature was explained by Hefzy and Grood,[24] who noted that ligament length patterns depend strongly on the location of the femoral attachment. They used this finding to show how differences among results of prior studies[41-45] could be caused by small differences in the femoral attachment locations used.

Regions of Fiber Lengthening and Shortening

A number of investigators have more thoroughly studied how femoral attachment location affects length patterns of both the ACL[4,10,46,47] and the PCL.[3,10] These investigators found, for each cruciate ligament, that the femoral surface could be divided into two regions. Within one region the primary fiber response was lengthening so that fibers were longer in flexion than extension. The reverse occurred for the other region. Fibers that attach at the boundary where the two regions meet have the same length in extension as in flexion. Bradley and associates[46] further subdivided each region, based on whether the initial length change with flexion was shortening or lengthening.

The line dividing the primary shortening and lengthening regions has a different orientation for the two cruciate ligaments (Fig. 10). The line for the ACL is oriented primarily in the proximodistal direction, so that anterior fibers are longer in flexion while posterior fibers are shorter.[4,10,24] The line for the PCL is oriented primarily in the anteroposterior direction. Fibers proximal to the line are shorter in flexion while those distal to the line are longer in flexion.

The amount of fiber lengthening and shortening was found to depend strongly on the distance between the fiber's origin and the line that separated the shortening and lengthening regions. This can be appreciated from the contour plots in Figure 4. The further the attachment is from this line, the greater the length change. In contrast, fibers attached along the line separating the regions had the smallest changes in length.

These findings are important to surgical reconstruction, because they show that the effect of an error in placement depends on the direction of the error. An error in placement perpendicular to the line will have much greater effect than the same error made in the direction of the line. For ACL grafts, placement errors in the femur's anteroposterior direction have the largest effect. Similarly, placement errors for PCL grafts are largest if the error is in the femur's proximodistal direction.

Similar rules for other ligaments of the knee, and for the ligaments of other joints can easily be obtained. All that is needed is to determine the orientation of the line that separates regions of fiber lengthening from regions of shortening. This is obtained from the orientation of the line connecting the average center of rotation and the center of the ligament's tibial attachment when the knee is midway in its range of flexion.

Studies on Intra-Articular Graft Placement

The last two sections discussed studies conducted on intact knees. This section deals with placement studies in which the anterior cruciate ligament was removed and reconstructed. Surprisingly, there are relatively few such studies. In these, the effect of femoral attachment location is considered first, followed by the effect of tibial attachment location.

Femoral Attachment Location   There are two basic approaches to the femoral attachment of grafts. The graft can be fixed within a femoral tunnel or it can be pulled over the top of the lateral femoral condyle and fixed to the femur extra-articularly. Several investigators and clinical experience have shown that over the top reconstructions become slack with flexion, causing excessive anterior translation.[1,6,13] As a result, many clinicians place a trough in the femoral condyle so the graft passes closer to the ACL's anatomic insertion. This technique has been shown to be more isometric than over the top alone and, also, to eliminate excessive anterior translation with flexion. At the same time the technique eliminates two advantages of the over the top alone approach: (1) the lack of rough bone edges that can cause abrasion, and (2) the lower sensitivity of the result to surgical technique.[13] Instead of the reproducible and consistent graft shortening with flexion, the length pattern will depend on the variable depth of the trough. As a result, there is proba-

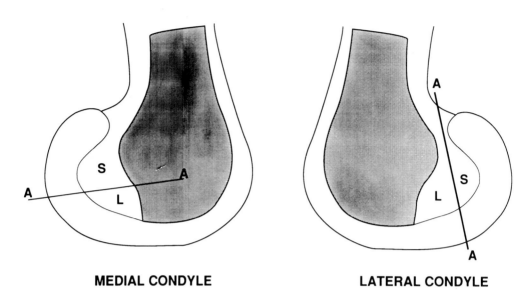

MEDIAL CONDYLE   **LATERAL CONDYLE**

Fig. 10   *The division of the femoral surface into shortening and lengthening regions. The line, A-A, dividing the regions has a different orientation for the two cruciate ligaments. Small errors in placement along the direction of the line have only small effects on length patterns. In contrast, placement errors perpendicular to the line cause large changes in length patterns.*

bly little difference between using the over the top technique with a trough and a properly placed femoral tunnel.

Melhorn and Henning,[1] in a retrospective clinical review, showed that the pattern of anteroposterior translation correlated with the graft's femoral attachment location. Twelve previously reconstructed knees were divided into three groups, based on femoral attachment location as determined from radiographs: anterior tunnel, over the top, and over the top with a deep bone trough. Anterior laxity of each group was measured in extension (20 degrees) and flexion (90 degrees). The authors found that (1) the anterior placement group was loose in extension but tight in flexion; (2) the over the top group showed the opposite pattern, being tight in extension and lax in flexion; and (3) only the deep bone trough group was tight at both flexion angles.

Penner and associates[7] showed that changes in the distance between graft attachments were associated with changes in graft tension. The greater the distance between attachments, the greater the tension. Tension was measured during knee flexion in four groups differing in femoral placement: anterior tunnel, posterior tunnel, over the top, and over the top plus trough. For each route, they determined how much of the graft had to be withdrawn (or inserted) into the tibial tunnel to maintain a constant graft tension. Large tension changes were associated with the anterior tunnel and over the top groups. In the over the top group, the graft had to be with-drawn from the tunnel as the knee was flexed to maintain a constant tension. The anterior tunnel group exhibited the opposite behavior, with the extra-articular part of the graft having to be inserted into the tibial tunnel as the knee was flexed to maintain a constant tension. The smallest changes occurred for the over the top plus trough and the posterior tunnel groups. Unfortunately, the precise location of the femoral tunnels was not clearly described.

The results of these studies are, for the most part, consistent with each other and with the results of Bylski-Austrow and associates,[13] who measured length patterns and anteroposterior translation in the intact knee and graft tension and anteroposterior translation in the reconstructed knee. Three tunnel locations, anterior, distal, and posterior, were studied along with an over the top routing combined with four extra-articular attachment locations. Once the graft was passed over the top, the results did not depend on where it was fixed to bone. Further, the variation in results for all over the top groups combined was much less than for any of the femoral tunnel locations. This suggests the outcome of over the top reconstructions may be more consistent and reproducible than femoral tunnel reconstructions.

Overall, Bylski-Austrow and associates[13] found that the knee had the least anterior translation and the graft the largest tensions under conditions where the distance between attachments was longest. The only significant difference with the results of Penner and associates[7] was for the posterior tunnel. Where Penner and associates[7] found little change in tension with knee flexion, Bylski-Austrow and associates[13] found both decreased tension and increased anterior translation with flexion. This disagreement might be due to differences in the location of the posterior tunnel used or to Bylski-Austrow's use of a fine cable substitute and Penner's use of The Kennedy Ligament Augmentation Device as a substitute.

Schutzer and associates[9] measured the length patterns in knees reconstructed with a 6-mm diameter synthetic replacement. They investigated the intact knee and reconstructions at three femoral attachments: anatomic, over the top, and anterior. The length pattern most similar to that of the intact knee was the anatomic tibial attachment combined with the anatomic femoral attachment. Over the top femoral attachment produced significant shortening with flexion, while the anterior tunnel produced significant lengthening.

Tibial Attachment Location   Schutzer and associates[9] also reported on three tibial attachments: anterior, anatomic, and posterior. Although none of the effects were statistically significant, there were a few possible trends. With an anteriorly placed femoral graft, a smaller length change could be obtained by moving the tibial attachment posterior. With an over the top placement, moving the tibial attachment posterior had the opposite effect and increased the length change. The effect of a posterior tibial attachment combined with an over the top placement was also noted by Penner and associates.[7] Their observations, however, were based on only a few specimens, and the statistical significance of the results was not tested.

Graf[2] also reported an effect of tibial attachment based on measurement made in cadaveric knees using a clinical isometer. A nearly isometric femoral attachment was used. A tunnel at the anterior edge of the ACL's tibial attachment resulted in about 2 mm of shortening with flexion. In contrast, a central tibial tunnel produced 4 mm of shortening, and the posterior tunnel just over 8 mm of shortening.

Overall, the data on the effect of tibial attachment are sparse, and the effects produced are much smaller than those produced by similar changes in the femoral attachment location. Based on the available data, it does not appear that a significant error in femoral placement can be completely compensated for by changing the tibial attachment.

Intraoperative Determination of Isometric Attachments

A number of commercial devices are now available to assist the surgeon in determining the location of isometric femoral and tibial tunnels.[2,48] Typically, these devices allow the surgeon to measure how the intra-articular distance between potential attachment points changes with knee flexion. Any pair of points for which the distance between attachments changes less than 2 mm over a full range of motion is considered clinically acceptable. Clancy and associates[49] noted that bone tunnels should be drilled eccentric to these points because grafts, once implanted, lie along one edge of the tunnel.

Existing commercial devices use one of three methods to determine isometric attachments intraoperatively. The first method is to pass a suture through small diameter trial holes in each bone. The proximal end of the suture is attached to the femur, and the distal end is attached to an isometer that measures relative motion between the suture and the tibia as the knee is flexed and extended. The isometer applies a small force to the suture to ensure that all slack is removed. The surgeon applies an external force to the tibia to ensure it is fully reduced. If the relative motion between suture and tibia is too large, the location of the pilot hole is changed and the measurements repeated.

The second method is to use a six degree-of-freedom instrumented spatial linkage that measures both the intra-articular distance between selected attachments and the knee flexion angle. This approach is considerably more expensive than isometers because it requires, in addition to the instrumented linkage, a dedicated computer to collect and display the measurements.

The third approach is to use the drill guide developed by Odensten and Gillquist.[50] The design of this guide is based on the authors' observations that isometric attachments have an intra-articular distance of 32 mm.[6] When compared to visualization and hand drilling, this drill guide reduced the variability of locating isometric attachments.[51]

Recent evidence shows that the use of isometers does not guarantee restoration of normal knee motion. Galloway and associates[11,12] found that using an intraoperative isometer for determination of placement in PCL reconstruction resulted in poor control of posterior translation at 90 degrees of flexion. In contrast, a nonisometric placement restored normal posterior translation in both extension and flexion.

There are several possible explanations for these findings. A likely one is that intraoperative use of isometers might yield bad estimates of the isometric region for the intact or the reconstructed knee.

Factors Affecting Isometric Attachments

Blankevoort[52] noted that the isometric point may change postoperatively because the reconstruction itself alters knee motions. Many other factors affect knee motion, so it is reasonable to expect that these factors also affect length patterns and the location of the isometric region. Hefzy and Grood[24] stated that ACL length patterns should be determined in the intact knee while applying an anterior force to the tibia to ensure that the ligament is always under tension. Unfortunately, this is not possible at the time of reconstruction because the ligament has been ruptured.

Both Sidles and associates[10] and Hefzy and associates[4] found the location of the most isometric region for the ACL depended on whether an anterior or posterior shear force was applied to the tibia. Posterior forces, like those used to reduce the joint at surgery, caused the proximal portion of the isometric region to move anteriorly.

Sapega and associates[8] measured length patterns under operative conditions when both gravity and the surgeon applied a posterior shear force to the tibia. Three ACL bands were studied: anteromedial, central, and posterior. Corresponding femoral insertions were aligned from proximal (anterior band) to distal (posterior band). They concluded the most isometric femoral attachment was located just superior to the origin of the anteromedial fibers. However, they stated that these fibers will not appear isometric intraoperatively because the posterior shear force causes the fibers of the ACL to slacken during early knee flexion.[8] Finally, Schutzer and associates[9] found that length patterns are affected by other injuries. This effect was minimized when these injuries were repaired before testing for isometry.

Pre-tensioning

Once placement is selected, proper pre-tensioning is required to ensure elimination of abnormal joint laxity. Because some joint laxity returns postoperatively, there is a tendency to obtain maximal reduction and tensioning at the time of surgery. However, excessive pre-tensioning might overconstrain the knee, producing high-graft tensions that can stretch the graft, and thereby contribute to the return of knee laxity.

Bylski-Austrow and associates[13] found ACL graft tensions depended on the femoral attachment site, the tensioning angle, and the amount of pre-tension applied. No single level of pre-tension was found appropriate for restoring normal limits to anterior translation. Further, these authors found that the tensioning angle was as important as the amount of pre-tension in obtaining full reduction of the knee.[13] Both the tensioning angle and the amount of pre-tension also affected graft tension when an anterior force was applied to the tibia. The highest graft tensions occurred when the knee was overconstrained and laxity was less than normal. An overconstrained condition was easiest to create (lowest pre-tension) at 30 degrees of flexion. This is where the intact knee has its greatest physiologic anteroposterior translation. Bylski-Austrow and associates[13] hypothesized that both tensioning angle and pre-tension magnitude exerted their influence by changing the ligament graft's initial intra-articular length.

Burks and Leland[53] found that the tissue used as a graft also affected the amount of pre-tension needed to obtain a normal 20-pound KT-1000 test. The stiffest tissue used, patellar tendon, required the least pre-tension (3.6 lbs). The least stiff tissue used, iliotibial band, required the largest pre-tension (13.6 lbs). Lewis and associates[14] found that joint position and graft force were highly variable, even when one surgeon performed all reconstructions and a constant 67-N (16-lb) pre-tension was used.

Ligament Load Sharing

Lewis and associates[15-17,54] have suggested that the primary goal of placement and pre-tensioning is not only to restore laxity to normal, but also to restore the forces in all joint tissues to normal. They noted that large changes in ACL graft force are associated with only small changes in knee laxity.[14] Thus, even if the joint laxity returns to normal, ligament forces may be abnormal. To obtain surgical control of graft force, Hunter and associates[17] developed a new tensioning device that enabled the adjustment of graft pre-tension while an anterior force of 90 N was applied to the tibia. When compared to pre-tensioning with no anterior force applied to the tibia, they found pre-tensioning with an anterior force returned all ligament forces closer to normal and also reduced the variability from knee to knee.

Bone Impingement

A major goal of proper placement is to avoid deleterious impingement of the ligament substitute by bone. Impingement becomes deleterious when it excessively stretches the graft, causes abrasion, or induces fibrocartilaginous remodeling as a result of compressive stresses. There are two primary locations of impingement. The first is against the roof and walls of the intercondylar fossa. The second is at the intra-articular exits of bone tunnels.

Impingement With the Intercondylar Roof   A normal ACL lies along the roof of the intercondylar fossa when the knee is fully extended. The distal portion of the ACL fans out, and the most anterior fibers appear to curve around the junction of the fossa and trochlear groove prior to insertion into the tibia (Butler DL, personal communications, 1991). The fiber curvature just before the tibial insertion does not exist in grafts or synthetic replacements. Therefore, a graft placed at the anterior edge of the ACL's tibial attachment can impinge on the roof of the intercondylar fossa at full extension. Impingement can also occur with the wall of the intercondylar fossa. The extent of this impingement is affected by the shape of the fossa, the presence of osteophytes, and the size of the ligament graft.

Impingement at Tunnel Exits   Impingement also occurs at the intra-articular exit of bone tunnels, and is probably not completely avoidable at this location. This is an area of potential severe abrasion because knee flexion causes the graft to bend and rub at the tunnel exit. Clinically, this impingement problem is reduced by putting a generous radius at the tunnel exit. Drill guides have also been developed[50] that allow the surgeon to drill both tunnels at once so they align with each other. Odensten and Gillquist[50] recommended drilling the tunnels with the knee at 90 degrees of flexion. Doing so would avoid impingement at the posterior exit of the tibial tunnel because the graft will pull away from this edge as the knee extends. The interaction between grafts and the tunnel edges has nearly been ignored by basic scientists. The only work to date on this subject appears to be that of Sidles and associates,[55,56] who have measured large pressures within the graft at the tunnel exits. This pressure is induced by curvature of fibers as they wrap around the bone edge at the tunnel exit.

Biologic Effects of Impingement   In addition to large internal pressures, a lateral compressive stress applied to tendons has been shown to induce a fibrocartilaginous response.[57,58] Proteoglycan (aggrecan) content increases, and the cells become more rounded and appear to live in lacuna-like chondrocytes.[57,58] Recently, Howell and associates[59] reported radiographic changes in ACL grafts that impinge the roof of the intercondylar notch. The significance of these changes to the long-term viability of the graft remains to be determined.

Summary

Graft placement is one of many factors under direct control of the surgeon that affects treatment outcome. The often stated goal of using isometric placement is an oversimplification that does not always provide optimal restoration of the knee. Normal ligaments are not isometric and errors occur when isometric locations in injured knees are determined intraoperatively. Although they are not optimal, isometric attachments provide a guide that avoids large deleterious errors in placement. In selecting attachments, the surgeon must also consider impingement of the graft with bone. In addition, the surgeon must select both the flexion angle at which the graft is tensioned and the amount of tension applied. These factors depend on the graft's femoral attachment, which determines its length pattern and degree of isometricity. In general, it is easiest to overconstrain the knee if tensioning is done at the flexion angle where the graft length pattern is largest and the knee has the most physiologic laxity.

References

1. Melhorn JM, Henning CE: The relationship of the femoral attachment site to the isometric tracking of the anterior cruciate ligament graft. *Am J Sports Med* 1987;15:539-542.

2. Graf B: Isometric placement of substitutes for the anterior cruciate ligament, in Jackson DW, Drez D Jr (eds): *The Anterior Cruciate Deficient Knee: New Concepts in Ligament Repair.* St. Louis, CV Mosby, 1987, pp 102-113.

3. Grood ES, Hefzy MS, Lindenfield TN: Factors affecting the region of most isometric femoral attachments: Part I. The posterior cruciate ligament. *Am J Sports Med* 1989;17:197-207.

4. Hefzy MS, Grood ES, Noyes FR: Factors affecting the region of most isometric femoral attachments: Part II. The anterior cruciate ligament. *Am J Sports Med* 1989;17:208-216.

5. Hoogland T, Hillen B: Intra-articular reconstruction of the anterior cruciate ligament: An experimental study of length changes in different ligament reconstructions. *Clin Orthop* 1984;185:197-202.

6. Odensten M, Gillquist J: Functional anatomy of the anterior cruciate ligament and a rationale for reconstruction. *J Bone Joint Surg* 1985;67A:257-262.

7. Penner DA, Daniel DM, Wood P, et al: An in vitro study of anterior cruciate ligament graft placement and isometry. *Am J Sports Med* 1988;16:238-243.

8. Sapega AA, Moyer RA, Schneck C, et al: Testing for isometry during reconstruction of the anterior cruciate ligament: Anatomical and biomechanical considerations. *J Bone Joint Surg* 1990;72A:259-267.

9. Schutzer SF, Christen S, Jakob RP: Further observations on the isometricity of the anterior cruciate ligament: An anatomical study using a 6-mm diameter replacement. *Clin Orthop* 1989;242:247-255.

10. Sidles JA, Larson RV, Garbini JL, et al: Ligament length relationships in the moving knee. *J Orthop Res* 1988;6:593-610.

11. Galloway MT, Mehalik JN, Grood ES, et al: Posterior tibial translation following PCL reconstruction. *Transactions of the Combined Meeting of the Orthopaedic Research Societies, U.S.A., Japan and Canada.* Banff, Canada, Organizing Committee of the Orthopaedic Research Societies, 1991, p 263.

12. Grood ES, Mehalik JN, Galloway MT, et al: Posterior cruciate ligament reconstruction: Effect of femoral attachment site location of posterior tibial translation. Transactions of the First European Orthopaedic Research Society, 1991.

13. Bylski-Austrow DI, Grood ES, Hefzy MS, et al: Anterior cruciate ligament replacements: A mechanical study of femoral attachment location, flexion angle at tensioning, and initial tension. *J Orthop Res* 1990;8:522-531.

14. Lewis JL, Lew WD, Engebretsen L, et al: Factors affecting graft force in surgical reconstruction of the anterior cruciate ligament. *J Orthop Res* 1990;8:514-521.

15. Lewis JL, Lew WD, Hill JA, et al: Knee joint motion and ligament forces before and after ACL reconstruction. *J Biomech Eng* 1989;111:97-106.

16. Lew WD, Engebretsen L, Lewis JL, et al: Method for setting total graft force and load sharing in augmented ACL grafts. *J Orthop Res* 1990;8:702-711.

17. Hunter RE, Lew WD, Lewis JL, et al: Graft force-setting technique in reconstruction of the anterior cruciate ligament. *Am J Sports Med* 1990;8:12-19.

18. Fick R: Anatomie und mechanik der gelinke unter berucksichtigung der bewegenden muskelen. Band II, Teil III, in *Handbuch der Anatomie des Menschen*. Karl von Bardeleben, 1911.

19. Butler DL, Kay MD, Stouffer DC: Comparison of material properties in fascicle-bone units from human patellar tendon and knee ligaments. *J Biomech* 1986;19:425-432.

20. Crowninshield R, Pope MH, Johnson RJ: An analytical model of the knee. *J Biomech* 1976;9:397-405.

21. Howe JG, Wertheimer C, Johnson RJ, et al: Arthroscopic strain gauge measurement of the normal anterior cruciate ligament. *Arthroscopy* 1990;6:198-204.

22. Krackow KA, Brooks RL: Optimization of knee ligament position for lateral extraarticular reconstruction. *Am J Sports Med* 1983;11:293-302.

23. Bartel DL, Marshall JL, Schieck RA, et al: Surgical repositioning of the medial collateral ligament: An anatomical and mechanical analysis. *J Bone Joint Surg* 1977;59A:107-116.

24. Hefzy MS, Grood ES: Sensitivity of insertion locations on length patterns of anterior cruciate ligament fibers. *J Biomech Eng* 1986;108:73-82.

25. Menschik A: Mechanik des kniegelenks. Teil 3. *Z Orthop* 1974:3-24.

26. Menschik A: The basic kinematic principle of the collateral ligaments, demonstrated on the knee joint, in Chapchal G (ed): *Injuries of the Ligaments and Their Repair: Hand, Knee, Foot.* Stuttgart, Georg Thieme Publishers, 1977, pp 9-16.

27. Strasser H: *Lehrbuch der Muskel- und Gelenkmechanik.* Berlin, Springer, 1913.

28. Burmester L: *Lehrbuch der Kinematik.* Leipzig, Germany, A Felix Verlag, 1888.

29. Mueller W: *The Knee: Structure, Function, Injury, and Repair.* Berlin, Springer-Verlag, 1983.

30. Engebretsen L, Lew WD, Lewis JL, et al: The effect of an iliotibial tenodesis on intraarticular graft forces and knee joint motion. *Am J Sports Med* 1990;18:169-176.

31. Girgis FG, Marshall JL, Al Monajem ARS: The cruciate ligaments of the knee joint: Anatomical, functional and experimental analysis. *Clin Orthop* 1975;106:216-231.

32. Kennedy JC, Weinberg HW, Wilson AS: The anatomy and function of the anterior cruciate ligament. *J Bone Joint Surg* 1974;56A:223-235.

33. Furman W, Marshall JL, Girgis FG: The anterior cruciate ligament: A functional analysis based on postmortem studies. *J Bone Joint Surg* 1976;58A:179-185.

34. Norwood LA, Cross MJ: Anterior cruciate ligament: Functional anatomy of its bundles in rotatory instabilities. *Am J Sports Med* 1979;7:23-26.

35. Arnoczky SP: Anatomy of the anterior cruciate ligament. *Clin Orthop* 1983;172:19-25.

36. Fuss FK: Anatomy of the cruciate ligaments and their function in extension and flexion of the human knee joint. *Am J Anat* 1989;184:165-176.

37. Clark JM, Sidles JA: The interrelation of fiber bundles in the anterior cruciate ligament. *J Orthop Res* 1990;8:180-188.

38. Amis AA, Dawkins GPC: Functional anatomy of the anterior cruciate ligament: Fibre bundle actions related to ligament replacements and injuries. *J Bone Joint Surg* 1991;73B:260-267.

39. Kurosawa H, Yamakoshi K-I, Yasuda K, et al: Simultaneous measurement of changes in length of the cruciate ligaments during knee motion. *Clin Orthop* 1991;265:233-240.

40. Blankevoort L, Huiskes R, de Lange A: Recruitment of knee joint ligaments. *J Biomech Eng* 1991;113:94-103.

41. Edward RG, Lafferty JF, Lange KO: Ligament strain in the human knee joint. *Trans Am Soc Mech Eng* 1970;92:133-136.

42. Wang C-J, Walker PS: The effects of flexion and rotation on the length patterns of the ligaments of the knee. *J Biomech* 1973;6:587-596.

43. Kennedy JC, Hawkins RJ, Willis RB: Strain gauge analysis of knee ligaments. *Clin Orthop* 1977;129:225-229.

44. Dorlot JM, Christel P, Meunier A, et al: The displacement of the bony insertion sites of the anterior cruciate ligament during the flexion of the knee, in Huiskes R, van Campen DH, de Wijn JR (eds): *Biomechanics: Principles and Applications*. The Hague, Martinus Nijhoff Publishers, 1982, pp 185-190.

45. Van Dijk R: *The Behaviour of the Cruciate Ligaments in the Human Knee*, thesis. Amsterdam, Rodopi, 1983.

46. Bradley J, FitzPatrick D, Daniel D, et al: Orientation of the cruciate ligament in the sagittal plane: A method of predicting its length-change with flexion. *J Bone Joint Surg* 1988;70B:94-99.

47. O'Connor J, Shercliff T, FitzPatrick D, et al: Geometry of the knee, in Daniel DM, Akeson WH, O'Connor JJ (eds): *Knee Ligaments: Structure, Function, Injury, and Repair*. New York, Raven Press, 1990, pp 163-199.

48. Raunest J: Application of a new positioning device for isometric replacement in anterior cruciate ligament repair and reconstruction. *J Trauma* 1991;31:223-229.

49. Clancy WG Jr, Nelson DA, Reider B, et al: Anterior cruciate ligament reconstruction using one-third of the patellar ligament, augmented by extra-articular tendon transfers. *J Bone Joint Surg* 1982;64A:352-359.

50. Odensten M, Gillquist J: A modified technique for anterior cruciate ligament (ACL) surgery using a new drill guide for isometric positioning of the ACL. *Clin Orthop* 1986;213:154-158.
51. Good L, Odensten M, Gillquist J: Precision in reconstruction of the anterior cruciate ligament: A new positioning device compared with hand drilling. *Acta Orthop Scand* 1987;58:658-661.
52. Blankevoort L: ACL reconstruction: Simply a matter of isometry?, in *Passive Motion Characteristics of the Human Knee: Experiments and Computer Simulation*, thesis. Nijmegen, Catholic University of Nijmegen, 1991.
53. Burks RT, Leland R: Determination of graft tension before fixation in anterior cruciate ligament reconstruction. *Arthroscopy* 1988;4:260-266.
54. Hanley P, Lew WD, Lewis JL, et al: Load sharing and graft forces in anterior cruciate ligament reconstructions with the Ligament Augmentation Device. *Am J Sports Med* 1989;17:414-422.
55. Sidles JA, Clark JM, Huber JD: Large internal pressures occur in ligament grafts at bone tunnels. *Trans Orthop Res Soc* 1990;15:81.
56. Sidles JA, Clark JM, Garbini JL: A geometric theory of equilibrium mechanics of fibers in ligaments and tendons. *J Biomech* 1991;24:943-950.
57. Gillard GC, Reilly HC, Bell-Booth PG, et al: The influence of mechanical forces on the glycosaminoglycan content of the rabbit flexor digitorum profundus tendon. *Conn Tissue Res* 1979;7:37-46.
58. Vogel K: Proteoglycans accumulate in a region of human tibialis posterior tendon subjected to compressive force in vivo and in ligaments. *Transactions of the Combined Meeting of the Orthopaedic Research Societies, U.S.A., Japan and Canada*. Banff, Canada, Organizing Committee of the Orthopaedic Research Societies, 1991, p 58.
59. Howell SM, Berns GS, Farley TE: Unimpinged and impinged anterior cruciate ligament grafts: MR signal intensity measurements. *Radiology* 1991;179:639-643.

Chapter 21

Mathematical Modeling of the Knee

Rik Huiskes, PhD

Introduction

A model is a representation of reality that emphasizes its most important characteristics. By concentrating on the essentials, the complex reality becomes surveyable, controllable, and comprehensible. Models are indispensable tools for understanding the knee joint, where subtle interplay between anatomic structures determines complicated motion patterns. The history of modeling human joints is as old as the study of these structures themselves. Most of the models used were based on analogies. Examples are the ball-in-socket model of the hip joint, the hinge model of the elbow joint, and the four-bar-linkage model of the knee joint.[1] The beauty of these models is that they relate the complex joint motions directly to relatively simple engineering mechanisms that are well understood; can actually be fabricated, manipulated, and tested; and, indeed, mimic some of the most essential kinematic characteristics of the real joints. The kinematic characteristics of these engineering mechanisms can also be described mathematically, resulting in a mathematical model of a physical analogy of a joint. Because the analogies in these examples are relatively simple, the mathematical models can be very precise, and can, in fact, replace the physical analogy. The mathematical model then has the advantages of flexibility and quantifiability but, because it is abstract, does not provide the possibilities for manipulations and visual confirmation, which are the assets of the physical model.

Because the analogy between the knee joint and a four-bar-linkage mechanism is limited to some of these essential kinematic characteristics, the applicability of this model for the understanding of the knee mechanism also is limited. This does not imply that there is something wrong with it. Limitation of analogy is the central asset of any model. Without such a limitation, the model would not be a model, but a reproduction as complex as reality itself, and as difficult to comprehend. The problem with the four-bar-linkage model is that, although it does provide answers to important questions of functional anatomy, its limitations prevent our answering some important questions about diagnosis and surgical reconstruction of knee disabilities. To answer many of these questions we must have quantitative understanding of the complex relationships between joint structures, forces, and motions that cannot be provided by simple models, nor by experiments alone.

Although there is no obvious mechanical analogy of the knee beyond the four-bar-linkage mechanism, the possibilities for mathematical modeling are not exhausted. In fact, owing to the development of computers, these possibilities have become almost limitless, or appear limitless at this point. These possibilities were first recognized about 15 years ago, in a few groups active in biomechanical analysis using finite element methods. In the finite element methods, a structure is divided in parts, the mechanical behavior of which can be mathematically described with reasonable accuracy. A computer is used to solve the interrelationships between the elements (parts) to evaluate the mechanical behavior of the structure as a whole. This approach implied that the geometric and material properties of the relevant substructures of the knee, such as ligaments, menisci, and articular surfaces, would be described mathematically in a computer program that could simulate their mechanical interrelationships. Although the mathematical equations that govern these interrelationships had not yet been developed, and the geometric and material properties of the substructures had not been determined, the groups concerned were optimistic about the time and efforts required to develop a realistic computer-simulation model. Once developed, this model (or numeric analogy) was expected to provide complete understanding of the complex knee mechanism and to be useful in solving an almost unlimited number of practical problems relative to criteria for diagnosis and treatment for knee disabilities.

Fifteen years later, it is evident that the difficulties to be overcome for the realization of these goals were grossly underestimated. The efforts were not appreciated all that much by orthopaedists in clinical practice or in research, and many groups have abandoned this approach. Although the original vision has not yet been realized, progress was made; a number of knee-joint computer-simulation models are now in working condition and are used to address practical, clinical problems.

In this chapter, I discuss the philosophy and the principles on which these mathematical models are based and present a brief historical overview, followed by a discourse on experimental verification. The applicabilities of the models are discussed relative to their characteristics and limitations. Finally, a critical assessment concludes that these models must actually be used and further developed, proven by corroborating experimental data, and fueled by clinical interest.

The Characteristics of Mathematical Knee Models

Mathematical knee model is a generic term. Persons not familiar with the mathematics by which models are defined may well be confused about their similarities and differences. The literature will not be helpful, because although models are actually characterized by their practical limitations, authors usually emphasize the beauty of the mathematics and the models' potential applicabilities. To start from a common ground, I will introduce a conceptual model of the passive knee joint as a mechanical control mechanism, activated by forces. The model is limited to the tibiofemoral articulation, although this is a practical, rather than a principle choice. According to the conceptual model (Fig. 1), knee motions are caused by forces that are either internal or external. The relationship between forces and motion, signified by conversions in Figure 1, can be described by the Newtonian dynamic equilibrium equations. The external forces, applied to the tibia and femur, may be caused by gravity, by accelerations of the bones, and by muscles or outside manipulation. This conceptual model assumes that these external forces have independent, given (variable) characteristics. Because the model does not account for the relationships between knee motions and external forces through the nervous system, it is called a model of the passive knee joint. The internal forces, however, do depend on the motions, via the geometry and mechanical properties of the ligaments, capsular structures, menisci, and articular surfaces. Hence, a number of feedback loops in the force-motion relationship are apparent (Fig. 1).

This conceptual model is a generic one, relative to which the characteristics of all actual mathematical models can be explained. These characteristics depend on the limitations, simplifications, and assumptions on which a model is based. They may relate to the formulation of the dynamic equilibrium equations used in the model, or to the precision and degree of complexity by which the anatomic structures are mathematically described.

Two-Dimensional (2-D) Models

A 2-D model assumes that the motion and loading characteristics of the knee can be represented in one plane. Hence, for a model describing the knee mechanisms in the sagittal plane, internal-external rotation, varus-valgus rotation, and mediolateral translation are neglected. An example is the four-bar-linkage model[1,2] extended by O'Connor and associates[3] in a mathematical sense by including elastic, instead of rigid ligaments. Although simple, 2-D models provide insight in the generic relationship between condylar shape and ligament properties.

Quasi-Static Versus Dynamic Models

The knee joint is a dynamic system in the sense that the external forces and the motions vary in time. Because variation of motion

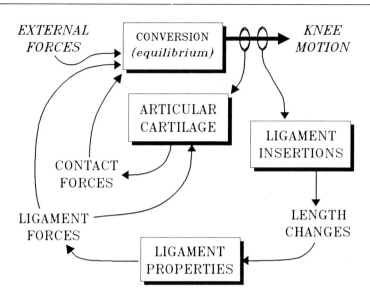

Fig. 1 *Conceptual model of the knee joint as a mechanical system. Knee motion occurs as a result of dynamic equilibrium between external and internal forces. The latter depend on the motion characteristics, fed-back via the anatomic knee-joint structures. (Reproduced with permission from Blankevoort L:* Passive Motion Characteristics of the Human Knee Joint, *thesis. The Netherlands, University of Nijmegen, 1991.)*

implies accelerations and decelerations, the dynamic equations of force equilibrium (Fig. 1) have terms representing the forces caused by the mass inertia of the elements involved, such as the bones. If the mass of an element is relatively small, or if its accelerations and decelerations are relatively small, the contributions of these inertia forces are also relatively small and could, potentially, be neglected. This underlying assumption of quasi-static (sometimes called kinetic) knee-joint models does not imply that forces and motions are constant; it only means that their variations occur relatively slowly, in the sense that the inertia forces are negligible relative to the other external forces. In practice it implies that quasi-static models cannot be used to study the effects of impact forces. The force and motion variations involved in normal walking can be considered as being relatively slow, as probably, can those involved in running. There is no clear dividing line; the faster the motion variations occur, the less precise a quasi-static model becomes.

Most of the knee-joint models hitherto developed were quasi-static ones. Moeinzadeh and Engin[4] developed the mathematical formulation for a three-dimensional (3-D) dynamic model; however, actual calculations were presented relative only to a 2-D model.

Elastic Versus Time-Dependent Properties

The equations of dynamic equilibrium also contain terms that account for the force variations resulting from time-dependent behavior of the joint structures (viscoelasticity). For instance, these terms describe the loading-rate dependency in the responses of ligaments and articular cartilage. These effects usually are neglected in mathematical knee-joint models; the only model known to me in which they are not neglected is that of Moeinzadeh and Engin.[4] The characterization dynamic often is assumed to include this time-dependent behavior, whereas quasi-static is assumed to imply that properties are purely elastic and, thus, time independent.

Contrary to the above difference between a quasi-static and a dynamic model, there is very little explicit justification for neglecting the time-dependent effects of the knee-joint structures. Results of experiments with cartilage and ligaments indicate that under normal, physiologic conditions, time-dependent behavior does play a role.[5,6] Hence, the response of the joint to external forces is loading-rate dependent. As long as the loading rate is relatively slow, such as in diagnostic manipulation, the rate dependency in the motion characteristics is probably of minor consequence.[5] A much more important effect is that of preconditioning of the ligaments; because the ligaments are stretched after a period of rest, they are much stiffer after they have been stretched (or preconditioned) a number of times consecutively.[5] When the knee is loaded in a knee-laxity tester, its response to the first loading cycle is significantly different from responses to the consecutive cycles.[7]

Inverse Versus Direct Dynamics Models

In mechanics, forces are causes and motions are effects. Without force, there is no motion. According to the conceptual model of Figure 1, the knee system is activated by external forces, which produce motions. The kind of motions (or joint positions) that will actually result depends on the characteristics of the external forces, but also on the internal forces, which again depend on the motions. In fact, the motion characteristics will be such as to satisfy dynamic (or quasi-static) equilibrium between internal and external forces. In direct dynamics models, this process is stimulated. Hence, in the mathematical solution procedure, those motions or positions are sought that satisfy the equilibrium between external and internal forces, just as it occurs in reality. The mathematical complexity is introduced because of the nonlinear feedback loop in the system. As a result, the relationship between forces and motions is not explicit.

Reversing causes and effects in the mathematical analysis produces inverse dynamics models. In that case, the motion characteristics are given quantities, and the forces are determined. To determine the internal forces in this way is relatively simple, at least mathematically, because a particular given position of the tibia relative to the femur uniquely determines, for example, the amount of elongation in a ligament or the amount of compressive strain in the articular cartilage. Therefore, assuming that the force/length relationships (the elastic characteristics) of the knee-joint structures are known, the internal forces in each structure can be directly calcu-

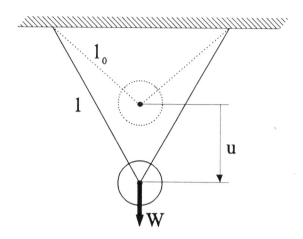

Fig. 2 *Illustration of the difference between a direct and an inverse dynamics model, using a ball hung from the ceiling by two equal rubber bands.*

lated from its deformation, which is uniquely and explicitly determined by the relative positions of the bones.

The difference between a direct and an inverse dynamics model may be illustrated by an example (Fig. 2): Assume a ball is hung from the ceiling by two rubber bands of equal thickness. The nonlinear force/elongation characteristics of the bands are given, as well as the position of the ball in which each band is straight but unloaded (the unloaded reference position). The variables of interest are the weight of the ball, the forces in the bands, and the ultimate, equilibrium position of the ball when it hangs free, relative to the initial, unloaded reference position. In a direct dynamics problem, the weight of the ball (W) is given, while the forces in the bands must be determined. In an inverse dynamic problem, the equilibrium position of the ball (u) is given, while the forces in the bands must be determined. Few readers will be able to solve the first problem, and no one will solve it easily. All readers who can read a nonlinear force/elongation graph and know Pythagoras' theorem will be able to solve the second problem.

Understanding the differences between these two approaches is important, because it separates the two main classes of knee-joint models in the present literature. Examples of inverse dynamics models are those of Crowninshield and associates[8] and Grood and Hefzy,[9] who modeled the 3-D ligament configuration around the knee to determine the ligaments' relative contribution to knee stiffness, using prescribed motion characteristics as input. A similar approach was taken by Walker and associates,[10] who included the average 3-D shape of the articular surfaces in a geometric model to determine ligament-length changes and contact areas for given motion patterns. Because no forces were determined in this model, and constitutive properties of the ligaments were not considered, it was rightfully named a computer-graphics model.[11]

Direct dynamics models were reported by Wismans and associates,[12,13] Andriacchi and associates,[14] Moeinzadeh and Engin,[4] Essinger and associates,[15] and Blankevoort and associates.[16-18] Except for the model of Moeinzadeh and Engin,[4] discussed above, all these models are 3-D and quasi-static. These models are similar in the sense that they describe the 3-D shape of the articular surfaces mathematically and represent the ligaments and capsule structures with one or more line elements (or springs) with particular elastic properties (Fig. 3). In all cases, a particular flexion angle and an arbitrary system of external forces must be prescribed. Therefore, knee function is simulated as a series of flexion steps. After each step, the equilibrium positions of the bones are determined from the quasi-static equilibrium equations and the equations describing the contact conditions between the condyles. Andriacchi and associates[14] used an indirect finite element approach for the mathematical solution strategy. Wismans and associates[12,13] introduced an iterative solution procedure based on the Newton-Raphson method, which is more computer efficient and solves the equations directly. The same approach was followed by Blankevoort and associates.[16-18] Essinger and associates[15] used the principle of minimum potential energy, which has an effect similar to that of the direct iterative procedures.

Because the direct dynamics models are intended to describe the knee mechanism as it works in reality (Fig. 1), they may be rightfully called computer simulation models. Instead of external forces, motions (3 rotations and 3 translations) may also be prescribed in these models. Hence, these direct dynamics models also can be used as inverse ones. The opposite is not possible.

Representation of Articular Shape and Contact

Direct dynamics models must always include descriptions of articular shape and contact conditions. Huiskes and associates[19] developed an effective and accurate method to measure and describe articular geometry, using stereophotogrammetry and polynomial interpolation. This method was later enhanced, both in accuracy and efficiency, by Ateshian and associates.[20] It was used by Blankevoort and associates[16] to measure four knee-joint specimens, each of which was analyzed individually. Essinger and associates[15] used femoral and tibial condylar shapes from 10 knee-joint specimens, determined from sagittal and frontal sections.[10] Wismans and associates[12] measured the articular surfaces of knee-joint specimens with a dial gauge and also used polynomial interpolation. Andriacchi and associates[14] took geometric data from the literature.

Of the four computer-simulation models reported in the literature, only Andriacchi and associates[14] included a representation of the

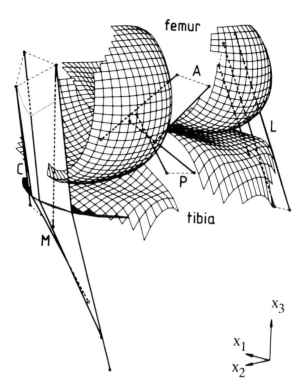

Fig. 3 *Graphic representation of the computer-simulation model of Blankevoort and associates seen from medioposterior with the knee in extension. (Reproduced with permission from Blankevoort L, Huiskes R: Ligament bone interaction in a three dimensional model of the knee.* J Biomech Eng *1991;113:263-269.)*

menisci. They did this by using a shear beam element in the FE-model, the precise characteristics and justification of which are not entirely clear to me. Certainly, modeling the meniscus remains an unsolved problem. The contact elements used in the model of Andriacchi and associates[14] were nonlinear elastic. Wismans and associates[12] assumed rigid joint surfaces; hence, contact points rather than contact areas were represented in the model. Essinger and associates[15] used a rigid femoral surface against a deformable tibial one; the cartilage of the tibia was assumed to be linear elastic. Blankevoort and associates[16] included thin, nonlinear elastic layers on both femur and tibia to represent the articular cartilage, assuming uniaxial stress within the layers. None of the models included surface friction, and in all cases the cartilage properties (stiffness values) were estimated based on the literature.

In fact, articular cartilage is a biphasic material, displaying complex nonlinear and time-dependent mechanical properties.[6] Blankevoort and associates[16] investigated the consequences of a simplified deformable contact formulation in their model by varying cartilage stiffness values in both linear and nonlinear elastic models. The

int/ext. [deg.]

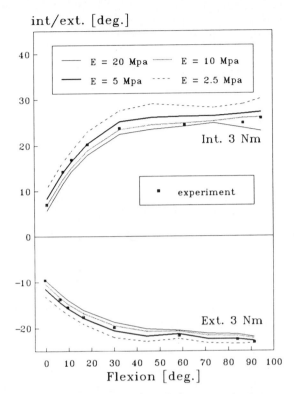

Fig. 4 *Internal and external rotation laxity for torques of ±3 N·m as functions of flexion, as determined with the computer simulation model.[16] In the model, the elastic modulus of cartilage was varied between 2.5 and 20 MPa. The effects on the laxity are relatively small. Also shown are the experimental findings for the same knee-joint specimen from which the model geometry was derived. (Reproduced with permission from Blankevoort L, Kuiper JH, Huiskes R, et al: Articular contact in a three-dimensional model of the knee. J Biomechanics 1991;24:1019-1031.)*

effects on the knee-motion patterns, ligament forces, and contact forces were very small for moderate axial loading conditions (Fig. 4). It must be expected, however, that larger axial forces, such as occur during walking, will have more significant effects, making the simplified representations used in the models less precise in that case. In addition, the simplified models would not be very precise for the investigation of the local stress distribution in the cartilage. Of course, the lack of menisci in the model also reduces precision in this respect.

Representation of Ligament Function

In all knee-joint models presently known, the ligaments are represented by one or more line elements that run from tibial to femoral insertions (Fig. 3). These line elements are assigned particular elastic properties in the sense of force-elongation characteristics. Wis-

mans and associates,[12,13] Essinger and associates,[15] and Blankevoort and associates[16-18] assumed nonlinear elastic force-elongation
characteristics, whereby the parameter values describing the stiffness characteristics were estimated from the literature. Andriacchi
and associates[14] assumed linear elastic properties. The number of
line elements used per ligament varied from one to four in the different models, whereas in some cases capsule structures also were
taken into account by additional line elements.

In fact, the knee-joint ligaments are complex 3-D structures of
which different parts are tensed in the various knee-joint motions.[2]
The choice for one, two, or more line elements per ligament seems
to have been made rather arbitrarily; at least it was not based on
rigorous analyses of the ligaments themselves. The ligament properties are nonlinear and time-dependent.[5] The latter aspect is neglected in all models. Another important parameter to be included in
the models is the prestrain existing in the ligaments, which depend
on the unloaded (or zero-force) length, about which, in fact, nothing
is known. Andriacchi and associates[14] did not include prestrain.
Wismans and associates[12] and Essinger and associates[15] selected
prestrain values on rather arbitrary grounds. Blankevoort and
Huiskes[18] assess prestrain value from comparisons between experimental and model results.

Finally, the medial collateral ligament, in particular, does not run
straight from its tibial to its femoral insertion, but wraps around the
tibial condylar edge, whereby mechanical ligament-bone interaction
occurs. This is accounted for only in the model of Blankevoort and
associates.[17] The effects of this phenomenon were investigated relative to a line-element representation without bone interaction. It
turned out that it had a minor effect on the knee-motion parameters,
but did cause the medial collateral ligament to counterbalance
forced valgus rotations more effectively.[17]

Experimental Verification

The 3-D direct dynamics models have been verified experimentally only to a certain extent. Wismans and associates[12] and Andriacchi and associates[14] have compared knee stiffness values determined by their models to experimental results published in the
literature.[21,22] Essinger and associates[15] used experimental data on
articular geometry and ligament insertion geometry, measured in 10
knee-joint specimens.[10] Ten knees were modeled such that ligament
stiffness parameters, prestrains, and articular stiffness were equal in
each case. In each analysis, a flexion motion from 0 to 120 degrees
was simulated by quadriceps pull. Internal-external rotations,
varus-valgus rotations, translations in the three perpendicular directions, ligament length patterns, and tibiofemoral contact patterns as
functions of flexion were determined and averaged for the series of
10 simulations. These average results were similar to average experimental results reported in the literature.[10,23,24]

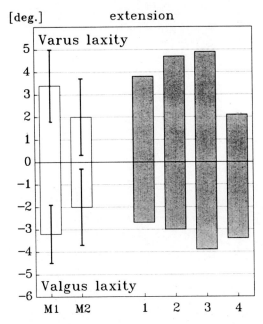

Fig. 5 *The varus and valgus laxities determined in computer-simulation models of four different knee-joint specimens[18] compared to in vitro experimental data (M_1)[21,22] and in vivo experimental data (M_2).[26] (Reproduced with permission from Blankevoort L: Passive Motion Characteristics of the Human Knee Joint, thesis. The Netherlands, University of Nijmegen, 1991.)*

Blankevoort and Huiskes[18] simulated individual experiments with four knee-joint specimens. In each case, the knee was moved through an internally and an externally rotated motion pathway, and internal-external rotations, varus-valgus rotations, and translation in the three perpendicular directions were measured as functions of flexion.[25] The knees were then dissected, and the articular surface and ligament insertion geometries were measured and used in four simulation studies. In each of these studies, the ligament stiffness parameters were equal, and their prestrain values were chosen from experimental ligament-length patterns. Experimental results and numerical predictions were compared for each knee specimen separately (Fig. 4). In addition, the four simulation models were subjected to anteroposterior-laxity tests in 20 and 90 degrees of flexion, and to varus-valgus-laxity tests in extension and 20 degrees of flexion. The results were compared with those obtained experimentally and reported in the literature (Fig. 5).[21,22,26] The similarities were quite satisfactory. Simulations were repeated with adjusted prestrain values per line element and per specimen, based on a numeric optimization procedure in which the individual prestrain values were optimized relative to requirements of minimal deviation between experimental and predicted motion patterns.[18] This improved the similarity with the experimental results. The articular contact-

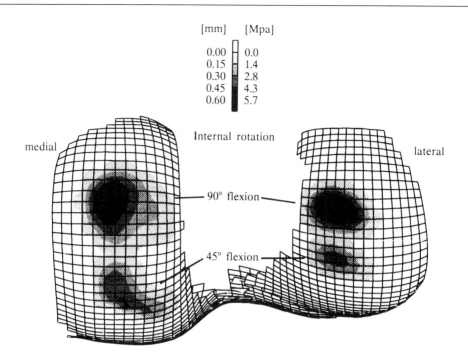

Fig. 6   *Contact-stress distribution on the femoral condyles, for 45 and 90 degrees of flexion during an internally rotated flexion pathway, as determined in the computer-simulation model. (Reproduced with permission from Blankevoort L, Kuiper JH, Huiskes R, et al: Articular contact in a three-dimensional model of the knee.* J Biomechanics *1991;24:1019-1031.)*

area locations, magnitudes, and contact-stress values obtained in the simulations (Fig. 6) were also compared with experimental results,[27,28] and, finally, the ligament forces predicted for internal and external rotation were compared with experimental values.[29]

Attempts at validation of the models have been directed predominantly at the general motion patterns and the general laxity patterns. In most cases, the model results were compared with average experimental data reported in the literature. Only Blankevoort and Huiskes[18] have compared experimental and numeric results for individual knee specimens, at least where 3-D motion patterns were concerned. In all cases, authors reported the results of confrontations with experimental data to be satisfactory. The question is, however, what is satisfactory. This question cannot be answered without considering the inherent limitations of the models and their uses.

First, the models are limited in their scopes; dynamic and time-dependent effects are neglected, limiting the validity of the models to relatively slow (quasi-static) loading rates. The simplified representation of articular cartilage, the neglect of friction, and the absence of the menisci restrict use of the models to moderate articular contact loads, that is, moderate axial knee forces. The absence of the menisci also implies that important secondary restraints to internal-external rotations and anteroposterior laxity are missing.[30] The same is true for the absence of some of the capsule structures. Thus, the models are probably less suitable to study the knee without the ligaments as primary stabilizers. Or, in a more general sense, the models are valid particularly for configurations as near to the normal knee as possible. Validation studies have not yet established precisely what slow loading rates, moderate forces, and 'as near to the normal knee as possible' mean in a quantitative sense.

Second, there are limitations to the degree of valid details. As noted, the simplified cartilage representation precludes an accurate, detailed analysis of local cartilage stresses, and the same is true for the ligaments. However, the detail to which, in a quantitative sense, the model results can be trusted, if only as reasonable approximations, is still uncertain.

Third, there is the problem of validation. If results of the simulation of an experiment are in excellent agreement with the results of the experiment itself, for example, the 3-D motion patterns for a particular loading case, it can be concluded only that the model, as a whole, behaves similarly to the knee-joint specimen as a whole. The agreement does not prove, for example, that all ligaments were modeled correctly. A deficiency in the model of one ligament may compensate for the deficiency in another. This problem has not yet been addressed sufficiently in validation studies.

An important question is what kind of a model is actually required: one of an average knee, of a particular knee, or of a typical knee. An average-knee model would not display only average 3-D motion patterns in one particular flexion-extension movement, as in the validation study of Essinger and associates.[15] It also would require average articular surface and ligament geometries, and average ligament and cartilage properties. And, of course, an average knee has two menisci. None of the four models discussed can meet these requirements, and none of the authors have really attempted to model a particular knee. Although Blankevoort and Huiskes[18] have included articular surface shapes and ligament geometries of particular knees and experimented with the same knees, their ligament stiffness parameters were average ones, taken from the literature, not from the particular knees. However, it is probably fair to say that, within the inherent limitations discussed above, the models of Essinger and associates[15] and Blankevoort and associates[16-18] have been validated as typical knee models in the sense that the differences in overall behavior between the models and an arbitrary knee joint are no more extensive than those between two arbitrary knee joints where it concerns geometric and mechanical properties and mechanical behavior.

Applications

Different applications of knee-model studies must be recognized. First, these studies can be conducted to investigate the models themselves. Such an objective may sound trivial or superfluous to some, but it is extremely important to assess the sensitivity in the behavior of a complex mathematical model to its particular characteristics or parameter values. Investigating the model points out, for example, if the results are very susceptible to a particular parameter, that is, if that parameter should be measured very precisely, or if the parameter's influence is only small and its precise assessment should be of lesser priority. Extensive sensitivity analyses of this kind were published by Wismans and associates[12,13] and by Blankevoort and associates[16-18] relative to ligament stiffness parameters (Fig. 4), prestrains in ligaments, amount and placement of line elements representing the ligaments, variations of articular-surface geometry, and articular cartilage properties.

A second objective is to obtain information about the mechanical interrelationships in the knee. Applications of this kind have been reported by Andriacchi and associates,[14] relative to the 3-D stiffness characteristics of the knee, and by Blankevoort,[31] relative to the contribution of the articular surfaces to resistance against internal-external rotation torques.

A third objective is the analysis of clinical problems. In this category, Essinger and associates[15] reported studies of contact-area locations, magnitudes, and contact stresses in different types of knee prostheses, and Blankevoort[31] applied his model to the problem of femoral placement and prestress of anterior cruciate ligament reconstructions.

For the last two classes of objectives, additional examples are briefly discussed.

Articular Surface Contribution to Rotary Laxity

When the tibia is rotated relative to the femur, internal forces develop in ligaments and between condylar contact regions. For a particular torque applied to the tibia, it will rotate until the internal forces balance the applied torque. Ahmed and associates[29] performed tests of this kind with a large number of knee-joint specimens. For increasing torque values they used buckle transducers to measure the amount of internal and external rotation and the forces developed in the ligaments. They then estimated the contributions of the ligaments to the restraining torque to find that the ligament forces could nicely balance the torque when applied to the tibia towards external rotation, but not when applied towards internal rotation. These authors concluded that "restraining mechanisms [other than tension in the ligaments] must be involved in resisting internal rotation."[29]

This test was simulated with the computer-simulation models of four knee-joint specimens.[31] Other than during the experiments, the model could also determine the articular contact forces. These contact forces were found to increase to about 100 N laterally and 200 N medially when the tibia was externally rotated to 25 degrees, and to

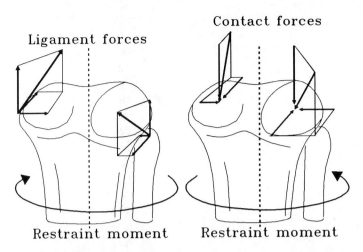

Fig. 7   *The ligament forces and the contact forces in the knee both have horizontal components, depending on the obliqueness of the ligaments and the inclinations in the plateaus. These horizontal force components contribute to the balance of the applied torque. (Reproduced with permission from Blankevoort L: Passive Motion Characteristics of the Human Knee Joint, thesis. The Netherlands, University of Nijmegen, 1991.)*

about 40 N laterally and 250 N medially when the tibia was internally rotated to 25 degrees. This increase, of course, is caused by the increase of ligament forces while the tibia rotates. As a result of the inclination of the tibial plateaus, these contact forces (perpendicular to the contact surfaces) have components in the horizontal plane that may contribute to resisting the applied torque (Fig. 7). Because of tibial articular geometry, this actually does occur in internal rotation, but does not in external rotation. Thus, it was found that, in internal rotation, the articular surfaces contribute an average of 50% to 85% (depending on the flexion angle) to the restraining torque (Fig. 8).

This is an example of the kind of information about biomechanical interrelationships in the knee-joint that is quite difficult to establish with experiments alone. The example also shows how experimental results can be better understood and generalized by using mathematical knee models.

Effects of Anterior Cruciate Ligament (ACL) Reconstruction on Knee Motion and Ligament Forces

It has often been suggested in the literature that the femoral and tibial insertions of an ACL reconstruction should be isometric, that is, that the graft length preferably should remain constant, at least by approximation, throughout the flexion range. Several authors have reported experimental studies in which isometric femoral insertion locations were determined in normal knee-joint speci-

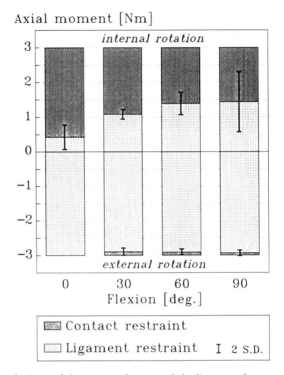

Fig. 8 *Contributions of the contact forces and the ligament forces to the balance of the applied torques of ±3 N·m. Averages and standard deviations were determined in the computer-simulation models based on the geometries of four knees. (Reproduced with permission from Blankevoort L: Passive Motion* Characteristics of the Human Knee Joint, *thesis. The Netherlands, University of Nijmegen, 1991.)*

mens.[32,33] The question is, however, will an isometric location still be isometric after the normal ACL is replaced by a graft? According to the scheme of Figure 1, this is very unlikely. Because of the interrelationships between internal forces, ligament properties and insertion locations, and motions, it is highly likely that the answer is negative.

ACL replacement was simulated in the model of a particular knee-joint specimen,[31] in which 11 alternative femoral insertion locations were tried (Fig. 9). Beside the different insertion locations, all other parameters were kept as constant as possible by assuming a graft with the same force-elongation characteristics as the original ACL and by using a consistent amount of pre-tension. In the normal case and in each of the 11 reconstruction cases, a full flexion motion was simulated, whereby the graft tension was calculated. In addition, anterior laxity and internal-external rotation laxity tests were simulated for the knee in 20 and in 90 degrees of flexion, whereby the anterior displacement and the internal-external rotation were determined. It was also found that after the reconstruction, the relative anteroposterior position of the tibia relative to the femur

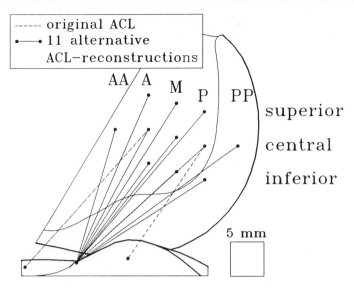

Fig. 9 *The 11 alternative femoral insertion locations tested in the simulation of ACL reconstruction. (Reproduced with permission from Blankevoort L:* Passive Motion Characteristics of the Human Knee Joint, *thesis. The Netherlands, University of Nijmegen, 1991.)*

changes in comparison with the normal situation. This shift, or anteroposterior position error, was determined as well, in 20 and 90 degrees of flexion (Fig. 10).

It is evident from the results that an isometric location will not remain isometric after normal ACL is replaced by a graft. The change in relative position of the femur and tibia indicates that the interrelationships of all the ligaments change as well. Thus, the motion characteristics are different after the reconstruction. The anteroposterior-laxity characteristics changed up to 36% relative to the normal situation in 20 degrees of flexion, and up to 93% in 90 degrees of flexion. For internal-external rotation laxity these changes were maximally 12% and 73%. Scoring the alternative insertion locations relative to normality of anteroposterior position (minimal anteroposterior error), anterior laxity, and internal-external laxity, and on minimal graft tension during flexion, it was concluded that locations A-central and A-superior (Fig. 9) provided the best options, and location AA-central the worst.

Applying a computer-simulation model is probably the only way in which this kind of information can be obtained. It would be almost impossible to perform the same experiments on knee-joint specimens because of variability in individual knee-joint specimens, the impossibility of performing multiple reconstructions in the same specimen, and the inaccessibility of the knee to a variety of measurement gauges. Of course, the simulation was performed relative to the geometry of a single knee-joint, and the simulation model is a simplified representation of reality. Therefore, it would be foolish

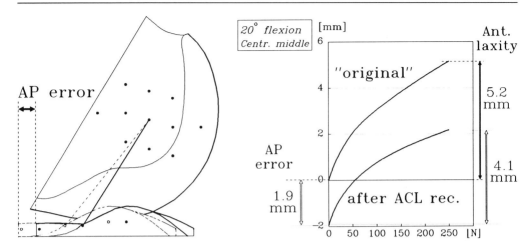

Fig. 10 *Left, If the ACL is replaced, an anteroposterior error usually occurs as a posterior shift of the tibia relative to femur. Right, A comparison of anterior laxity tests is shown between original and reconstructed cases. The anteroposterior error causes an adjustment of the ligament interrelationship and, thus, a change in the motion characteristics. (Reproduced with permission from Blankevoort L: Passive Motion Characteristics of the Human Knee Joint, thesis. The Netherlands, University of Nijmegen, 1991.)*

for clinicians to navigate solely on simulation results. Before definite conclusions with respect to optimal graft location can be drawn, the theoretical results must be confirmed experimentally, or at least corroborated by other experiences. But the model results do provide an excellent starting point for further experimentation.

Discussion

Many authors used knee-joint models in the past. These included simple mechanical analogies, 2-D mathematical models, geometric models, computer-graphics models, and inverse dynamics and direct dynamics mathematical models. This review was focused mainly on 3-D direct dynamics (quasi-static) models, which are, without doubt, the most complex and sophisticated ones, and which are rightfully called computer simulation models. That does not mean that these models are considered better than the others. In mathematical modeling, good is whatever does the job. There are many examples in the literature in which simpler models were successfully applied to clarify anatomic relationships, to generate useful information for the solution of clinical problems, or to determine mechanical variables based on experimental information. The limitation to computer simulation models is merely a matter of scope, not of quality.

In the early, optimistic years, when the development of these models started, much effort was put into the derivation of the mathematical equations and into the development of the numeric solution techniques. Owing to advances in mechanics and informatics in general, to the pioneering work of Wismans and associates[12] and Andriacchi and associates,[14] and to the exponential growth of computer capacity, these problems have now become much less important. In fact, if the mechanical characteristics of an anatomic knee-joint structure can be described mathematically, its inclusion in the computer-simulation models no longer presents major problems. Description of those mechanical characteristics, however, has turned out to be a far greater problem than originally anticipated. For example, the menisci are not excluded from these models because they are not believed to have a function, but simply because not enough is known about their mechanical behavior to model them mathematically. The same is true for the relatively primitive way in which the ligaments are represented; not enough experimental information exists about their time-dependent mechanical characteristics as 3-D structures for a more sophisticated representation. The lack of experimental information is why the first five years of development were focused on the mathematics, and the next ten years were devoted primarily to the collection of experimental data for the triggering of model parameters and for the validation procedures.

Presently, two 3-D direct dynamics models are actively used: one in Nijmegen, The Netherlands,[16-18] and one in Lausanne, Switzerland.[15] Both are of similar scope and subject to similar limitations. These limitations include predominantly a restriction to moderate loading cases, to relatively slow loading rates, to situations near to the normal knee configuration (but including total knee replacement), and to the level of detail for which realistic results can be expected. Both models have been subjected to extensive validation procedures, but, as discussed above, this process has not yet been completed. Therefore, important conclusions of practical or scientific significance, based on the results of the models, should be corroborated by experimental verification. Or, in other words, these models are excellent tools to generate hypotheses that can be used to direct and target experimental protocols in the laboratory, in animals, and in the clinic, and they also are great assets for explaining, extrapolating, and generalizing experimental and clinical findings.

In addition to further validation, application and improvement of the models should be emphasized in the coming years. Application could be in the areas of ligament reconstruction, analyses of manual and instrumented knee-laxity tests, analyses of intra-individual variability in knee-joint mechanical behavior, and development of artificial knee joints. Other applications may be in the area of teaching or instruction for orthopaedic residents, in which interactive and animated computer programs could be applied. Improvements are possible in accuracy and in scope. For more accuracy, ligament representation in the models should be improved as a first priority. Scope should be enlarged by including the time-dependent behavior of ligaments, particularly the effects of preconditioning, and by the inclusion of the menisci. However, for validation studies, applications, and improvement of the models, the objectives must be defined precisely in order to obtain useful results within a reasonable time period. This implies that these efforts would be enhanced by the active interest and participation of clinicians. It is interesting to note that most development of computer-simulation models has taken place outside the United States and in the periphery of orthopaedic and sports medicine research. There is no question in my mind, however, that these tools deserve a wider interest.

References

1. Strasser H: *Lehrbuch der Muskel und Gelenkmechanik: III*. Berlin, Springer, 1917.
2. Muller W: *The Knee: Form, Function, and Ligament Reconstruction*. Berlin, Springer-Verlag, 1983.
3. O'Connor J, Shercliff T, FitzPatrick D, et al: Geometry of the knee, in Daniel DM, Akeson WH, O'Connor JJ (eds): *Knee Ligaments: Structure, Function, Injury, and Repair*. New York, Raven Press, 1990, pp 163-199.
4. Moeinzadeh MH, Engin AE: Dynamic modelling of the human knee joint, in Spilker RL, Simon BR (eds): *Computational Methods in Bioengineering*. New York, The American Society of Mechanical Engineers, vol 9, pp 145-156.
5. Woo SL-Y, Gomez MA, Seguchi Y, et al: Measurement of mechanical properties of ligament substance from a bone-ligament-bone preparation. *J Orthop Res* 1983;1:22-29.
6. Mak AF, Lai WM, Mow VC: Biphasic indentation of articular cartilage: I. Theoretical analysis. *J Biomechanics* 1987;20:703-714.
7. Edixhoven P, Huiskes R, de Graaf R, et al: Accuracy and reproducibility of instrumented knee-drawer tests. *J Orthop Res* 1987;5:378-387.
8. Crowninshield R, Pope MH, Johnson RJ: An analytical model of the knee. *J Biomechanics* 1976;9:397-405.
9. Grood ES, Hefzy MS: An analytical technique for modeling knee joint stiffness: Part I: Ligamentous forces. *J Biomech Eng* 1982;104:330-337.
10. Walker PS, Rovick JS, Robertson DD: The effects of knee brace hinge design and placement on joint mechanics. *J Biomechanics* 1988;21: 965-974.
11. Garg A, Walker PS: Prediction of total knee motion using a three-dimensional computer-graphics model. *J Biomechanics* 1990;23:45-58.
12. Wismans J, Veldpaus F, Janssen J, et al: A three-dimensional mathematical model of the knee-joint. *J Biomechanics* 1980;13:677-685.
13. Wismans J: *A Three-Dimensional Mathematical Model of the Human Knee Joint*, thesis. Eindhoven, The Netherlands, Eindhoven University of Technology, 1980.
14. Andriacchi TP, Mikosz RP, Hampton SJ, et al: Model studies of the stiffness characteristics of the human knee joint. *J Biomechanics* 1983;16:23-29.
15. Essinger JR, Leyvraz PF, Heegard JH, et al: A mathematical model for the evaluation of the behaviour during flexion of condylar-type knee prostheses. *J Biomechanics* 1989;22:1229-1241.
16. Blankevoort L, Kuiper JH, Huiskes R, et al: Articular contact in a three-dimensional model of the knee. *J Biomechanics* 1991;24:1019-1031.

17. Blankevoort L, Huiskes R: Ligament bone interaction in a three dimensional model of the knee. *J Biomech Eng* 1991;113:263-269.

18. Blankevoort L, Huiskes R: Parametric validation of a three-dimensional model of the knee. *J Biomechanics*, in press.

19. Huiskes R, Kremers J, de Lange A, et al: Analytical stereophoto-grammetric determination of three-dimensional knee-joint geometry. *J Biomechanics* 1985;18:559-570.

20. Ateshian GA, Soslowsky LJ, Mow VC: Quantitation of articular surface topography and cartilage thickness in knee joints using stereophotogrammetry. *J Biomechanics* 1991;24:761-776.

21. Markolf KL, Mensch JS, Amstutz HC: Stiffness and laxity of the knee: The contributions of the supporting structures. *J Bone Joint Surg* 1976;85A:583-594.

22. Markolf KL, Graff-Radford A, Amstutz HC: *In vivo* knee stability. A quantitative assessment using an instrumented clinical testing apparatus. *J Bone Joint Surg* 1978;60A:664-674.

23. Rovick JS, Reuben JD, Schrager RJ, et al: The influence of the ACL on the motion of the knee. Presented at American Orthopaedic Society for Sports Medicine, Sun Valley, ID, July 14-17, 1986, pp 34-36.

24. Reuben JD, Rovick JS, Walker PS, et al: Three-dimensional kinematics of normal and cruciate deficient knees: A dynamic in-vitro experiment. *Trans Orthop Res Soc* 1986;11:385.

25. Blankevoort L, Huiskes R, de Lange A: The envelope of passive knee joint motion. *J Biomechanics* 1988;21:705-720.

26. Markolf KL, Kochan A, Amstutz HC: Measurement of knee stiffness and laxity in patients with documented absence of the anterior cruciate ligament. *J Bone Joint Surg* 1984;66A:242-253.

27. Fukubayashi T, Kurosawa H: The contact area and pressure distribution pattern of the knee: A study of normal and osteoarthrotic knee points. *Acta Orthop Scand* 1980;51:871-879.

28. Ahmed AM, Burke DL: In-vitro measurement of static pressure distribution in synovial joints: Part I: Tibial surface of the knee. *J Biomech Eng* 1983;105:216-225.

29. Ahmed AM, Hyder A, Burke DL, et al: In-vitro ligament tension pattern in the flexed knee in passive loading. *J Orthop Res* 1987;5: 217-230.

30. Butler DL, Noyes FR, Grood ES: Ligamentous restraints to anterior-posterior drawer in the human knee. *J Bone Joint Surg* 1980;62A: 259-270.

31. Blankevoort L: *Passive Motion Characteristics of the Human Knee Joint*, thesis. The Netherlands, University of Nijmegen, 1991.

32. Hefzy MS, Grood ES: Sensitivity of insertion locations on length patterns of anterior cruciate ligament fibers. *J Biomech Eng* 1986;108:73-82.

33. Sidles JA, Larson RV, Garbini JL, et al: Ligament length relationships in the moving knee. *J Orthop Res* 1988;6:593-610.

Future Directions

Determine the mechanism of load sharing and force transmission by ligaments over the functional ranges of knee motion.

Ligament reconstruction is done to restore the normal structural function of ruptured ligaments. The ability to reach this goal is limited by incomplete knowledge of how ligament collagen fibers share and transmit loads and of how their function depends on joint position. Specifically, little is known about the transmission of loads between ligament fascicles resulting from shear interaction. Dissection studies are needed to determine the trajectories of collagen fascicles and the nature of their branching and interconnections. Additional studies must be done to determine the three-dimensional (3-D) mechanical properties of ligament fascicles and the regional variation of those mechanical properties. Experimental and mathematic models are needed to show how the tension of whole ligaments is shared among the fascicles and how load sharing depends on joint position. This research would provide a basic understanding of collagen fiber function and of the morphology of the various ligamentous structures of the knee joint.

Determine how the initial mechanical state of the reconstructed knee depends on placement, tensioning, and graft mechanical properties.

A major goal of ligament reconstruction is to eliminate the mechanical and kinematic abnormalities in joints caused by ligament disruption. The final mechanical state of the joint following reconstruction depends on the immediately postoperative tension and length state of the ligament graft established by the surgeon. The initial state of the ligament graft is controlled by the surgeon through the specific replacement tissue used, and the way the tissue is placed within the knee, tensioned, and fixed to bone. The relationship between surgically controlled variables and the joint's initial mechanical state must be determined experimentally and through modeling methods to determine the forces and strains in the graft and other joint structures after surgical implantation. The goal is to develop surgical recommendations for graft tensioning and placement that promote healing and graft maturation, and to identify undue graft forces and strain in order to reduce graft stretch-out and failure.

Determine the effect of spatial distribution and time history of load and strain on the biology and remodeling of the graft tissue.

There is convincing evidence that graft mechanical properties decrease soon after surgery and then gradually increase with time. It is not known if the rate of increase or maximum value attained is influenced by the spatial distribution or time history of load and strain in the tissue. If this relationship were known, surgical and rehabilitation methods could be devised to achieve better graft healing and remodeling.

This should be studied in animal models in which known loads are applied to graft tissue, and mechanical properties of this tissue are measured at various times. When optimal conditions are known, clinical trials in humans should be performed to demonstrate improvement in outcome.

Obstacles to achieving the goal are suitable animal models, methods for controlling graft loads in animals, and methods for measuring graft force histories in humans.

Determine the cause of joint degeneration after ligament injuries resulting in instability.

Joint degeneration often occurs after anterior cruciate ligament (ACL) rupture because of repetitive giving-way reinjuries. In contrast, knees with posterior cruciate ligament (PCL) deficiency rarely have giving-way episodes, but experience over time in many instances a progressive articular cartilage deterioration, principally of the medial tibiofemoral compartment and patellofemoral joint. At present there are no reliable clinical means to assess which knees will deteriorate and, therefore, require early reconstruction. Factors that may be important in joint degeneration include altered kinematics caused by the instability, biomechanical factors, genetic factors, and damage to cartilage and subchondral bone at the initial injury. The relative importance of these factors is unknown. This question should be studied in animal models in which the individual factors are varied independently. Obstacles include potential difficulties in identifying an animal model in which mechanical and biological effects could be varied independently and differences among animal models' responses to ligament injury and specific instability states.

Develop improved transducers and instrumentation for measuring in vivo tissue forces and strains.

There is an almost complete lack of knowledge of the forces and strains in normal ligaments and tendons during activities of daily living and various sporting activities. Little also is known about the forces imposed on grafts during rehabilitative activities. This knowledge is needed to understand the normal homeostatic state, to design prosthetic devices, and to determine the mechanical state during graft healing and remodeling. Measurement of in vivo forces and strains is difficult because of transducer failures, leadwire breakage, and other measurement problems. New transducers need to be de-veloped that are smaller and less intrusive, that have a longer in vivo life, that minimally affect the system being measured, and that use telemetry for the transcutaneous transmission of information. This can be accomplished by taking advantage of newly developed micromachining and existing microelectronic circuit fabrication technologies. New and innovative transducer configurations also need to be designed.

Develop and experimentally validate 3-D computer-simulated models of the knee joint.

Mathematic knee-joint models provide analytic support and provide explanations for experimental and clinical findings. Computer simulation models can be used to explain, interrelate, and generate experimental findings relative to the biomechanical behavior of the knee and its relationship with the anatomic structures that form it. Models also help generate hypotheses that can be used to formulate experimental protocols for use in laboratory, animal, and clinical studies. Because the applicability of mathematic models is limited, their use should be documented in extensive experimental validation studies. Models limited to quasi-static conditions should be developed to include dynamic loading and time-dependent properties. Representation of ligament geometry and properties should be improved, and more precise representation of meniscal function should be included.

Determine the variability among animal models with regard to their mechanics, biochemistry, graft remodeling, and response to injury and surgery.

Many animal models used to evaluate ligament reconstruction have been inadequately characterized with regard to their unique biomechanical and biologic characteristics. This hinders the generalization of results and makes it difficult to compare results obtained using different models and results of studies from different laboratories. The kinematics and kinetics of animal joints used in experimental studies should be measured under well-defined laboratory conditions. Differences in blood and neural supply tissues, tissue composition, the time course of healing, and the biologic and inflammatory response to injury and surgery are just a few of the variables to consider. Questions arise as to the differing effects of meniscectomy and ligament deficiency on the mechanical and biologic response of the joint. Until such cross-comparison studies are performed, observations will remain model-specific, preventing important summary conclusions that would apply to more than one animal model.

Determine the effectiveness of surgical reconstructive procedures to restore lower limb function and provide knee joint stability and function.

Well-controlled randomized clinical studies should be done to define the ability of selected surgical procedures to restore lower limb function after serious ligament injury. Given the frequency of ligament injuries and knee ligament surgery, the effectiveness and stated outcomes of surgical procedures should be documented.

Sufficient clinical information and experience in using knee rating systems exist to study and validate clinical assessment methods that yield the most reliable data in surgical outcome studies. Specific tests of lower extremity function should be developed to provide more objective assessment techniques. Future research should be done to validate techniques for assessing knee joint displacement before and after surgical reconstruction. The postoperative serial assessment of knee joint stability allows determination of whether ligament stretch-out in unsuccessful cases is related to postoperative rehabilitation phases. This information is needed to provide recommendations for improved postoperative programs designed to restore lower limb function in a safe manner without subjecting the knee ligament reconstruction to excessive loads that may result in failure. Future studies should involve long-term follow-up to assess if ligament reconstructive procedures significantly forestall future development of joint arthrosis. Long-term clinical studies are required in which outcomes are assessed at two, five, and ten years after surgery to determine what happens to an active athletic population over time.

Determine the natural history of ligament deficiency states in well-defined patient populations.

The risk factors that result in joint deterioration in young athletically active individuals with ACL, PCL, or other ligamentous injuries are poorly understood and have not been studied in well-defined populations. Every year many hundreds of thousands of individuals sustain ligament injuries. Criteria have not been adequately determined for which patients require surgery and which do not. Giving-way injuries in athletically active subjects with ACL ruptures are an obvious indication for surgical reconstruction. However, patients with reduced activity demands may function without symptoms. Subjects with posterolateral complex injuries and subjects with PCL ruptures may also be asymptomatic for many years, although other subjects may develop an articular cartilage deterioration within a year of the injury.

There now exist epidemiologic and statistical methods to define injury populations and study the risk factors that may be operative both in subjects that adapt to ligament injury and do not require intervention and in subjects who progress to joint deterioration. This research would provide data needed for physicians to develop more rational treatment programs for ligament injuries. These data also will allow the analysis of surgical outcomes based on the natural history of these injury states. The use of functional tests in these populations may allow prediction as to which subjects with ligamentous injuries will go on to have joint deterioration. Genetic factors may also need to be assessed.

Determine gait parameters and gait adaptations in patients with ligament deficiencies, and the changes that occur after ligament reconstructive surgery.

It is known that significant gait adaptations occur in the lower extremity after ligament injury. The altered gait patterns are thought to be a neuromuscular adaptation to knee joint instability. The effect of altered gait patterns may not be uniformly beneficial. Excessive knee adduction moments may result in abnormally high medial compartment loadings. Large external knee extension moments may lessen anterior tibial displacement after ACL disruption, but may also cause large tibiofemoral contact stresses caused by excessive muscle forces. Decreased external knee flexion moments, caused by quadriceps avoidance type response, may result in long-term quadriceps atrophy.

A sufficient body of control subject data and proven gait analysis methods exist to do research in these areas. Future work should include assessment of gait adaptations in PCL and posterolateral ligament-deficient patients. The results of these studies may lead to conclusions regarding the risk for joint deterioration in subjects with defined knee ligament injuries. The data on the external moments that occur with gait adaptations provides information needed for knee models that predict medial and lateral tibiofemoral compartment contact forces and ligament tensile forces. Most importantly, future work should assess the ability of surgical reconstructive procedures to correct abnormal gait adaptations so as to return knee joint moments and articular cartilage joint loadings to normal states.

Develop methods to accurately quantitate in vivo motion limits and abnormal tibiofemoral subluxations after ligament injury and surgical repair.

Accurate quantitative measurement of knee motion is needed to aid in the diagnosis of ligament injury, to study the natural history of complex instabilities, and to evaluate and compare the effectiveness of surgical procedures.

Clinical examination of the knee joint for abnormal position (subluxation) and increased motion limits currently is qualitative at best with large variations found between examiners. While arthrometers are available to measure anteroposterior translation of the midline of the tibia, accurate measurement of tibial rotation and the separate anteroposterior translation of the medial and lateral plateaus is not yet possible.

Precise methods should be developed for measuring the motion limits and tibiofemoral subluxations in patients in order to diagnose the more complex instabilities and to document surgical outcomes. Strategies for successful development of joint arthrometer devices should include stress radiography techniques, computerized tomography, and stress magnetic resonance imaging. The development of these techniques will allow better characterization of the natural history of ligament deficiencies such as PCL and associate posterolateral ligament complex injuries. Accurate measurements of joint subluxations will also allow better assessment of ligament reconstructive procedures to restore joint stability.

Section Six
Clinical Investigations of Ligament Reconstruction

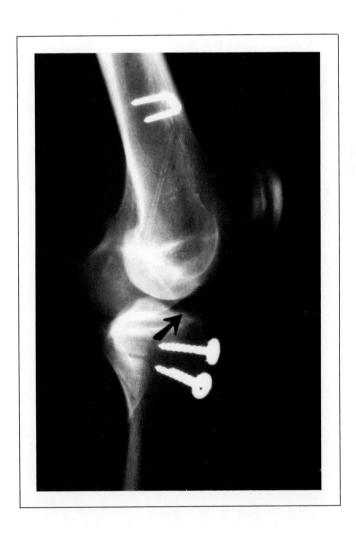

Overview

The knee ligaments guide and limit joint motion. A knee ligament disruption results in an alteration in the normal motion limits, that is, joint instability. The resulting alteration in joint kinematics and mechanics may result in giving-way episodes, repeated injury, and joint arthrosis.

Clinical investigations should include measures of patient outcome. Is the patient satisfied with the treatment? Has the patient been able to return to preinjury activity? Is the patient disabled? Performance indicators of knee function, range of motion, measurement of knee motion limits, and limb girth and strength measurements, are of value only if they can be related to patient outcome. For a period of years after ligament disruption, the patient with knee instability may return to full work and sporting activity with only an occasional giving-way episode or injury. Years may pass before the joint pathomechanics result in disabling arthrosis. Can ligament surgery alter this course of events? The patient may be satisfied with knee function after ligament surgery despite abnormal joint mechanics. Over a period of time the function may deteriorate because of the abnormal joint mechanics of a successful ligament reconstruction or graft failure. A period of five to ten years after the index injury or treatment may be required before outcome measures can be used to evaluate the patient's treatment. For the 20-year-old, it is inappropriate to classify an evaluation done when the patient is 25 as a "long-term" follow-up. For the investigator who tries to minimize the "lost to follow-up" column, a five- to ten-year follow-up of a population of high school and college-age students will seem like an eternity. Performance indicators must be identified and validated that will predict long-term outcomes from two-year follow-ups.

Because of the variability of study populations and designs in knee evaluation systems, the information gained from uncontrolled studies is limited. To improve the usefulness of clinical investigations, the investigator should develop detailed study admission criteria, document carefully the makeup of the study population, and use standardized knee evaluation systems. Inclusion of a prospective control group that meets the study admission criteria and is evaluated with a common knee evaluation system will greatly enhance the scientific value of the report. Figure 1 summarizes how systematic error (bias) may result from the design or conduct of a study.

The opening two chapters in this section discuss evaluation of the knee. The middle four chapters discuss ligament reconstructive surgery using various graft sources. The final chapter presents an overview of the posterior cruciate ligament-injured knee.

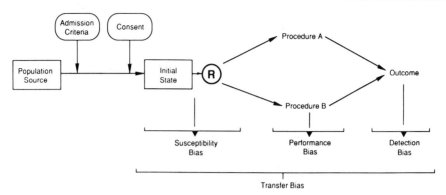

Fig. 1   *A summary of where, in a randomized clinical trial, potential biases may occur. Susceptibility bias is bias that occurs from contrasting the results of therapy for two prognostically dissimilar groups. Performance bias is bias resulting from dissimilar levels of skill in performing the procedures. Detection bias occurs when outcomes are not measured in a comparable manner. Transfer bias occurs when differential loss to follow-up occurs in the two treatment groups. R indicates the point when patients are randomized. (Reproduced with permission from Rudicel S: How to avoid bias. AJSM Suppl 1988;16:48-52.)*

Chapter 22

The Clinical Application of Allografts in the ACL-Deficient Knee

Frank R. Noyes, MD

Introduction

A variety of operative reconstructions for the treatment of acute and chronic ruptures of the anterior cruciate ligament (ACL) have been reported in the orthopaedic literature in the past decade. Intra-articular replacement with a graft and extra-articular procedures, either alone or in combination, have been used with differing results. The use of allograft tissue to reconstruct ACL ruptures has been reported recently by a few authors.[1-11] The first clinical follow-up study was published in 1986 by Shino and associates,[3] who reported results of patients with chronic ACL ruptures who had undergone allograft reconstruction. A variety of fresh-frozen tendons were used, and the authors reported favorable results because 24 of 31 patients were able to return to full sports activities with no or only mild symptoms. Shino and associates[4-6] have since published three more studies documenting the gross appearance, histologic findings, and surface blood flow of allografts during follow-up arthroscopy. The studies conclude that allografts reach gross maturity at 12 months following implantation, with histologic maturity occurring at approximately 18 months.

Wainer and associates[7] and Indelicato and associates[9] reported favorable results of allografts used for patients with both acute and chronic ACL ruptures. Jackson and associates[8] and Roberts and associates[10] recently described clinical studies in which the potentially deleterious effects of using ethylene oxide as a sterilizing agent were discussed.

In 1981, I began to use intra-articular allografts as replacements for the ACL in patients with chronic ruptures whose own tissues had been compromised by previous operations. In 1982, I initiated the use of an allograft to augment the repair of an acutely injured ACL. The rationale for the use of allograft tissue was that it offered advantages over autogenous tissue in patients who had a narrow patellar ligament, malalignment of the extensor mechanism, a previous failed reconstruction of the ACL with an autogenous graft, or patellofemoral or tibiofemoral osteoarthrosis.

Two prospective studies, which are described in detail elsewhere,[1,2] were performed to determine the effectiveness of allografts for acute and chronic ruptures of the ACL. This chapter provides and compares the results of these two studies and provides recommendations for the role of allografts in ligament reconstructive procedures.

Clinical Experience: Acute ACL Ruptures

Purpose

This study was undertaken to determine the short-term results of two types of allograft procedures for acute ruptures of the ACL.

Subjects

Forty-seven consecutive patients (34 male, 13 female) who had an acute complete rupture of the ACL were operated on between October 1983 and April 1987. All had ACL surgery within six weeks of the injury, and none had a history of previous trauma or injury to the involved knee. The mean age at the time of the surgery was 22 years (range, 14 to 39 years); the mean time from surgery to the most recent follow-up was 40 months (range, 25 to 67 months). The injury occurred during sports activities in 42 patients and during work-related activities in five patients. All patients returned for evaluations, providing a 100% rate of follow-up

Evaluation

The objective evaluation consisted of a KT-1000 arthrometer test[12] at 89 N of total anteroposterior force performed by one technician, an isokinetic test at speeds of 60 and 300 degrees per second, and two one-legged hop function tests.[13] Five patients with a previous ACL reconstruction on the contralateral limb were excluded from all tests; ten additional patients with demonstrable patellofemoral crepitus were excluded from the isokinetic and function tests. All were examined radiographically. Subluxation was classified in accordance with a previously published system.[14] A comprehensive knee examination was performed, which rated general, tibiofemoral, patellofemoral, and alignment-related factors.[1]

The Cincinnati knee rating system[1,15] was used to determine the results of treatment. This rating system assesses symptoms (Table 1), functional limitations during sports activities and activities of daily living (Table 2), level of sports activity (Table 3), and changes in the level of activity, and it provides an overall rating (Table 4). The overall rating is determined on the basis of 20 factors, including subjective ratings (20 points), levels of activity (15 points), the re-

Table 1 Symptom rating scale

Description	Points
Normal knee, able to do strenuous work/sports with jumping, hard pivoting	10
Able to do moderate work/sports with running, turning, twisting; symptoms* with strenuous work/sports	8
Able to do light work/sports with no running, twisting, jumping; symptoms with moderate work/sports	6
Able to do activities of daily living alone; symptoms with light work/sports	4
Moderate symptoms (frequent, limiting) with activities of daily living	2
Severe symptoms (constant, not relieved) with activities of daily living	0

*Symptoms rated are pain, swelling, partial giving-way, and full giving-way. (Reproduced with permission from Noyes FR, Barber SD, Mangine RE: Bone-patellar ligament-bone and fascia lata allografts for reconstruction of the anterior cruciate ligament. *J Bone Joint Surg* 1990;72A:1125-1136.)

Table 2 Assessment of Function

Activities of Daily Living Functions	Points	Sports Functions	Points
Walking		Straight Running	
Normal, unlimited	40	Fully competitive	100
Some limitations	30	Some limitations, guarding	80
Only 3 to 4 blocks possible	20	Run half-speed, definite limitations	60
Less than 1 block, cane, crutch	0	Not able to do	40
Stairs		Jumping/Landing on Affected Leg	
Normal, unlimited	40	Fully competitive	100
Some limitations	30	Some limitations, guarding	80
Only 11 to 30 steps possible	20	Definite limitations, half speed	60
Only 1 to 10 steps possible	0	Not able to do	40
Squatting/Kneeling		Hard Twists/Cuts/Pivots	
Normal, unlimited	40	Fully competitive	100
Some limitations	30	Some limitations, guarding	80
Only 6 to 10 possible	20	Definite limitations, half speed	60
Only 0 to 5 possible	0	Not able to do	40

(Reproduced with permission from Noyes FR, Barber SD, Mangine RE: Bone-patellar ligament-bone and fascia lata allografts for reconstruction of the anterior cruciate ligament. *J Bone Joint Surg* 1990;72A:1125-1136.)

sults of examination (25 points), instability (20), radiographic findings (10 points), and the results of functional tests (10 points). The rating can be expressed either as the difference between the total number of preoperative points and the total at the most recent follow-up examination, or as excellent, good, fair, or poor. For a patient to achieve a final rating of excellent, at least 19 of the 20 factors must be classified as excellent. Patients with a good result have scores in both the excellent and good categories and none in the fair or poor categories. A fair result is assigned when any one score is fair and a poor result, when any one score is poor.

Operative Procedure

The operative procedure has been described in detail.[1] A limited medial arthrotomy was performed just adjacent to the patellar ligament to allow placement of the allograft and direct repair of the ruptured ACL fibers without dislocation of the patella. Eighteen

Table 3 Sports activities rating scale

Activity	Points
Level I (Participates 4 to 7 days/week)	
Jumping, hard pivoting, cutting	
(basketball, volleyball, football, gymnastics, soccer)	100
Running, twisting, turning	
(tennis, racquetball, handball, baseball, ice hockey, field hockey, skiing, wrestling)	95
No running, twisting, jumping	
(cycling, swimming)	90
Level II (Participates 1 to 3 days/week)	
Jumping, hard pivoting, cutting	
(basketball, volleyball, football, gymnastics, soccer)	85
Running, twisting, turning	
(tennis, racquetball, handball, baseball, ice hockey, field hockey, skiing, wrestling)	80
No running, twisting, jumping	
(cycling, swimming)	75
Level III (Participates 1 to 3 times/month)	
Jumping, hard pivoting, cutting	
(basketball, volleyball, football, gymnastics, soccer)	65
Running, twisting, turning	
(tennis, racquetball, handball, baseball, ice hockey, field hockey, skiing, wrestling)	60
No running, twisting, jumping	
(cycling, swimming)	55
Level IV (No sports)	
Performs activities of daily living without problems	40
Has moderate problems with activities of daily living	20
Has severe problems with activities of daily living—on crutches, full disability	0

(Reproduced with permission from Noyes FR, Barber SD, Mangine RE: Bone-patellar ligament-bone and fascia lata allografts for reconstruction of the anterior cruciate ligament. *J Bone Joint Surg* 1990;72A:1125-1136.)

patients had an associated meniscal repair performed using an arthroscopically-assisted approach through an accessory posteromedial or posterolateral incision. No other operative procedure, such as reconstruction of the medial collateral or lateral collateral ligament, was performed.

Twenty-two patients received a fascia lata allograft and 25 patients a bone-patellar ligament-bone allograft. The allograft was selected, based on the tissue available at the time of the operation. All grafts were obtained from tissue banks certified by the American Association of Tissue Banks. Eighteen of the fascia allografts were freeze-dried and sterilized with ethylene oxide. The remaining four were freeze-dried only. All bone-patellar ligament-bone allografts were deep-frozen.

Postoperative Rehabilitation

All patients were enrolled in a postoperative program for immediate motion and rehabilitation.[1,16,17] Continuous passive motion was begun immediately following surgery and active-assisted motion, isometric quadriceps-sets, straight-leg raises, electrical muscle

Table 4 Scheme for final rating

	Excellent		Good		Fair		Poor	
	Level	Points	Level	Points	Level	Points	Level	Points
Pain*	10	5	8	3	6-4	1	2-0	0
Swelling	10	5	8	3	6-4	1	2-0	0
Partial giving-way	10	5	8	3	6-4	1	2-0	0
Full giving-way	10	5	8	3	6-4	1	2-0	0
Walking**	40	3	30	2	20	1	0	0
Stairs (score lowest)	40	3	30	2	20	1	0	0
Squatting (score lowest)	40	3	30	2	20	1	0	0
Running	100	3	80	2	60-40	1-0		0
Jumping	100	3	80	2	60-40	1-0		0
Hard twists, cuts, pivots	100	3	80	2	60-40	1-0		0
Effusion	NL	5	<25 cc	4	26 to 60 cc	2	>60 cc	0
Lack of flexion	0 to 5°	5	6 to 15°	4	16 to 30°	2	>30°	0
Lack of extension	0 to 3°	5	4 to 5°	4	6 to 10°	2	>10°	0
Tibiofemoral crepitus+	NL	5			Moderate	2	Severe	0
Patellofemoral crepitus	NL	5	Moderate	2			Severe	0
Anterior displacement (KT-1000)	<3 mm	10	3-5 mm	7	6 mm	4	>6 mm	0
Pivot shift	Negative	10	Slip	7	Definite	4	Severe	0
Medial tibio-femoral (radiographs)++	NL	10	Mild	7	Mod	4	Severe	0
Lateral tibio-femoral (radiographs)	NL		Mild		Mod		Severe	0
Patellofemoral (radiographs)	NL		Mild		Mod		Severe	0
Function Testing‡ (% limb symmetry)	100-85	10	84-75	7	74-65	4	<65	0

* Rating for pain, swelling, partial giving way and full giving-way (see Table 1).
** Rating for walking, stairs, squatting, running, jumping, hard twists, cuts, pivots (see Table 2).
+ Crepitus: Moderate indicates definite fibrillation, cartilage abnormality 25 to 50 degrees; severe, >50 degrees.
++ Radiographs: Moderate indicates narrowing <½ joint space; severe >½ joint space.
‡ Function testing, use average of at least two one-legged hop type tests.
(Reproduced with permission from Noyes FR, Barber SD, Mangine RE: Bone-patellar ligament-bone and fascia lata allografts for reconstruction of the anterior cruciate ligament. *J Bone Joint Surg* 1990;72A:1125-1136.)

stimulation, and patellar mobilization were begun the day following surgery. Partial weightbearing was begun at the end of the first post-operative week and was gradually increased to full weightbearing by the fourth to eighth weeks. A swimming program and a progressive-resistance exercise program were initiated in the third postoperative month. Running was begun by the tenth to twelfth postoperative month. The program was monitored with the KT-1000 to assess changes in anteroposterior displacement.

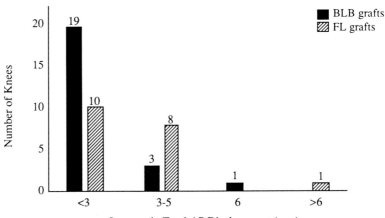

Fig. 1 *Graph showing the results of postoperative arthrometric testing for increased total anteroposterior displacement for the bone-patellar ligament-bone allografts (black bars) and the fascia lata allografts (hatched bars) in the acute ACL rupture population. (Redrawn with permission from Noyes FR, Barber SD, Mangine RE: Bone-patellar ligament-bone and fascia lata allografts for reconstruction of the anterior cruciate ligament.* J Bone Joint Surg *1990;72A:1125-1136.)*

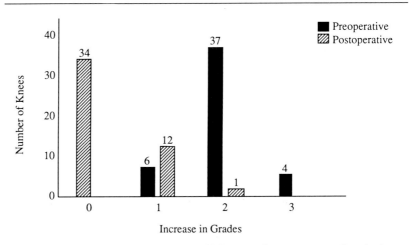

Fig. 2 *Graph showing preoperative (black bars) and postoperative (hatched bars) increases in grades for the pivot shift test in the acute ACL rupture population. (Redrawn with permission from Noyes FR, Barber SD, Mangine RE: Bone-patellar ligament-bone and fascia lata allografts for reconstruction of the anterior cruciate ligament.* J Bone Joint Surg *1990;72A:1125-1136.)*

Results

On KT-1000 testing, knees that had a bone-patellar ligament-bone allograft had significantly lower values for anteroposterior displacement than those that had a fascia lata allograft ($p < 0.05$) (Fig. 1). All patients except one showed major improvement in the pivot shift test (Fig. 2).

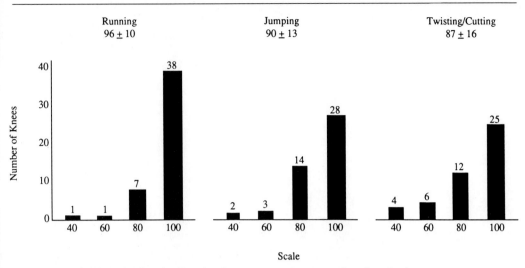

Fig. 3   *Graphs showing distributions for the postoperative sports functions in the acute ACL rupture population. Scale: 40, not able to perform; 60, definite limitations, half speed; 80, some limitations, guarding; 100, fully competitive. (Reproduced with permission from Noyes FR, Barber SD, Mangine RE: Bone-patellar ligament-bone and fascia lata allografts for reconstruction of the anterior cruciate ligament.* J Bone Joint Surg *1990;72A:1125-1136.)*

A mild effusion was found in the joint in four patients; it was barely noticeable and aspiration was not required. Moderate patellofemoral crepitus was found in ten patients. No significant correlations were found between patellofemoral crepitus and pain scores or postoperative problems regaining full knee motion that necessitated additional treatment. A full range of knee motion (0 to 135 degrees) was present in all knees.

Isokinetic testing was performed on 29 patients. At 300 degrees per second, the quadriceps strength-deficit rating showed that 20 patients had no deficit; four, a mild deficit; and five, a moderate deficit. For the hamstrings, 15 patients had no deficit; 11, a mild deficit; and three, a moderate deficit. Similar findings were noted for the 60 degrees per second test.

Function testing was performed on 32 patients; all had normal symmetry on the one-legged timed-hop test and 28 had normal symmetry on the one-legged single-hop test.

The follow-up mean symptom scores (scale, 0 to 10) were as follows: pain, 9 ± 1.6 points; swelling, 9 ± 1.8 points; and full and partial giving-way, 9 ± 0.9 points. Only one patient reported giving-way, which occurred with activities of daily living.

Forty-five patients stated that they could run normally or with only slight limitations, 42 could jump on the involved limb with no or slight limitations, and 37 could perform twisting and cutting activities with no or slight limitations (Fig. 3).

Twenty-two patients returned to the same level of sports activity, 17 had a one-level decrease due to the knee condition but were

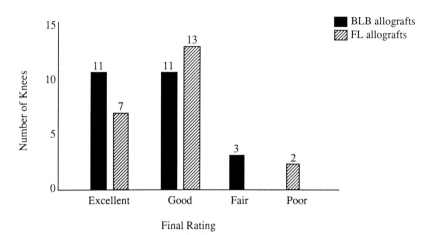

Fig. 4 *Graphs showing the results of the final rating for the two allograft tissue groups in the acute ACL rupture population. Black bars indicate bone-patellar ligament-bone allografts and hatched bars, fascia lata allografts. (Redrawn with permission from Noyes FR, Barber SD, Mangine RE: Bone-patellar ligament-bone and fascia lata allografts for reconstruction of the anterior cruciate ligament. J Bone Joint Surg 1990;72A:1125-1136.)*

asymptomatic, and six did not return to sports as a result of factors not related to the knee. Only two patients did not return to sports because of knee-related problems.

Eighteen patients had a final rating of excellent; 22, good; three, fair; and two, poor (Fig. 4). There was no significant difference in the overall rating between patients who received a fascia lata allograft and those who received a bone-patellar ligament-bone allograft. There was no difference in the overall rating between the 18 patients who had a fascia lata graft that had been sterilized with ethylene oxide and the four patients who had a fascia lata graft that was freeze-dried only.

Stepwise linear regressions were performed between the overall rating scores and 20 variables. The results, shown in Table 5, demonstrate that only a few variables are required to predict the overall rating score. In fact, the combination of only two variables (pain and KT-1000) resulted in the ability to predict the overall rating in 91% of the population. The failure rate was 2%, as only one allograft failed (see Complications).

Clinical Experience: Chronic ACL Ruptures

Purpose

This study was undertaken to compare, in patients with a chronic ACL rupture, the results of an intra-articular allograft replacement performed alone with the results of a combined intra-articular allograft replacement and extra-articular iliotibial band procedure.

Table 5 Results of stepwise linear regression analyses

Step No.	Variable	R	R^2
	Acute ACL Rupture Population, N = 47		
1	Pain	0.91	0.82
1 + 2	KT-1000	0.95	0.91
1 + 2 + 3	Jump	0.98	0.95
1 + 2 + 3 + 4	Patellofemoral crepitus	0.98	0.98
1 + 2 + 3 + 4 + 5	Pivot shift	0.99	0.99
	Chronic ACL Rupture Population, N = 109		
1	Pivot Shift	0.51	0.26
1 + 2	Radiographs	0.64	0.41
1 + 2 + 3	Swelling	0.72	0.52
1 + 2 + 3 + 4	Patellofemoral crepitus	0.75	0.56
1 + 2 + 3 + 4 + 5	KT-1000	0.77	0.59
1 + 2 + 3 + 4 + 5 + 6	Kneeling	0.79	0.62
1 + 2 + 3 + 4 + 5 + 6 + 7	Tibiofemoral crepitus	0.81	0.65

Subject

One-hundred and four consecutive patients who had a chronic complete ACL rupture were operated on between August 1985 and September 1987. All had failed a conservative program of rehabilitation and were either participating in sports activities with symptoms and major functional limitations or had substantially decreased or ceased participation in sports activities because of the knee condition. The patients were sorted into two groups based on the surgical procedures that were performed.

Group 1 was composed of 64 patients (41 male, 23 female) in whom only an intra-articular bone-patellar ligament-bone allograft replacement was performed. The mean age at surgery was 24 years (range, 14 to 40 years). Fifty-seven injured the knee during sports activities. A total of 83 operations, including nine failed ACL reconstructions, had been performed before this procedure. All patients returned for follow-up evaluations a mean of 34 months (range, 23 to 53 months) after the operation.

Group 2 was composed of 40 patients (36 male, 4 female) in whom both an intra-articular replacement with a bone-patellar ligament-bone allograft and an extra-articular procedure involving tenodesis of the iliotibial band were done. The mean age at surgery was 23 years (range, 14 to 36 years). Thirty-seven patients injured the knee during sports activities. A total of 60 operations, including eight failed ACL reconstructions, were performed before the combined procedure. All returned for follow-up evaluations a mean of 36 months (range, 23 to 54 months) after the operation.

This was not a randomized study; in fact, a selection bias was present in that those patients who demonstrated a strong desire to return to competitive sports activities usually received the combined procedure. However, there were no statistically significant differences found between the two groups for 20 variables including age, number of additional injuries, time from the original injury to operation, number of previous operations, duration of follow-up, results on pivot shift and arthrometer testing, symptoms, functional limitations in sports or activities of daily living, or radiographic changes. This allowed a valid comparison to be made between the two operative procedures.

Evaluation

The objective evaluation consisted of a KT-1000 arthrometer test at 89 N total anteroposterior force and an isokinetic test at either 60 or 450 degrees per second or in an isometric mode. Eight patients who had ACL involvement of the contralateral limb were excluded from the arthrometer test.

A comprehensive examination of the knee was performed as previously described.[1] Subluxation was recorded in accordance with a previously published system.[14] During the surgical procedure, the appearance of the articular cartilage was classified according to the previously described system.[18]

The subjective analysis and overall rating were performed as described for the acute population. The only difference was the interpretation of the overall rating, which was assessed in terms of the difference in points achieved preoperatively and at follow-up rather than assignment into an excellent, good, fair, or poor category. This rating method was used because many patients with chronic ACL ruptures have factors existing preoperatively (such as moderate patellofemoral crepitus, tibiofemoral osteoarthrosis, or radiographic changes) that do not allow an improvement in the descriptive categories at follow-up.

Operative Procedure

An intra-articular arthroscopically-assisted replacement with a bone-patellar ligament-bone allograft was performed in all patients. All of the allografts were obtained from tissue banks certified by the American Association of Tissue Banks, and were fresh-frozen at the time of procurement. Ten grafts in group 1 and two grafts in group 2 were also sterilized with 2.5 Mrads of gamma irradiation.

Concomitant medial meniscus repairs were performed in 23 patients; lateral meniscus repairs were also done in eight patients. The meniscus repairs were arthroscopically-assisted, and the sutures were placed with an inside-out technique and tied through an accessory posteromedial or posterolateral incision. No other operative procedures were performed at the time of the operation.

The extra-articular procedure has been described in detail.[2] A Losee-type[19] tenodesis of the iliotibial band was performed, modified by insertion of the proximal part of the strip of the iliotibial band, approximately 12 mm wide, through an osseous tunnel in the lateral femoral condyle only, and not through the gastrocnemius tendon or beneath the lateral collateral ligament. The postoperative rehabilitation program closely matched that described for the acute population.[1,16,17]

Results

A statistically significant difference ($p<0.01$) existed between the two groups for the KT-1000 arthrometer test at follow-up (Fig. 5). More patients in group 2 (74%) had a difference of 2.5 mm or less between the displacements of the two limbs than did the patients in group 1 (54%). The rate of failure due to displacement (6 mm or more) was higher in group 1 (12%) than in group 2 (4%). There was no statistically significant relationship, preoperatively or at follow-up, for either group between the amount of displacement and symptoms, functional limitations, deterioration of articular cartilage, or the overall score.

Preoperatively, all patients except one with physiologic laxity in the contralateral limb had at least a two-grade increase in the pivot shift test compared with the contralateral limb. The increase in grade compared with the contralateral limb was significantly larger in group 2 than in group 1 ($p<0.05$), as shown in Figure 6. At follow-up, there was no significant different between the two groups, and all but four patients showed major improvement on this test.

Isokinetic testing was performed on 39 patients (61%) in group 1 and on 30 patients (75%) in group 2. There was no statistically significant difference between the two groups in terms of deficits of the quadriceps or hamstrings as compared between limbs. Overall, normal quadriceps or only a mild deficit of the quadriceps was found in 70% of group 1 and in 83% of group 2. Similar percentages were found for the deficits of the hamstrings.

At follow-up, normal or mild patellofemoral crepitus had become moderate in nine patients (14%) in group 1 and eight (20%) in group 2. No statistically significant difference was found between the groups in terms of the percentage of patients who had moderate crepitus at follow-up. There was also no statistically significant relationship in either group between crepitus and symptoms, functional limitations, or deterioration of articular cartilage.

A mild joint effusion was detected in five patients in group 1 and in three patients in group 2; aspiration was not required. All but four patients had a normal range of knee motion (0 to 135 degrees) at follow-up; four lacked 5 degrees of full extension.

There was no statistically significant difference between the two groups in terms of the percentage of patients with abnormal articular cartilage surfaces recorded during the operation (Table 6). Positive relationships were found in group 1 between the detection of one abnormal surface and difficulty in stair-climbing ($p<0.05$), difficulty in kneeling ($p<0.05$), and partial giving-way ($p<0.05$). The detection of two or more abnormal surfaces positively correlated with patellofemoral compression pain in group 1 ($p<0.01$) and with a decreased ability to walk in group 2 ($p<0.01$).

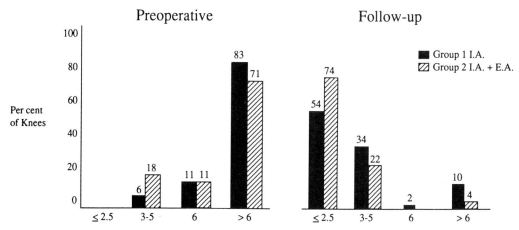

Fig. 5   *Preoperative and follow-up results of testing with the KT-1000 arthrometer for anteroposterior displacement at 89 N of total force for group 1 (allograft alone) and group 2 (allograft and extra-articular procedure) in the chronic ACL rupture population. (Reproduced with permission from Noyes FR, Barber SD: The effect of an extra-articular procedure on allograft reconstructions for chronic ruptures of the anterior cruciate ligament.* J Bone Joint Surg *1991;73A:882-892.)*

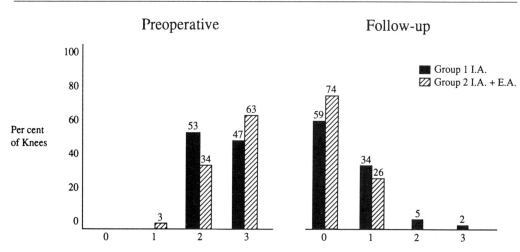

Fig. 6   *Preoperative and follow-up results of pivot shift testing, as measured by the increase in grade compared with that of the contralateral, normal knee, for group 1 (allograft alone) and group 2 (allograft and extra-articular procedure) in the chronic ACL rupture population. (Reproduced with permission from Noyes FR, Barber SD: The effect of an extra-articular procedure on allograft reconstructions for chronic ruptures of the anterior cruciate ligament.* J Bone Joint Surg *1991;73A:882-892.)*

Table 6 Articular cartilage appearance at index procedure

	Patellofemoral		Lateral Tibiofemoral		Medial Tibiofemoral	
	Normal	Abnormal*	Normal	Abnormal*	Normal	Abnormal*
Group 1+	53	11**	51	13	47	17
Group 2++	39	1**	32	8	32	8

*   Abnormal = fissuring, fragmentation of 15 mm or more of the surface or subchondral bone exposed.
+   Intra-articular bone-patellar ligament-bone allograft replacement
++ Intra-articular bone-patellar ligament-bone allograft replacement plus extra-articular procedure involving
     tenodesis of the iliotibial band
** Statistically significant difference between groups (p<0.05).
(Reproduced with permission from Noyes FR, Barber SD: The effect of an extra-articular procedure on allograft reconstructions for chronic ruptures of the anterior cruciate ligament. *J Bone Joint Surg* 1991;73A:882-892.)

Table 7 Subjective assessment of symptoms

Symptom	Points*	Percent Preoperative			Percent Follow-up		
		Group 1+	Group 2	P value	Group 1	Group 2	P value
Pain	10	9	10	0.25	34	40	0.16
	8	5	10		33	50	
	6	2	10		17	8	
	4	65	50		9	2	
	0-2	19	20		7	—	
	Mean	4.2	4.8		7.7**	8.6**	
Swelling	10	21	18	0.55	57	67	0.23
	8	5	8		25	30	
	6	2	8		8	—	
	4	67	63		8	3	
	0-2	5	3		2	—	
	Mean	5.4	5.4		8.6**	9.3**	
Partial	10	6	13	0.22	84	100	0.08
giving-way	8	6	3		2	—	
	6	2	8		2	—	
	4	73	58		12	—	
	0-2	13	18		—	—	
	Mean	4.3	4.7		9.8**	10**	
Full	10	16	8	0.08	95	100	0.38
giving-way	8	5	4		2	—	
	6	—	10		3	—	
	4	63	65		—	—	
	0-2	16	13		—	—	
	Mean	4.8	4.6		9.8**	10**	

*Point scale:
  10 = normal knee, able to do strenuous work/sports with jumping, hard pivoting.
  8 = able to do moderate work/sports with running, twisting, turning; symptoms with strenuous work/sports.
  6 = able to do light work/sports with no running, twisting, jumping; symptoms with moderate work/sports.
  4 = able to do activities of daily living alone; symptoms with light work/sports.
  2 = moderate symptoms (frequent, limiting) with activities of daily living.
  0 = severe symptoms (constant, not relieved) with activities of daily living.
  Group 1 had intra-articular bone-patellar ligament-bone allograft replacement; group 2 had intra-articular bone-patellar ligament-bone allograft replacement plus an extra-articular procedure involving tenodesis of the iliotibial band.
**Statistically significant changes from preoperative values (P <0.05).
(Reproduced with permission from Noyes FR, Barber SD: The effect of an extra-articular procedure on allograft reconstructions for chronic ruptures of the anterior cruciate ligament. *J Bone Joint Surg* 1991;73A:882-892.)

In group 1, statistically significant improvements from the preoperative scores were found at follow-up for walking, running, jumping, twisting, and all symptoms (Table 7) (p<0.01). In group 2, significant improvements were found for walking, stair-climbing, running, jumping, twisting, and all symptoms (p<0.05). A higher

Table 8 Change in sports activities from preoperative levels

Change in Activities	Group 1* (%)	Group 2 (%)
Increased level, no symptoms	65	68
Same level, no symptoms	2	13
Decreased level, no symptoms	6	1
Playing with symptoms	13	10
Not participating because of knee condition	11	8
Not participating because of nonknee-related reasons	3	0

*Point scale:
  10 = normal knee, able to do strenuous work/sports with jumping, hard pivoting.
  8 = able to do moderate work/sports with running, twisting, turning; symptoms with strenuous work/sports.
  6 = able to do light work/sports with no running, twisting, jumping; symptoms with moderate work/sports.
  4 = able to do activities of daily living alone; symptoms with light work/sports.
  2 = moderate symptoms (frequent, limiting) with activities of daily living.
  0 = severe symptoms (constant, not relieved) with activities of daily living.
Group 1 had intra-articular bone-patellar ligament-bone allograft replacement; group 2 had intra-articular bone-patellar ligament-bone allograft replacement plus an extra-articular procedure involving tenodesis of the iliotibial band.
(Reproduced with permission from Noyes FR, Barber SD: The effect of an extra-articular procedure on allograft reconstructions for chronic ruptures of the anterior cruciate ligament. *J Bone Joint Surg* 1991;73A:882-892.)

distribution of patients in group 1 were still experiencing functional limitations and symptoms than in group 2; however, this difference was not significant.

A significant difference was found at follow-up between the two groups in terms of the frequency with which they participated in sports activities. In group 2, 81% were participating in sports activities on a weekly basis compared to 63% of group 1.

At follow-up, 65% of group 1 and 68% of group 2 had increased the level of sports activity compared with preoperative levels and were playing with no or mild symptoms (Table 8). This improvement was highly significant ($p<0.001$). Seven patients in group 1 and four patients in group 2 were participating despite moderate symptoms and limitations.

Preoperatively, the overall score was 58.1 ± 7.2 points for group 1 and 60.1 ± 8.9 points for group 2; this difference was not statistically significant (Fig. 7). At follow-up, the overall score was 85.8 ± 11.1 points for group 1 and 91.4 ± 6.8 points for group 2; this difference was significant ($p<0.01$). However, in both groups, the improvement from the preoperative score was highly significant ($p<0.001$). Fifty-eight percent of the patients in group 2 had at least a 31-point increase from the preoperative score, and 38% of those in group 1 had a similar increase (Table 9). Only one patient in group 1 had a decrease in the overall score.

The nine patients in group 1 in whom a previous ACL reconstruction had failed had an overall score of 79.6 ± 9.2 points at follow-up; the overall score for the rest of the group was 86.9 ± 11.1 points. In group 2, the overall score for the eight patients in whom such an operation had failed was 88.3 ± 0.1 points; the score for the rest of the group was 92.2 ± 5.9 points. These differences were not significant.

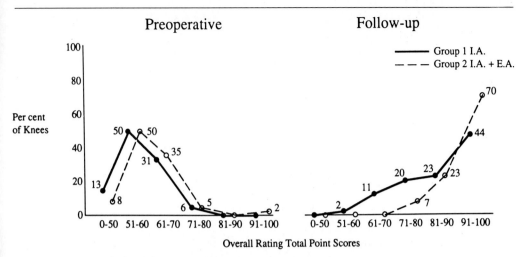

Fig. 7   *Preoperative and follow-up distributions of overall rating scores for group 1 (allograft alone) and group 2 (allograft and extra-articular procedure) in the chronic ACL rupture population. (Reproduced with permission from Noyes FR, Barber SD: The effect of an extra-articular procedure on allograft reconstructions for chronic ruptures of the anterior cruciate ligament.* J Bone Joint Surg *1991;73A:882-892.)*

Table 9 Increase in total points from preoperative score

Increase in Points	Group 1* (%)	Group 2 (%)
<10	3	2
11-20	20	2
21-30	39	38
31-40	28	43
41-50	8	15
>50	2	0
mean	27.8	31.3

*Point scale:
10 = normal knee, able to do strenuous work/sports with jumping, hard pivoting.
8 = able to do moderate work/sports with running, twisting, turning; symptoms with strenuous work/sports.
6 = able to do light work/sports with no running, twisting, jumping; symptoms with moderate work/sports.
4 = able to do activities of daily living alone; symptoms with light work/sports.
2 = moderate symptoms (frequent, limiting) with activities of daily living.
0 = severe symptoms (constant, not relieved) with activities of daily living.
Group 1 had intra-articular bone-patellar ligament-bone allograft replacement; group 2 had intra-articular bone-patellar ligament-bone allograft replacement plus an extra-articular procedure involving tenodesis of the iliotibial band.
(Reproduced with permission from Noyes FR, Barber SD: The effect of an extra-articular procedure on allograft reconstructions for chronic ruptures of the anterior cruciate ligament. *J Bone Joint Surg* 1991;73A:882-892.)

   In group 1, patients who were 30 years old had significantly lower overall scores (p<0.05) than patients less than 30 years old. No difference was found between these two subgroups in group 2.
   Stepwise linear regressions were performed between the overall rating scores and twenty variables. The results, shown in Table 5, demonstrate that many variables are required to predict the overall rating score, and that even a combination of up to seven variables

will result in the ability to predict the final score in only 65% of the population.

Complications

There were no instances of infection, clinical evidence of rejection of the allografts, or, at the time of writing, transmission of disease in either study.

In the study of acute ACL ruptures only one allograft failed. Three years after surgery, the patient had moderate pain, swelling, and giving-way with activities of daily living. Arthroscopy showed that the fascia lata allograft was intact but lax; it allowed 8 mm of increased anteroposterior translation in comparison with the contralateral knee on arthrometer testing. This patient also had significant fibrillation of the articular cartilage throughout the knee joint. The allograft was removed and the patient does not participate in any athletic activities.

In the study of acute ACL ruptures, the immediate motion program was effective in restoring normal motion of the knee in all patients. Three patients required an arthroscopic release for peripatellar soft-tissue contractures between 12 and 20 weeks postoperatively. These patients demonstrated normal knee motion at follow-up. Twenty-seven patients in the study of acute ACL ruptures required follow-up arthroscopy when the prominent staples that were used for graft fixation required removal. It was noted that the sutured fibers of the ACL, which easily could be distinguished from the allograft, were lax, representing poorly oriented collagenous tissue. The underlying allograft had a well organized, longitudinally oriented, collagenous fiber-bundle appearance and provided resistance to an applied anterior displacement. Because of the poor appearance of the sutured ACL fibers, I no longer perform the repair but use a replacement alone.

Three allografts failed in the study of chronic ACL ruptures. Two of these allografts failed in the early postoperative period: one was replaced in the sixteenth postoperative week with a second allograft and the other was successfully reattached at the osseous component in the tibial tunnel during the twelfth postoperative week. Both of these reoperations were successful and the results were included in the study. A third allograft failed in a 36-year-old woman who had undergone four arthroscopies and a proximotibial osteotomy prior to the allograft surgery. The allograft gradually stretched to a nonfunctioning status over the postoperative course; the pivot shift and Lachman tests showed two grades of increase compared with the contralateral limb. The patient is no longer involved in sports activities, but is asymptomatic during activities of daily living.

In the study of chronic ACL ruptures, 64 of the 104 patients required removal of prominent tibial fixation. During the period of both studies, tibial fixation was achieved with one or two small staples and a 6-mm diameter cancellous-bone screw. Sutures from the osseous portion of the allograft were attached to the distal staple. In late 1987, the introduction of a larger 9-mm diameter interference cancellous-bone screw allowed the use of the staples to be discontinued; this reduced the number of patients requiring removal of the tibial fixation.

In the study of chronic ACL ruptures, the immediate motion program restored normal motion in 93 (89%) of the 104 knees. All of the patients regained at least 135 degrees of flexion; the remaining 11 knees had limitations of extension that required treatment, which has been described in detail.[1,17] At follow-up, only four still lacked 5 degrees of extension.

Discussion

There are four areas of concern in considering the use of allografts: immunogenicity, preservation and secondary sterilization, remodeling and its effects on mechanical properties, and disease transmission. In the clinical trials described in this chapter, no deleterious effects were found in any of these areas to contraindicate the use of allografts.

There was no evidence of rejection of the allografts in either clinical trial. This finding is in agreement with other published studies; in fact, there have been no reports of rejection of ACL ligament allograft replacements to date.[3,7,9,10] The allografts used in these published clinical studies have either been freeze-dried or frozen; the hypothesis that these processing techniques partially destroy the antigenicity of cells has been supported by several reports. Friedlaender[20] and Czitrom and associates[21] each reported that fresh bone allografts are the most immunogenic, frozen allografts are less immunogenic, and freeze-dried grafts are the least immunogenic. Fresh bone-patellar ligament-bone allografts invoked an inflammatory response in the Arnoczky and associates[22] dog model, with infiltration of lymphocytes observed during the fourth postoperative week. However, frozen grafts showed no evidence of rejection and, at one year after surgery, they resembled a normal ACL both grossly and histologically. Shino and associates[23] also transplanted frozen bone-tendon-bone allografts in dogs and found no histologic evidence of an immune rejection.

The effects of various secondary sterilization techniques on allograft properties have been examined by several studies. Freeze-drying markedly reduces the mechanical properties of the bone component of allografts;[24,25] few or no deleterious effects are caused by freezing and low-dose (less than 2.5 Mrads) gamma irradiation.[26-28] Freezing and low-dose irradiation also are not deleterious to the mechanical properties of the collagen component of allografts.[27,28] Ethylene oxide is not advocated as a safe method of sterilization as a result of recent reports of recurrent postoperative synovitis and the formation of tibial and femoral bone cysts in knees that received allograft tissue sterilized with this agent.[8,10]

Allograft remodeling and its effect on mechanical properties are still under investigation. Animal studies suggest that allografts and autogenous grafts undergo significant reductions in strength and stiffness following implantation.[23,29-36] A gradual increase in these mechanical properties occurs over many months, but even at one year after surgery the properties remain below normal values. Sabiston and associates[35] found that the strength and stiffness of medial collateral ligament allografts in rabbits were less than 50% of normal 48 weeks after implantation. There is insufficient evidence to determine if a delay exists in maturation of allografts compared with autogenous grafts. There may be certain areas in the collagenous portion of the allograft that remain nonviable for many months following implantation. Histologic studies of human allografts have examined only the surface portion of the graft.[4-6]

Concern exists among all individuals involved with allografts regarding the possibility of transmission of the human immunodeficiency virus (HIV) from infected donors who test negative for the antibody in the time period prior to the production of antibodies. The need for rigorous selection criteria for donors, antibody and antigen screening for HIV, and detailed histologic examination of donor tissues has been advocated by Buck and associates.[37,38] These authors estimated that, given the current donor screening procedures, the risk of HIV transmission from an undetected donor is less than one in one million. The use of secondary gamma irradiation would be expected to reduce the risk even further. The effect of gamma irradiation on inactivation of HIV is, however, dependent on the bioburden of the virus and the dose of irradiation used. The exact dose-response curve to inactivate HIV has not been established. Although the American Association of Tissue Banks[39] currently recommends 2.5 Mrads (with the provision that some resistant viruses may survive this dose), Conway and associates[40] presented calculations that hypothesized that higher levels (4 Mrads) would be required to inactivate HIV in grafts from donors with higher levels of HIV bioburden. The dose of 2.5 Mrads would be expected to inactivate the virus in the infected donor in the window period that precedes production of antibodies because the HIV bioburden is not at the higher concentration levels. I advise my patients that there is a risk of disease transmission with any transplant procedure; however, with all of the precautions taken and with the addition of secondary sterilization with irradiation, this risk is so slight that it is difficult to calculate with any accuracy. In short, the risk is next to zero, but it is not zero.

Tissue banking may still be considered to be in an inchoate state, and it is uncertain that existing banks can maintain a sufficient supply of tissue for all orthopaedic needs. I strongly advocate that surgeons obtain grafts only from tissue banks certified by the American Association of Tissue Banks. Kateley[41] recommended that all banks incorporate various screening and serologic studies, including those for HIV antibody, hepatitis-B core antibody and surface antigen, hepatitis-C antibody, herpes virus, antinuclear antibody, and rheumatoid factor. Surgeons should be aware that not all tissue banks have adopted these recommendations, and should be fully familiar with the protocols of the tissue banks that are used to provide grafts for operations.

The results of patients operated on for acute and chronic ACL ruptures should be analyzed separately. These two clinical studies show that differences exist in a number of variables that do not allow these populations to be combined in a single study. One important example is the results of the KT-1000 arthrometer data. Although 83% of the patients with acute ACL rupture who received bone-patellar ligament-bone allografts had less than 3 mm of anteroposterior displacement (compared with the opposite knee), only 54% (allograft alone) and 74% (combined procedure) of patients with chronic ACL rupture had this desirable amount of displacement at follow-up. One also cannot assess the overall results of acute and chronic populations in the same manner; the majority of patients with chronic ACL ruptures will have preoperative problems, such as moderate or severe patellofemoral crepitus or radiographic evidence of arthrosis, that cannot be corrected by surgery. The results of the stepwise linear regression analyses provide statistical support to this concept. The results of only a few variables were required in the study of acute ACL rupture to predict the overall result. However, in the study of chronic ACL rupture, the combination of several variables was necessary to predict the overall result, and the percentage of accuracy was significantly lower than that obtained in the acute population. Thus, according to the rating system, one must adopt separate strategies for assessing treatment programs for studies of acute and chronic ACL ruptures.

In the study of acute ACL ruptures, the majority of patients were young athletic individuals who wished to return to competitive sports. All were counseled regarding a conservative program of rehabilitation and activity modification for the ACL rupture.[42,43] These individuals elected to undergo reconstruction to avoid the potential complications of returning to competitive sports with a chronic ACL-deficient knee. The short-term results presented in this study showed that all but two patients returned to sports activities, and that nearly half were able to return to the same level of activity as before their ACL injury. Considering that the criteria for the determination of the overall rating are among the strictest that have been published to date, I was pleased that 89% in the acute study had an excellent or good overall rating. I feel that this type of strict rating is justified for acute knee studies, and that to achieve an excellent result a patient must have a near normal knee and be able to perform twisting, turning, pivoting, and jumping activities with no or only slight limitations.

In the study of chronic ACL ruptures, both the intra-articular alone and intra-articular and extra-articular combined procedures proved to be effective in decreasing functional limitations and symptoms and in improving the level of sports activity and the overall scores. The use of an extra-articular procedure affected the outcome, however, because those patients had significantly better results in reduced abnormal anteroposterior displacement, level of sports activity, overall score, and failure rate. A potential bias did exist in this study, because all of the patients in the combined group demonstrated a strong desire to return to competitive sports activities. This was not as strong a factor in the decision to undergo surgery in the other group, in which other problems such as symptoms during activities of daily living, and associated with meniscal loss and articular cartilage deterioration constituted the main reasons for undergoing reconstruction. Patients who wish to return to sports activities often are more motivated during the rehabilitation program and have a better functional result, hence the potential for higher overall scores at follow-up.

It is interesting that no statistically significant relationships were found in the study of chronic ACL rupture between abnormal articular cartilage surfaces and pain, swelling, or level of sports activity. These results present a dilemma in that the surgery successfully restabilizes the knee, allowing the patient to return to sports activities, and the presence of arthrosis does not necessarily correlate with symptoms or functional limitations. The patient may feel free to return to competitive sports activities that may be deleterious to the joint over the long-term. Although no correlation was found between symptoms and articular cartilage deterioration in the study of chronic ACL rupture, I still advise patients of the potential for further deterioration of the joint with strenuous activities and advise reduction of sports that require heavy twisting, turning, jumping, and pivoting. The need clearly exists for a long-term study of the natural history of knees in which a chronic ACL rupture is successfully restablilized and the patient returns to sports activities.

The results of the study of chronic ACL ruptures support the use of allografts in knees in which prior autogenous ACL reconstructions have failed. In the subgroup of 17 patients, all but one had a significant increase in the overall score from preoperative to follow-up. The severe symptoms and instability that had been found prior to surgery had resolved in all of these individuals.

Any limitation in knee motion should be treated early (within weeks) in the postoperative period to avoid a serious contracture. The immediate motion and rehabilitation program used for the two study groups is a critical part of these studies and has been described in detail.[1,16,17] Of the 151 patients studied in both groups, only three required early arthroscopic lysis of adhesions as a result of motion limitations. I am concerned about the high percentage of combined-procedure patients in the study of chronic ACL rupture who experienced difficulty regaining full extension of the knee (18%). Surgeons and therapists should be aware that patients who undergo a combined intra-articular and extra-articular procedure may have greater difficulty regaining full extension than those who have only an intra-articular procedure.

I am also concerned about the high percentage of patients in whom normal or mild preoperative patellofemoral crepitus had become moderate at follow-up. In the study of acute ACL ruptures, 21% had increased crepitus, and, in the other study, 20% of the patients with the combined procedure and 14% of the patients with the allograft alone had increased crepitus. Although no significant relationships were found between patellofemoral crepitus and symptoms or functional limitations, the rehabilitation program is continually monitored, and exercises that place large forces on the patellofemoral joint are modified when crepitus is detected.

The displacement data showed two major conclusions: (1) Allografts are not as effective when they are used alone in the treatment of chronic ACL ruptures as when they are used in combination with the described extra-articular procedure. (2) Although the combined procedure significantly reduced displacements in the study of chronic ruptures, the results were not equal to those of the study of acute ruptures. These conclusions are drawn from the percentage of patients with less than 3 mm of anteroposterior displacement. There are some knees that show 3 to 5 mm of increased anteroposterior displacement in which the pivot shift test is negative and the patients are able to function without limitations. This amount of increased displacement represents an area in which it is difficult to assess the true functional capacity of the ligament replacement. I believe that knees in this displacement range, which have a negative pivot shift, do have a partially functioning ligament replacement. Additionally, I agree with Daniel and Stone[44] that performing the test at a higher force level (30 lbs) will help to distinguish those replacements that are truly functioning. The 30-lb total anteroposterior test is preferred over the manual maximum test because of possible inherent reliability problems with the latter. The variability from one examiner to another in performing the manual maximum test makes comparison between studies impossible.

Summary

In the two clinical studies presented in this chapter, allografts are shown to be effective in reducing symptoms, functional limitations, and anteroposterior displacements in knees with acute and chronic ACL tears. Bone-patellar ligament-bone allografts had significantly lower anteroposterior displacement measurements at follow-up than fascia lata allografts and are recommended for acute ACL tears. In chronic ACL tears, a combined allograft and extra-articular procedure resulted in significantly lower anteroposterior displacement measurements at follow-up than an allograft used alone. However, surgeons and therapists need to be aware of the increased morbidity of an extra-articular procedure in terms of limitations in regaining full knee extension postoperatively. Moreover, the combined procedure still did not provide anteroposterior displacement values equal to those provided by allografts used in acute ACL injuries. The combined procedure appears to provide results comparable to autogenous bone-patellar ligament-bone grafts, but more data are needed before final conclusions can be reached.

Allografts continue to offer advantages in select patients who have a narrow patellar ligament, malalignment of the extensor mechanism, a previously failed reconstruction of the ACL with an autogenous graft, or patellofemoral or tibiofemoral osteoarthrosis. As such, the use of allografts represents an important adjunct to the surgeon performing knee reconstructive procedures. Still, I believe a central one-third bone-patellar tendon-bone autograft placed in an arthroscopically-assisted manner is the best procedure at the present time, particularly in routine situations in which no special circumstance warrants the allograft procedure. The risk of morbidity from the autograft procedure is believed to be very low when immediate motion programs are carefully instituted postoperatively.

As stated in previous reports, the clinician faces many obstacles when using allografts. These include the need for careful supervision of grafts obtained for transplant to ensure that they have been correctly processed, secondarily sterilized, and are free of transmittable disease. Because the underlying responsibility for prevention of disease transmission rests with the surgeon, I advocate that personnel be specifically trained in these areas so that current and future knowledge in transplantation and graft procurement and sterilization are readily available. For these reasons, I caution against the widespread use of allografts at the present time and continue to recommend that they be used only at centers that have the necessary trained personnel available.

References

1. Noyes FR, Barber SD, Mangine RE: Bone-patellar ligament-bone and fascia lata allografts for reconstruction of the anterior cruciate ligament. *J Bone Joint Surg* 1990;72A:1125-1136.
2. Noyes FR, Barber SD: The effect of an extra-articular procedure on allograft reconstructions for chronic ruptures of the anterior cruciate ligament. *J Bone Joint Surg* 1991;73A:882-892.
3. Shino K, Kimura T, Hirose H, et al: Reconstruction of the anterior cruciate ligament by allogeneic tendon graft: An operation for chronic ligamentous insufficiency. *J Bone Joint Surg* 1986;68B:739-746.
4. Shino K, Inoue M, Horibe S, et al: Maturation of allograft tendons transplanted into the knee: An arthroscopic and histological study. *J Bone Joint Surg* 1988;70B:556-560.
5. Shino K, Inoue M, Nakamura H, et al: Arthroscopic follow-up of anterior cruciate ligament reconstruction using allogeneic tendon. *Arthroscopy* 1989;5:165-171.
6. Shino K, Inoue M, Horbie S, et al: Surface blood flow and histology of human anterior cruciate ligament allografts. *Arthroscopy* 1991;7:171-176.

7. Wainer RA, Clarke TJ, Poehling GG: Arthroscopic reconstruction of the anterior cruciate ligament using allograft tendon. *Arthroscopy* 1988;4:199-205.

8. Jackson DW, Windler GE, Simon TM: Intraarticular reaction associated with the use of freeze-dried, ethylene oxide-sterilized bone-patella tendon-bone allografts in the reconstruction of the anterior cruciate ligament. *Am J Sports Med* 1990;18:1-11.

9. Indelicato PA, Bittar ES, Prevot TJ, et al: Clinical comparison of freeze-dried and fresh frozen patellar tendon allografts for anterior cruciate ligament reconstruction of the knee. *Am J Sports Med* 1990;18:335-342.

10. Roberts TS, Drez D Jr, McCarthy W, et al: Anterior cruciate ligament reconstruction using freeze-dried, ethylene oxide-sterilized, bone-patellar tendon-bone allografts: Two year results in thirty-six patients. *Am J Sports Med* 1991;19:35-41.

11. Jackson DW, Kurzweil PR: Allografts in knee ligament surgery, in Scott WN (ed): *Ligament and Extensor Mechanism Injuries of the Knee: Diagnosis and Treatment.* St. Louis, Mosby Year Book, 1991, pp 349-360.

12. Daniel DM, Malcom LL, Losse G, et al: Instrumented measurement of anterior laxity of the knee. *J Bone Joint Surg* 1985;67A:720-726.

13. Barber SD, Noyes FR, Mangine RE, et al: Quantitative assessment of functional limitations in normal and anterior cruciate ligament-deficient knees. *Clin Orthop* 1990;255:204-214.

14. Noyes FR, Grood ES: Diagnosis of knee ligament injuries: Clinical concepts, in Feagin JA Jr (ed): *The Crucial Ligaments: Diagnosis and Treatment of Ligamentous Injuries About the Knee.* New York, Churchill Livingstone, 1988, pp 261-285.

15. Noyes FR, Barber SD, Mooar LA: A rationale for assessing sports activity levels and limitations in knee disorders. *Clin Orthop* 1989;246:238-249.

16. Noyes FR, Mangine RE, Barber S: Early knee motion after open and arthroscopic anterior cruciate ligament reconstruction. *Am J Sports Med* 1987;15:149-160.

17. Noyes FR, Mangine RE, Barber SD: The early treatment of motion complications following anterior cruciate ligament reconstruction. *Clin Orthop,* in press.

18. Noyes FR, Stabler CL: A system for grading articular cartilage lesions at arthroscopy. *Am J Sports Med* 1989;17:505-513.

19. Losee RE, Johnson TR, Southwick WO: Anterior subluxation of the lateral tibial plateau: A diagnostic test and operative repair. *J Bone Joint Surg* 1978:60A:1015-1030.

20. Friedlaender GE: Immune responses to osteochondral allografts: Current knowledge and future directions. *Clin Orthop* 1983;174:58-68.

21. Czitrom AA, Langer F, McKee N, et al: Bone and cartilage allotransplantation: A review of 14 years of research and clinical studies. *Clin Orthop* 1986;208:141-145.

22. Arnoczky SP, Warren RF, Ashlock MA: Replacement of the anterior cruciate ligament using a patellar tendon allograft: An experimental study. *J Bone Joint Surg* 1986;68A:376-385.

23. Shino K, Kawasaki T, Hirose H, et al: Replacement of the anterior cruciate ligament by an allogeneic tendon graft: An experimental study in the dog. *J Bone Joint Surg* 1984;66B:672-681.

24. Pelker RR, Friedlaender GE, Markham TC: Biomechanical properties of bone allografts. *Clin Orthop* 1983;174:54-57.

25. Triantafyllou N, Sotiropoulos E, Triantafyllou JN: The mechanical properties of the lyophylized and irradiated bone grafts. *Acta Orthop Belg Suppl* 1975;41:35-44.

26. Bright RW, Smarsh JD, Gambill VM: Sterilization of human bone by irradiaton, in Friedlaender GE, Mankin J, Sell KW (eds): *Osteochondral Allografts: Biology, Banking, and Clinical Applications.* Boston, Little Brown, 1981, pp 223-232.

27. Butler DL, Noes FR, Walz KA, et al: Biomechanics of human ligament allograft treatment. *Trans Orthop Res Soc* 1987;12:128.

28. Gibbons MJ, Butler DL, Grood ES, et al: Effects of gamma irradiation on the initial mechanical and material properties of goat bone-patellar tendon-bone allografts. *J Orthop Res* 1991;9:209-218.

29. Ballock RT, Woo SL-Y, Lyon RM, et al: Use of patellar tendon allograft for anterior cruciate ligament reconstruction in the rabbit: A long-term histologic and biomechanical study. *J Orthop Res* 1989;7: 474-485.

30. Butler DL, Hulse DA, Kay MD, et al: Biomechanics of cranial cruciate ligament reconstruction in the dog: II. Mechanical properties. *Vet Surg* 1983;12:113-118.

31. Butler DL, Grood ES, Noyes FR, et al: Mechanical properties of primate vascularized vs nonvascularized patellar tendon grafts: Changes over time. *J Orthop Res* 1989;7:68-79.

32. Clancy WG Jr, Narechania RG, Rosenberg TD, et al: Anterior and posterior cruciate ligament reconstruction in rhesus monkeys: A histological, microangiographic, and biomechanical analysis. *J Bone Joint Surg* 1981;63A:1270-1284.

33. Jackson DW, Grood ES, Arnoczky SP, et al: Freeze dried anterior cruciate ligament allografts: Preliminary studies in a goat model. *Am J Sports Med* 1987;15:295-303.

34. Jackson DW, Grood ES, Arnoczky SP, et al: Cruciate reconstruction using freeze dried anterior cruciate ligament allograft and a ligament augmentation device (LAD): An experimental study in a goat model. *Am J Sports Med* 1987;15:528-538.

35. Sabiston P, Frank C, Lam T, et al: Transplantation of the rabbit medial collateral ligament: II. Biomechanical evaluation of frozen solidus thawed allografts. *J Orthop Res* 1990;8:46-56.

36. Webster DA, Werner FW: Freeze-dried flexor tendons in anterior cruciate ligament reconstruction. *Clin Orthop* 1983;181:238-243.

37. Buck BE, Balinin TI, Brown MD: Bone transplantation and human immunodeficiency virus: An estimate of risk of acquired immunodeficiency syndrome (AIDS). *Clin Orthop* 1989;240:129-136.

38. Buck BE, Resnick L, Shah SM, et al: Human immunodeficiency virus cultured from bone: Implications for transplantation. *Clin Orthop* 1990;251:249-253.

39. American Association of Tissue Banks: *Technical Manual for Surgical Bone Banking.* McLean, VA, American Association of Tissue Banks, 1987, p 8.

40. Conway B, Tomford WW, Hirsch MS, et al: Effects of gamma irradiation on HIV-1 in a bone allograft model. *Trans Orthop Res Soc* 1990;15:225.

41. Kateley JR: Establishing a tissue bank, in Fawcett K, Barr AR (eds): *Tissue Banking.* Arlington, VA, Amercan Association of Blook Banks, 1987, pp 17-27.

42. Noyes FR, Mooar P, Matthews DS, et al: The symptomatic anterior cruciate-deficent knee: Part I. The long-term functional disability in athletically active individuals. *J Bone Joint Surg* 1983;65A:154-162.

43. Noyes FR, Matthews DS, Mooar PA, et al: The symptomatic anterior cruciate-deficient knee: Part II. The results of rehabilitation, activity modification, and counseling on functional disability. *J Bone Joint Surg* 1983;65A:163-174.
44. Daniel DM, Stone ML: KT-1000 anterior-posterior displacement measurements, in Daniel DM, Akeson WH, O'Connor JJ (eds): *Knee Ligaments: Structure, Function, Injury, and Repair*. New York, Raven Press, 1990, pp 427-447.

Chapter 23

The Clinical Measurement of Knee Instability

Dale M. Daniel, MD
Mary Lou Stone, RPT
Christopher Rangger, MD

Introduction

Joint motion is determined by external loads, muscle forces, joint surface contours, and the soft-tissue restraints. The articular surfaces hold the bones apart and are loaded in compression. Because the joint surfaces covered with hyaline cartilage have a very low coefficient of friction, there is negligible joint surface resistance to shear. The soft tissues that cross the joint (ligaments, tendons, and capsular structures) hold the joint together and are loaded in tension. The muscles, with their tendons, stabilize the skeleton in the presence of gravitational forces and other loads; they also initiate and maintain movements. The ligaments, capsular structures, and bony architecture limit the joint motions, preventing joint subluxation and dislocation.

The motion of the knee or any other joint can be described in terms of rotations about or translations along three mutually perpendicular axes. Rotation means to turn about an axis; translation means to slide along an axis. Free motion about or along these axes that is used to define a space represents six degrees of freedom. Figure 1 shows the three axes. Evaluations of flexion/extension about the mediolateral axis, abduction/adduction about the anteroposterior axis, and anteroposterior translation along the anteroposterior axis are part of the routine clinical examination, and the technique for motion evaluation is well described.[1] Medial/lateral and penetration/distraction translations are not routinely evaluated. Internal/external rotation has been evaluated,[2-6] but clinical measurement has shown poor reproducibility.[7,8] "Pivot shift" tests that produce complex motions have been used to evaluate axial rotation.[3,6,9]

It is rare for any anatomic movement to require only one degree of freedom. Knee flexion is associated primarily with rotation about the y axis (Fig. 1), but the tibia also translates along the x axis and rotates about the z axis during flexion. Motions such as these are referred to as coupled motions. Equally, it is rare that the external

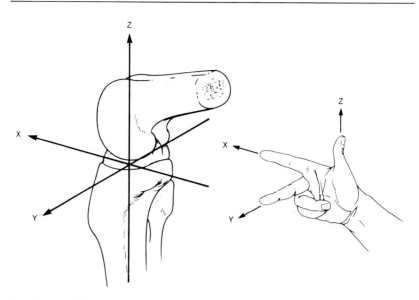

Fig. 1 *Left, Diagram of the knee with axes superimposed. **Right**, The axes form a "right-hand" system. The axis system can be thought of as attached or embedded in the tibia. Motion of the femur with respect to the tibia consists of three translations and three rotations. Translation along the x axis is anteroposterior movement, along the y axis is mediolateral inducement, and along the z axis is distraction or interpenetration of the femur; tibia rotation about the x axis is abduction or adduction, about the y axis is flexion or extension, and about the z axis is tibial rotation. (Reproduced with permission from Biden E, O'Connor J: Experimental methods used to evaluate knee ligament function, in Daniel DM, Akeson WH, O'Connor JJ (eds):* Knee Ligaments: Structure, Function, Injury, and Repair. *New York, Raven Press, 1990, pp 135-151.)*

loads are such that only one component of force or moment is transmitted across the joint (Fig. 2). In Figure 2, when an anteriorly-directed force is applied to the tibia, lateral to the axis of tibial rotation, internal rotation is produced as well as anterior translation of the tibia relative to the femur. When the force is applied medial to the axis, external rotation is produced as well as translation. Only when the load is applied through the axis and has zero moment about the axis is the resulting motion one of pure translation without coupled rotation. When motions are linked or coupled to one another, constraint of one motion will limit the other motion as illustrated in Figure 3. Thus, the displacement measured along one axis may depend on the testing systems' constraints of motions around or along other axes.

The evaluation of joint instability has been used to diagnose a knee ligament disruption, plan surgical procedures, predict functional outcomes, and evaluate surgical results.[1-3,10-15] The relationship between functional outcome and measured instability is yet to be documented.

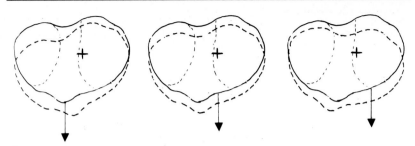

Fig. 2   *Left*, *Anterior force applied to the tibia lateral to axis of rotation produces internal rotation as well as anterior translation.* ***Center***, *Anterior force applied through axis of rotation produces only anterior translation.* ***Right***, *Anterior force applied medial to axis of rotation produces external rotation as well as anterior translation (Reproduced with permission from Biden E, O'Connor J: Experimental methods used to evaluate knee ligament function, in Daniel DM, Akeson WH, O'Connor JJ (eds):* Knee Ligaments: Structure, Function, Injury, and Repair. *New York, Raven Press, 1990, pp 135-151.)*

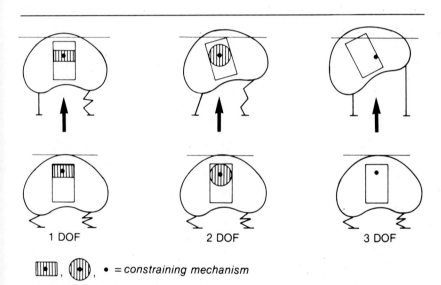

Fig. 3   *Influence of motion constraints on anterior translation in structures with two restraining tethers of different lengths. A structure shaped like the surface of the tibia is drawn with a central rectangular window. When the structure is placed over a rectangular peg the same width as the window, the structure can only translate anteriorly and posteriorly, and there is one degree of freedom. When the structure is placed over a large circular peg, it has two degrees of freedom, anteroposterior translation, and rotation about the peg. When the structure is placed over a small peg, there is anteroposterior translation, mediolateral translation and rotation around the peg (three degrees of freedom). The anterior translation of the structure is restrained by two tethers of different lengths. When there is only one degree of freedom, the structure can move only as far as the shorter tether will allow. When the structure has two degrees of freedom, the anterior translation increases; when there are three degrees of freedom, the structure can move forward until the two tethers are taut. (Reproduced with permission from Daniel DM, Stone ML: Instrumented measurement of knee motion, in Daniel DM, Akeson WH, O'Connor JJ (eds):* Knee Ligaments: Structure, Function, Injury, and Repair. *New York, Raven Press, 1990, pp 421-426.)*

Manual Examination

The clinical evaluation of joint motion produced by external forces has been the basis for the diagnosis of ligament injuries. The clinician moves the normal limb to determine the patient's normal limb motion, and then moves the injured limb in a similar manner to estimate the amount of motion and the "end point stiffness" of the joint motion limits. Careful manual examination of joint motion will reveal most ligament disruptions.

The patient should lie supine on a firm but comfortable examining table with the limb supported. Patient relaxation is important for accurate results. The motion resulting from a clinical test depends on the limb's position at the beginning of the test, the force applied, point of application of the force, and point of detection of the displacement. Joint motion varies considerably within the normal population, but there is little right-left variation in a normal subject. Therefore, in a patient with a unilateral knee injury, the motion of the injured knee should be compared with that of the normal knee. To compare the two limbs, especially if comparing the results of different examiners or serial examinations, the following examination conditions must be constant: starting position, applied force, and site of motion measurement.

Several tests have been described to detect pathologic motion in the knee. The pathologic motion resulting from certain tests is associated with a specific ligament or ligament complexes (Table 1). Primary tests render pathologic motion only if the ligament in question is injured. The injury of other ligaments may increase the pathologic motion being tested, provided that the primary ligament is disrupted.[16] With all displacement measurements, the femur is held constant and tibial translation or joint space opening is measured. The starting position is the neutral resting position with the joint surfaces in contact. The variability of manual clinical test measurements by experienced examiners has recently been reported.[7-9]

Instrumented Measurement of Knee Motion

Motion measurements are determined by: (1) positioning the limb in a specified manner; (2) applying a displacing force; and (3) measuring the resultant joint motion or position. The testing devices may perform one, two, or all of the above tasks; however, the early reports of instrumented testing indicated that all of these tasks were performed. Change in joint position was documented by comparing photographs[17] or radiographs[4,18-21] of the unstressed and stressed knee. Stress radiography has not been widely used in North America. This may be because of concern about the resultant radiation exposure, the expense of multiple roentgenogram examinations, and the attention to detail needed when positioning the patient and when measuring the films.

Table 1 Primary clinical limits of motion tests

Test	Ligament/ligament complex isolated injury*				
	ACL	PCL	MCC	LCC	PLC
Lachman	X				
Pivot shift	X				
Tibia posterior subluxation		X			
Abduction (25 degrees)			X		
Adduction (25 degrees)				X	
Reverse pivot shift					X

*ACL, anterior cruciate ligament; PCL, posterior cruciate ligament; MCC, medial collateral complex; LCC, lateral collateral complex; PLC, posterior lateral complex. (Reproduced with permission from Daniel DM: Diagnosis of a ligament injury, in Daniel DM, Akeson WH, O'Connor JJ (eds): *Knee Ligaments: Structure, Function, Injury, and Repair.* New York, Raven Press, 1990, pp 3-10.)

Instrumented measurement systems that document anteroposterior tibial displacement by tracking the tibial tubercle in relation to the patella have been widely reported. Markolf,[22] Shino,[23] and Edixhoven[24] and their associates developed stationary testing systems. Commercially available portable testing systems were developed by Cannon and Lamoreux (Knee Laxity Tester, Stryker Ligament Tester) and Malcolm and Daniel (KT-1000).[25,26] More recently, commercial devices have been introduced that simultaneously measure motion in several directions.

Testing Variables

Motion measurements depend on the following factors; (1) joint position at the initiation of the test; (2) motion constraints imposed by the testing system; (3) displacing force; (4) measurement system; (5) muscle activity; and (6) passive motion constraints. The role of the testing device is to minimize the variability between the first five factors so that the difference in measurements between one or both knees tested at time intervals indicates a true change in the passive motion constraints. Examples of how the first five factors may affect the displacement measurements are given next.

Joint Starting Position

Flexion   The joint flexion angle will affect the orientation of the ligament with respect to the applied force and may affect the distance between the ligament's attachment sites.[27] When the anterior cruciate ligament (ACL) is disrupted, there is a greater increase in anterior displacement with the knee in 30 degrees of flexion than in 90 degrees of flexion.[28-30] When the posterior cruciate ligament is disrupted, there is a greater increase in displacement at 90 degrees of flexion than at 30 degrees of flexion.[31] With the cruciates sectioned, other structures become the primary anteroposterior displacement constraints. The effects of joint position on these structures vary.

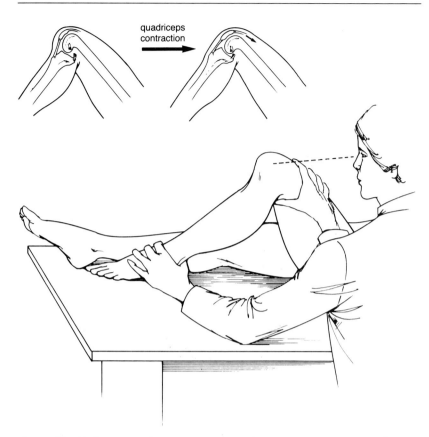

Fig. 4   *The 90-degree quadriceps active test. Keeping the eyes level with the subject's flexed knee, the examiner rests the elbow on the table and uses the ipsilateral hand to support the subject's thigh and to confirm that the thigh muscles are relaxed. The foot is stabilized by the examiner's other hand, and the subject is asked to slide the foot gently down the table. Tibial displacement resulting from the quadriceps contraction is noted. (Reproduced with permission from Daniel DM, Stone ML: KT-1000 anterior-posterior displacement measurements, in Daniel DM, Akeson WH, O'Connor JJ (eds): Knee Ligaments: Structure, Function, Injury, and Repair. New York, Raven Press, 1990, pp 427-447.)*

Axial Rotation   Rotation of the tibia affects the distance between the ligament's attachment sites and anteroposterior displacement measurements.[28,32,33] Markolf and associates[22,28] reported that 15 degrees of external rotation results in the greatest anterior knee laxity in vivo.

Sagittal Plane Displacement   Flexion of the knee relaxes the posterior capsule. In a patient lying supine, the posterior cruciate partially supports the weight of the leg. If the posterior cruciate ligament is disrupted, the tibia will sag posteriorly (Fig. 4). When the patient is in the prone position, the ACL partially supports the weight of the leg. If the ACL is disrupted, the tibia will sag anteriorly. Sagittal plane motion is the measured displacement between posterior and anterior displacing forces.

Motion Constraints Imposed by the Tester or the Testing System

An unconstrained testing system allows six degrees of freedom, that is, rotation around and translation along each of the three axes (Fig. 1). Anterior translation and internal rotation are normally paired, as are posterior translation and external rotation. When motions are coupled, constraint of one of the motions will limit the other. This concept is illustrated in Figure 3. In the modestly constrained anteroposterior testing system reported by Edixhoven and associates,[24] pulling the tibia anteriorly resulted in 11 to 13 degrees of internal tibial rotation. Pushing posteriorly resulted in 2 to 6 degrees of external tibial rotation. The KT-1000 testing system was designed to provide minimal constraint to knee motion while measuring anteroposterior translation. Perhaps one of the reasons that Sherman and associates[34] measured greater displacements with the KT-1000 arthrometer than with the UCLA testing device is because the UCLA device provides greater limb constraint.

Displacement Force

Magnitude   When loaded, the soft-tissue constraints of the knee are lengthened. The greater the displacement force, the greater the displacement. Figure 5 illustrates factors to consider when calculating the displacing force. Because the ligaments are viscoelastic tissues, the rate of load application will affect joint displacement. However, Markolf and associates[22] and Edixhoven and associates[24] have reported that the rate of load application in clinical testing did not affect the force/displacement curve. Edixhoven and associates[24] recommend that one testing cycle be performed to condition the joint before measuring displacement.

Greater displacement forces reveal a greater incidence of pathologic motion. The manual maximum force that does not extend the knee, cause patient discomfort, or induce muscle contraction has been more diagnostic of a cruciate ligament disruption than a measured 89-N (20-lb) force. Because the manual force (estimated to be from 30 to 40 lbs) is applied more proximally on the leg than the force through the force handle of the KT-1000 arthrometer, a higher load can be applied without extending the knee. While watching the instrument dial, a force is applied until the displacement stops. Although the force used by different examiners undoubtedly varies, in our clinic displacement measured with the manual maximum test reveals the greatest incidence of pathologic motion (Tables 2 and 3) and has proved to be a measurement that can be repeated between examiners.[35] Therefore, in addition to a measured 89-N and a 134-N

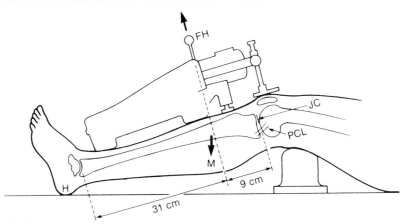

Fig. 5   *The patient is supine. The testing instrument is mounted on the front of the leg. The mass of the leg and testing device (M) is supported by tension in the soft tissues, represented by the posterior cruciate ligament (PCL), compression force at the joint surface (JC), and compression at the heel (H). When an anterior force is applied through the force handle (FH), the weight of the leg and testing device is first lifted to unload the joint structures and then, as further force is applied, the anterior constraining soft tissues are placed under tension. (Reproduced with permission from Daniel DM, Stone ML: Instrumented measurement of knee motion, in Daniel DM, Akeson WH, O'Connor JJ (eds):* Knee Ligaments: Structure, Function, Injury, and Repair. *New York, Raven Press, 1990, pp 421-426.)*

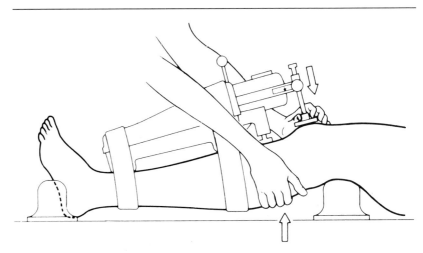

Fig. 6   *Manual maximum test. The limbs are positioned with the support system, the arthrometer is applied, and the testing reference position is obtained in the standard way. While the patellar sensor pad is stabilized with one hand, the other hand applies a strong anterior displacement force directly to the proximal calf to produce the maximum anterior displacement. Care is taken that the knee is not extended. The tibial displacement is read off the dial. (Reproduced with permission from Daniel DM, Stone ML: KT-1000 anterior-posterior displacement measurements, in Daniel DM, Akeson WH, O'Connor JJ (eds):* Knee Ligaments: Structure, Function, Injury, and Repair. *New York, Raven Press, 1990, pp 427-447.)*

Table 2 Anterior displacement measurements

	Mean	Range	Standard
Normal Subjects (N = 120)			
89 N Test			
Right	7.1	3.0 - 13.0	1.94
Left	7.3	4.0 - 14.5	1.90
R minus L	-0.2	-2.0 - 3.5	1.07
Manual Maximum Test			
Right	8.5	5.0 - 14.5	2.23
Left	8.8	5.0 - 15.0	2.12
R minus L	-0.3	-3.0 - 4.0	1.09
Quadriceps Active Test			
Right	5.4	2.0 - 12.5	1.8
Left	5.9	2.0 - 13.5	1.85
R minus L*	-0.5	-2.0 - 3.0	0.94
Acute Unilateral ACL Disruption (N = 105)			
89 N Test - No Anesthesia			
Noninvolved	7.8	3.0 - 13.0	1.76
Involved	11.5	5.0 - 18.0	2.59
I minus N*	3.6	0.0 - 13.0	2.12
89 N Test - With Anesthesia			
Noninvolved	7.3	3.5 - 13.0	2.04
Involved	11.5	5.0 - 18.0	2.88
I minus N*	4.4	0.0 - 11.5	2.45
Manual Maximum Test - No Anesthesia			
Noninvolved	9.1	3.5 - 13.0	1.77
Involved	15.2	10.1 - 21.0	2.50
I minus N*	6.1	1.0 - 12.0	2.22
Manual Maximum Test - With Anesthesia			
Noninvolved	9.0	3.5 - 13.0	2.12
Involved	16.3	6.0 - 20.0	2.83
I minus N*	7.3	0.0 - 11.5	2.48
Quadriceps Active Test - No Anesthesia			
Noninvolved	6.5	1.0 - 11.0	1.80
Involved	8.5	2.0 - 20.0	2.45
I minus N*	2.0	-3.5 - 9.0	2.31
Chronic Unilateral ACL Disruptions (N = 159)			
89 N Test - No Anesthesia			
Noninvolved	7.7	2.5 - 13.5	1.97
Involved	13.0	4.0 - 25.0	3.51
I minus N*	5.4	0.0 - 13.5	2.89
89 N Test - With Anesthesia			
Noninvolved	7.3	3.0 - 14.0	2.08
Involved	13.1	5.0 - 23.0	3.40
I minus N*	5.9	-1.0 - 15.0	3.14
Manual Maximum Test - No Anesthesia			
Noninvolved	9.1	4.0 - 15.0	2.08
Involved	17.7	10.0 - 28.0	3.94
I minus N*	8.6	2.5 - 20.0	3.28
Manual Maximum Test - With Anesthesia			
Noninvolved	9.3	4.0 - 15.0	2.32
Involved	18.7	10.0 - 28.0	3.89
I minus N*	9.4	1.0 - 20.0	3.65
Quadriceps Active Test - No Anesthesia			
Noninvolved	6.4	2.0 - 13.0	2.37
Involved	10.8	3.0 - 21.0	3.44
I minus N*	4.4	-1.0 - 16.0	3.04

* p <0.001

Table 3 Comparison of displacement measurements

Test	F-Value	P-Level	Group Comparisons*
89 N noninvolved	4.76	0.091	Ch = Ac = No
89 N involved	136.57	<0.0001	Ch > Ac > No
89 N side-to-side difference	183.03	<0.0001	Ch > Ac > No
Manual noninvolved	3.02	0.051	Ch = Ac = No
Manual involved	290.38	<0.0001	Ch > Ac > No
Side-to-side difference	391.86	<0.0001	Ch > Ac > No
Active noninvolved	11.19	0.1	Ch = Ac = No
Active involved	111.02	<0.0001	Ch > Ac > No
Side-to-side difference	100.72	<0.0001	Ch > Ac > No

* Ch = Chronic, Ac = Acute, No = Normal, assuming left leg for normal group was uninvolved and right leg was involved.

force, we routinely perform a manual maximum test (Fig. 6) because it has proved to be a more diagnostic test of pathologic motion.

Direction   If the displacement load is directed so that in addition to imparting an anterior force, a joint distraction or compression force or a rotational movement is applied, the resulting anterior displacement will be affected. An internal rotational moment on the tibia will increase anterior joint displacement, and an external rotational moment will increase posterior joint displacement. A joint compression force will increase joint stiffness.[34,36,37]

To evaluate instrument rotation during testing, a KT-100 arthrometer was modified to include a pendulum inside the instrument that recorded rotation around the longitudinal axis. Ten experienced examiners tested the same patient. The examiners did not know that instrument rotation was being measured. Instrument rotation during a complete anteroposterior cycle varied from 0 to 7 degrees, with a mean of 2 degrees. One examiner tested 45 patients. Instrument rotation varied from 0 to 10 degrees, with a mean of 1.7 degrees.

Point of Application   The anterior force applied to a proximal point on the leg results in a moment that rotates the leg about the heel and ankle. The rotational moment depends on the distance of the point of force application from the ankle. In Figure 5, the rotational moment about the ankle is applied through a 31-cm moment arm. The closer the applied load is to the knee joint, the greater the moment and, therefore, the greater the anterior displacement.

Measurement System

Measurement Display   The measurement may be indicated on a digital readout, dial display, or printed copy as a displacement number; it may also be displayed on hard copy or a video display monitor as a force displacement diagram. The force displacement curve gives the examiner information about the joint's stiffness or compliance and the absolute displacement;[38] however, it increases the cost of the testing device and renders the device less portable.

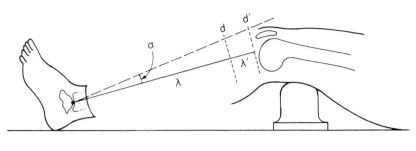

$$tangent\ a \cdot \lambda = d$$
$$tangent\ a\ (\lambda + \lambda') = d'$$

Fig. 7   *An anterior force applied to the proximal tibia rotates the tibia about the ankle. The anterior tibial displacement is dependent on the change in flexion angle and on the distance from the ankle that the displacement is measured. The greater the distance, the greater the measured displacement. (Reproduced with permission from Daniel DM, Stone ML: Instrumented measurement of knee motion, in Daniel DM, Akeson WH, O'Connor JJ (eds):* Knee Ligaments: Structure, Function, Injury, and Repair. *New York, Raven Press, 1990, pp 421-426.)*

Measurement Location   Anteroposterior knee displacement has been evaluated by stabilizing the femur and measuring anteroposterior displacement of the tibial tubercle,[22,34,39] or by measuring the differential displacement between the patella and the tibial tubercle.[23,24,26,38] During a standard anteroposterior displacement test, the patella and femur are maintained in a constant position and the foot rests on the examining table. When a displacement force is applied to the proximal segment of the leg, the leg rotates about the heel and ankle. The displacement measurement depends on the distance at which the measurement is taken with respect to the ankle (Fig. 7). Most devices display the displacement at the tibial tubercle (D. Cannon personal communication, 1985).[22-24,34] The KT-1000 arthrometer indicates the displacement occurring at the site of the arrow that should be placed on the joint line. In a subject with a tibia 40 cm in length, the anteroposterior displacement measurement at the tibial tubercle 5 cm distal to the joint line will be 15% less than the displacement measured at the joint line.[40]

The precision of anteroposterior displacement measurements with the KT-1000 arthrometer depends on a standardized method of placing the measuring device on the leg and securely stabilizing the patella in the femoral trochlea. With adequate patellar stabilization, tibial tubercle motion relative to the patella accurately reflects the motion of the tibia relative to the femur. It is necessary to flex the knee 20 to 30 degrees in order to engage the patella in the femoral trochlea. In patients with patella alta or lateral tracking patella, the knee may need to be flexed to 40 or more degrees (Fig. 8). The patella is stabilized in the femoral trochlea by direct pressure that should be oriented to seat the patella.

485

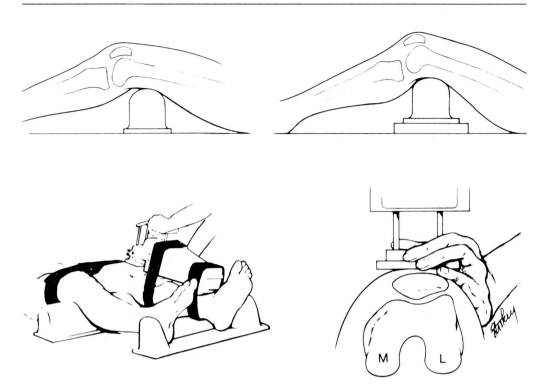

Fig. 8   *The knee is supported in a flexed position to engage the patella in the femoral trochlea (**top left**). In some patients the thigh support must be raised an additional 3 to 6 cm to provide sufficient knee flexion to engage the patella in the femoral trochlea. This may be done by placing a board under the thigh support (**top right**). The thigh should be supported so the patella is facing up. Occasionally a thigh strap is used to accomplish this task (**bottom left**). The foot support is not used to internally rotate the limb, but simply to support the feet. The examiner stabilizes the patellar sensor with manual pressure. Prior to establishing the testing reference position, sufficient pressure should be applied to the patella to press it firmly into the femoral trochlea (2 to 6 lbs), so the increase in pressure on the patella pad that will inevitably occur while stabilizing the instrument and limb during testing will not change the position of the patella and patella sensor. The hand stabilizing the patellar sensor should rest against the lateral thigh to help stabilize the testing instrument and prevent instrument rotation during testing (**bottom right**).*

A recent evaluation in which seven examiners used a KT-1000 arthrometer that was modified to include a patellar pad pressure sensor revealed that all examiners increased the patellar pad pressure as they increased force through the force handle. The examiners did not know that patellar pad pressure was being measured during the test. Patellar pad pressure changed from 5 N to 75 N in most patients. If the patellofemoral geometry and condition of the subject's two knees are symmetrical and the same examiner tests both knees with a similar technique, patellar depression during the test, with increasing patellar pressure, will have a negligible effect

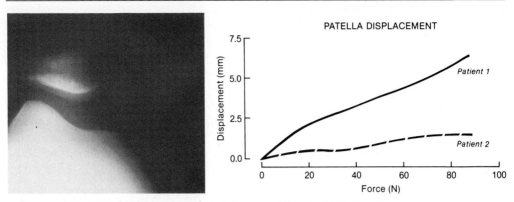

Fig. 9   *Left, Radiograph with the knees in 45 degrees of flexion.* **Right,** *Patellar pad posterior displacement versus patellar pad force. Patient 1, patient with lateral patella subluxation (Fig. 9, **left**). Patient 2, patient with normal patella position.*

on the right/left displacement differences. However, if the patella is not well seated in the femoral trochlea as shown in Figure 9, *left*, varying the patellar pad pressure may have a significant effect on the patella sensor position (Patient 1, Fig. 9, *right*).

For the 30-degree test, we have measured the displacement from the limb resting position to the anterior load position.[38] The posterior force in the resting position results from the weight of the leg and the weight of the testing device. Some investigators have begun their measurement while applying an 89-N posterior force.[41,42] To compare the two measurement techniques, we used a KT-1000 arthrometer to perform measurements on 200 patients, five years after unilateral ACL injury. Seventy-four patients had undergone ACL reconstruction; 126 patients had not. All patients had a negative 90-degree quadriceps active test for posterotibial subluxation (Fig. 4). We measured the anterior displacement from the testing reference position, and we measured the displacement with an applied 89-N anteroposterior force. In the normal and injured nonreconstructed knees, the measurements by both tests gave similar results (paired t test results: $p = 0.85$). In the ACL-reconstructed knee, the injured-minus-normal-knee difference by the 89-N anteroposterior test was 1.7 ± 2.1 mm, slightly less than the anterior displacement measurement of 1.9 ± 1.9 mm (paired t test results: $p = 0.006$).

Testing Technique, 30-Degree Test, KT-1000 Arthrometer   The knee is supported in a flexed position to engage the patella in the femoral trochlea. To stabilize the instrument on the limb, the hand stabilizing the patella in the femoral trochlea should rest on the thigh and prevent the instrument from rotating during the test (Fig. 8). The patient should be comfortable and relaxed. Gentle, manual anteroposterior oscillation may assist in relaxing the muscle. The arthrometer is applied to the leg and positioned so that pressure on the patellar sensor pad will stabilize the patella within the femoral trochlea. This usually places the force handle parallel to the foot axis. Patellar pressure should be applied until the dial motion stops. If the patella cannot be securely stabilized, the knee should be flexed to bring the patella farther down into the femoral trochlea. An 89-N anteroposterior cycle is performed to condition the joint. The measurement reference position is then obtained by repeatedly applying and releasing an 89-N posterior load until a reproducible unloaded knee position is obtained. The instrument dial is then set at zero. After each anterior load cycle is performed, an 89-N posterior force is applied and released. Return of the dial to 0 ± 0.5 mm confirms that the instrument orientation on the leg has not been altered and the quadriceps is relaxed. Confirmation of a stable reference position should be performed after each test. The mean of three tests rounded to 0.5 mm is recorded as the actual measurement.

Soft-Tissue Motion

Anteroposterior displacement measurements are performed by tracking the tibial tubercle motion in relation to the patella. There is a relatively thin layer of soft tissue between these structures and the skin. Daniel and associates[38,40] and Edixhoven and associates[24] found little discrepancy between in vitro measurement of displacements by skeletal pin motion[38] or radiographic techniques.[24] In contrast, Shino and associates[23] reported relatively large measurement errors secondary to soft-tissue deformation. The measurement of varus-valgus and internal-external rotations with surface-placed testing devices is subject to a significantly greater potential error from soft-tissue motion. The technique used by the Genucom system[39] to deal with the soft-tissue deformation is to measure the stiffness of the soft-tissue sleeve of the thigh and then, with computer assistance, subtract the predicted soft-tissue motion from the measured motion.

Muscle Activity

Muscle activity is probably the most significant variable in the measurement of motion limits.[22-24,31] Activity in muscles crossing the joints not only increases the joint stiffness, but also affects the joint resting position.[24,31] Testing should be comfortable and conducive to muscle relaxation. The tester should continually monitor muscle tone and encourage patient relaxation.

Testing the Testing System

There are several ways that accuracy of the testing system can be evaluated. Using the KT-1000 arthrometer as an example, instrument evaluation will be discussed. Instrument force and displace-

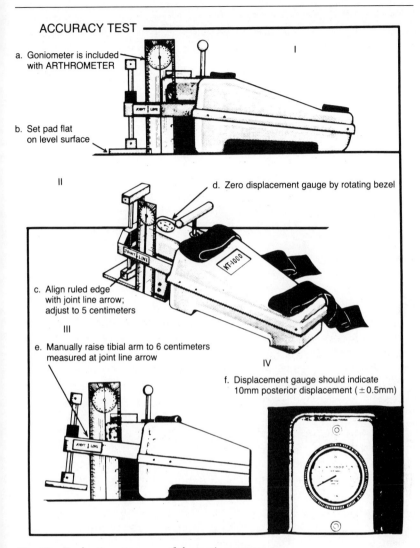

ACCURACY TEST

a. Goniometer is included with ARTHROMETER

I

b. Set pad flat on level surface

II

d. Zero displacement gauge by rotating bezel

c. Align ruled edge with joint line arrow; adjust to 5 centimeters

III

e. Manually raise tibial arm to 6 centimeters measured at joint line arrow

IV

f. Displacement gauge should indicate 10mm posterior displacement ($\pm$0.5mm)

Fig. 10 *Evaluating accuracy of the testing system.*

ment calibration may be evaluated as illustrated in Figure 10. Displacement measurements recorded by the instrument and by an independent skeletally-mounted measurement device in human knee cadaver specimens may be compared.[38,40] Instrumented measurement may also be compared with measurements from simultaneous radiographs.[43] Testing precision, or repeatability, may be evaluated between examinations by the same or different examiners with the same testing device,[35,44,45] or with different testing devices (Table 4). Testers should document their own test/retest repeatability and include these data in published reports.

The sensitivity of instrumented measurement in diagnosis of cruciate ligament disruption has been reported by several au-

Table 4 Chronic unilateral ACL disruption (N = 50)

Test	KT-1000	Stryker	DCT	KSS	Genucom
20 lb Posterior					
Normal	2.7	2.3	1.9	6.0	
Injured	2.9	2.4	1.7	6.7	
20 lb Anterior					
Normal	8.0	6.1	3.7	4.8	9.9
Injured	13.0	10.4	6.9	7.9	13.9
Difference	5.0	4.3	3.2	3.1	4.0
≤3 mm (%)	82	82	76	52	76
Manual Maximum					
Normal	8.2	7.2	5.2	7.2	
Injured	16.8	13.1	11.0	12.7	
Difference	8.6	5.9	5.8	5.5	
≤3 mm (%)	100	92	86	82	

(Reproduced with permission from Anderson A, Snyder R: Instrumented evaluation of anterior knee laxity: A comparison of five devices. *Orthop Trans* 1990;14:586.)

thors.[25,26,31,34,35,38,44,46-52] With the exception of Forster,[51] all authors have reported accurate diagnosis in 70% to 95% of cases. The right/left displacement differences are more diagnostic than the absolute displacement difference. A 3-mm right/left difference is considered pathologic. Data from 120 normal subjects, 105 patients with an acute unilateral ACL disruption, and 159 patients with a chronic unilateral ACL disruption who have asked for an ACL reconstruction are presented in Tables 3 and 4 and Figure 11. The right/left difference in the normal subjects was 97% with the manual maximum test, and 99% with the quadriceps active test.

Instrument Testing in Clinical Practice

The KT-1000 arthrometer has been used routinely at the Kaiser Hospital in San Diego to diagnose ligament disruptions, make treatment decisions, evaluate surgical procedures, and document the evolution of pathologic states. Staff using the device include the treating physician, a physical therapist, and an office nurse. Examinations are performed on patients with acute injuries and chronic problems, and in the clinic and operating room. At the time of ligament surgery, joint measurements are performed in the operating room to confirm that the desired joint stability is obtained. After surgery, examinations are performed at 6, 12, 26, 52, and 104 weeks.

We recently reviewed 292 patients who had an acute knee hemarthrosis between 1981 and 1986. Initial arthrometer examination showed that results in 56 of the patients were stable when tested with the KT-1000 arthrometer (all KT-1000 measurements showed an injury-minus-normal difference of <3mm and 236 were unstable. Eighty-eight of the early unstable patients and two of the early stable patients had ACL reconstructions (45 within 90 days of injury and 45 after more than 90 days after injury). At the follow-up evaluation the patients were divided into four groups: (1) early stable, no reconstruction; (2) early unstable, no reconstruction; (3) early reconstruction; and (4) late reconstruction. Serial anterior displace-

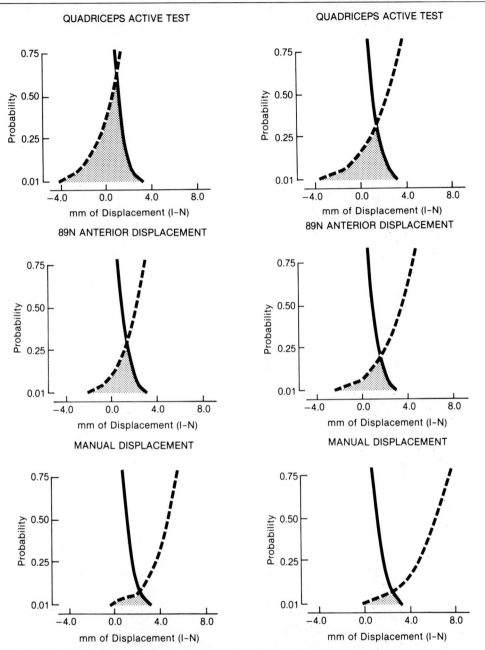

Fig. 11   *Probability distributions for side-to-side difference for each test. The solid line indicates the probability that a normal subject would have measurements to the right of the line. The hatched line indicates the probability that a patient with a unilateral ACL injury would have a measurement to the left of the line. The shaded area represents measurements where patients in the normal group could be incorrectly classified as injured and the patients in the injured group be incorrectly classified as normal. Figures on the left compare patients with acute unilateral ACL injury (N = 105) to normal patients (N = 120) and those on the right compare patients with chronic unilateral ACL injury (N = 159) to normal patients (N = 120).*

Table 5 Arthrometer measurements

Group*	I Early Stable		II Early Unstable No Recon.		III Early Recon.		IV Late Recon. +	
Displacement Force	20 lb	MM**	20 lb	MM	20 lb	MM	20 lb	MM
Acute Injury								
Clinic (N)		27		115		36		37
I-N	-0.0	0.2	3.4	6.0	4.1	6.5	3.7	6.1
Anesthesia (N)		5		58		31		28
I-N	-1.1	0.2	3.9	6.6	4.8	7.2	3.6	5.7
Postinjury 3 months								
Clinic (N)		8		58				20
I-N	0.3	-0.1	3.8	5.3	—	—	4.6	6.6
Postinjury 12 months								
Clinic (N)		20		91		33		22
I-N	0.6	0.7	3.6	4.9	2.2	3.0	5.0	6.7

* Millimeters of injured minus normal difference (I-N) in all groups
** Manual maximum
 + Measurements prior to ligament surgery

Table 6 Arthrometer measurements for reconstructed patients tested under anesthesia

Group	Before Repair		After Repair	
Group III (N = 33)	Mean*	N <3 +	Mean	N <3
20 lb	4.8	4	-1.5	33
MM**	7.4	0	—	—
Group IV (N = 40)				
20 lb	4.6	7	-1.5	36
MM	7.4	1	—	—

* Millimeters of injured minus normal differences (I-N)
** Manual maximum
 + Number of patients with difference <3 mm

Table 7 Motion measurements follow-up evaluation

Group	I Early Stable	II Early Unstable No Recon.	III Early Recon.	IV Late Recon.
Arthrometer* (No.)	54	135	43	36
Quadriceps Active	0.5	3.0	2.4	2.5
mean <3 mm (%)	89	44	49	53
20 lb	0.5	2.3	1.7	2.4
mean <3 mm (%)	93	55	63	61
30 lb	0.6	3.2	2.3	2.8
mean <3 mm (%)	92	39	49	49
Man Max	0.7	5.0	3.7	4.2
mean <3 mm (%)	91	16	33	30
Pivot Shift (No.)	51	121	36	32
% = 0	92	16	64	50

* Millimeters of injured minus normal difference

ment measurements are presented in Tables 5 and 6, and follow-up measurements are presented in Table 7. Note that the patients with ACL injury who do not seek reconstruction have less pathologic motion than those seeking surgery and only slightly more pathologic motion than those who have had ligament surgery.

At the time of the follow-up evaluation (64 ± 9 months), 238 of the patients had radiographs of their knees and 168 had bone scans. The incidence of degenerative disease diagnosed by radiograph and bone scan correlated with the injured-minus-normal knee displacement differences on the manual maximum and quadriceps active examinations ($p < 0.05$).

Conclusion

Instrumented measurement may be used to document anteroposterior instability. The measurement procedure consists of positioning the limb in a specific manner, applying a designated displacement force, and measuring the resultant motion. The precision and accuracy of the tests depend on the examiner's technique. A normal subject's two knees will have similar displacement measurements. An anteroposterior displacement difference of <3 mm was recorded in 97% of normal subjects. A high force displacement test, the manual maximum test, revealed the greatest incidence of abnormal motion in the patients with ACL injury. An injured-minus-normal knee anterior displacement difference of ≤3 mm is considered pathologic in a previously-injured knee.

References

1. Daniel DM: Diagnosis of a ligament injury, in Daniel DM, Akeson WH, O'Connor JJ (eds): *Knee Ligaments: Structure, Function, Injury, and Repair*. New York, Raven Press, 1990, pp 3-10.
2. Müller W, Biedert R, Hefti F, et al: OAK knee evaluation: A new way to assess knee ligament injuries. *Clin Orthop* 1988;232:37-50.
3. Noyes FR, Grood ES: Diagnosis of knee ligament injuries: Clinical concepts, in Feagin JA Jr (ed): *The Crucial Ligaments: Diagnosis and Treatment of Ligamentous Injuries About the Knee*. New York, Churchill Livingstone, 1988, pp 261-285.
4. Stäubli H-U: Stressradiography: Measurements of the knee motion limits, in Daniel DM, Akeson WH, O'Connor JJ (eds): *Knee Ligaments: Structure, Function, Injury, and Repair*. New York, Raven Press, 1990, pp 449-459.
5. Stäubli H-U, Jakob RP: Posterior instability of the knee near extension: A clinical and stress radiographic analysis of acute injuries of the posterior cruciate ligament. *J Bone Joint Surg* 1990;72B:225-230.
6. Jakob RP, Stäubli H-U, Deland JT: Grading the pivot shift: Objective tests with implications for treatment. *J Bone Joint Surg* 1987;69B:294-299.
7. Daniel DM: Assessing the limits of knee motion. *Am J Sports Med* 1991;19:139-147.
8. Noyes FR, Cummings JF, Grood ES, et al: The diagnosis of knee motion limits, subluxations, and ligament injury. *Am J Sports Med* 1991;19:163-171.

9. Noyes FR, Grood ES, Cummings JF, et al: An analysis of the pivot shift phenomenon: The knee motions and subluxations induced by different examiners. *Am J Sports Med* 1991;19:148-155.

10. Noyes FR, Grood ES, Torzilli PA: Current concepts review: The definitions of terms for motion and position of the knee and injuries of the ligaments. *J Bone Joint Surg* 1989;71A:465-472.

11. Hughston JC, Andrews JR, Cross MJ, et al: Classification of knee ligament instabilities: Part I. The medial compartment and cruciate ligaments. *J Bone Joint Surg* 1976;58A:159-172.

12. Hughston JC, Andrews JR, Cross MJ, et al: Classification of knee ligament instabilities: Part II. The lateral compartment. *J Bone Joint Surg* 1976;58A:173-179.

13. Warner JP, Warren RF, Cooper DE: Management of acute anterior cruciate ligament injury, in American Academy of Orthopaedic Surgeons *Instructional Course Lectures, XL*. Park Ridge, IL American Academy of Orthopaedic Surgeons, 1991, pp 219-232.

14. Hirshman HP, Daniel DM, Miyasaka K: The fate of unoperated knee ligament injuries, in Daniel DM, Akeson WH, O'Connor JJ (eds): *Knee Ligaments: Structure, Function, Injury, and Repair*. New York, Raven Press, 1990, pp 481-503.

15. Daniel DM, Stone ML, Riehl B: Ligament surgery: The evaluation of results, in Daniel DM, Akeson WH, O'Connor JJ (eds): *Knee Ligaments: Structure, Function, Injury, and Repair*. New York, Raven Press, 1990, pp 521-534.

16. Shoemaker SC, Daniel DM: The limits of knee motion: *In vitro* studies, in Daniel DM, Akeson WH, O'Connor JJ (eds): *Knee Ligaments: Structure, Function, Injury, and Repair*. New York, Raven Press, 1990, pp 153-161.

17. Sprague RB, Asprey GM: Photographic method for measuring knee stability: A preliminary report. *Phys Ther* 1965;45:1055-1058.

18. Jacaobsen K: Stress radiographical measurement of the anteroposterior, medial and lateral stability of the knee joint. *Acta Orthop Scand* 1976;47:335-344.

19. Kennedy JC, Fowler PJ: Medial and anterior instability of the knee An anatomical and clinical study using stress machines. *J Bone Joint Surg* 1971;53A:1257-1270.

20. Torzilli PA, Greenberg RL, Hood RW, et al: Measurement of anterior-posterior motion of the knee in injured patients using a biomechanical stress technique. *J Bone Joint Surg* 1984;66A:1438-1442.

21. Torzilli PA, Greenberg RL, Insall J: An *in vivo* biomechanical evaluation of anterior-posterior motion of the knee: Roentgenographic measurement technique, stress machine, and stable population. *J Bone Joint Surg* 1981;63A:960-968.

22. Markolf KL, Graff-Radford A, Amstutz HC: *In vivo* knee stability: A quantitative assessment using an instrumented clinical testing apparatus. *J Bone Joint Surg* 1978;60A:664-674.

23. Shino K, Inoue M, Horibe S, et al: Measurement of anterior instability of the knee: A new apparatus for clinical testing. *J Bone Joint Surg* 1987;69B:608-613.

24. Edixhoven P, Huiskes R, de Graaf R, et al: Accuracy and reproducibility of instrumented knee-drawer tests. *J Orthop Res* 1987;5:378-387.

25. Daniel DM, Stone ML, Sachs R, et al: Instrumented measurement of anterior knee laxity in patients with acute anterior cruciate ligament disruption. *Am J Sports Med* 1985;13:401-407.

26. Malcom LL, Daniel DM, Stone ML, et al: The measurement of anterior knee laxity after ACL reconstructive surgery. *Clin Orthop* 1985;196: 35-41.

27. O'Connor J, Shercliff T, FitzPatrick D, et al: Geometry of the knee, in Daniel DM, Akeson WH, O'Connor JJ (eds): *Knee Ligaments: Structure, Function, Injury, and Repair*. New York, Raven Press, 1990, pp 163-199.

28. Markolf KL, Kochan A, Amstutz HC: Measurement of knee stiffness and laxity in patients with documented absence of the anterior cruciate ligament. *J Bone Joint Surg* 1984;66A:242-253.

29. Nielsen S, Kromann-Andersen C, Rasmussen O, et al: Instability of cadaver knees after transection of capsule and ligaments. *Acta Orthop Scand* 1984;55:30-34.

30. Sullian D, Levy IM, Sheskier S, et al: Medial restraints to anterior-posterior motion of the knee. *J Bone Joint Surg* 1984; 66A:930-936.

31. Daniel DM, Stone ML, Barnett P, et al: Use of the quadriceps active test to diagnose posterior cruciate-ligament disruption and measure posterior laxity of the knee. *J Bone Joint Surg* 1988;70A:386-391.

32. Bargar WL, Moreland JR, Markolf KL, et al: The effect of tibia-foot rotatory position on the anterior drawer test. *Clin Orthop* 1983;173: 200-203.

33. Noyes FR, Keller CS, Grood ES, et al: Advances in the understanding of knee ligament injury, repair, and rehabilitation. *Med Sci Sports Exerc* 1984;16:427-443.

34. Sherman OH, Markolf KL, Ferkel RD: Measurements of anterior laxity in normal and anterior cruciate absent knees with two instrumented test devices. *Clin Orthop* 1987;215:156-161.

35. Daniel DM, Stone ML: KT-1000 anterior-posterior displacement measurements, in Daniel DM, Akeson WH, O'Connor JJ (eds): *Knee Ligaments: Structure, Function, Injury, and Repair*. New York, Raven Press, 1990, pp 427-447.

36. Hsieh H-H, Walker PS: Stabilizing mechanisms of the loaded and unloaded knee joint. *J Bone Joint Surg* 1976;58A:87-93.

37. Markolf KL, Bargar WL, Shoemaker SC, et al: The role of joint load in knee stability. *J Bone Joint Surg* 1981;63A:570-585.

38. Daniel DM, Malcom LL, Losse G, et al: Instrumented measurement of anterior laxity of the knee. *J Bone Joint Surg* 1985;67A:720-726.

39. Baxter MP: Assessment of normal pediatric knee ligament laxity using the Genucom. *J Pediatr Orthop* 1988;8:546-550.

40. Daniel DM, Stone ML: Instrumented measurement of knee motion, in Daniel DM, Akeson WH, O'Connor JJ (eds): *Knee Ligaments: Structure, Function, Injury, and Repair*. New York, Raven Press, 1990, pp 421-426.

41. Sommerlath K, Lysholm J, Gillquist J: The long-term course after treatment of acute anterior cruciate ligament ruptures: A 9 to 16 year followup. *Am J Sports Med* 1991;19:156-162.

42. Noyes FR, Barber SD: The effect of an extra-articular procedure on allograft reconstructions for chronic ruptures of the anterior cruciate ligament. *J Bone Joint Surg* 1991;73A:882-892.

43. Stäubli H-U, Jakob RP: Anterior knee motion analysis: Measurement and simultaneous radiography. *Am J Sports Med* 1991;19:172-177.

44. Steiner ME, Brown C, Zarins B, et al: Measurement of anterior-posterior displacement of the knee: A comparison of the results with instrumented devices and with clinical examination. *J Bone Joint Surg* 1990;72A:1307-1315.

45. Wroble RR, Van Ginkel LA, Grood ES, et al: Repeatability of the KT-1000 arthrometer in a normal population. *Am J Sports Med* 1990;18:396-399.

46. Sommerlath K, Gillquist J: Instrumented testing of sagittal knee laxity in stable and unstable knees: A clinical comparison of simple and computerized devices. *Am J Knee Surg* 1991;4:70-78.

47. Anderson A, Snyder R: Instrumented evaluation of anterior knee laxity: A comparison of five devices. *Orthop Trans* 1990;14:586.

48. Bach BR Jr, Warren RF, Flynn WM, et al: Arthrometric evaluation of knees that have a torn anterior cruciate ligament. *J Bone Joint Surg* 1990;72A:1299-1306.

49. Dahlstedt LJ, Dalén N: Knee laxity in cruciate ligament injury: Value of examination under anesthesia. *Acta Orthop Scand* 1989;60:181-184.

50. Daniel DM, Stone ML: Diagnosis of knee ligament injury: Tests and measurements of joint laxity, in Feagin JA Jr (ed): *The Crucial Ligaments: Diagnosis and Treatment of Ligamentous Injuries About the Knee*. New York, Churchill Livingstone, 1988, pp 287-300.

51. Forster IW, Warren-Smith CD, Tew M: Is the KT-1000 knee ligament arthrometer reliable? *J Bone Joint Surg* 1989;71B:843-847.

52. Biden E, O'Connor J: Experimental methods used to evaluate knee ligament function, in Daniel DM, Akeson WH, O'Connor JJ (eds): *Knee Ligaments: Structure, Function, Injury, and Repair*. New York, Raven Press, 1990, pp 135-151.

Chapter 24

Reconstruction of the Anterior Cruciate Ligament With Autografts

Robert J. Johnson, MD

There are several surgical and nonsurgical treatment options available for management of anterior cruciate ligament (ACL) injuries. The types of surgical repair include repair with augmentation, reconstruction using autografts, autografts with prosthetic augmentation, allografts or prostheses, and extra-articular reconstructions (alone or in combination with other procedures) that attempt to eliminate the functional disability caused by the loss of the ACL. This chapter will discuss the following autograft procedures: extra-articular reconstruction, repair of the ACL with autograft augmentation, intra-articular autograft with ligament augmentation device (LAD) augmentation, and intra-articular autograft reconstruction, which attempts to replace the ACL.

Studies of the surgical procedures documented in the literature are often preliminary, of short duration, and poorly designed; therefore, their results must be interpreted carefully. The biases generated in such reports may completely mask factors such as rehabilitation and postoperative management which, in at least some instances, were most important in attaining the apparently successful results.[1] Various surgical procedures may produce equally satisfactory results. During the past 20 years, most surgeons have performed a variety of procedures, changing frequently from one to another in the hope that by changing one or several variables, the results will be improved even before the long-term outcome of the previously used procedure is known. From this information, it is not surprising that no single management program has been clearly identified as superior. Certainly no single treatment approach will satisfactorily meet every patient's needs. Thus, the physician must have several options from which to choose so that each patient with an ACL injury can be managed with the best available approach.

Surgical Restoration of the ACL

Presently, the most successful method of surgical restoration of the ACL is intra-articular reconstruction using a bone-patellar tendon-bone autograft.[2,3] Although many would argue that this is probably true, it is wise to continue to seek a better method. Still others would undoubtedly argue that other procedures are in fact better than the bone-patellar tendon-bone autograft procedure. However, the published results of patellar tendon autografts are numerous, and the procedure has been performed long enough to establish a basis for future comparison.[4-16] Thus, any procedure being advocated should be at least as effective and preferably better than patellar tendon autograft procedures before it is assumed to be adequate for treating most patients. Unfortunately, the means of establishing the most effective current or future procedure is not readily available. Not only do most presently available follow-up study designs frequently produce biases that render the information attained relatively questionable, but they also do not use standardized evaluation techniques.[1,17,18]

Rating systems used to evaluate the outcome of ACL surgery are simply not comparable, and defects in the various systems tend to over- or underestimate the actual results.[18,19] Therefore, the ability to accurately establish which procedure(s) are superior to any other is at best flawed. The American Orthopaedic Society for Sports Medicine (AOSSM) and the European Society of Knee Surgery and Arthroscopy (ESKSA) have made a major effort through the Knee Documentation Committee to develop consistent and repeatable means of subjective and objective evaluation of patients with ACL injuries.[17] Their goal is to develop protocols that will be acceptable to all surgeons performing ACL surgery, so that results of studies from all over the world can be truly comparable. If successful, this will be a major step toward establishing the natural history of the ACL-deficient knee as well as that of the surgical treatment of ACL injuries. When such protocols are coupled with prospective, randomized, carefully controlled studies comparing various means of treating ACL ruptures, there is a greater possibility of truly establishing the most effective or ideal ACL therapy.

Surgical Repair With Augmentation

The literature contains reports of satisfactory outcomes following suturing of acutely injured ACL ligaments.[20,21] However, the majority opinion now appears to be that when compared with other procedures discussed in this chapter, suturing alone leads to inferior results.[22-27]

Several studies have reported good results with intra-articular autograft augmentation in addition to suture repair of the torn ACL.[22,26,28-30] The major disadvantage of such procedures is that the relatively poor fixation of the suture repair necessitates very stringent postoperative protection. Thus, the potential advantage of retaining the original ligamentous material and perhaps some of the innervation and blood supply may well be outweighed by the profound muscle atrophy and fibrosis that accompany such prolonged disuse. For these reasons, surgical repair with augmentation has been performed less frequently than it was a few years ago.

Extra-articular Reconstructions

Extra-articular reconstructions designed for tenodesis of the posterolateral aspect of the knee using a portion of the iliotibial tract became popular in the 1970s.[31-45] They were performed to eliminate the functional instability caused by the absence of the ACL without actually replacing the ligament. Several papers have been published supporting the use of these procedures, but the number of cases was small and the length of follow-up was short in almost all of the papers.[31-33,35,36,38,39,43,44] Several other studies revealed a high rate of failure.[40,41,45] It now appears that the majority of physicians have abandoned the option of lateral replacement reconstruction as the way to restore function following disruption of the ACL.[34] These extra-articular procedures have very limited indications as noted in a consensus conference on this subject sponsored by the Foundation for Sports Medicine Education and Research of the American Orthopaedic Society of Sports Medicine.[34] A minority of the attendees of that conference believed that such procedures may have a limited role in the treatment of very young patients with open epiphyses, as an adjunct to intra-articular reconstructions and in older, more sedentary patients with chronic ACL dysfunction. These procedures can only succeed in reducing the abnormal anterior translation of the tibia from beneath the femur by tenodesing the posterolateral aspect of the joint.[46] They are unable to constrain the central or medial aspects of the knee and therefore are subject to gradual failure because of stretching of the reconstruction.

Engebretsen and associates[47] have shown that iliotibial band tenodesis used in combination with an intra-articular autograft can significantly decrease the force generated within an ACL reconstruction and thus potentially protect it during rehabilitation. However, they warned that the tenodesis caused the tibia to be externally rotated, which could interfere with the screw home mechanism. O'Brien, Strum, and their associates could demonstrate no benefit from an extra-articular tenodesis in addition to their intra-articular autograft reconstruction in their follow-up studies.[14,48] For that reason, O'Brien and associates[14] no longer use a lateral sling procedure to protect their central third patellar tendon autografts. Interestingly, in a similar study comparing the use of intra-articular allografts alone with a combination of intra-articular allografts and an extra-articular procedure, Noyes and Barber[49] observed that the combination procedure appeared to be necessary to satisfactorily reduce anteroposterior displacement in all knees.

Intra-articular Autogenous Reconstructions

Presently, the majority of orthopaedic surgeons who surgically restore the function of the ACL perform an intra-articular autograft, in an attempt to replace anatomically the destroyed ACL. The material selected for the graft is harvested locally from the ACL-deficient knee. Through the years, several structures have been used, including menisci, the iliotibial band, various combinations of hamstring tendons, and a portion of the patellar tendon. The relative strength of these materials was documented by Noyes and associates[50] in 1984. A 14-mm wide bone-patellar tendon-bone graft was 168% as strong as the normal ACL; all other materials were weaker than the ACL. Recently, it has been shown that the normal tensile strength of the ACL is as high as 2,500 N, not the 1,750 N that was the standard for many years.[50,51] This has caused several surgeons to use combinations of graft sources in an attempt to increase the strength of their grafts, but no studies are yet available to show that such combinations are truly additive.[52-54] It is well documented that the initial failure strength and other mechanical properties of any autograft or allograft undergo profound and rapid degradation during the first six to eight weeks following implantation.[55,56] For a time it was hoped that this problem could be prevented by using vascularized patellar tendon grafts, but Butler and associates[55,56] demonstrated in cynomolgus monkeys that the mechanical properties of free grafts were not inferior to those of similar vascularized patellar tendon grafts.

The normal anatomic details of the ACL, with fibers that vary in length and tension as knee flexion angle changes, are impossible to reproduce with any of the autografts now in use.[57] The present autograft procedures, with a few exceptions, attempt to replace only the anteromedial band of the ACL, which has been identified as the most nearly isometric portion of the normal structure. Clearly there are no fibers within any ACL that are isometric; attempts to identify positions of attachment that allow no change in graft length during range of motion of the knee are impossible. However, placement of the graft as closely as possible to the centers of the tibial and femoral attachments of the anteromedial band will result in the least amount of strain (change in length of the ACL during the complete range of motion of the knee). Devices called isometers have been developed to identify the center of these attachment points by passing a suture through small guide pin tracts entering into the center of the suspected correct site of attachment.[58] Fixation of one end of the suture to the femoral attachment site and a compliant, spring-loaded scale to the suture extending from the trial tibial tunnel allows the operator to confirm that the guide pins are in the correct position by passively moving the knee through a full range of motion and measuring the excursion of the suture through the tibial tunnel. If the excursion measured is 2 mm or less, the position of the pins is deemed acceptable. If pin movement is more than 2 mm, then the pins need to be repositioned. Also, the normal anteromedial band fibers are strained as the knee goes into extension, and loosen during flexion.[59,60] The isometer measurement must duplicate this pattern as well as not exceed 2 mm in total excursion. Isometer findings must be carefully interpreted because the measurement is being made in an ACL-deficient knee with abnormal kinematics, and the results have been shown to correlate poorly with the load measured in an ACL substitute after it had been fixed in the tibial tunnel.[61] Thus, isometers can be of some help in identifying the proper placement of attachment sites, but relying on them alone may produce variable results. Full understanding of the three-dimensional anatomy of the attachment sites has allowed very accurate placement of the bone tunnels without using an isometer. Therefore, exact femoral attachment is very important, because anterior placement of the graft into the femur results in high strain and loads within the graft, which results in restriction of knee flexion if the graft survives, or elongation of the graft if the range of motion is restored.[62,63] Placement posterior or inferior to the normal attachment site will result in excessive tightening of the graft when the knee is extended. The "over-the-top position" results in this anatomic variation, and some surgeons have created a trough in the femur to bring the graft more closely into an anatomic position or fix the graft in place with the knee in full extension. Although tibial attachment of the graft is not considered as important as the femoral placement, it should be positioned so as to avoid impingement on the roof of the outlet of the intracondylar notch when the knee is fully extended.[62,63]

Tensioning of the graft within the properly placed tunnels is also extremely important. If the initial tension is too great, the knee will be overconstrained, leading to decreased anteroposterior laxity and/or an increase in the load within the graft.[63] This also has been shown to result in focal degeneration and failure of the graft.[64] Grood and associates,[63] using a flexible cable to replace human cadaveric ACLs, found that normal joint kinematics was restored when the cable tension was between 4.5 and 9 N with the knee at 90 degrees of flexion. Burks and Leland[65] measured the initial graft tension required to restore normal anterior joint laxity for three types of autograft: bone-patellar tendon-bone, iliotibial band, and semitendinosus. They found that the initial tension required for an autograft was tissue-specific. In a series of studies from the University of Minnesota, buckle gauge transducers were used to compare ligament tension on normal and ACL-reconstructed human cadaver knees.[66-68] The authors of these studies adjusted the initial length of the intra-articular grafts until the graft tension was equal to that previously measured in the normal ACL when an anterior shear load of 90 N was applied to the tibia with the knee positioned at 30 degrees of flexion. They then found, however, that the graft force measured by this same technique was significantly higher than normal when the knee was tested in extension and at 60 and 90 degrees of flexion. Although these studies demonstrate that tensioning of the graft is important, they do not currently provide enough information to make specific recommendations about the exact tension and how it is to be applied in procedures that are now being performed to replace the ACL.

Another variable that is important to the success of any reconstruction of the ACL is the method of fixation of the graft to the host bone. Kurosaka and Robertson and their associates have shown that the initial weak link in any tibia-graft-femur construct in reconstruction of ligaments is the fixation of the graft to bone, not the strength of the graft material itself.[69,70] In their studies of fixation of bone and soft-tissue grafts, interference fit screws that secured bone plugs within the tunnels, and screw and spiked washer fixation of soft tissue were superior to staple and suture fixation. Not all means of fixation have been studied, and further investigations are necessary before the ideal means of fixation is identified. However, the surgeon must understand that the strength of the initial graft fixation is weaker than the graft material itself to allow rational planning for the postoperative rehabilitation program.

Intra-articular reconstruction of the ACL can be performed with many types of autogenous grafts; however, it appears that the majority of surgeons now prefer the patellar tendon with a significant minority using one or two hamstring tendons.[2,3] The second most popular autograft involves one or more of the hamstring tendons.[26,71-75] The meniscus is probably not an option for use as a graft, it should be retained within the joint in its original role if it is undamaged or repairable.[76-79] The iliotibial band and tract appear to be a poor choice as an intra-articular autograft because of their inadequate strength and great compliance.[80,81] Despite these disadvantages, several authors have reported successful outcomes using this procedure,[82-86] while others have thought the failure rate was unacceptably high.[81]

The primary advantages of the bone-patellar tendon-bone graft appear to be its great strength and availability, the ease of attaining immediate high strength fixation with interference screws or heavy suture fixations, the theoretical advantage of rapid healing of the bone plugs within the tibial and femoral tunnels, and the allowance of early vigorous rehabilitation.[53] The use of the hamstring tendon as the graft source instead of the patellar tendon enables the surgeon to avoid the following: sacrifice of a portion of the extensor mechanism; a high incidence of postoperative parapatellar pain; quadriceps weakness; and the occasionally reported fracture of the patella or disruption of the patellar tendon following surgery.[53,57] Also, Warner and associates[53] believed that harvesting of the hamstring tendons is technically less difficult than preparing bone-patellar tendon-bone grafts. Disadvantages of using hamstring tendons include their greater elasticity,[50] the less secure fixation of these tendons to bone,[69,70] and their increased likelihood to fail postoperatively when used in reconstructions associated with chronic ACL insufficiency.[87] The reported slower healing of hamstring tendons compared to bone blocks within the bone tunnels has not yet been proven. Warner and associates[53] advocate the use of hamstring tendons (gracilis and semitendinosus) in reconstruction of the ACL in association with repair of the residual ligament in acute cases of less than three weeks' duration, but prefer bone-patellar tendon-bone grafts in cases of chronic ACL deficiency. Although it has been assumed that hamstring tendon grafts are less frequently associated with postoperative parapatellar pain than patellar tendon grafts, this condition cannot be totally eliminated by any intraoperative reconstruction of the ACL.[28,88] Marder and associates[89] found no difference in the incidence of postoperative patellofemoral pain in two groups of patients who underwent patellar tendon or semitendinosus and gracilis autografting of their ACLs.

Both patellar tendon and hamstring grafting procedures can be done with small arthrotomies as well as with arthroscopic techniques.[90] The proponents of arthroscopic surgery believe that they can better visualize the intra-articular anatomy and more meticulously position their bone tunnels, while those preferring the open procedures believe that they can do just as well with less demanding and time-consuming techniques. Of course, surgeons using either procedure can consistently attain excellent results. However, the use of large parapatellar incisions with dislocation of the patella to attain good visualization is not only unnecessary, but dramatically increases the morbidity of ACL surgery and thus is to be avoided.

My interpretation of the factors presented in this chapter leads me to believe that at present, the most efficacious procedure for the surgical treatment of chronic ACL deficiency is reconstruction with a bone-patellar tendon-bone autograft. Acute injuries, where secondary stabilizing ligament and capsular structure are intact, can be treated just as well with appropriately performed hamstring or patellar tendon autografts. Patients with acute injuries and injured secondary stabilizers and those whose lifestyles make them more at risk for injury are probably also better served by patellar autografts.

Ligament Augmentation Devices

Ligament augmentation devices (LAD) have been studied on a limited basis, and although early results indicate that they can be associated with successful outcomes, no study has yet revealed that they are clearly superior to present autograft techniques.[91,92] The concept of load sharing with autograft-graft material during the early phases of rehabilitation when the biomechanical properties of the autograft deteriorate markedly is enticing. However, the amount of load sharing and for how long it is necessary are not known. Hanley and associates[93] showed that load sharing occurs immediately after surgery in fresh cadaver knees. The amount of load borne by the autograft and that by the LAD was widely variable and not reproducible. They concluded that further work is required to clarify the source of the variability observed in total graft force and the load sharing. Thus, the ultimate place for LADs in the armamentarium of treatment options is yet to be established.

Rehabilitation Following ACL Surgery

Rehabilitation following ACL surgery is universally accepted as being very important to the final outcome of the treatment. However, the performance of such rehabilitation programs is tempered by one of the most frustrating dilemmas faced by any knee surgeon. On the one hand is the need to protect the repaired or reconstructed ACL so that it can heal without further injury. On the other hand are the numerous problems resulting from immobilizing the joint while healing occurs. In the past, protection by prolonged casting or splinting was common, but during the last decade the majority of physicians have begun to allow immediate motion following surgery. How such motion is performed (passively administered by a therapist or patient, continuous passive motion (CPM), or with active muscle control) varies. The advocates of CPM machines have stated that swelling and pain are minimized in the early postoperative phase, but those who question the cost effectiveness of this treatment point out that there is no difference in the degree of swelling and pain in groups of patients treated with or without CPM machines within a few weeks of the surgery.[94]

Quadriceps muscle activity was often advocated in an unlimited fashion as soon as it was practical after ligament surgery, until several studies revealed that the quadriceps acts antagonistically to the ACL between approximately 50 degrees of flexion and full extension.[59,95-97] Many surgeons have recently suggested that isotonic quadriceps loading be avoided into full extension until several months after ACL reconstruction.[98] Several muscle rehabilitation programs are recommended following knee ligament surgery. Isokinetic, eccentric, closed kinetic chain, and sports-specific training are popular choices, but the timing and safety of these programs must be carefully considered for the patient's well-being. Advocates of aggressive rehabilitation do not report detrimental effects from early quadriceps activity, but repaired, reconstructed, or even injured ligaments are more susceptible to overloading if rehabilitation programs are too aggressive.[99]

Rehabilitation braces allowing gradually increasing knee motion during the first few weeks are now often used, but some surgeons use no immobilization following surgery. In recent years with stronger graft material and fixation techniques, the need for prolonged immobilization with casts and braces has become unnecessary. In the past, prolonged avoidance of weightbearing for up to four months following ligament injury or surgery was often suggested. As recently as 1981, the majority of surgeons questioned by Paulos and associates[97] did not allow weightbearing until eight or more weeks following their ACL repairs or reconstructions.

Shelbourne and Nitz[99] now allow their patients to begin weightbearing as tolerated immediately after bone-patellar tendon-bone grafts.

As patients increase their activity following ACL surgery, the question of whether or not to prescribe a functional knee brace is often considered. Although much anecdotal information concerning their effectiveness exists, very little hard data has been published that proves that these devices can adequately stress-shield repaired or reconstructed ligaments.[100,101] Much more investigation is necessary before the final role of functional braces in postoperative management can be determined.

The question of when to return an athlete to sports activity has remained controversial. During the 1950s and 1960s, the main criteria for success following ligament surgery appeared to be how quickly the athlete could return to sports. In the 1970s and 1980s, a much more conservative approach was advocated as more was learned about the healing properties of repaired and reconstructed ligaments and the potentially dangerous effects of early muscle activity.[97] During that time many investigators were not advocating return to full activities for a year or longer. In recent years, a definite trend toward more rapid rehabilitation and return to full activities has been advocated by several investigators,[99] who stressed that a bone-patellar tendon-bone graft placed isometrically and firmly fixed can probably tolerate vigorous early rehabilitation and early return to sports activity, but this same rapid rehabilitation may not be successful with other surgical procedures.

There can be no standard approach for rehabilitation programs following ACL surgery. The trend toward aggressive advances in weightbearing, range of motion, muscle exercises, and return to functional activities has potential dangers. Decisions must be based on the development of individual rehabilitation programs and scientific fact rather than anecdotal statements of how rapidly someone else's patients were able to return to sports. Each surgeon should carefully weigh all the data presently available and be prepared to improve his/her own rehabilitation programs as the results of long-term, randomized, controlled studies clearly show that one program is superior to another. Such outcome studies are not yet available.

Conclusions

The management of ACL injuries is complex and still unclear. Patients who have low-risk lifestyles can be adequately managed nonsurgically. Younger, more energetic patients who wish to maintain active lifestyles and perform high-risk activities, both recreationally and occupationally, probably are best served by surgery to restore the function of the ACL. Most present procedures do not even attempt to reproduce the exact anatomy of the ACL and, likewise, are totally incapable of completely replacing the fine-tuned function of these structures. The surgical techniques necessary to attain good results are demanding and meticulous. Surgeons who do not apply the presently available knowledge of anatomy and biomechanics to their approach to this problem will certainly not succeed in attaining consistent results. Although there is good evidence that surgical reconstructions or repairs with augmentation can allow patients to return to vigorous sports, there is no assurance that this type of outcome will be associated with avoidance of future damage to articular cartilages and menisci. Each surgeon must have available several different procedures that can be applied to patients of various ages and with different needs.

The knowledge of the basic mechanics and kinematics of the knee joint and the healing processes necessary to attain good results from ACL surgery are increasing. Thus, the dramatic changes in protocols and procedures will probably continue to evolve and provide the means of further improvement in treatment techniques. Each physician and surgeon treating ACL injuries must keep abreast of the ever-expanding literature concerning this complex subject. Carefully designed, prospective randomized studies with long-term follow-up comparing one treatment technique with another must be produced before the best treatment for ACL injury can be determined.

References

1. Kannus P, Järvinen M: Conservatively treated tears of the anterior cruciate ligament: Long-term results. *J Bone Joint Surg* 1987;69A:1007-1012.

2. Amiel D, Kleiner JB, Akeson WH: The natural history of the anterior cruciate ligament autograft of patellar tendon origin. *Am J Sports Med* 1986;14:449-462.

3. Sperner G, Benedetto KP, Glötzer W, et al: Regeneration of patellar tendon following graft dissection for ACL reconstruction. *SOT* 1991;14:179-181.

4. Broström L, Gillquist J, Liljedahl SO, et al: Behandling au inerad ruptur au frame korsbanet (Treatment of old ruptures of the anterior cruciate ligament). *Lakartidmingen* 1968;65:4479-4487.

5. Clancy WG Jr, Nelson DA, Reider B, et al: Anterior cruciate ligament reconstruction using one-third of the patellar ligament, augmented by extra-articular tendon transfers. *J Bone Joint Surg* 1982;64A:352-359.

6. Clancy WG Jr, Ray JM, Zoltan DJ: Acute tears of the anterior cruciate ligament: Surgical versus conservative treatment. *J Bone Joint Surg* 1988;70A:1483-1488.

7. Eriksson E: Reconstruction of the anterior cruciate ligament. *Orthop Clin North Am* 1976;7:167-179.

8. Fried JA, Bergfreld JA, Weiker G, et al: Anterior cruciate reconstruction using the Jones-Ellison procedure. *J Bone Joint Surg* 1985;67A:1029-1033.

9. Gillquist J, Liljedahl SO, Lindvall H: Reconstruction for old rupture of the anterior cruciate ligament: A follow-up study. *Injury* 1971;2:271-278.

10. Johnson RJ, Eriksson E, Haggmark T, et al: Five- to ten-year follow-up evaluation after reconstruction of the anterior cruciate ligament. *Clin Orthop* 1984;183:122-140.

11. Jones KG: Reconstruction of the anterior cruciate ligament using the central one-third of the patellar ligament. *J Bone Joint Surg* 1970;52A:1302-1308.

12. Jones KG: Results of use of the central one-third of the patellar ligament to compensate for anterior cruciate ligament deficiency. *Clin Orthop* 1980;147:39-44.

13. Lambert KL: Vascularized patellar tendon graft with rigid internal fixation for anterior cruciate ligament insufficiency. *Clin Orthop* 1983;172:85-89.

14. O'Brien SJ, Warren RF, Pavlov H, et al: Reconstruction of the chronically insufficient anterior cruciate ligament with the central third of the patellar ligament. *J Bone Joint Surg* 1991;73A:278-286.

15. Paulos LE, Butler DL, Noyes FR, et al: Intra-articular cruciate reconstruction: II. Replacement with vascularized patellar tendon. *Clin Orthop* 1983;172:78-84.

16. Shelbourne KD, Whitaker HJ, McCarroll JR, et al: Anterior cruciate ligament injury: Evaluation of intraarticular reconstruction of acute tears without repair: Two to seven year followup of 155 athletes. *Am J Sports Med* 1990;18:484-489.

17. Feagin JA Jr: The office diagnosis and documentation of common knee problems. *Clin Sports Med* 1989;8:453-459.

18. Howe JG, Johnson RJ, Kaplan MJ, et al: Anteror cruciate ligament reconstruction using quadriceps patellar tendon graft: Part I. Long-term followup. *Am J Sports Med* 1991;19:447-457.

19. Harter RA, Osternig LR, Singer KM, et al: Long-term evaluation of knee stability and function following surgical reconstruction for anterior cruciate ligament insufficiency. *Am J Sports Med* 1988;16:434-443.

20. Sherman MF, Lieber L, Bonamo JR, et al: The long-term followup of primary anterior cruciate ligament repair: Defining a rationale for augmentation. *Am J Sports Med* 1991;19:243-255.

21. Theodorou BC, Miliotis E, Syrmalis L, et al: Acute ruptures of the cruciate ligaments: Outcome of primary repair. *Injury* 1989;20:281-283.

22. Andersson C, Odensten M, Good L, et al: Surgical or non-surgical treatment of acute rupture of the anterior cruciate ligament: A randomized study with long-term follow-up. *J Bone Joint Surg* 1989;71A:965-974.

23. Cabaud HE, Feagin JA, Rodkey WG: Acute anterior cruciate ligament injury and augmented repair: Experimental studies. *Am J Sports Med* 1980;8:395-401.

24. Feagin JA Jr, Curl WW: Isolated tear of the anterior cruciate ligament: 5-year follow-up study. *Am J Sports Med* 1976;4:95-100.

25. Kaplan N, Wickiewicz TL, Warren RF: Primary surgical treatment of anterior cruciate ligament ruptures: A long-term follow-up study. *Am J Sports Med* 1990;18:354-358.

26. Sgaglione NA, Warren RF, Wickiewicz TL, et al: Primary repair with semitendinosus tendon augmentation of acute anterior cruciate ligament injuries. *Am J Sports Med* 1990;18:64-73.

27. Weaver JK, Derkash RS, Freeman JR, et al: Primary knee ligament repair: Revisited. *Clin Orthop* 1985;199:185-191.

28. Jonsson T, Peterson L, Renström P, et al: Augmentation with the longitudinal patellar retinaculum in the repair of an anterior cruciate ligament rupture. *Am J Sports Med* 1989;17:401-408.

29. Larson RL: Augmentation of acute rupture of the anterior cruciate ligament. *Orthop Clin North Am* 1985;16:135-142.

30. Straub T, Hunter RE: Acute anterior cruciate ligament repair. *Clin Orthop* 1988;227:238-250.

31. Andrews JR, Sanders RA, Morin B: Surgical treatment of anterolateral rotatory instability: A follow-up study. *Am J Sports Med* 1985;13:112-119.

32. Arnold JA, Coker TP, Heaton LM, et al: Natural history of anterior cruciate tears. *Am J Sports Med* 1979;7:305-313.

33. Bertoia JT, Urovitz EP, Richards RR, et al: Anterior cruciate reconstruction using the MacIntosh lateral-substitution over-the-top repair. *J Bone Joint Surg* 1985;67A:1183-1188.

34. Bergfeld JA, Pearl A (eds): *Extraarticular Reconstruction in the Anterior Cruciate Ligament Deficient Knee*. Champaign, IL, Human Kinetics Publishers, 1992.

35. Durkan JA, Wynne GF, Haggerty JF: Extraarticular reconstruction of the anterior cruciate ligament insufficient knee: A long-term analysis of the Ellison procedure. *Am J Sports Med* 1989;17:112-117.

36. Ellison AE: Distal iliotibial-band transfer for anterolateral rotatory instability of the knee. *J Bone Joint Surg* 1979;61A:330-337.

37. Ellison AE: The pathogenesis and treatment of anterolateral rotatory instability. *Clin Orthop* 1980;147:51-55.

38. Hanks GA, Joyner DM, Kalenak A: Anterolateral rotatory instability of the knee: An analysis of the Ellison procedure. *Am J Sports Med* 1981;9:225-232.

39. Ireland J, Trickey EL: MacIntosh tenodesis for anterolateral instability of the knee. *J Bone Joint Surg* 1980;62B:340-345.

40. Kalenak A: An analysis of the Ellison procedure: An 11 year follow-up. Presented at the American Academy of Orthopaedic Surgeons. The Athlete's Knee, Washington, DC, November 4-6, 1991.

41. Kennedy JC, Stewart R, Walker DM: Anterolateral rotatory instability of the knee joint: An early analysis of the Ellison procedure. *J Bone Joint Surg* 1978;60A:1031-1039.

42. Lemaire M: Ruptures anciennes du ligament croisé antéreur du genou. *J Chir* 1967;93:311-320.

43. Losee RE, Johnson TR, Southwick WO: Anterior subluxation of the lateral tibial plateau: A diagnostic test and operative repair. *J Bone Joint Surg* 1978;60A:1015-1030.

44. MacIntosh DL, Darby TA: Lateral substitution reconstruction. *J Bone Joint Surg* 1976;58B:142.

45. Odesten M, Lysholm J, Gillquist J: Long-term follow-up study of a distal iliotibial band transfer (DIT) for anterolateral knee instability. *Clin Orthop* 1983;176:129-135.

46. Draganich LF, Reider B, Ling M, et al: An in vitro study of an intraarticular and extraarticular reconstruction in the anterior cruciate ligament deficient knee. *Am J Sports Med* 1990;18:262-266.

47. Engebretsen L, Lew WD, Lewis JL, et al: The effect of an iliotibial tenodesis on intraarticular graft forces and knee joint motion. *Am J Sports Med* 1990;18:169-176.

48. Strum GM, Fox JM, Ferkel RD, et al: Intraarticular *versus* intraarticular and extraarticular reconstruction for chronic anterior cruciate ligament instability. *Clin Orthop* 1989;245:188-198.

49. Noyes FR, Barber SD: The effect of an extra-articular procedure on allograft reconstructions for chronic ruptures of the anterior cruciate ligament. *J Bone Joint Surg* 1991;73A:882-892.

50. Noyes FR, Butler DL, Grood ES, et al: Biomechanical analysis of human ligament grafts used in knee-ligament repairs and reconstructions. *J Bone Joint Surg* 1984;66A:344-352.

51. Woo SL-Y, Hollis JM, Adams DJ, et al: Tensile properties of the human femur-anterior cruciate ligament-tibia complex: The effects of specimen age and orientation *Am J Sports Med* 1991;19:217-225.

52. Lipscomb AB, Johnston RK, Snyder RB, et al: Evaluation of hamstring strength following use of semitendinosus and gracilis tendons to reconstruct the anterior cruciate ligament. *Am J Sports Med* 1982;10:340-342.

53. Warner JJP, Warren RF, Cooper DE: Management of acute anterior cruciate ligament injury, in Tullos HS (ed): American Academy of Orthopaedic Surgeons *Instructional Course Lectures, XL*. Park Ridge, IL, American Academy of Orthopaedic Surgeons, 1991, pp 219-232.

54. Zarins B, Rowe CR: Combined anterior cruciate-ligament reconstruction using semitendinosus tendon and iliotibial tract. *J Bone Joint Surg* 1986;68A:160-177.

55. Butler DL: Anterior cruciate ligament: Its normal response and replacement. *J Orthop Res* 1989;7:910-921.

56. Butler DL, Grood ES, Noyes RD, et al: Mechanical properties of primate vascularized vs. nonvascularized patellar tendon grafts; changes over time. *J Orthop Res* 1989;7:68-79.

57. Johnson RJ: Anatomy and biomechanics of the knee, in Chapman MW, Madison M (eds): *Operative Orthopaedics*. Philadelphia, JB Lippincott, 1988, vol 3, pp 1617-1631.

58. Daniel DM: Principles of knee ligament surgery, in Daniel DM, Akeson WH, O'Connor JJ (eds): *Knee Ligaments: Structure, Function, Injury, and Repair*. New York, Raven Press, 1990, pp 11-29.

59. Arms SW, Pope MH, Johnson RJ, et al: The biomechanics of anterior cruciate ligament rehabilitation and reconstruction. *Am J Sports Med* 1984;12:8-18.

60. Beynnon BD, Fleming BC, Pope MH, et al: An in-vivo study of the ACL strain biomechanics in the normal knee. *Trans Orthop Res Soc* 1989;14:324.

61. Fleming B, Beynnon B, McLeod W, et al: Comparison of a tensiometer and isometer for implantaton of a prosthetic anterior cruciate ligament. *J Biomech* 1990;23:718.

62. Hefzy MS, Grood ES: Sensitivity of insertion locations on length patterns of anterior cruciate ligament fibers. *J Biomech Eng* 1986;108:73-82.

63. Hefzy MS, Grood ES, Noyes FR: Factors affecting the region of most isometric femoral attachments: Part II. The anterior cruciate ligament. *Am J Sports Med* 1989;17:208-216.

64. Yoshiya S, Andrish JT, Manley MT, et al: Graft tension in anterior cruciate ligament reconstruction: An in vivo study in dogs. *Am J Sports Med* 1987;15:464-470.

65. Burks RT, Leland R: Determination of graft tension before fixation in anterior cruciate ligament reconstruction. *Arthroscopy* 1988;4:260-266.

66. Hunter RE, Lew WD, Lewis JL, et al: Graft force-setting technique in reconstruction of the anterior cruciate ligament. *Am J Sports Med* 1990;18:12-19.

67. Lewis JL, Lew WD, Engebretsen L, et al: Factors affecting graft force in surgical reconstruction of the anterior cruciate ligament. *J Orthop Res* 1990;8:514-521.

68. Lewis JL, Lew WD, Hill JA, et al: Knee joint motion and ligament forces before and after ACL reconstruction. *J Biomech Eng* 1989;111:97-106.

69. Kurosaka M, Yoshiya S, Andrish JT: A biomechanical comparison of different surgical techniques of graft fixation in anterior cruciate ligament reconstruction. *Am J Sports Med* 1987;15:225-229.

70. Robertson DB, Daniel DM, Biden E: Soft tissue fixation to bone. *Am J Sports Med* 1986;14:398-403.
71. Barber FA, Small NC, Click J: Anterior cruciate reconstruction by semitendinosus and gracilis tendon autograft. *Am J Knee Surgery* 1991;4:84-93.
72. Cho KO: Reconstruction of the anterior cruciate ligament by semitendinosus tenodesis. *J Bone Joint Surg* 1975;57A:608-612.
73. Lipscomb AB, Johnston RK, Synder RB, et al: Secondary reconstruction of anterior cruciate ligament in athletes by using the semitendinosus tendon. *Am J Sports Med* 1979;7:81-84.
74. Mott HW: Semitendinosus anatomic reconstruction for cruciate ligament insufficiency. *Clin Orthop* 1983;172:90-92.
75. Moyer RA, Betz RR, Iqquinto J, et al: Arthroscopic anterior cruciate reconstruction using the semitendinosus and gracilis tendons: Preliminary report. *Cont Orthop* 1986;12:17-23.
76. Reichelt A: Klinische und röntgenologische Spätergebnisse nach Kreuzbandersatzplastiken mit dem Meniskus, English abstract. *Arch Orthop Unfallchir* 1977;88:37-48.
77. Collins H, Hughston JC, DeHaven K, et al: The meniscus as a cruciate ligament substitute. *Am J Sports Med* 1974;2:11-21.
78. Tillberg B: The late repair of torn cruciate ligaments using menisci. *J Bone Joint Surg* 1977;59B:15-19.
79. Walsh JJ Jr: Meniscal reconstruction of the anterior cruciate ligament. *Clin Orthop* 1972;89-171-177.
80. Holden JP, Grood ES, Butler DL, et al: Biomechanics of fascia lata ligament replacements: Early postoperative changes in the goat. *J Orthop Res* 1988;6:639-647.
81. Hooper GJ, Walton DI: Reconstruction of the anterior cruciate ligament using the bone-block iliotibial-tract transfer. *J Bone Joint surg* 1987;69A:1150-1154.
82. Insall J, Joseph DM, Aglietti P, et al: Bone-block iliotibial-band transfer for anterior cruciate insufficiency. *J Bone Joint Surg* 1981;63A:560-569.
83. Nicholas JA, Minkoff J: Iliotibial band transfer through the intercondylar notch for combined anterior instability (ITPT Procedure). *Am J Sports Med* 1978;6:341-353.
84. Scott WN, Ferriter P, Marino M: Intra-articular transfer of the iliotibial tract: Two to seven-year follow-up results. *J Bone Joint Surg* 1985;67A:532-538.
85. Windsor RE, Insall JN: Bone-block iliotibial band reconstruction for anterior cruciate insufficiency: Follow-up note and minimum five-year follow-up period. *Clin Orthop* 1990;250:197-206.
86. Yost JG, Chekofsy K, Schoscheim, et al: Intraarticular iliotibial band reconstructon for anterior cruciate ligament insufficiency. *Am J Sports Med* 1981;9:220-224.
87. Holmes PF, James SL, Larson RL, et al: Retrospective direct comparson of three intraarticular anterior cruciate ligament reconstructions. *Am J Sports Med* 1991;19:596-600.
88. Sachs RA, Daniel DM, Stone ML, et al: Patellofemoral problems after anterior cruciate ligament reconstruction. *Am J Sports Med* 1989;17:760-765.
89. Marder RA, Raskin JR, Carroll M: Prospective evaluation of arthroscopically assisted anterior cruciate ligament reconstruction: Patella tendon versus semitendinosus and gracilis tendons. *Am J Sports Med* 1991;19:478-484.
90. Gillquist J, Odensten M: Arthroscopic reconstruction of the anterior cruciate ligament. *Arthroscopy* 1988;4:5-9.

91. Fowler PJ, Capra SW: Anterior cruciate ligament reconstruction with the Kennedy ligament augmentation device, in Scott WN (ed): *Ligament and Extensor Mechanism Injuries of the Knee*. St. Louis, Mosby Year Book, 1991, pp 301-310.

92. Engebretsen L, Benum P, Fasting O, et al: A prospective, randomized study of three surgical techniques for treatment of acute ruptures of the anterior cruciate ligament. *Am J Sports Med* 1990;18:585-590.

93. Hanley P, Lew WD, Lewis JL, et al: Load sharing and graft forces in anterior cruciate ligament reconstructions with the Ligament Augmentation Device. *Am J Sports Med* 1989;17:414-422.

94. Noyes FR, Mangine RE, Barber S: Early knee motion after open and arthroscopic anterior cruciate ligament reconstruction. *Am J Sports Med* 1987;15:149-160

95. Henning CE, Lynch MA, Glick KR Jr: An in vivo strain gage study of elongation of the anterior cruciate ligament. *Am J Sports Med* 1985;13:22-26.

96. Maltry JA, Noble PC, Woods GW, et al: External stabilization of the anterior cruciate ligament deficient knee during rehabilitation. *Am J Sports Med* 1989;17:550-554.

97. Paulos L, Noyes FR, Grood E, et al: Knee rehabilitaton after anterior cruciate ligament reconstruction and repair. *Am J Sports Med* 1981;9:140-149.

98. Huegel M, Idelicato PA: Trends in rehabilitation following anterior cruciate ligament reconstruction. *Clin Sports Med* 1988;7:801-811.

99. Shelbourne KD, Nitz P: Accelerated rehabilitation after anterior cruciate ligament reconstruction. *Am J Sports Med* 1990;18:292-299.

100. Beynnon B , Wertheimer C, Fleming B, et al: An in-vivo study of the anterior cruciate ligament strain biomechanics during functional knee bracing. *Trans Orthop Res Soc* 1990;15:223.

101. Cawley PW, France EP, Paulos LE: The current state of functional knee bracing research: A review of the literature. *Am J Sports Med* 1991;19:226-233.

Chapter 25

The Use of Soft-Tissue Allografts in Knee Ligament Reconstruction

Lonnie E. Paulos, MD
John L. Pinkowski, MD
Charles L. Beck, MD

The Clinical Use of Allograft Tissue

Soft-tissue allografts have several applications in orthopaedic surgery (Outline 1). Perhaps one of the most common uses for soft-tissue allografts involves ligament reconstruction of the knee, particularly the anterior cruciate ligament (ACL). In this chapter, we highlight the current basic science and clinical knowledge regarding the use of allograft tissues.

Currently, the most popular methods of ACL reconstruction use autogenous tissue,[1] but significant complications can occur.[2-9] Weakening of the donor muscle group can occur by violating the normal extensor mechanism or harvesting one or two hamstring tendons. With patellar tendon autografts, patellar fracture or infrapatellar tendon rupture is possible.[3] The incidence of chondrosis of the patellofemoral joint may be higher after harvesting the patellar tendon.[3,7] In addition, the donor site is compromised during the process of harvesting autogenous tissue.

Other methods of ACL reconstruction use two basic types of allograft tissue. One is composed of soft tissue alone; the other contains a bony block on one or both ends. The most popular allografts currently in use are the bone-patellar tendon-bone and bone-Achilles tendon grafts. Other grafts used include the fascia lata, semitendinosus, gracilis, flexor tendons of the hand, anterior or posterior tibialis tendons, peroneal tendons, and ACL allograft.

The use of allograft tissue for ACL reconstruction is advantageous because the graft reproduces the bundle arrangement of the damaged ACL. Another advantage is that compromise of the donor site is avoided, in contrast to using autografts.

It is well known that any biologic substitute loses some of its initial strength during incorporation. Being able to use larger cross-sectional areas of allograft tissue leads to a potentially hither ultimate yield than could be obtained for a smaller autograft. As public awareness of donor programs increases, allograft tissue has the po-

Outline 1 Clinical uses of allograft tissue

Isolated anterior cruciate ligament reconstruction
Isolated posterior cruciate ligament reconstruction
Medial collateral ligament augmentation
Lateral collateral ligament augmentation
Combined ligament injuries of the knee
Rotator cuff tears in the shoulder
Shoulder ligament reconstruction
Wrist tendon reconstruction
Others

tential for unlimited availability and sizes. However, problems exist with sizing and the amount of strength that is lost with revascularization and remodeling. Controversy exists regarding immunology, disease transmission, remodeling, vascularity, viability, inflammation caused by secondary sterilization, contributions to degenerative arthritis, and biomechanical function and strength; many questions remain unanswered.

Current Controversies

Immunologic Rejection

The possibility of recipient rejection of donor tissue is a concern when large organs are transplanted, but its true impact on ligamentous transplantation is unclear. The basic pathways of immunologic response are the humoral and the cellular immunity sequences. The humoral response causes lymphocytes to produce antibodies, while cellular immunity involves a direct cytotoxic reaction. The cellular immunity sequence is the major pathway of transplantation rejection, so studies using this type of assay would appear to be more representative of the actual fate of the soft-tissue allograft.

Most immunologic studies involve animal experimentation, while a few others have examined the human response. Animal studies must be carefully interpreted because they cannot be rigidly extrapolated to humans. There are several different methods of assaying the immunologic response that vary in sensitivity and specificity and make comparison difficult. These include measurement of antibodies and of T-lymphocyte activity in cytotoxicity tests and the lymphoblast transformation test. Those studies using histology as the only criteria for immune response are flawed by low specificity and the assumption that the biopsy site represents the entire ligament structure.

Potential sources of antigenicity include the major histocompatibility antigens on the cell surface; matrix[10,11] and collagen are sources of weak antigenicity.[12] However, the preservation process may alter these areas and change the antigenicity.

Authors writing on immunologic topics in orthopaedics should distinguish between bone and soft-tissue allografts. The literature must also stipulate the type of bone present, such as cortical, cancellous, or both.[13]

Fresh allograft bone has been shown to be extremely immunogenic.[10,14-17] Frozen bone is less able to stimulate immune response; this quality appears to be dose related.[15,17,18] In one investigation, a significant difference in immunogenicity between fresh and frozen bone tissue was not found. Instead, varying degrees of immunogenicity in both types of grafts occurred theoretically because of blocking factors in the serum.[16,18] Friedlaender and associates,[11] using humoral antibody and lymphocytotoxic assays, showed that freeze-dried cortical allogeneic bone in rabbits was not antigenic, whereas both freeze-dried and frozen cancellous allogeneic transplants evoked an immunologic response.[11] The retained marrow elements or the larger surface area of cancellous bone compared with cortical bone are possible explanations for this response.[11,19] Later, in 1977, these same researchers reported that 20% of those receiving freeze-dried bone produced anti-HLA antibodies to freeze-dried bone receptors.[20] Studies done by Burchardt and associates[21,22] indicate that freeze-drying does not protect cortical allogeneic grafts from immunologic rejection in dogs, but rejection can be suppressed with azathioprine.

Soft-tissue studies have shown that fresh tendon allografts elicit an immune response,[4,23,24] but the response is weakened by deep-freezing (-70 or -80 C), the use of paraformaldehyde, or lyophilization (freeze-drying).[4,22,25,26] In a more recent study examining the response to ethylene oxide sterilized, freeze-dried bone-patellar tendon-bone allografts used in ACL reconstruction, Pinkowski and associates[8] found that 50% of their patients had an immunologic sensitization. In one patient, synovial fluid obtained 9 months after ACL reconstruction showed an intense immunologic response. Histologically, the fluid contained lymphocytes and plasma cells and was extremely reactive to the lymphoblast transformation test. The exact antigen causing this response was not identified but could be cell surface antigens, collagen, or matrix. One proposed hypothesis was that the ethylene-oxide sterilization process altered the graft structure or acted as a hapten to elicit this response. Pinkowski and Paulos and their associates,[7,8] in a continuing experiment, have found that to date none of the patients receiving deep-frozen bone-patellar tendon-bone or Achilles tendon allografts elicited any immunologic response during the lymphoblast transformation test. Presently, there are no persistent effusions and no clinical failures in this group.

Disease Transmission

The first step in avoiding disease transmission is donor screening. The American Association of Tissue Banks has developed criteria to minimize the risk of transmission of neoplastic or infectious disease. Concern about the risk of transmission of diseases such as hepatitis B, non-A, non-B hepatitis, HIV, syphilis, and hairy cell leukemia affects patients' willingness to accept allografts. Screening assays exist for many of these diseases but these assays are not completely reliable. Furthermore, current HIV testing may allow a window of up to several months, during which time a person could be infected with HIV but not yet test positive for the presence of antibodies.

Tissue retrieval is a key step in maintaining graft sterility. Sterile harvesting does not require secondary sterilization with gamma irradiation, ethylene oxide, or other processes. These secondary sterilization processes lead to other problems. Gamma irradiation in doses above 2.5 Mrads can alter the tissue biomechanically; also, spore-forming viruses in ligamentous tissue may survive this treatment. Ethylene oxide sterilization reportedly causes inflammation[7] and may contribute to immunologic responses in the host.[8] Total incorporation of ethylene oxide-preserved tissue is also in question.[27,28]

Vascularity, Viability, and Remodeling

Knowledge of the process by which autogenous tissue is incorporated[2,9,14,29,30] is important in understanding the response to allogeneic tissue. Autogenous free graft tissue is implanted as a non-vascularized structure, with a few viable intrasubstance cells.[24] Incorporation involves necrosis, revascularization, cellular repopulation, new matrix and collagen formation, then remodeling. The initially disorganized new collagen bundles are rearranged in longitudinal bundles.

Except for initial cell viability, incorporation of allograft tissue proceeds along a course similar to that of autografts.[31,32] Differences do exist in the timing of certain stages and the source of repopulating cells. Stability of tissue structure takes longer in allografts but the final structure does resemble that of autografts. Various animal studies, including primate research,[33] confirm the incorporation of allograft tissue in reconstructive surgery.[26]

Levitt and associates[34] compiled data from studies of allograft biopsies, taken from 8 weeks to 5 years after implantation in 30 patients. The initially acellular graft developed a synovial covering within 2 months. Cellularity increased from the periphery and spread centrally; the entire graft achieved cellularity by 9 months. Vascularity increased within the first few months and subsided between 9 and 15 months. At one year, collagen patterns were seen, but it took from 18 to 24 months before a more normal orientation of collagen bundles and normal cellular patterns were evident, twice the time it takes for autograft incorporation.

In 1991, Shino and associates[35] reported on the histologic structure and surface blood flow of allografts, from six to 89 months after implantation. In the 53 patients studied, six-month grafts had significantly higher blood flow than grafts at 12 months, the point of surface blood flow stabilization. Histologic examination confirmed that the allograft tissue remodeled in essentially the same sequence as the autografts. Microscopic morphologic stability was reached at 18 months,[35] confirming earlier histologic reports.[36,37] Shino and associates[38] are currently evaluating flowmetry on their autograft patients, and their preliminary data have indicated no difference between surface blood flow in autografts as compared with allografts.

In a study currently being conducted by Beck and Paulos, successful allografts in stable knees and failed allograft reconstructions are being examined histologically. Grafts have been examined at periods ranging from 3 to 36 months after implantation. Biopsies have been obtained in both superficial and deep portions of the reconstructed ligament in an attempt to ascertain the degree of healing in each portion of the graft. Initial results indicate a time scale similar to that noted by Shino and associates[36] and Levitt and associates[34] for morphologic stability of the superficial portions of the graft. However, there are striking differences in graft cellularity and vascularity between superficial and deep portions of the graft, even at 36 months (Figs. 1 thru 6).

Preliminary indications are that graft viability is not uniform and varies from patient to patient as well as from superficial to deep portions of the graft. Also noted in the allograft tissue is a tendency toward metaplasia (fibrocartilage and calcification) with increasing duration of implantation (Fig. 6). These grafts were 1.5 to 2.0 times larger than the autograft tissue available for harvest would have been in these patients and perhaps were significantly larger than the grafts used in the studies of Levitt and associates[34] and Shino and associates.[36] Nevertheless, Beck and Paulos' study shows that acellularity may persist much longer in these larger grafts than it does in a smaller graft or a graft composed of multiple fascicles, such as in the study reported by Shino and associates. These large allografts may possibly function as a bioprosthesis for an extended period, much longer than previously suspected. Furthermore, the preliminary results of this study agree with the results of Shino's study that there is no apparent correlation between histologic appearance and short-term clinical results for allografts or autografts (Fig. 4). A long-term follow-up period of at least 3 years, and preferably as long as 10 years, is required to confirm the durability of allograft ligament reconstructions. Further studies should be done in the areas of promotion of vascular access to the deeper portions of the graft, biochemical augmentation of fibroblast ingrowth and collagen organization, and elucidation of the biomechanical characteristics of these grafts over time.

Function and Strength

Biomechanical studies have been performed on allograft tissue prior to implantation to determine the effects of processing and sterilization. Other studies have examined allograft tissue implanted in

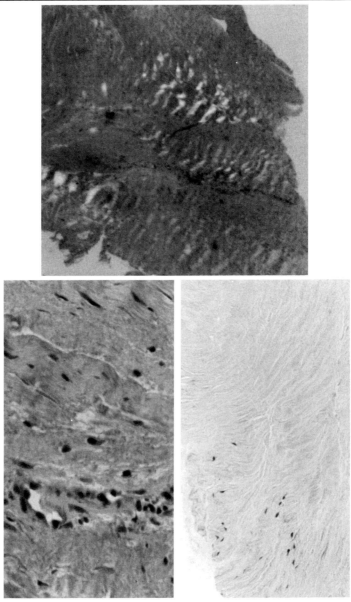

Fig. 1   *Patellar tendon allograft biopsy at 12 months postimplantation. **Top**, Low-powered view demonstrating excellent collagen organization in superficial portion of graft. **Bottom left**, High-powered view showing vascular ingrowth, maintenance of ligament-like collagen crimp pattern, and hypercellularity in superficial portion of graft. **Bottom right**, Deep portion of the graft showing cellularity in a small section, but near-total acellularity in a large segment of this biopsy section.*

animals to determine its strength after incorporation. France and associates[15] biomechanically tested several tissues prior to implantation. They found that in deep-frozen allograft tissue, the patellar

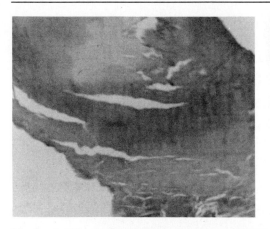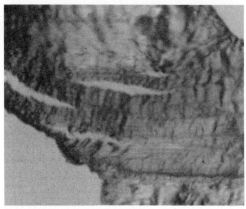

Fig. 2   *Achilles tendon at 7 months after implantation. Deep biopsy shows maintenance of collagen organization, but with acellularity at 7 months (**left**),(hematoxylin-eosin, x 100).* **Right**, *Same view polarized.*

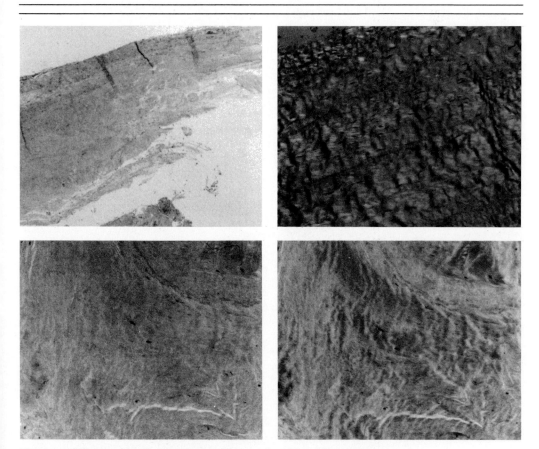

Fig. 3   *Achilles tendon allograft failed at 21 months after reinjury.* **Top left**, *Torn end of graft with excellent cellularity and collagen organization.* **Top right**, *Polarized higher powered view of top left.* **Bottom left**, *Deep portion of ligament showing hypocellularity.* **Bottom right**, *Same as bottom left polarized.*

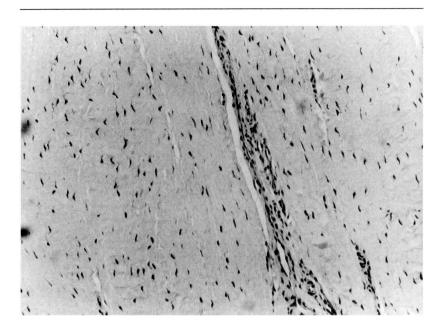

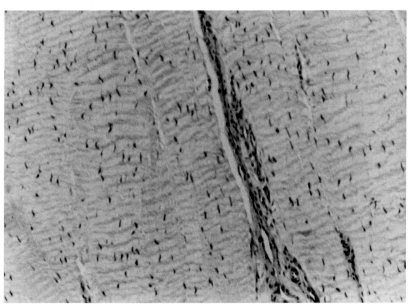

Fig. 4 *Patellar tendon autograft at 21 months after implantation, high power view. Note vascularity, hypercellularity, and excellent microscopic organization. However, this graft was a failed, "stretched-out" graft removed for histologic examination at the time of second reconstruction. This sample illustrates the poor correlation between histologic and clinical results.*

tendon was stronger in ultimate stress testing than the Achilles tendon or fascia lata. However, although no statistically significant

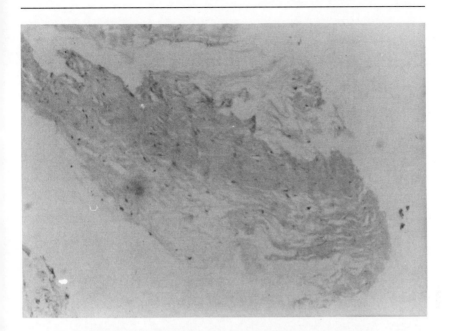

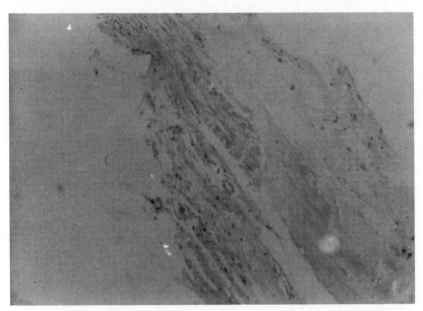

Fig. 5 *Patellar tendon allograft deep biopsy 16 months after implementation; polarized views.* **Top**, *Organization and collagen crimp pattern maintained with good cellularity.* **Bottom**, *Sections showing area of hypercellularity enveloping remnant of original acellular allograft tissue.*

difference existed between the freeze-dried and deep-frozen allografts, the lyophilized allografts had a general tendency toward slightly decreased ultimate strength. It was also determined that the

521

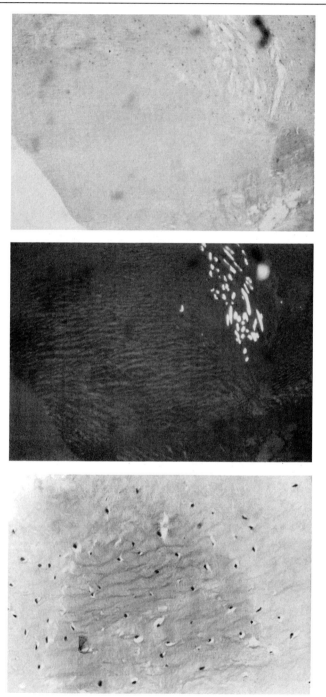

Fig. 6   *Fascia lata graft removed 3 years after implantation. Graft was successful and maintained stability; however, it was removed because of arthrofibrosis secondary to overtensioning of the graft at time of implantation. **Top**, Nonpolarized view, low power. **Center**, Polarized view of graft with collagen crimp pattern apparent but with areas of calcification. **Bottom**, High power view of metaplastic area (fibrocartilage transformation).*

freeze-dried irradiated grafts had the most significant reduction in ultimate strength compared with either deep-frozen or freeze-dried patellar tendon, Achilles tendon, or fascia lata. Another study has shown that the order of irradiation and freeze-drying of tissue has a significant effect on ultimate strength. There was more biomechanical deterioration when tissue was dehydrated prior to irradiation, indicating that water content appears to have a protective effect on final strength. Maeda and associates[39] investigated the effects on flexor tendons of organic solvents, currently used in preservation and viral sterilization of dural allograft tissue, combined with 2.5 Mrads of irradiation. They found that the tissue became weaker if subjected to gamma irradiation after the use of organic solvents, rather than the reverse. It was concluded that the irradiation had more detrimental effects on the tissue after the organic solvents decreased its water content.

Various biomechanical studies[1,14,15,20,27,40-42] of autograft and allograft incorporation have determined that during the incorporation process, the graft tissue loses a significant amount of its original ultimate strength. Autografts tested between three and four months after implantation retained an average of 26% of their original strength (range 15% to 40%), grafts tested between six and seven months averaged 25% (range 13% to 30%), and those tested between one and two years retained 32% (range 11% to 52%). Allografts tested between three and four months after implementation retained 26% (range 17% to 35%) of their strength, those tested between six and seven months averaged 34% (range 14% to 63%), and allografts tested between one and two years retained 30% (25% to 35%). There appears to be no significant difference in final ultimate strength between allografts and autografts.[2,4,5,14,15,20,24,29,39,41-52]

Although histologic studies determine when the transplanted tissue resembles the microstructure of the ACL morphologically, Shino and associates[37] have shown in animal experiments that there is no strong correlation between the structure of grafts and their mechanical properties.

Degenerative Arthritis

Although the trauma from the initial injury may lead to future hyaline cartilage degeneration, recurrent laxity or altered kinematics of the knee after reconstruction may also contribute to arthritis. A recent finding by Silvaggio and associates[53] was the production of interleukin-1 (IL-1) from wear particles of various synthetic or biologic grafts. In an in vitro study, freeze-dried ethylene oxide-sterilized patellar tendon allografts promoted a significant increase in IL-1, compared with deep-frozen tissue. The production of this substance induces synoviocytes and chondrocytes to produce prostaglandins, collagenase, and phospholipase A2. The IL-1 inhibits matrix synthesis and mediates connective tissue destruction and inflammation.

Chemical Inflammation

Paulos and associates[7] reported on two types of ethylene oxide-sterilized, freeze-dried allograft reactions. One was an acute synovial reaction 5 to 18 months after surgery. This degenerative process within the ligament, in which the allograft has been described as resembling applesauce, occurred in 15% of patients either intra-articularly or at the attachment sites. The hypothetical cause of this response is related to the ethylene oxide residues and by-products, ethylene glycol and ethylene chlorhydrin. The second reaction was a late, gradual failure from 9 to 24 months after implantation. Incorporation of the graft appeared to be unsuccessful, with increased laxity. Second-look arthroscopy revealed an "empty sock" of synovial tissue, with no reaction or scarification present.[7]

Animal and Clinical Studies

Many animal studies have been conducted using rabbits, dogs, goats, and primates. Fewer studies of clinical trials have been published. Investigations by Cordrey and associates[20] in 1963 compared autogenous and preserved homogenous tendon grafts in rabbit Achilles tendons. All allograft tissue became viable and incorporated, as did autogenous grafts, regardless of how the allograft was preserved. Preservation materials/methods included ethanol, Merthiolate (thimerosal), and freeze-drying. Revascularization was noted in autografts and in allografts after approximately one week and three weeks, respectively. This corroborated Graham and associates'[54] earlier research in rabbits, in which 13 of 14 Achilles tendon allografts procedures were successful.

Webster and Werner[52] evaluated freeze-dried flexor tendon allografts and fresh autografts in dogs and demonstrated that they did not differ in tensile strength three to six months after transplantation. In another study,[42] these authors found no appreciable difference in mechanical properties of allograft or autograft after incorporation.

Curtis and associates[47] performed ACL reconstructions in dogs using freeze-dried fascia lata allografts. The allografts remained intact in all knees, with only mild instability. No evidence of rejection was observed.

In the study by Drez and associates,[27] 28 goats were evaluated at 6, 12, 26, and 52 weeks after freeze-dried bone-patellar tendon-bone allograft ACL reconstruction. The allografts were revascularized in 12 weeks, and matured and resembled normal connective tissue at 26 weeks. The graft stiffness and maximum force to failure were 29% and 43% of the control value, respectively, at 52 weeks. They concluded that freeze-dried bone-patellar tendon-bone allografts are biomechanically and biologically similar to patellar tendon autografts.

McCarthy and associates[55] have implanted cryopreserved primate ACL allografts in primates and compared these with patellar tendon autografts. The allografts were found to have increased calcification and necrosis and decreased fibrosis, compared with autografts of the same age. The laxity patterns and biomechanical testing performed indicated that the two types of grafts were otherwise comparable.

Kirkpatrick and associates[40] compared cryopreserved canine allografts and fresh canine autografts and found no significant difference in the clinical outcome. When several biomechanical tests were performed, only the maximal load to failure and the slope of the deformation curve showed any significant difference. The histologic comparison yielded more advanced cellularity in the autografts than the allografts.

Meyers[56] had an opportunity to evaluate 54 patients who had undergone freeze-dried patellar tendon allograft ACL reconstruction with a minimum two-year follow-up. Overall success was 78% good or excellent, with 87% of the patients satisfied with the results. In 28 patients, second-look arthroscopy revealed 18 normal-appearing grafts, six with intercondylar notch scarring in stable knees, two with slight fraying along the lateral femoral condyle, and two that had failed completely. The lateral compartment hyaline cartilage surfaces remained normal in all 28 patients. There were three instances of patellofemoral deterioration, and six cases of medial compartment deterioration, four of which had previous medial meniscectomy.

In another review of patients receiving freeze-dried, ethylene oxide-sterilized bone-patellar tendon-bone allografts for ACL reconstruction, less than optimal results were found. Only 47% (17 of 36) of the patients had functional knees and 22% had complete dissolution of allograft associated with large femoral cysts.[9] Indelicato and associates[4] compared their experience using sterile freeze-dried patellar tendon allografts (no ethylene oxide treatment) with sterile deep-frozen allografts. The patients receiving deep-frozen allografts were more satisfied with their results (93% versus 79%), but objective testing revealed no significant difference (84% versus 85%). None of the patients in this study demonstrated any clinical signs of an immune reaction or graft rejection, but no assays were performed to check for a response. Four biopsy specimens were obtained from the surface of the reconstructed ligament and none showed any lymphocytic infiltrate or giant cell reaction.

Shino and associates[35] compared 40 patients who underwent middle-third patellar tendon autograft reconstruction with 49 patients in whom reconstruction was done with various allograft tissue. The allografts included fresh-frozen Achilles, tibialis, or peroneus tendons without bony attachments. The patients were studied for a period of 18 to 36 months. The autograft tissue showed a side-to-side laxity difference of 1.9 mm, compared with 0.9 mm for the allograft reconstructions, which proved to be statistically significant. They concluded that in terms of restored anterior stability, the allograft ACL reconstruction is significantly better than that using the central third of the autogenous patellar tendon.

Conclusions

Safe and effective use of allograft tissue in knee ligament reconstruction is an obtainable goal. Current research indicates that allograft tissue is similar to autograft tissue with regard to incorporation and joint stability and does not violate normal tissues. However, no long-term studies are yet available.

Few, if any, immunologic reactions have occurred clinically when using deep frozen, soft-tissue allografts. Many earlier problems (incorporation and inflammation) noted with allograft reconstruction seem to have been eliminated by avoiding secondary sterilization with ethylene oxide.

Vascularity, viability, remodeling, function, and strength are similar in allograft and autograft tissues. Ligamentization takes longer in allografts; however, no significant alteration in joint stability or function has been documented because of this. Long-term studies examining bone tunnel healing, late graft rupture, joint laxity patterns, and meniscal survival will be necessary before allographic tissues can be used with impunity.

With continued improvement of the screening and sterilization process, transmission of infectious disease will become less of a factor in the decision-making process.

References

1. Noyes FR, Butler DL, Grood ES, et al: Biomechanical analysis of human ligament grafts used in knee-ligament repairs and reconstructions. *J Bone Joint Surg* 1984;66A:344-352.

2. Arnoczky SP, Tarvin GB, Marshall JL: Anterior cruciate ligament replacement using patellar tendon: An evaluation of graft revascularization in the dog. *J Bone Joint Surg* 1982;64A:217-224.

3. Bonamo JJ, Krinick RM, Sporn AA: Rupture of the patellar ligament after use of its central third for anterior cruciate reconstruction: A report of two cases. *J Bone Joint Surg* 1984;66A:1294-1297.

4. Indelicato PA, Bittar ES, Prevot TJ, et al: Clinical comparison of freeze-dried and fresh frozen patellar tendon allografts for anterior cruciate ligament reconstruction of the knee. *Am J Sports Med* 1990;18:335-342.

5. Jackson DW, Windler GE, Simon TM: Intraarticular reaction associated with the use of freeze-dried, ethylene oxide-sterilized bone-patella tendon-bone allografts in the reconstruction of the anterior cruciate ligament. *Am J Sports Med* 1990;18:1-11.

6. Nikolaou PK, Seaber AV, Glisson RR, et al: Anterior cruciate ligament allograft transplantation: Long-term function, histology, revascularization, and operative technique. *Am J Sports Med* 1986;14:348-360.

7. Paulos LE, Rosenberg TD, Gurley WD: Anterior cruciate ligament allografts, in Friedman MJ, Ferkel RD (eds): *Prosthetic Ligament Reconstruction of the Knee*. Philadelphia, WB Saunders, 1988, pp 186-192.

8. Pinkowski JL, Reiman PR, Chen S-L: Human lymphocyte reaction to freeze-dried allograft and xenograft ligamentous tissue. *Am J Sports Med* 1989;17:595-600.

9. Roberts TS, Drez D Jr, McCarthy W, et al: Anterior cruciate ligament reconstruction using freeze-dried, ethylene oxide-sterilized, bone-patellar tendon-bone allografts: Two year results in thirty-six patients. *Am J Sports Med* 1991;19:35-41.

10. Burchardt H: The biology of bone graft repair. *Clin Orthop* 1983;174:28-42.

11. Friedlaender GE, Strong DM, Sell KW: Studies on the antigenicity of bone: I. Freeze-dried and deep-frozen bone allografts in rabbits. *J Bone Joint Surg* 1976;58A:854-858.

12. Trentham DE, Townes AS, Kang AH, et al: Humoral and cellular sensitivity to collagen in type II collagen-induced arthritis in rats. *J Clin Invest* 1978;61:89-96.

13. Mankin HJ, Doppelt S, Tomford W: Clinical experience with allograft implantation: The first ten years. *Clin Orthop* 1983;174:69-86.

14. Ballock RT, Woo SL-Y, Lyon RM, et al: Use of patellar tendon autograft for anterior cruciate ligament reconstruction in the rabbit: A long-term histologic and biomechanical study. *J Orthop Res* 1989;7:474-485.

15. France EP, Paulos LE, Rosenberg TD, et al: The biomechanics of anterior cruciate allografts, in Friedman MJ, Ferkel RD (eds): *Prosthetic Ligament Reconstruction of the Knee*. Philadelphia, WB Saunders, 1988, pp 180-185.

16. Langer F, Czitrom A, Pritzker KP, et al: The immunogenicity of fresh and frozen allogeneic bone. *J Bone Joint Surg* 1975;57A:216-220.

17. Lee EH: The immunology of osteochondral and massive bone allografts. *Trans Orthop Res Soc* 1979;4:61.

18. Langer F, Gross AE, West M, et al: The immunogenicity of allograft knee joint transplants. *Clin Orthop* 1978;132:155-162.

19. Muscolo DL, Kawai S, Ray RD: Cellular and humoral immune response analysis of bone-allografted rats. *J Bone Joint Surg* 1976;58A:826-832.

20. Cordrey LJ, McCorkle H, Hilton E: A comparative study of fresh autogenous and preserved homogenous tendon grafts in rabbits. *J Bone Joint Surg* 1963;45B:182-195.

21. Burchardt H, Jones H, Glowczewskie F, et al: Freeze-dried allogeneic segmental cortical-bone grafts in dogs. *J Bone Joint Surg* 1978;60A:1082-1090.

22. Burchardt H, Glowczewskie FP, Enneking WF: Allogeneic segmental fibular transplants in azathioprine-immunosuppressed dogs. *J Bone Joint Surg* 1977;59A:881-884.

23. Amiel D, Kleiner JB, Akeson WH: The natural history of the anterior cruciate ligament autograft of patellar tendon origin. *Am J Sports Med* 1986;14:449-462.

24. Arnoczky SP, Warren RF, Ashlock MA: Replacement of the anterior cruciate ligament using a patellar tendon allograft: An experimental study. *J Bone Joint Surg* 1986;68A:376-385.

25. Minami A, Usui M, Ishii S, et al: The in vivo effects of various immunoreactive treatments on allogeneic tendon grafts. *J Hand Surg* 1983;8:888-893.

26. Potenza AD, Melone C: Evaluation of freeze-dried flexor tendon grafts in the dog. *J Hand Surg* 1978;3:157-162.

27. Drez DJ Jr, DeLee J, Holden JP, et al: Anterior cruciate ligament reconstruction using bone-patellar tendon-bone allografts: A biological and biomechanical evaluation in goats. *Am J Sports Med* 1991;19: 256-263.

28. Jackson DW, Grood ES, Wilcox P, et al: The effects of processing techniques on the mechanical properties of bone-anterior cruciate ligament-bone allografts: An experimental study in goats. *Am J Sports Med* 1988;16:101-105.

29. Clancy WG Jr, Narechania RG, Rosenberg TD, et al: Anterior and posterior cruciate ligament reconstruction in rhesus monkeys: A histological, microangiographic, and biomechanical analysis. *J Bone Joint Surg* 1981;63A:1270-1284.

30. McFarland EG, Morrey BF, An KN, et al: The relationship of vascularity and water content to tensile strength in a patellar tendon replacement of the anterior cruciate in dogs. *Am J Sports Med* 1986;14:436-448.

31. Liu TK: Transplantation of preserved composite tendon allografts: An experimental study in chickens. *J Bone Joint Surg* 1975;57A:65-70.

32. McMaster WC, Kouzelos J, Liddle S, et al: Tendon grafting with glutaraldehyde fixed material. *J Biomed Mater Res* 1976;10:259-271.

33. Cameron RR, Conrad RN, Sell KW, et al: Freeze-dried composite tendon allografts: An experimental study. *Plast Reconstr Surg* 1971;47:39-46.

34. Levitt RL, Malinin T, Michalow A: Serial histologic evaluation of human ACL allograft tissue over a five year period. Presented at the Seventeenth Annual Meeting of the American Orthopaedic Society for Sports Medicine, Orlando, FL, July 1991.

35. Shino K, Inoue M, Nakata K, et al: Laxity measurement following arthroscopic ACL reconstruction: Autograft vs. allograft. Presented at the Seventeenth Annual Meeting of the American Orthopaedic Society for Sports Medicine, Orlando, FL, July 1991.

36. Shino K, Inoue M, Horibe S, et al: Maturation of allograft tendons transplanted into the knee: An arthroscopic and histological study. *J Bone Joint Surg* 1988;70B:556-560.

37. Shino K, Kawasaki T, Hirose H, et al: Replacement of the anterior cruciate ligament by an allogeneic tendon graft: An experimental study in the dog. *J Bone Joint Surg* 1984;66B:672-681.

38. Shino K, Inoue M, Horibe S, et al: Surface blood flow and histology of human anterior cruciate ligament allografts. *Arthroscopy* 1991;7: 171-176.

39. Maeda A, Inoue M, Nakata K, et al: Changes in mechanical properties after solvent preservation and/or gamma irradiation for tendon allografts. *Trans Orthop Res Soc* 1991;16:201.

40. Kirkpatrick JS, Glisson RR, Seaber AV, et al: Biomechanical, histological, and microvascular properties of cryopreserved ACL allografts 9 months post-transplantation. *Trans Orthop Res Soc* 1991;16:183.

41. Turner WD, Vasseur P, Gorek JE, et al: An in vitro study of the structural properties of deep-frozen versus freeze-dried, ethylene oxide-sterilized canine anterior cruciate ligament bone-ligament-bone preparations. *Clin Orthop* 1988;230:251-256.

42. Webster DA, Werner FW: Mechanical and functional properties of implanted freeze-dried flexor tendons. *Clin Orthop* 1983;180:301-309.

43. Barad S, Cabaud HE, Rodrigo JJ: Effects of storage at -80 C as compared to 4 C on the strength of Rhesus monkey anterior cruciate ligaments. *Trans Orthop Res Soc* 1982;7:378.

44. McCarthy JA, Blomstrom G, Shively RL, et al: Maturation of biologic ACL reconstructions: The effect of augmentation over time. *Trans Orthop Res Soc* 1991;16:202.

45. Butler DL, Noyes FR, Grood ES, et al: The effects of vascularity on the mechanical properties of primate anterior cruciate ligament replacements. *Trans Orthop Res Soc* 1983;8:93.

46. Butler DL, Noyes FR, Walz KA, et al: Biomechanics of human knee ligament allograft treatment. *Trans Orthop Res Soc* 1987;12:128.

47. Curtis RJ, DeLee JC, Drez DJ Jr: Reconstruction of the anterior cruciate ligament with freeze dried fascia lata allografts in dogs: A preliminary report. *Am J Sports Med* 1985;13:408-414.

48. Jackson DW, Grood ES, Arnoczky SP, et al: Cruciate reconstruction using freeze dried anterior cruciate ligament allograft and a ligament augmentation device (LAD): An experimental study in a goat model. *Am J Sports Med* 1987;15:528-538.

49. Jackson DW, Grood ES, Arnoczky SP, et al: Freeze dried anterior cruciate ligament allografts: Preliminary studies in a goat model. *Am J Sports Med* 1987;15:295-303.

50. Thorson EP, Rodrigo JJ, Vasseur PB, et al: Comparison of frozen allograft versus fresh autogenous anterior cruciate ligament replacement in the dog. *Trans Orthop Res Soc* 1987;12:65.

51. Vasseur PB, Rodrigo JJ, Stevenson S, et al: Replacement of the anterior cruciate ligament with a bone-ligament-bone anterior cruciate ligament allograft in dogs. *Clin Orthop* 1987;219:268-277.

52. Webster DA, Werner FW: Freeze-dried flexor tendons in anterior cruciate ligament reconstruction. *Clin Orthop* 1983;181:238-243

53. Silvaggio VJ, Fu FH, Georgescu HI, et al: The induction of IL-1 by freeze dried ethylene oxide treated bone-patellar tendon-bone allograft wear particles: An in vitro study. *Trans Orthop Res Soc* 1991;16:207.

54. Graham WC, Smith DA, McGuire MP: The use of frozen stored tendons for grafting: An experimental study. *J Bone Joint Surg* 1955;37A:624.

55. McCarthy JA, Blomstrom G, Steadman JR, et al: Cryopreserved allogenic ACL reconstruction, biomechanics and histology. *Trans Orthop Res Soc* 1991;16:182.

56. Meyers JF: Arthroscopic evaluation of allograft anterior cruciate ligament reconstruction. Presented at the Ninth Annual Meeting of the Arthroscopy Association of North America, Orlando, FL, April 1990.

Chapter 26

Posterior Cruciate Ligament Insufficiency and Reconstruction

Marc T. Galloway, MD
Edward S. Grood, PhD

Introduction

The posterior cruciate ligament (PCL) is a primary stabilizer of the knee and important determinant of normal knee kinematics.[1-12] Despite the ligament's role in normal knee function, the consequences following PCL disruption remain unclear, as does the optimal manner in which to treat patients sustaining these injuries. Poor clinical outcomes observed in patients treated nonoperatively for PCL injury have lead some surgeons to advocate early ligament reconstruction or repair.[13-22] Other studies report acceptable knee function without surgery and recommend nonoperative management of these injuries.[14,23-25] In this chapter, we will review the normal structure and function of the PCL. Moreover, we will examine the reported natural history of PCL injury as well as clinical and biomechanical evaluations following attempts at repair or reconstruction of this ligament.

Anatomy

The PCL develops during the eighth week of gestation and is both longer and wider than the anterior cruciate ligament (ACL).[5,9,26,27] The ligament arises from a semicircular configuration on the distal aspect of the medial wall of the intercondylar notch and inserts onto a rectangular area on the posterior aspect of the tibia (Fig. 1).[5,9,27] With flexion, the PCL becomes oriented along the anteroposterior axis of the knee, allowing it to better resist posterior displacement of the knee in this position.

Though no distinct anatomic divisions are present, the PCL is often described as composed of two functional bands.[5,9,27] The anterior fibers are observed to tighten with knee flexion, whereas the more posterior fibers become taut with knee extension (Fig. 2). An oblique reinforcing band that is present in some knees also becomes taut with knee extension,[5,9,27] and may add to knee stability in this position.

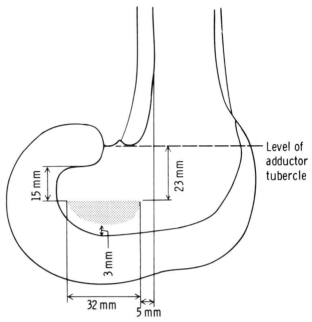

Fig. 1   *Femoral insertion of the posterior cruciate ligament. (Reproduced with permission from Girgis FG, Marshall JL, Al Monajem ARS: The cruciate ligaments of the knee joint: Anatomical, functional and experimental analysis. Clin Orthop 1975;106:216-231.)*

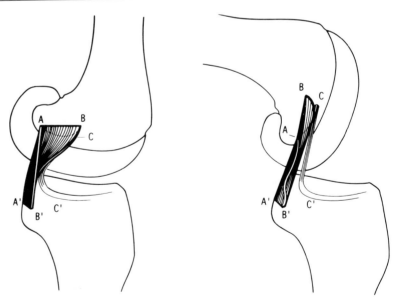

Fig. 2   *Reciprocal function of the PCL fiber bundles. The anterior fibers tense as the knee is flexed. Tension develops in the posterior fibers with progressive knee extension. (Reproduced with permission from Girgis FG, Marshall JL, Al Monajem ARS: The cruciate ligaments of the knee joint: Anatomical, functional and experimental analysis. Clin Orthop 1975;106:216-231.)*

The lateral meniscofemoral ligaments of Humphrey and Wrisberg vary in both their size and incidence. When present, the anterior meniscofemoral ligament of Humphrey can be up to one half the diameter of the PCL.[9] The posterior meniscofemoral ligament of Wrisberg is usually smaller; it extends from either the posterior horn of the lateral meniscus, tibia, or posterior capsule to attach to the femur along with the posteromedial fiber bundle band.[9,27]

Biomechanics

Fiber Length Patterns

The PCL provides knee stability throughout a full range of flexion by behaving as independent fiber bundles that experience relative tension as the knee is flexed.[6,9,28-33] Grood and associates[34] and Sidles and associates[12] used computer modeling of the bony landmarks to calculate the changes in distance that developed between different pairs of attachment points on the femur and tibia. No part of the PCL was totally isometric.[34] In separate studies, they concluded that the femoral attachment site was a more significant factor than the tibial attachment site in determining the resulting length patterns and described maps of isometry on the medial wall of the intercondylar notch. Grood described the most isometric region as a bullet-shaped region that extended in an anteroposterior direction from the intercondylar notch (Fig. 3). This region was 3-mm wide and extended 11 mm along the anteroposterior axis of the knee.[34]

Knee Motion Limits

Many investigators have believed the PCL to be the primary stabilizer of the knee.[3-5] Butler and associates[7] showed that the PCL provides 95% of the restraint to posterotibial translation. Fukubayashi and associates[8] reported a threefold increase in posterotibial translation following PCL transection, which was greatest with the knee flexed 70 and 90 degrees (Fig. 4). In addition, the PCL is responsible for the coupled external tibial rotation that accompanies a posteriorly directed tibial load, resists mediolateral tibial translation, and is an important secondary restraint to external tibial rotation.[8,11,35]

The secondary restraints to posterotibial displacement include the arcuate complex, the posteromedial capsule, and the meniscofemoral ligaments.[7,10,11,34] Posterolateral instability of the knee is increased following PCL disruption (Fig. 5).[11]

Articular Cartilage Contact Pressures

When present, long-term disability following PCL disruption has most often been attributed to ensuing osteoarthritis. The patel-

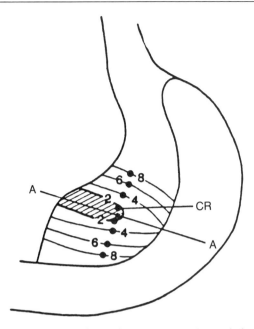

Fig. 3 *Isometry map for femoral attachment sites on the medial wall of the intercondylar notch. The area that produces a 2 mm or less change in tibiofemoral separation distance measures 3 mm x 11 mm and is angled slightly distal to the anteroposterior axis of the knee. (Reproduced with permission from Grood ES, Hefzy MS, Lindenfield TN: Factors affecting the region of most isometric femoral attachments: Part I. The posterior cruciate ligament.* Am J Sports Med *1989;17:197-207.)*

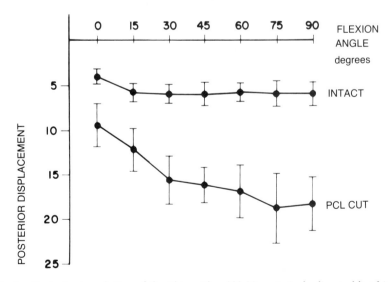

Fig. 4 *Posterior translation of the tibia with a 100-N posteriorly directed load in place following transection of the PCL.*

POSTEROLATERAL STRUCTURES CUT FIRST

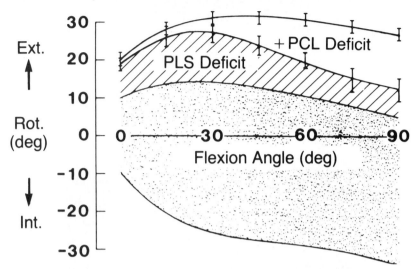

Fig. 5 *Effect of sectioning the posterolateral complex on knee stability after PCL transection. Posterior tibial displacement is greater following injury to the PCL and the posterolateral complex than is noted after isolated PCL disruption. (Reproduced with permission from Grood ES, Stowers SF, Noyes FR: Limits of movement in the human knee: Effect of sectioning the posterior cruciate ligament and posterolateral structures.* J Bone Joint Surg *1988;70A:88-97.)*

lofemoral and medial tibiofemoral compartments are common sites of radiographic change.[17,36] Kennedy and Grainger[17] observed arthritic changes at an average of 61 months in 25 of 57 PCL-deficient knees. Skyhar and associates[37] have confirmed elevated patellofemoral and medial tibiofemoral contact pressures following transection of the PCL in cadaveric knees.

PCL Injury

The incidence of PCL injury has been reported to range from 1% to 30% of knee ligament injuries.[13,14,18,23,24,38,39] Motor vehicle accidents account for over 50% in most series.[39] Sports-related injuries are involved in approximately 45% of PCL disruptions.[39]

Isolated PCL disruption commonly occurs as the result of a blow to the anterior aspect of the flexed knee (Fig. 6).[17,24,25,40] Hyperflexion, hyperextension, and combinations of flexion-abduction-external rotation have also been implicated as potential injury mechanisms.[41,42]

Clinical Findings

Subjective complaints and physical findings following acute disruption of the PCL depend on the mechanism of injury as well as on

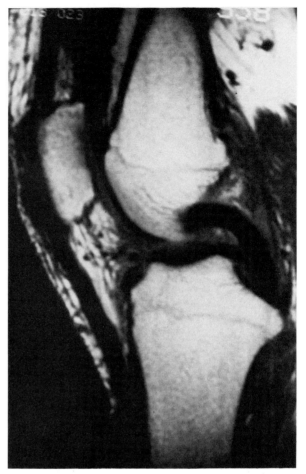

Fig. 6   *Posteriorly directed blow to the flexed knee; a common mechanism of PCL injury. (Reproduced with permission from Kennedy JC, Grainger RW: The posterior cruciate ligament.* J Trauma *1967;7:367-377.)*

the severity of associated ligament disruptions. Sports-related PCL injuries are frequently isolated and may result in little more than transient knee swelling and stiffness. Those injured in motor vehicle accidents most often incur combined ligament injuries (knee dislocations), and their symptoms include swelling, pain, and limited knee motion. In one series, the significance of associated ligamentous injuries was missed in 42% of patients with PCL involvement.[18]

Diagnostic Tests

A variety of clinical maneuvers have been proposed to evaluate the integrity of the PCL.[16,18,43-48] The widely practiced posterior drawer test measures posterotibial translation with the knee in 90 degrees of flexion. Hughston[44] has emphasized the importance of differentiating the posterior translation of the lateral tibial plateau (posterolateral drawer) that is seen in posterolateral rotatory instability from straight posterior translation observed with isolated PCL injury.[47]

Daniel and associates[45] have shown the quadriceps active test to be useful in detecting PCL injuries. They observed anterior translation of the tibia with forceful quadriceps contracture in 41 of 42 patients with confirmed PCL disruptions. The test was not positive in patients with normal or anterior cruciate ligament deficient knees.

Radiographic evaluation can demonstrate avulsion of the PCL tibial origin but may be normal following midsubstance injury. Magnetic resonance imaging (MRI) is useful in detecting PCL disruption.[49] The orientation and size of the PCL within the intercondylar notch make it easily visualized on MRI (Fig. 7). MRI is helpful not only in determining the presence of a lesion but also in characterizing its location and thereby guiding therapy (Fig. 8).

Objective Measurement of Knee Stability

Joint arthrometers and stress radiographs can be used for objective documentation of the degree of posterior or posterolateral instability. Although used primarily for confirmation of anterior cruciate ligament disruption, the KT-1000 arthrometer can detect abnormal tibial displacement following injuries to the PCL.[45] The arthrometer documents the extent of abnormal anterior translation present with the quadriceps active test and characterizes the increase in posterior compliance present in patients with PCL-deficient knees. Daniel and associates[45] have described an average anterotibial shift of 6 mm in chronic PCL-deficient knees and of 4.2 mm following acute PCL injuries.

Stäubli and Jakob[46] have shown that stress radiography is useful in diagnosing PCL and posterolateral complex injuries. Stress radiographs in PCL-deficient knees demonstrated mean posterotibial translation of 10.4 mm, compared with 3.7 mm seen in uninjured knees. In addition, lateral stress radiographs can be used to discern rotational instabilities by detecting differences between the extent of translation of the tibial plateaus.[46]

Natural History

The sequelae of injuries to the PCL are difficult to discern from published reports. Clinical series are frequently composed of heterogeneous patient populations from whom it is difficult to derive conclusions. Often, a converse conclusion can be drawn from the data presented. Reports of the results following surgical reconstruction are usually derived from groups of patients with multiple ligament injuries or use subjective rating criteria that do not allow comparison with other series. To date, the management of PCL injuries

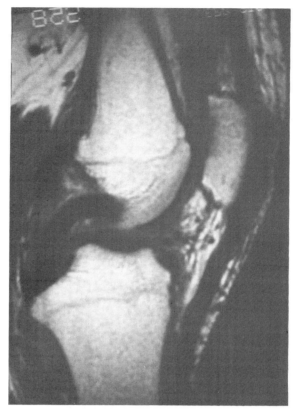

Fig. 7   *Magnetic resonance image demonstrating normal PCL.*

has depended on whether the ligament was avulsed, was an isolated injury, or was combined with other ligamentous disruptions.

PCL Avulsions

Numerous authors have confirmed that although patients with nondisplaced PCL avulsions maintain joint stability with nonoperative management, displaced tibial fragments can lead to nonunion, subsequent instability, and functional compromise.[17,22,42,43,50-54] Trickey[43] described resulting stability in only two of five patients with displaced PCL avulsions and in two of three patients with nondisplaced PCL avulsions. He observed a 100% return of stability in eight patients that underwent repair of the ligament. Others have reported similar findings.[15,50,52-54]

These studies suggest that displaced PCL avulsions and those that involve large bony fragments should be repaired. Nondisplaced or smaller PCL avulsions may be amenable to nonoperative management but must be followed closely, with thought given to repair if instability should develop.

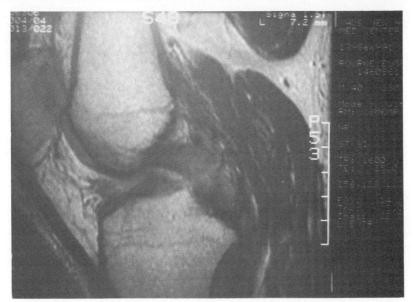

Fig. 8   *Magnetic resonance image demonstrating midsubstance PCL disruption.*

Isolated Midsubstance PCL Injuries

The natural history of isolated PCL disruption is not clear.[14,15,23,25,34,42,43,52] Parolie and Bergfeld[23] reported that 80% of patients managed nonoperatively were satisfied and 68% returned to their previous activity despite a 36% incidence of arthritis. These findings have been echoed by others.[24,25,42] In general, improved function has been correlated with quadriceps strength, leading many to advocate quadriceps rehabilitation as crucial in the nonoperative management of these injuries. Torg and associates[14] reported good functional return in 12 of 14 patients despite radiographic evidence of arthritis in 60% of those treated nonoperatively. Balkfors[55] reported that 10 of 19 patients were able to return to sports after isolated PCL injury.

Conversely, Clancy and associates[13] noted moderate to severe osteoarthritic changes of the patella and medial femoral condyle in 90% of patients examined more than four years after PCL injury; these were present in knees without meniscal injury. Insall and Hood[56] and Kennedy and Galpin[57] have also reported patellar and condylar lesions in chronically PCL-deficient knees. Trickey[16] has concluded that the results of early PCL repair were superior to those following late reconstruction and recommended repair if greater than 1 cm of posterior displacement is present on posterior drawer testing.

At present, it is difficult to predict which patients will remain asymptomatic following PCL injury and which will develop progressive osteoarthritic changes. Patients with isolated PCL injuries that are managed nonoperatively should be followed closely for symptoms related to degenerative arthritis. PCL reconstruction should be considered in those demonstrating findings of arthritis as well as those with a 3 + increase in the posterior drawer test.

Combined Ligamentous Injuries Including the PCL

PCL tears commonly accompany other ligament injuries such as are seen with knee dislocations. An associated tear of the anterior cruciate may exist in 65% of knees with PCL injuries.[18] As with isolated PCL disruptions, no controlled long-term studies exist that examine the natural history of nonoperatively treated knees or the results of surgical management. This, in part, is a consequence of the rarity of these injuries. Moreover, the diversity of combined ligament injuries does not allow for standardized treatment regimens. As a result, the literature reflects primarily anecdotal accounts of the success of various treatment strategies.

Numerous authors have cited improved results with operative management of combined ligament injuries.[17-21] Meyers and associates[22] reported better functional results in patients undergoing ligament repair than in those treated with immobilization; however, no objective results were reported. Hughston and associates[19] observed a good subjective rating in 90% of patients following repair or reconstruction of the PCL using a medial meniscal graft. Persistent objectively measured instability did not correlate with the patients' perception of their results.[19]

Torg and associates[14] noted that 44% of their patients with combined ligament injuries that were treated nonsurgically had good or excellent outcomes. Good to excellent outcomes were seen in 85% of patients with isolated PCL injuries. Patients with multiple ligament injuries that included the PCL were twice as likely to develop patellofemoral chondromalacia as were patients with isolated PCL tears.[14] Conversely, Cross and Powell[25] were unable to distinguish differences in results of surgical and nonsurgical management of combined ligament injuries.

The literature would seem to suggest that combined ligament injuries that include the PCL place the patient at significant risk for permanent instability and progressive arthritic changes. Theoretically, surgical management of these injuries could improve initial knee stability and reduce the period of required immobilization. However, it remains to be determined if primary PCL repair or reconstruction in this setting offers significant benefit over nonsurgical therapy.

Surgical Reconstructions

A wide variety of procedures have been advocated for reconstruction of the PCL-deficient knee.[13,36,56-62] Most authors have reported a high percentage of good to excellent functional and subjective results, although patient follow-up has usually been insufficient to establish the long-term benefits of the procedures. Objective postoperative knee evaluation is commonly omitted in reports of results after surgery, and when included frequently demonstrates persistent instability. The unpredictable outcome following PCL reconstruction has in large part contributed to the hesitancy that many express in recommending these procedures.

The finding of acceptable knee function despite continued objective instability has led many to conclude that the creation of a dynamic support is sufficient for improved knee function.[36,57,60] Others have challenged this concept and have advocated restoration of objective stability as the goal of surgery.[13] Posterior cruciate ligament reconstructions can, therefore, be categorized into those designed to create a dynamic restraint to tibial motion and those that restore static knee stability.

Dynamic Reconstructions

Early attempts to reconstruct the PCL sought to create a dynamic restraint to posterotibial translation.[36,56-62] Hughston and Degenhardt[36] reported functional improvement in 25 of 29 patients following intra-articular transfer of the medial head of the gastrocnemius muscle, despite residual posterior instability in 67%. Insall and Hood[56] modified Hughston's technique by retaining the bony attachment of the gastrocnemius origin and including it in the transfer. Objective stability was improved in all patients but never was returned to normal. Kennedy and Galpin[57] noted similar results with 80% demonstrating good and excellent functional results despite residual objective instability in all patients. Tibone and associates[63] observed marked posterior instability in patients having undergone medial gastrocnemius transfer. Gait analysis demonstrated increased knee flexion during midstance phase of the gait cycle in both the PCL-deficient and reconstructed groups.

Roth and associates[60] retrospectively analyzed their results in 31 patients followed for an average of 53 months after medial gastrocnemius tendon transfer for symptomatic chronic PCL insufficiency. They compared the outcomes of the surgically managed groups with those of patients managed nonsurgically. Although subjective improvement was observed in 69% of patients, 91% had painful knees and 59% experienced continued instability. In addition, no significant change in anteroposterior translation was evident on KT-1000 evaluation, and isokinetic strength profiles were better in the control group. Many patients in the surgically treated group described deteriorating knee function with time.[60]

Static Reconstructions

Reconstructions designed to restore static restraint to the PCL-deficient knee are more physiologic in their design. Initial efforts to restore knee stability were described by Hey Groves,[1] who used intra-articular transfer of the semitendinosus for PCL reconstruction. He later modified his technique to include both semitendinosus and gracilis, which he left intact distally and attached to the medial tibial plateau/capsule after routing them through the femur.[1] Gallie and LeMesurier[61] and Lipscomb and associates[64] have reported good results using this technique.

Campbell[65] described PCL reconstruction using a distally attached strip of patella tendon and parapatella retinaculum that he passed through drill holes in the femur and tibia. Eriksson and associates[66] reported no excellent, six acceptable, and four unchanged results with this technique. Clancy and associates[13] have modified this technique by including the bony attachments from the tibia and patella. The inclusion of bone blocks improved the initial stability of the construct, and they observed good to excellent subjective and objective results in 21 of 23 patients who were followed for at least two years.[13] A higher percentage of improved stability was observed in patients with acute PCL injuries.

Tillberg[67] used the medial or lateral meniscus to reconstruct the PCL in 43 patients with chronic disability secondary to PCL deficiency. Follow-up evaluation ranged from one to 30 years. Forty-one patients returned to work and all had pain-free joints. The posterior drawer sign was 5 mm or less in 43 of these 45 knees. Tillberg considered this technique effective in the management of chronic PCL insufficiency.[67]

Experimental Models of PCL Reconstruction

Restoration of the normal limitation to posterior translation of the tibia following PCL reconstruction has proven to be a challenge. Persistent posterior tibial drop back following PCL reconstruction could represent either an intrinsic inadequacy of the procedure or, possibly, postsurgical changes in the mechanical properties of the substitute. The clinical implications of mild to moderate instability following reconstruction, as well as the ability of PCL reconstruction to prevent the type of degenerative joint changes observed following ligament transection in animal models[68,69] remain to be determined. To date, few studies have been performed that address these issues.

Noguchi[70] performed PCL reconstructions in rabbits using the medial meniscus as a graft. Incomplete incorporation of the grafts was observed at two years after surgery. In addition, the mechanical strength of the transferred menisci was only 26% of that of the PCL. Noguchi[70] concluded that the meniscus was not an appropriate substitute for use in PCL reconstruction. Mitsou and associates[71] also described findings using this animal model.

Clancy and associates[72] performed PCL reconstructions in Rhesus monkeys, using the medial one third of the patella tendon. The histologic, vascular, and biomechanical properties of the substitute were determined at three, six, nine, and 12 months. They reported complete revascularization at eight weeks and a return to 71% of the tensile strength of the implanted structure at one year. Histologically, the reconstructed ligament remained hypercellular at one year. Mature collagen bundles were noted to be present at this time. Objective knee stability testing demonstrated differences of less than 1 mm between tibial translation of reconstructed and control knees.

Factors important to successful cruciate ligament reconstruction include substitute strength, initial graft fixation technique, attachment site location, and the position of the limb at graft fixation.[73,74] Clancy and associates[72] emphasized the importance of an "off-center" placement of the femoral and tibial tunnels. They contend that this placement allows the substitute to remain under tension throughout a full range of knee motion. Conversely, Daluga and associates[75] advocated isometric placement of PCL substitutes in order to obtain a "more predictable reconstruction." Bomberg and associates[76] evaluated knee stability following in vitro PCL reconstruction. They reported that placing the femoral tunnel slightly anterior to the femoral isometric point produced the most "satisfactory" reconstruction, resulting in a nearly normal strain pattern in the knee.

We measured resulting tibial displacement patterns in six cadaveric limbs following PCL reconstructions using a flexible wire substitute.[77] With the wire through the center of the tibial origin, a spring-loaded tensiometer was used to identify an isometric position. The magnitude of posterior tibial displacement was then determined after reconstructions that were performed by placing the wire through the femoral isometric position and through points 3 mm anterior, posterior, proximal, and distal to the isometric position.

Marked variations in tibial displacement resulted from small alterations in attachment-site location. Significant changes occurred in the magnitudes and patterns of displacement when the femoral position was changed in the proximodistal direction (Fig. 9). Varying the femoral attachment site in the anteroposterior direction produced less dramatic motion pattern changes. Isometric substitute placement (central femoral location) produced displacement patterns characterized by overconstraint in extension and greater than normal displacement with progressive flexion. The most normal displacement patterns resulted when the reconstruction was placed 4 mm distal to the measured most isometric point. These findings validate previous studies that demonstrated the sensitivity of PCL-length patterns to femoral attachment site location.[12,34,75,76]

We next examined tibial motion patterns following biologic reconstructions in which 11-mm Achilles tendon grafts were used in 12 cadaveric whole lower limbs.[78,79] The effects of femoral placement and of knee flexion angle at the time of graft fixation were assessed using a six-degree-of-freedom instrumented spatial linkage. Reconstructions were performed through 11-mm bony tunnels

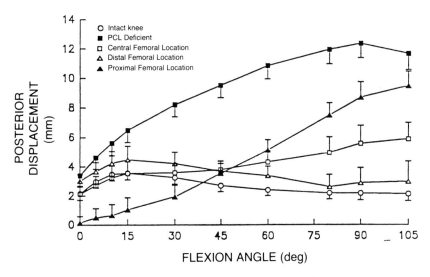

Fig. 9 *The effect of proximodistal variation of the femoral attachment site on posterior tibial displacement following PCL reconstruction using a 1.5-mm wire cable. (Mean ± SEM, n = 12 intact, n = 12 PCL cut, n = 6 femoral attachments.)*

that were centered on the PCL tibial origin in all limbs. The femoral attachment site was centered on an isometric position in six limbs and was placed at a position that produced a 4-mm length increase with knee flexion from 0 to 90 degrees in the others. Pistoning of the Achilles tendon graft in the tunnel was observed prior to fixation in all of the nonisometrically reconstructed knees. The graft was fixed using a 9-mm interference fit screw in the femur and a 15-mm soft-tissue washer and bicortical screw in the tibial side. A 100-N anteriorly directed load was applied to the tibia during graft fixation to ensure tibiofemoral reduction. Knees were tested with a 100-N posteriorly directed load in place. In addition, reconstructions were performed at 0, 30, and 90 degrees of knee flexion for each specimen to determine if the knee position at fixation, the tension angle, contributed to the magnitude of observed tibial displacement.

As was observed in the wire substitute model, a nonisometric graft placement resulted in a pattern of tibial displacement that more closely approximated that of the intact knee (Fig. 10). Isometric PCL reconstructions produced tibial displacement patterns that were characterized by overconstraint in the extended knee and excessive posterior translation in higher angles of knee flexion. The knee tension angle did not influence tibial displacement in the isometrically reconstructed knee, however significant differences in tibial displacement were produced by altering the tension in reconstructions using nonisometric graft placement (Fig. 11).

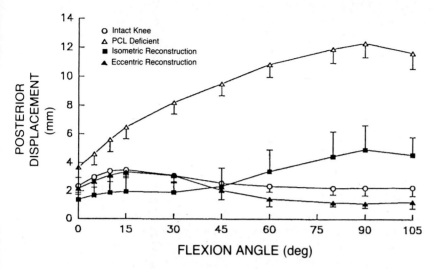

Fig. 10   *The effect of femoral attachment site on resulting tibial displacement following PCL reconstructions using an 11-mm Achilles tendon graft. (Mean ± SEM, n = 12 intact, n = 12 PCL cut, n = 6 isometric reconstruction, n = 6 eccentric reconstruction.)*

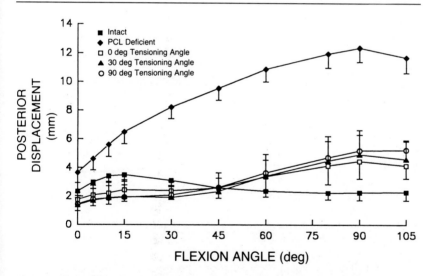

Fig. 11   *The effect of varying knee position during graft fixation in knee reconstructed with an isometrically placed 11-mm Achilles tendon. (Mean ± SEM, n = 12 intact, n = 12 PCL cut, n = 6 reconstruction.)*

These results suggest that an appropriate nonisometric PCL reconstruction results in a more physiologic pattern of knee motion than one in which the graft is placed isometrically. In particular, improved stability in higher angles of knee flexion was observed using this technique. However, further work is required before we advocate the use of this technique.

Summary

The PCL is the primary restraint to posterotibial translation at all angles of knee flexion. The ligament is not isometric but exists as two functional bands that undergo reciprocal length changes as the knee is flexed. Isolated PCL injuries are well tolerated by some patients while other patients will demonstrate progressive osteoarthritic changes. It is not clear which individuals are at risk. Combined ligament injuries may more adversely affect knee function.

Objective knee stability has been difficult to achieve following PCL reconstruction. The variable prognosis of patients with isolated PCL injuries combined with the uncertain outcome of reconstruction has made surgical management of these injuries controversial. Surgical reconstructions using the central one third of the patella tendon have been shown to improve objective knee stability. Centering PCL reconstructions on nonisometric positions may further improve these results.

References

1. Hey Groves EW: The cruciate ligaments of the knee-joint: Their function, rupture, and the operative treatment of the same. *Brit J Surg* 1920;7:505-515.
2. Palmer I: On the injuries to the ligaments of the knee joint: A clinical study. *Acta Chir Scand* 1938;81(suppl 53).
3. Cubbins WR, Callahan JJ, Scuderi CS: Cruciate ligaments: A resume of operative attacks and results obtained. *Am J Surg* 1939;43:481-485.
4. Abbott LC, Saunders JBDeCM, Bost FC, et al: Injuries to the ligaments of the knee joint. *J Bone Joint Surg* 1944;26A:503-521.
5. Girgis FG, Marshall JL, Al Monajem ARS: The cruciate ligaments of the knee joint: Anatomical, functional and experimental analysis. *Clin Orthop* 1975;106:216-231.
6. Trent S, Walker PS, Wolf B: Ligament length patterns, strength, and rotational axes of the knee joint. *Clin Orthop* 1976;117:263-270.
7. Butler DL, Noyes FR, Grood ES: Ligamentous restraints to anterior-posterior drawer in the human knee: A biomechanical study. *J Bone Joint Surg* 1980;62A:259-270.
8. Fukubayashi T, Torzilli PA, Sherman MF, et al: An *in vitro* biomechanical evaluation of anterior-posterior motion of the knee: Tibial displacement, rotation, and torque. *J Bone Joint Surg* 1982;64A:258-264.
9. Van Dijk R: The behavior of the cruciate ligaments in the human knee, dissertation. Rodopi, Amsterdam, Department of Orthopaedic Surgery, Catholic University, Nijmegin, The Netherlands, 1983.
10. Gollehon DL, Torzilli PA, Warren RF: The role of the posterolateral and cruciate ligaments in the stability of the human knee: A biomechanical study. *J Bone Joint Surg* 1987;69A:233-242.
11. Grood ES, Stowers SF, Noyes FR: Limits of movement in the human knee: Effect of sectioning the posterior cruciate ligament and posterolateral structures. *J Bone Joint Surg* 1988;70A:88-97.

12. Sidles JA, Larsen RV, Garbini JL, et al: Ligament length relationships in the moving knee. *J Orthop Res* 1988;6:593-610.

13. Clancy WG Jr, Shelbourne KD, Zoellner GB, et al: Treatment of knee joint instability secondary to rupture of the posterior cruciate ligament: Report of a new procedure. *J Bone Joint Surg* 1983;65A:310-322.

14. Torg JS, Barton TM, Pavlov H, et al: Natural history of the posterior cruciate ligament-deficient knee. *Clin Orthop* 1989;246:208-216.

15. Satku K, Chew CN, Seow H: Posterior cruciate ligament injuries. *Acta Orthop Scand* 1984;55:26-29.

16. Trickey EL: Injuries to the posterior cruciate ligament: Diagnosis and treatment of early injuries and reconstruction of late instability. *Clin Orthop* 1980;147:76-81.

17. Kennedy JC, Grainger RW: The posterior cruciate ligament. *J Trauma* 1967;7:367-377.

18. Loos WC, Fox JM, Blazina ME, et al: Acute posterior cruciate ligament injuries. *Am J Sports Med* 1981;9:86-92.

19. Hughston JC, Bowden JA, Andrews JR, et al: Acute tears of the posterior cruciate ligament: Results of operative treatment. *J Bone Joint Surg* 1980;62A:438-450.

20. Fleming RE Jr, Blatz DJ, McCarroll JR: Posterior problems in the knee: Posterior cruciate insufficiency and posterolateral rotatory insufficiency. *Am J Sports Med* 1981;9:107-113.

21. Moore HA, Larson RL: Posterior cruciate ligament injuries: Results of early surgical repair. *Am J Sports Med* 1980;8:68-78.

22. Meyers MH, Moore TM, Harvey JP Jr: Traumatic dislocation of the knee joint. *J Bone Joint Surg* 1975;57A:430-433.

23. Parolie JM, Bergfeld JA: Long-term results of nonoperative treatment of isolated posterior cruciate ligament injuries in the athlete. *Am J Sports Med* 1986;14:35-38.

24. Dandy DJ, Pusey RJ: The long-term results of unrepaired tears of the posterior cruciate ligament. *J Bone Joint Surg* 1982;64B:92-94.

25. Cross MJ, Powell JF: Long-term followup of posterior cruciate ligament rupture: A study of 116 cases. *Am J Sports Med* 1984;12:292-297.

26. Gray DJ, Gardner E: Prenatal development of the human knee and superior tibiofibular joints. *Am J Anat* 1950;86:235-287.

27. Van Dommelen BA, Fowler PJ: Anatomy of the posterior cruciate ligament: A review. *Am J Sports Med* 1989;17:24-29.

28. Kennedy JC, Hawkins RJ, Willis RB: Strain gauge analysis of knee ligament. *Clin Orthop* 1977;129:225-229.

29. Ahmed AM, Hyder A, Burke DL, et al: In-vitro ligament tension pattern in the flexed knee in passive loading. *J Orthop Res* 1987;5:217-230.

30. Dorlot J-M, Christel P, Sedel L, et al: The displacement of the bony insertion sites of the cruciate ligaments during the flexion of the knee. *Trans Orthop Res Soc* 1983;8:328.

31. Edwards RG, Lafferty JF, Lange KO: Ligament strain in the human knee. *J Basic Eng* 1970;92:131-136.

32. Arms SW, Pope MH, Johnson RJ, et al: The biomechanics of anterior cruciate ligament rehabilitation and reconstruction. *Am J Sports Med* 1984;12:8-18.

33. Crowninshield R, Pope MH, Johnson RJ: An analytical model of the knee. *J Biomech* 1976;9:397-405.

34. Grood ES, Hefzy MS, Lindenfield TN: Factors affecting the region of most isometric femoral attachments: Part I. The posterior cruciate ligament. *Am J Sports Med* 1989;17:197-207.

35. Piziali RL, Rastegar JC, Nagel DA: Measurement of the nonlinear, coupled stiffness characteristics of the human knee. *J Biomech* 1977;10:45-51.

36. Hughston JC, Degenhardt TC: Reconstruction of the posterior cruciate ligament. *Clin Orthop* 1982;164:59-77.

37. Skyhar MJ, Schwartz E, Warren RF, et al: The effects of posterior cruciate ligament and posterolateral complex laxity on articular contact pressures within the knee. Presented at the 56th Annual Meeting of the American Academy of Orthopaedic Surgeons, Las Vegas, NV, February 9-14, 1989.

38. O'Donoghue DH: Surgical treatment of fresh injuries to the major ligaments of the knee. *J Bone Joint Surg* 1950;32A:721-738.

39. Barton TM, Torg JS, Das M: Posterior cruciate ligament insufficiency: A review of the literature. *Sports Med* 1984;1:419-430.

40. Main WK, Scott WN: Posterior cruciate ligament insufficiency, in Scott WN (ed): *Ligament and Extensor Mechanism Injuries of the Knee.* St. Louis, Mosby Year Book, 1991, pp 361-372.

41. Clendenin MB, Delee JC, Heckman JD: Interstitial tears of the posterior cruciate ligament of the knee. *Orthopedics* 1980;3:764-772.

42. Fowler PJ, Messieh SS: Isolated posterior cruciate ligament injuries in athletes. *Am J Sports Med* 1987;15:553-557.

43. Trickey EL: Rupture of the posterior cruciate ligament of the knee. *J Bone Joint Surg* 1968;50B:334-341.

44. Hughston JC: The absent posterior drawer test in some acute posterior cruciate ligament tears of the knee. *Am J Sports Med* 1988;16:39-43.

45. Daniel DM, Stone ML, Barnett P, et al: Use of the quadriceps active test to diagnose posterior cruciate-ligament disruption and measure posterior laxity of the knee. *J Bone Joint Surg* 1988;70A:386-391.

46. Stäubli HU, Jakob RP: Posterior instability of the knee near extension: A clinical and stress radiographic analysis of acute injuries of the posterior cruciate ligament. *J Bone Joint Surg* 1990;72B:225-230.

47. Hughston JC, Norwood LA Jr: The posterolateral drawer test and external rotational recurvatum test for posterolateral rotatory instability of the knee. *Clin Orthop*1980;147:82-87.

48. Shelbourne KD, Benedict F, McCarroll JR, et al: Dynamic posterior shift test: An adjuvant in evaluation of posterior tibial subluxation. *Am J Sports Med* 1989;17:275-277.

49. Hughston JC, Andrews JR, Cross MJ, et al: Classification of knee ligament instabilities: Part I. The medial compartment and cruciate ligaments. *J Bone Joint Surg* 1976;58A:159-172.

50. Mandelbaum BR, Finerman GAM, Reicher MA, et al: Magnetic resonance imaging as a tool for evaluation of traumatic knee injuries: Anatomical and pathoanatomical correlations. *Am J Sports Med* 1986;14:361-370.

51. Meyers MH: Isolated avulsion of the tibial attachment of the posterior cruciate ligament of the knee. *J Bone Joint Surg* 1975;57A:669-672.

52. Torisu T: Isolated avulsion fracture of the tibial attachment of the posterior cruciate ligament. *J Bone Joint Surg* 1977;59A:68-72.

53. Torisu T: Avulsion fracture of the tibial attachment of the posterior cruciate ligament: Indications and results of delayed repair. *Clin Orthop* 1979;143:107-114.

54. Lee HG: Avulsion fracture of the tibial attachments of the crucial ligaments: Treatment by operative reduction. *J Bone Joint Surg* 1937;19A:460-468.

55. Balkfors B: The course of knee ligament injuries. *Acta Orthop Scand Suppl* 1982;198:1-99.

56. Insall JN, Hood RW: Bone-block transfer of the medial head of the gastrocnemius for posterior cruciate insufficiency. *J Bone Joint Surg* 1982;64A:691-699.

57. Kennedy JC, Galpin RD: The use of the medial head of the gastrocnemius muscle in the posterior cruciate-deficient knee: Indications—technique—results. *Am J Sports Med* 1982;10:63-74.

58. Bianchi M: Acute tears of the posterior cruciate ligament: Clinical study and results of operative treatment in 27 cases. *Am J Sports Med* 1983;11:308-314.

59. McCormick WC, Bagg RJ, Kennedy CW Jr, et al: Reconstruction of the posterior cruciate ligament: Preliminary report of a new procedure. *Clin Orthop* 1976;118:30-34.

60. Roth JH, Bray RC, Best TM, et al: Posterior cruciate ligament reconstruction by transfer of the medial gastrocnemuius tendon. *Am J Sports Med* 1988;16:21-28.

61. Gallie WE, LeMesurier AB: The repair of injuries to the posterior crucial ligament of the knee-joint. *Ann Surg* 1927;85:592-598.

62. Wirth CJ, Jager M: Dynamic double tendon replacement of the posterior cruciate ligament. *Am J Sports Med* 1984;12:39-43.

63. Tibone JE, Antich TJ, Perry J, et al: Functional analysis of untreated and reconstructed posterior cruciate ligament injuries. *Am J Sports Med* 1988;16:217-223.

64. Lipscomb AB, Johnston RK, Snyder RB: The technique of cruciate ligament reconstruction. *Am J Sports Med* 1981;9:77-81.

65. Campbell WC: Reconstruction of the ligaments of the knee. *Am J Surg* 1939;43:473-480.

66. Eriksson E, Haggmark T, Johnson RJ: Reconstruction of the posterior cruciate ligament. *Orthopedics* 1986;9:217-220.

67. Tillberg B: The late repair of torn cruciate ligaments using menisci. *J Bone Joint Surg* 1977;59B:15-19.

68. Pournaras J, Symeonides PP, Karkavelas G: The significance of the posterior cruciate ligament in the stability of the knee: An experimental study in dogs. *J Bone Joint Surg* 1983;65B:204-209.

69. Davis W, Moskowitz RW: Degenerative joint changes following posterior cruciate ligament section in the rabbit. *Clin Orthop* 1973;93:307-312.

70. Noguchi T: An experimental study on reconstruction of the posterior cruciate ligament using the medial meniscus. *Tokyo J Exp Clin Med* 1989;14:87-102.

71. Mitsou A, Vallianatos P, Piskopakis N, et al: Cruciate ligament replacement using a meniscus. *J Bone Joint Surg* 1988;70B:784-786.

72. Clancy WG Jr, Narechania RG, Rosenberg TD, et al: Anterior and posterior cruciate ligament reconstruction in Rhesus monkeys. *J Bone Joint Surg* 1981;63A:1270-1284.

73. Arnoczky SP: Basic science of anterior cruciate ligament repair and reconstruction, in Tullos HE (ed): American Academy of Orthopaedic Surgeons *Instructional Course Lectures, XL.* Park Ridge, IL, American Academy of Orthopaedic Surgeons, 1991, pp 201-212.

74. Bylski-Austrow DI, Grood ES, Hefzy MS, et al: Anterior cruciate ligament replacements: A mechanical study of femoral attachment location, flexion angle at tensioning, and initial tension. *J Orthop Res* 1990;8:522-531.

75. Daluga DJ, Bach BR Jr, Mikosz R, et al: Force displacement characteristics of the posterior cruciate ligament (PCL) with alterations of the femoral and tibial insertion sites. *Am J Sports Med* 1990;18:551.

76. Bomberg BC, Acker JH, Boyle J, et al: The effect of posterior cruciate ligament loss and reconstruction on the knee. *Am J Knee Surg* 1990;3:85-96.

77. Grood ES, Mehalik JN, Galloway MT, et al: Posterior cruciate ligament reconstruction: The effect of femoral attachment site on posterior translation. Presented at the European Orthopaedic Research Society Meeting, Paris, 1991.

78. Galloway MT, Mehalik JN, Grood ES, et al: Posterior tibial translation following PCL reconstruction: The effect of knee position at graft fixation. Presented at the American Orthopaedic Society for Sports Medicine, San Diego, CA, 1992.

79. Galloway MT, Mehalik JN, Grood ES, et al: Posterior tibial translation following PCL reconstruction, in *Transactions of the Combined Meeting of the Orthopaedic Research Societies, U.S.A., Japan, and Canada*. Banff, Canada, Organizing Committee of the Orthopaedic Research Societies, 1991, p 263.

Chapter 27

Artificial Ligaments

Jan Gillquist, MD, PhD

Introduction

Artificial ligaments are commonly used in anterior cruciate ligament (ACL) replacement, and may be indicated for use in replacing other ligaments as well. Injuries to the posterior cruciate ligament are often more complex, resulting in dependence on reconstructing surrounding structures.

Because almost all available information discusses replacement of the ACL, this chapter will be limited to that topic. The principles for artificial ligament design and the results with the presently available ligaments will be reviewed.

Basic Principles for Ligament Design

Augmentation Devices

Augmentation devices are intended to act as temporary supports for autologous tissue. The theory is that the strength of autologous tissue should increase while the augmentation protects it from overload.[1] Eventually, the autologous structure or the composite should take over the function completely. Presently, only one ligament augmentation device (LAD), the Kennedy LAD (3-M Co., St. Paul, MN), has been accepted for clinical use by the United States Food and Drug Administration (FDA), but other companies are working in the same area. Results of experimental studies have shown that augmentation provides stress shielding of the autologous structure.[2,3] Mäkisalo[4] also reported the presence of eosinophilia near intact LADs that may be a sign of an allergic reaction, which is believed to be caused by the material itself and not necessarily by wear particles. It seems that the theoretical principle of successive load transfer to the autologous tissue, although appealing, is not easily achieved. Because the augmentation devices are supposed to effect 100% host tissue, they are not discussed further.

Scaffolds

Scaffolds are designed to provide a basic structure into which collagen is supposed to grow and eventually become transformed into a neoligament under the influence of load and motion. Basically, allografts and autologous transplants function as scaffolds because the transferred tissue undergoes a cycle of necrosis and revascularization with cellular ingrowth.[5-7] Xenografts are also supposed to be scaffolds. Because they have been associated with high failure rates and severe joint reactions, xenografts are now obsolete.[8] Carbon fiber ligaments are also supposed to induce collagen ingrowth and form a neoligament. It has recently been shown that this neoligament consists of scar tissue of poor quality. Carbon ligaments are no longer used because clinical results have been insufficient,[9,10] and the ligaments were not accepted for clinical use by the FDA.

The Leeds-Keio Dacron ligament is also based on the scaffold principle. The inventors have claimed that ligament strength increases in proportion to collagen ingrowth. The special fixation to bone may facilitate bony ingrowth.[11] Clinical studies to date have not determined the value of this device. A Dacron tube (Stryker/Meadox coracoacromial cerclage) has been used as a scaffold by a few clinicians in Europe but no clinical studies are available. The Ligastic is a French device also based on the scaffold principle.[12] Clinical studies are ongoing, and no results are available to date.

Ingrowth Ligaments

The ingrowth ligaments induce collagen ingrowth into the ligament structure. This ingrowth may provide some ligament protection, but provides no strength, which comes totally from the artificial material. The Stryker/Meadox Dacron ligament allows ingrowth into the outer sheath of the ligament, but the central core, which provides ligament strength, is too dense for ingrowth (Fig. 1).[13] The effect of ingrowth in these ligaments is unknown, and the ligaments depend entirely on the artificial structure for their mechanical integrity. Other ligaments that are similar to the Stryker/Meadox Dacron prosthesis may also induce some collagen ingrowth (Protek: Proflex; Telos: Trevira Hochfest).

Noningrowth Ligaments

Other prostheses do not induce collagen ingrowth and remain the same from implantation to failure; there is no covering of scar tissue. Of the products now on the market, only the Gore-Tex ligament fits this description.[14] The Smith and Nephew Richards polyethyl-

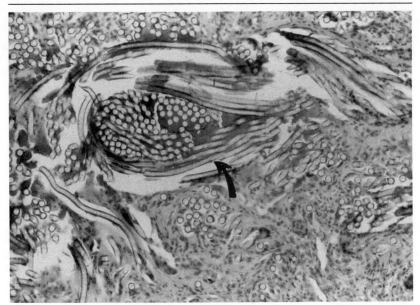

Fig. 1 *Ingrowth of scar tissue into the outer sheath of a Stryker/Meadox Dacron ligament. The central tapes (arrow) are too dense to allow any ingrowth.*

ene ligament, which is presently under clinical investigation, is another such prosthesis.[15]

Artificial Ligament Studies

Patients

In the United States, artificial ligaments have been used in preclinical trials under FDA control and clinically for salvage cases only. The most likely candidates for a salvage operation are usually 5 to 10 years older than patients with acute injuries of the ACL, and the knees of these candidates have been subjected to previous surgery and secondary injuries. Previous meniscectomy is common, and the cartilage surfaces are fractured or degenerated. Secondary restraints may have stretched out. In these patients, complex injuries to associated structures are also more common.[16]

In Europe, artificial ligaments have been used with more liberal indications in young patients with first-time reconstructions. The knees of these patients are usually in better condition; therefore, better results can be expected. The experiences in the United States and Europe may be different; however, one common characteristic is that patients with torn ACLs usually are very active in sports. A high activity level after surgery may increase the failure rate for an artificial ligament.

Evaluation Techniques

The evaluation of clinical results in ACL surgery has not been standardized. However, most clinical studies involving artificial ligaments have had similar evaluation criteria, and these studies can be carefully compared. It is important to remember that the characteristics of the patients are of the greatest importance in analyzing results. Important areas of evaluation are anteroposterior displacement, functional stability, activity, knee function, complications, and rupture rates.

Results

Stryker/Meadox Ligament   Results of a study of the Stryker/Meadox Dacron prosthesis in 70 cases included a 23% rupture rate in five years.[17] Stability was gradually lost and at five years, 55% of the initial group of patients had a 3 mm or less increase in anteroposterior displacement of the tibia at a 90-N load, satisfactory subjective knee function, and the desired activity level. Short-term follow-up (two years) results with this ligament have indicated significant improvement in knee function and stability in salvage cases.[18] Recently, López-Vázquez and associates[19] presented results from a two- to five-year follow-up study on 54 patients in whom the ACL had been reconstructed with a Stryker/Meadox ligament. This study demonstrates the catastrophic results that can be obtained with an artificial ligament if all other instabilities except that of the ACL are disregarded. According to the study by Gillquist and Odensten,[17] a patient with a badly placed ligament and nonrepaired medial instability had a 100% chance of failure within the first three years. In López-Vázquez and associates'[19] study, there was a failure rate of 48%; half of these were at the femoral insertion. There was also a 4% rate of infection (2/54); this rate is high for knee-ligament reconstructions.

Gore-Tex Ligament   Results with the Gore-Tex prosthesis have been presented after two and five years of follow-up.[20-22] Rupture rate and stability evaluated manually seem to be similar to those obtained with the Stryker/Meadox prosthesis.

Comparisons With Other Techniques   Allograft results have been presented by Noyes and associates.[23] In similar patients there seems to be no dramatic difference between their results and those obtained with the Stryker/Meadox Dacron ligament. Results are available of a five-year follow-up evaluation of patellar tendon reconstructions.[24] Generally, the results are very similar to those after prosthetic reconstruction except for a lower rupture rate; the number of unsatisfactory results seems to be the same. Zarins and

Rowe[25] published results of a more than three-year follow-up study of ACL reconstruction using the semitendinosus tendon and iliotibial tract. A critical review of the results reveals no significant differences from results reported for prosthetic reconstruction.

Summary of Results

The results obtained with artificial or other ACL reconstructions in general are not satisfactory. It is surprising that reconstructions, whether artificial or autologous, actually can survive and function rather well in a significant group of patients despite the complex mechanical and functional requirements of a knee ligament. Therefore, research should concentrate on the general problem of obtaining normal knee function after injury to major ligaments. This problem involves both surgical technique and materials.

Special Problems With Artificial Ligaments

Ingrowth

Presently, it is not known whether a prosthesis without collagen ingrowth or an ingrowth scaffold is preferable. In most artificial reconstructions with ingrowth, the tissue is of inferior quality with too little strength for normal use. Type III collagen is usually the main constituent of the neoligament[26,27] as opposed to the normal ACL, which is composed predominantly of type I collagen. The neoligament is usually characterized as scar tissue with inferior mechanical function.[13,28] One possible function of the scar tissue has not been investigated; it may offer some protection from abrasion and may diminish the shedding of particles into the joint cavity.

Ingrowth at the anchoring sites is another problem. It is usually very limited and parallels the intra-articular ingrowth.[28] Most artificial ligaments rely permanently on their anchoring devices (staples or screws). If the fixation devices are removed, it is usually possible to pull the ligament out by hand. The Leeds-Keio ligament has a special fixation technique. The loosely woven, tubular, Dacron ligament is fixed with an internal bone plug cut to fit the tunnel exactly. Ingrowth of bone into the ligament has been studied.[11] Clinically, the load to failure of this fixation is not known but the technique is theoretically appealing.

Debris Formation

The wear of the artificial structure produces particles. The size of the particles varies with the type of artificial material and influences the joint reaction.[29]

Synovitis

The most common type of reaction is synovitis with joint swelling, whether it is induced by pathologic motion, by particles from the ligament, or from the cartilage. This problem can have several clinical manifestations. The detailed mechanisms and preventive measures need to be researched further.

Stage 1 Synovitis The first manifestation is a subclinical type of synovitis that can be seen at arthroscopy and in synovial biopsies. The joint is not swollen but sometimes a thickened synovium can be felt. The patient experiences diffuse pain and stiffness during and after physical activity, and occasionally there is a trace of effusion. Arthroscopy usually reveals a thick, red, and irritated synovium in the center of the joint and in the posterior compartments. Synovial biopsies reveal mild or moderate chronic synovitis with or without visible foreign particles, depending on the type of artificial material. Particles within the synovium sometimes do not produce an inflammatory response.

Stage 2 Synovitis The patient experiences sudden, severe joint swelling associated with physical activity. The level of activity that provokes symptoms can vary from heavy sports activity to a one-day shopping tour in the city. The symptoms are usually infrequent and there may be months or a year between episodes. If there is frequent recurrence of synovitis symptoms, removal of the ligament may be considered.

Stage 3 Synovitis The final type of synovitis results in permanent swelling that usually starts during the rehabilitation period and continues through the first years after the artificial ligament is in place. In some cases, the swelling may eventually disappear but the patient usually requests treatment before that occurs. Microscopy reveals a severe foreign body reaction with giant cells (Fig. 2).

For stage 1 synovitis, nonsteroidal anti-inflammatory drugs (NSAIDs) may be used initially if the symptoms are pronounced. The preferred initial treatment for stages 2 and 3 is aspiration of the joint with analysis for particles and bacteria (aerobic and anaerobic cultures). The erythrocyte sedimentation rate is usually normal. The use of NSAIDs usually is more effective for pain relief than for decreasing the swelling. Recurrent or persistent problems are treated by arthroscopic lavage and synovectomy. In many cases this leads to at least an improvement in joint function. Should the condition become permanent, there is no alternative but to remove the ligament. This usually leads to resolution of the inflammatory symptoms.

The cause of the synovitis is not clear. There is a correlation to wear and fragmentation of the artificial ligament but complete ruptures can occur without any synovitis, even if synovial biopsies show a large number of particles.[29] The frequency of synovitis var-

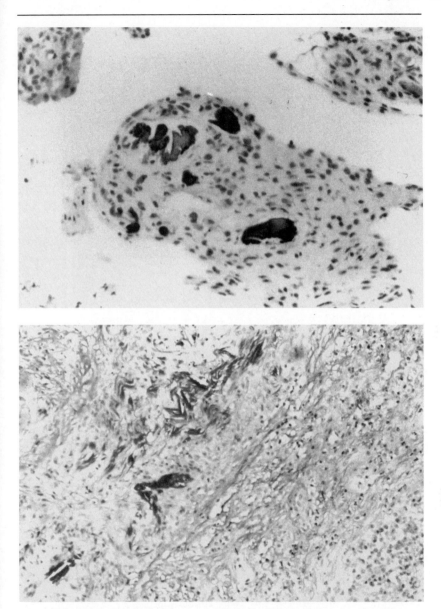

Fig. 2 *Top, Moderate synovitis with foreign particles.* **Bottom**, *Severe chronic synovitis with foreign body giant cells and fragments of xenograft.*

ies with different artificial materials and with the surgical technique. Susceptibility also seems to be different in each patient. Synovitis may occur even with pure autologous reconstructions, but the frequency is lower; Zarins and Rowe[25] reported an 8% incidence of effusion. The chemical and mechanical interactions leading to synovitis are an important area for research in order to improve the results of artificial ligament reconstructions.

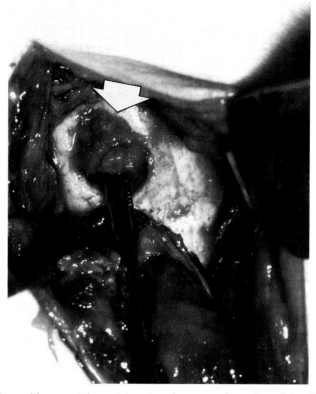

Fig. 3   *Grape-like synovial cyst (arrow) at the external opening of the tibial tunnel.*

Synovial Fistula   In a few patients, a synovial fistula may develop (Fig. 3). This is probably caused by a combination of chemical irritation and mechanical factors in the patient. Improper placement of the ligament and wide bony tunnels may lead to leakage of synovial fluid through the tunnels with the eventual development of a subcutaneous synovial cyst. In my experience, removal of the prosthesis is necessary to close the fistula. Synovial fistulas may also occur with autologous (patellar tendon) reconstructions.

Cartilage Degeneration

The clinical effects of chronic synovitis are muscle atrophy, cartilage degeneration, and sometimes, instability. Even if the ligament is not ruptured, the lower cartilage height will lead to instability. Other factors that may contribute to cartilage degeneration are overtensioning of the ligament and possibly improper placement of a strong and stiff prosthesis (overconstrained joint). Because the cartilage absorbs most of the preload and the functional loads caused by a badly placed ligament, poor placement will lead to abnormal loading of the joint.[30] Tibiofemoral loads in extension can be two to three times higher than normal with an improperly placed but well-fixed strong artificial substitute. There have been a few instances in which it seemed that high ligament loads led to fragmentation of the cartilage surface and early degeneration. The autologous reconstructions are more tolerant to improper placement because they simply stretch as necessary during the remodeling phase.

Infection

The implantation of prosthetic material always involves the risk of primary infection. Therefore, prophylactic antibiotics should be given immediately before surgery, before the tourniquet is inflated. Treatment should be continued for 24 to 48 hours after surgery, according to the surgeon's preference. Secondary infections may occur with artificial ligaments as with other prostheses. According to my studies, the frequency of infection is approximately 1%. After treatment with arthroscopic synovectomy and antibiotics, the artificial ligament is left in place, and the patient is able to maintain satisfactory knee function. Secondary infection may occur in connection with other remote infections, such as dental infections, an infected skin wound, and urinary or respiratory infection. The joint reaction (pain and swelling) usually occurs 3 to 14 days after the initiating event. The treatment consists of antibiotics after joint fluid culture, arthroscopic lavage, and synovectomy. Removal of the prosthesis is necessary if the infection recurs. The patient should be aware of the risk of this complication and advised to take antibiotics early if there is severe infection.

Instability

The aim of the reconstruction is to provide stability that will result in normal knee function. Stability is evaluated by manual tests such as the Lachman and Pivot shift tests. Objective measurement of the anteroposterior displacement of the tibia in 20 degrees of knee flexion using a laxity tester (Stryker/OSI laxity tester; KT-1000) is important. Both anterior and posterior tibial displacement at 90 N should be measured. The two values are added to obtain the total anteroposterior displacement. The total displacement of the injured minus that of the healthy knee equals the T-difference, which is an important measurement because it correlates with the manual tests and the functional end results.[17,31] Large T-differences (>3 mm) that occur early indicate an early failure.

It is difficult to set the anteroposterior displacement of the knee to normal values at surgery if a scaffold or autologous material is used. These substitutes depend on ingrowth that is supposed to increase their strength after surgery. With a true prosthesis it is easier to manipulate joint laxity by adjusting tension and placement. In these cases, the joint can be proved stable at the end of surgery. The question is how the stability should be set and if it remains unchanged after surgery. Follow-up studies of artificial ligaments have shown that immediate stability is gradually lost during the period after surgery.[17,32,33] The increase in anteroposterior displacement with time may eventually lead to subjective instability. Increased anteroposterior displacement after surgery may result in two different clinical presentations.

No Clinical Symptoms   The gradual anteroposterior displacement is usually not accompanied by any symptoms of instability until it reaches a T-difference of more than 3 mm. This level is correlated to the development of a 1+ positive pivot shift.[17]

Clinical Symptoms   Symptoms of instability usually occur when the T-difference reaches > +3 mm and when the pivot shift becomes positive. This usually happens with a failure of the prosthesis, which can occur in three different ways: by loosening, creep, or rupture.

Loosening is a failure of prosthesis fixation. A staple fixation may allow the prosthesis to slip at loads of 400 N or more.[34] This is the result of poor bone quality, improper application of the staple, or resorption of bone under the staple. A surgical technique in which the prosthesis bends over corners in the bone may also result in loosening because the bone under pressure is resorbed. The prosthesis gradually assumes a straight course between the attachments. Loosening by bone resorption occurs primarily during the first six months after surgery (Fig. 4). In some cases, high compressive loads generated by the prosthesis may cause cartilage degeneration. The diminished cartilage height will also lead to increased anteroposterior laxity.

Creep, a constant deformation of the prosthetic material, is device-dependent. Initially, some prostheses, such as Gore-Tex, undergo fiber settling, which may result in substantial elongation.[35] In other prostheses, creep occurs under a certain load at a certain number of cycles. With normal, daily ACL loads (estimated at 400 to 600 N) the typical cyclic creep is approximately 1% to 3%. Three percent elongation with a length of 14 cm between fixation points is quite substantial, and even if the tunnel-to-tunnel length is only 30 mm (the intra-articular distance) it can mean a 20% increase in anteroposterior displacement. With the Stryker/Meadox Dacron prosthesis, the annual increase in laxity was 11%.[17]

Rupture of the device represents the final event and occurs by three different mechanisms. Traumatic ruptures are the result of a significant accident with hemarthrosis, often during sports activity. This was the cause in 60% of the ruptures of the Stryker/Meadox Dacron ligament. A traumatic rupture occurs more easily if the ligament is abraded. Therefore, a combination with abrasion is common even if there is a final accident.

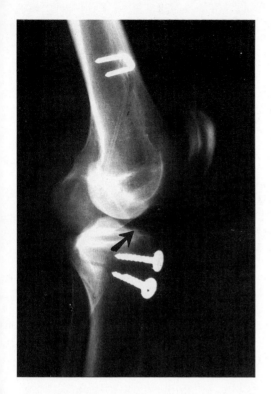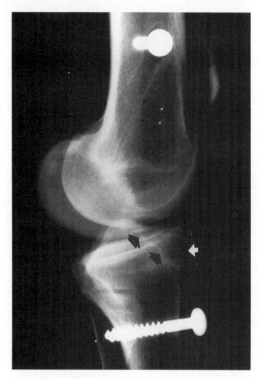

Fig. 4 *Drift of the tibial tunnel. **Left**, Initial tunnel placement too far anterior (arrow) at failure of a Dacron ligament. The ligament was replaced by a polyethylene ligament, and six months later this radiograph (**right**) was obtained because of increasing anteroposterior displacement. Note the more posterior position of the tibial tunnel (black arrows). The anterior aspect of the tibia is marked with a white arrow. At surgery the posterior drift of the posterior tunnel wall was found to be 1.5 cm.*

The second mechanism of rupture is abrasion, which will successively weaken the ligament and lead to failure, with a small overload. Abrasion is common and occurs most frequently close to the tibial surface in the intra-articular portion (Fig. 5). This results from contact between the roof of the notch and the anterior surface of the ligament with the knee in extension. Notchplasty is important but cannot compensate for a tibial tunnel that has been placed too far anteriorly. According to studies by Gillquist and Odensten,[17] placement of the tibial tunnel within the anterior third of the tibia increases the rupture rate ninefold. Another type of abrasion occurs at the femoral and the tibial tunnel openings because of increased pressure on the ligament at these points.[36] Rupture of the ligament at the femoral tunnel opening has been infrequent in my research, but may occur if the femoral tunnel deviates from the intra-articular axis of

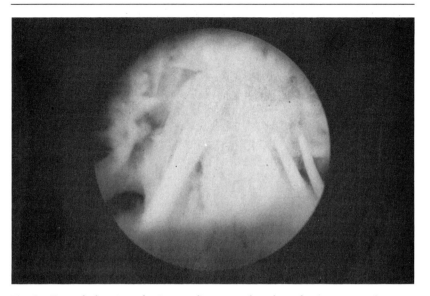

Fig. 5   *Typical abrasion of a Dacron ligament placed too far anterior in the tibia. The external Dacron sleeve is completely eroded.*

the ligament.[37] A multistrand ligament will also be subjected to internal abrasion because of internal friction between the strands of the ligament during motion.

Placement and design of the ligament are factors that can lead to abrasion, but the patient's activity level may also have an effect. Patients with a high activity level in sports may more often bring the joint into extreme positions, which leads to harmful contact between the bone and the prosthesis. Therefore, a prosthesis will survive longer in a patient with moderate physical demands.

The third mechanism of rupture is fatigue failure, a function of submaximal cyclic loading that depends on the patient's activity level. Clinical experience shows that abrasion and overload usually destroy the prosthesis before fatigue failure occurs.

Knee Motion

Effect on Sagittal Laxity   The interaction between load, anteroposterior displacement, stability, and stress relaxation of the knee needs to be investigated. The initially obtained anteroposterior displacement is obviously changed with time because of remodeling of the knee. For the clinical situation there is as yet no information available on the best preload for a certain substitute, and there is no consensus on where the best placement is.

Tibial Rotations   The effect on knee motion by an artificial ligament is important. The attachment configuration and the anatomic design of the ligament as well as its material characteristics play a role. These factors have not yet been studied.

Knee Load Patterns

Overtension in the Constrained Knee The effect of an overconstrained knee must be examined. It is not known what relation the anteroposterior displacement of the operated knee should have to normal knee motion. The general condition of the knee also plays a role. The effect of a certain preload on tibiofemoral load levels during knee motion seems to vary with the anatomic design of the knee as well as the status of the menisci and cartilage.[38]

Undertension in the Abnormally Lax Knee Low initial preload and stress relaxation lead to increased anteroposterior displacement. In a few years, anteroposterior displacement may reach the same magnitude as before surgery. Again, there is a relation between preload, ligament placement, anatomic factors, and stress relaxation of the knee.

Load Profile

The change in ligament load with knee motion is probably an important normal feature to stimulate the exchange of fluid in the cartilage surfaces. What deviations from that normal pattern that can be tolerated are not known. The load pattern, joint surface configuration, and degree of soft-tissue compensation will generally determine the extent of knee motion at certain knee positions. This is then important for the subjective feeling of stability. The absolute extent of the motion is probably less important than the extent relative to the motion of the normal knee.

Interaction With Other Structures

Other Ligaments The applied load and the change in load patterns of the knee during function affect the surrounding structures, menisci, ligaments, and cartilage. There is a compensatory function of the soft tissues that absorb the effects of improper ligament placement and abnormal loads, but the extent to which this is possible remains unknown.

Menisci The menisci are important stabilizing structures. Subjective knee function is improved and likelihood of ligament survival is increased if the menisci are intact.[25,31,39,40] The effect of ligament overtension and pathologic joint motions on the survival of the menisci is not known.

Important Factors for Artificial Ligaments

Design

Size   In order to minimize bony contact, an artificial ligament should fit the space in the intercondylar notch.

Configuration   The best design for an artificial ACL has not yet been determined. While the most common design is a single braided or rope-like structure, there have been experiments with two-bundle ligaments that imitate the anteromedial and anterolateral bundles.[41] More complex structures lead to more complex implantation techniques, and tensioning becomes a problem. In vitro experiments are needed to establish both the effect of multiple bundle ligaments and the best implantation technique before these ligaments can be tested in patients.

Material Characteristics

Biocompatibility   The prosthetic material possibly should induce tissue ingrowth but should not induce abnormal inflammatory reactions or synovitis.

Stiffness   The stiffness of the prosthesis is a complex matter. In function, the stiffness of the entire joint has to be calculated. A prosthesis that is too stiff may result in sharp changes in load levels in different joint positions. Abnormal transfer of load to the cartilage surface may eventually lead to osteoarthrosis.

Creep   Plastic deformation of the prosthesis is a negative factor that should be avoided. Creep is added to other laxity-increasing factors such as drift of the fixation, reduced cartilage height, and stretching of the secondary restraints.

Abrasion Resistance   All artificial materials used thus far in ligaments will suffer from abrasion by contact with the surrounding bone. The best solution today is to protect the ligament from bony contact. This is not always possible in extreme movements, but if the placement and diameter of the ligament are correct, abrasion can be minimized. An over-the-top placement will minimize bony contact but leads to abnormal joint mechanics.[42] The question of whether ingrowth into the surface of the ligament can protect it from abrasion has not been answered. This may diminish the problem with intraligament friction and abrasion.

Particle Formation   Abrasion leads to particle formation. The size, shape, and concentration of the particles depend on the prosthetic material, ligament placement, and patient activity. Particle formation induces a synovitis that may become symptomatic. In my experience, removal of the prosthesis leads to resolution of the symptoms.

Surgical Principles

Placement   Placement of the artificial ligament is one of the most important factors for abrasion reduction and ligament survival. Isometry is a popular concept but its importance is not known. It is quite clear that placing the tibial tunnel in the anterior half of the middle third of the tibia is desirable to avoid abrasion from the roof of the notch (Fig. 6).[17,43,44] With the same femoral position, this position will lead to more length change than anterior positioning of the tibial tunnel. It seems that the relative nonisometry is less important for ligament survival than bony contact. An anterior position on the femur relative to the normal attachment results in more failures, but it is not known whether an anatomic position is better than or inferior to an over-the-top placement. The over-the-top placement seems to be more flexible and easier to use clinically, but it leads to less control of tibial anteroposterior displacement in flexion.

Notchplasty   It is important to remove osteophytes that fill the anterior/distal opening of the femoral notch. Otherwise these osteophytes would increase the risk of abrasion. A large notchplasty may affect knee motion by moving the femoral attachment laterally. This will increase the external rotatory vector on the tibia;[42] its clinical importance is not known. Removal of the anterior part of the notch to make room for anterior placement of the tibial tunnel is advocated by some authors.[36] Even if part of the cause of abrasion is removed, its clinical effect is not known.

Orientation of Attachments   No artificial ligament can duplicate the normal ACL attachment. The attachment through drill holes is far from physiologic because the holes increase pressures on the ligament at the tunnel openings.[45] If the tunnels deviate from the long femoral axis there will also be torsion at the inner tunnel openings. A large angle between the femur tunnel and the femoral axis increases the risk of failure.[37,46] It is not possible to avoid torsion at the femoral insertion site but the situation can be improved significantly. The best approximation is to keep the angle between the tunnels and the femoral axis about 20 degrees in the frontal plane, which results in less torsion (Fig. 7). There will be bending at the femoral insertion in extension, which the ligament can tolerate better than torsion. The orientation in the frontal plane is changed with tibial rotation but the angles will not be excessive.

Tension   The best level of preload is not known. Slack in the ligament throughout the flexion range is usually avoided. Another

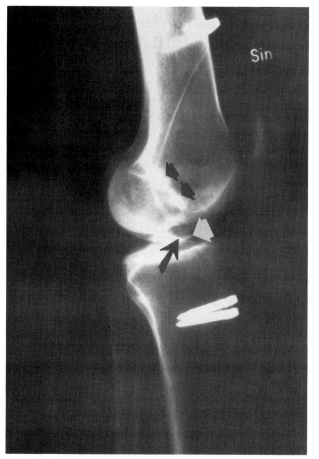

Fig. 6 *Proper placement of a Dacron ligament with an x-ray opaque marker. The roof of the notch (Blumensath's line) is marked with two black arrows. The ligament passes through the tibial surface between the black and the white arrows.*

effect of the preload is to determine the amount of sagittal displacement. The load always changes with the amount of flexion even if ideal isometry is supposed to mean no changes in length and load. Perfect isometry does not exist and is probably not desirable because it is not normal. In our series[17] there was a preload of about 40 N to restore the anteroposterior displacement of the knee to normal at 20 degrees of flexion. Because the load changes with knee flexion, ligament placement, and the condition of the knee, it is important to decide the angle of flexion at which to apply the preload.[47] The effect on the load of a change in flexion angle cannot be predicted in the individual case; the change in ligament load per degree of flexion change is different in every knee.[38] Right now it seems to be most important to ensure that the ligament is under some tension throughout the whole range of motion without reaching abnormal tension at

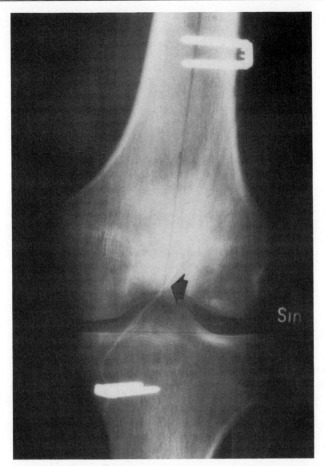

Fig. 7 *The same patient as in Figure 6, frontal view in extension. The bend in the ligament at the femoral tunnel opening (arrow) is visualized because the central beam is not along the sagittal plane of the ligament. The angle between the long axis of the femur and the femoral tunnel is 20 degrees, which is acceptable.*

full extension. The normal tension at full extension may be approximately 200 N.[48] Overtension will overconstrain the joint.[49] There are a few cases where it seems that an overconstrained joint may develop early cartilage degeneration. Another important goal may be to reestablish the normal pattern of anteroposterior displacement over the entire range of flexion; presently, this is difficult clinically.

Fixation and Preload   Fixation of the artificial ligament is important. If the normal anteroposterior displacement and preload are obtained during surgery, it is good to have the selected conditions remain over time. Therefore, a fixation that can tolerate high loads would be desirable. Even with a strong fixation, however, there is considerable change in the bone and the soft tissues of the knee with time. There is an immediate stress relaxation of the cartilage and the soft tissues when preload is applied to the ligament; therefore, the load is lost completely within a few seconds. More of the load remains after three or four cycles of tensioning, but the knee will relax, given enough time. The fixation is therefore of little importance for the persistence of the applied load and laxity over time. The importance of the fixation is to maintain the position and the intra-articular length of the ligament if the knee is subjected to abnormally high loads during rehabilitation. With a staple fixation there is always the risk that the ligament will slide if a high load is applied. In theory, the Leeds-Keio ligament seems to be more physiologic because it stimulates bony ingrowth.

Summary

A ruptured ACL with pathologic laxity may result in ruptured menisci and eventually osteoarthrosis in about 10 to 15 years.[31,50] A high activity level may accelerate degeneration so that the end result is reached in about five years. Long term follow-up must show that patients treated with surgery have better results than those treated nonsurgically. The implantation of a ligament prosthesis makes it possible to adjust the anteroposterior displacement and ligament loads to a desired level but also introduces several unknown, potentially harmful factors that need further research. An autologous reconstruction can avoid some of the problems by simply going into necrosis and adapting to the conditions. Of course, this leads to a less positive effect on the instability. Therefore, technical factors of importance for a successful ACL prosthesis may be equally applicable to the success of an autologous reconstruction.

References

1. McPherson GK, Mendenhall HV, Gibbons DF, et al: Experimental mechanical and histologic evaluation of the Kennedy ligament augmentation device. *Clin Orthop* 1985;196:186-195.
2. Yoshiya S, Andrish JT, Manley MT, et al: Augmentation of anterior cruciate ligament reconstruction in dogs with prostheses of different stiffnesses. *J Orthop Res* 1986;4:475-485.
3. McCarthy JA, Steadman JR, Dunlap J, et al: A nonparallel, nonisometric synthetic graft augmentation of a patellar tendon anterior cruciate ligament reconstruction: A model for assessment of stress shielding. *Am J Sports Med* 1990;18:43-49.
4. Mäkisalo S: *Carbon Fibers as an Alloplastic Implant*, thesis. Helsinki, Finland, University of Helsinki, 1991, pp 7-47.
5. Alm A, Gillquist J, Strömberg B: The medial third of the patellar ligament in reconstruction of the anterior cruciate ligament: A clinical and histologic study by means of arthroscopy or arthrotomy. *Acta Chir Scand Suppl* 1974;445:5-14.
6. Bosch U, Decker B, Kasperczyk W, et al: Biological aspects of long-term failure of autografts after cruciate ligament replacement. *Arch Orthop Trauma Surg* 1989;108:368-372.

7. Bosch U, Kasperczyk W: Healing of patellar tendon autograft after PCL reconstruction: A process of ligamentization? A biomechanical and histological study in a sheep model. *Am J Sports Med*, in press.

8. Good L, Odensten M, Pettersson L, et al: Failure of a bovine xenograft for reconstruction of the anterior cruciate ligament. *Acta Orthop Scand* 1989;60:8-12.

9. Bray RC, Flanagan JP, Dandy DJ: Reconstruction for chronic anterior cruciate instability: A comparison of two methods after six years. *J Bone Joint Surg* 1988;70B:100-105.

10. Rushton N, Dandy DJ, Naylor CPE: The clinical, arthroscopic and histological findings after replacement of the anterior cruciate ligament with carbon-fibre. *J Bone Joint Surg* 1983;65B:308-309.

11. Seedhom BB: The Leeds Keio ligament: Concepts and mechanical aspects of the device, abstract, in *Advances in Cruciate Ligament Reconstruction of the Knee: Autogenous vs Prosthetic*. Los Angeles, CA, Southern California Orthopedic Research and Education Center, 1990, pp 117-126.

12. Laboureau JP, Cazenave A: Presentation of the Ligastic ligament, in *Advances in Cruciate Ligament Reconstruction of the Knee: Autogenous vs Prosthetic*. Los Angeles, CA, Southern California Orthopedic Research and Education Center, 1990, pp 156-166.

13. Arnoczky SP, Warren RF, Minei JP: Replacement of the anterior cruciate ligament using a synthetic prosthesis: An evaluation of graft biology in the dog. *Am J Sports Med* 1986;14:1-6.

14. Bolton CW, Bruchman WC: The GORE-TEX expanded polytetrafluoroethylene prosthetic ligament: An in vitro and in vivo evaluation. *Clin Orthop* 1985;196:202-213.

15. McLeod W: Biomechanics of the Richards Prosthetic anterior cruciate ligament, abstract, in *Advances in Cruciate Ligament Reconstruction of the Knee: Autogenous vs Prosthetic*. Los Angeles, CA, Southern California Orthopedic Research and Education Center, 1990, p 155.

16. Andersson C, Gillquist J: Conservative treatment of acute ruptures of the anterior cruciate ligament: A prospective study with a long-term follow-up period. *Clin Orthop*, in press.

17. Gillquist J, Odensten M: Reconstruction of old anterior cruciate ligament tears with a dacron prosthesis: A prospective study. *Am J Sports Med*, in press.

18. Lukianov AV, Richmond JC, Barrett GR, et al: A multicenter study on the results of anterior cruciate ligament reconstruction using a Dacron ligament prosthesis in "salvage" cases. *Am J Sports Med* 1989;17:380-386.

19. López-Vázquez E, Juan JA, Vila E, et al: Reconstruction of the anterior cruciate ligament with a Dacron prosthesis. *J Bone Joint Surg* 1991;73A:1294-1300.

20. Ahlfeld SK, Larson RL, Collins HR: Anterior cruciate reconstruction in the chronically unstable knee using an expanded polytetrafluoro-ethylene (PTFE) prosthetic ligament. *Am J Sports Med* 1987;15:326-330.

21. Collins HR: Anterior cruciate ligament reconstruction using Gore Tex, abstract, in *Advances in Cruciate Ligament Reconstruction of the Knee: Autogenous vs Prosthetic*. Los Angeles, CA, Southern California Orthopedic Research and Education Center, 1990, pp 149-153.

22. Indelicato PA, Pascale MS, Huegel MO: Early experience with the GORE-TEX polytetrafluoroethylene anterior cruciate ligament prosthesis. *Am J Sports Med* 1989;17:55-62.

23. Noyes FR, Barber SD, Mangine RE: Bone-patellar ligament-bone and fascia lata allografts for reconstruction of the anterior cruciate ligament. *J Bone Joint Surg* 1990;72A:1125-1136.

24. Johnson RJ, Eriksson E, Haggmark T, et al: Five- to ten-year follow-up evaluation after reconstruction of the anterior cruciate ligament. *Clin Orthop* 1984;183:122-140.

25. Zarins B, Rowe CR: Combined anterior cruciate-ligament reconstruction using semitendinosus tendon and iliotibial tract. *J Bone Joint Surg* 1986;68A:160-177.

26. Mäkisalo SE, Paavolainen PP, Lehto M, et al: Collagen types I and III and fibronectin in healing anterior cruciate ligament after reconstruction with carbon fibre. *Injury* 1989;20:72-76.

27. Mendes DG, Angel D, Grishkan A, et al: Histological response to carbon fibre. *J Bone Joint Surg* 1985;67B:645-649.

28. Mäkisalo SE, Paavolainen P, Grönblad M, et al: Tissue reactions around two alloplastic ligament substitute materials: Experimental study on rats with carbon fibres and polypropylene. *Biomaterials* 1989;10:105-108.

29. Rodosky MW, Fu FH: Induction of synovial inflammation by matrix molecules, implant particles, and chemical agents, in Leadbetter WB, Buckwalter JA, Gordon SL (eds): *Sports-Induced Inflammation*. Park Ridge, IL, American Academy of Orthopaedic Surgeons, 1990, pp 357-381.

30. Schabus R, Fuchs M, Kwasny O: The effect of ACL-graft preload on the static pressure distribution in the knee joint. *Trans Orthop Res Soc* 1989;14:517.

31. Sommerlath K, Lysholm J, Gillquist J: The long-term course after treatment of acute anterior cruciate ligament ruptures: A 9 to 16 year follow-up. *Am J Sports Med* 1991;19:156-162.

32. Markolf KL, Patee G, Strum G, et al: Instrumented laxity measurements of patients receiving a Gore-Tex ACL substitute. *Trans Orthop Res Soc* 1988;13:132.

33. Stonebrook SN, Berman AB, Bruchman WC, et al: Functional biomechanics of the Gore-Tex cruciate-ligament prosthesis: Effects of implant tensioning, in Friedman MJ, Ferkel RD (eds): *Prosthetic Ligament Reconstruction of the Knee*. Philadelphia, WB Saunders, 1988, pp 140-148.

34. Good L, Tarlow SD, Odensten M, et al: Load tolerance, security, and failure modes of fixation devices for synthetic knee ligaments. *Clin Orthop* 1990;253:190-196.

35. More RC, Markolf KL: Measurement of stability of the knee and ligament force after implantation of a synthetic anterior cruciate ligament: In vitro measurement. *J Bone Joint Surg* 1988;70A:1020-1031.

36. Howell SM, Clark JA, Farley TE: A rationale for predicting anterior cruciate graft impingement by the intercondylar roof: A magnetic resonance imaging study. *Am J Sports Med* 1991;19:276-282.

37. Yosida S, Kurosaka M, Yamada M, et al: Optimal orientation of the bone tunnels in the anterior cruciate ligament reconstruction. *Trans Orthop Res Soc* 1991;16:602.

38. Gillquist J, Good L: Loads in artificial ACL substitutes during passive knee motion in vivo. *Clin Orthop*, in press.

39. Lysholm J, Gillquist J, Liljedahl SO: Arthroscopy in the early diagnosis of injuries to the knee joint: *Acta Orthop Scand* 1981;52:111-118.

40. Oretorp N, Gillquist J, Liljedahl SO: Long term results of surgery for non-acute anteromedial rotatory instability of the knee. *Acta Orthop Scand* 1979;50:329-336.

41. Veltri D, Fulkerson J: Isometricity of Y-graft replacement of the anterior cruciate ligament. *Trans Orthop Res Soc* 1989;14:518.

42. Good L, Askew MJ, Boom A, et al: An in vitro comparison between the normal knee and two techniques for reconstruction of the anterior cruciate ligament, using computerized analysis of knee kinematics. *Clin Biomech*, in press.

43. Clark JA, Howell SM: Tibial tunnel placement in isometric anterior cruciate ligament reconstruction and its role in producing graft impingement. American Academy of Orthopaedic Surgeons, abstracts, Park Ridge, IL, 1990, vol 57, p 86.

44. Norwood LA Jr, Cross MJ: The intercondylar shelf and the anterior cruciate ligament. *Am J Sports Med* 1977;5:171-176.

45. Sidles JA, Clark JM, Huber JD: Large internal pressures occur in ligament grafts at bone tunnels. *Trans Orthop Res Soc* 1990;15:81.

46. Gely P, Drouin G, Thiry PS, et al: Torsion and bending imposed on a new anterior cruciate ligament prosthesis during knee flexion: An evaluation method. *J Biomech Eng* 1984;106:285-294.

47. Bylski-Austrow DI, Grood ES, Hefzy MS, et al: Anterior cruciate ligament replacements: A mechanical study of femoral attachment location, flexion angle at tensioning, and initial tension. *J Orthop Res* 1990;8:522-531.

48. Markolf KL, Gorek JF, Kabo JM, et al: Direct measurement of resultant forces in the anterior cruciate ligament: An *in vitro* study performed with a new experimental technique. *J Bone Joint Surg* 1990;72A:557-567.

49. Amis AA: Anterior cruciate ligament replacement: Knee stability and the effects of implants. *J Bone Joint Surg* 1989;71B:819-824.

50. Jacobsen K: Osteoarthrosis following insufficiency of the cruciate ligaments in man. *Acta Orthop Scand* 1977;48:520-526.

Chapter 28

Evaluation of Treatment Results

Dale M. Daniel, MD
Allen F. Anderson, MD

Introduction

Disruption of a knee ligament alters the normal joint kinematics and mechanics. This may result in joint subluxation with symptoms of giving way and repeated joint injury. Over time the pathomechanics and repeated injuries may result in joint arthrosis. The short-term goal of treatment is to return the patient to preinjury activities without impairment or increased risk of additional injuries. The longer-term goal is to diminish the incidence of postinjury arthritis, which eventually may reduce the patient's ability to take part in recreational activities, work, or activities of daily living. Systems are needed that can be used to compare the abilities of different treatment methods to meet these goals.

Published Knee Evaluation Systems

Knee evaluation systems have been designed to document patient activity, symptoms and impairments, joint instability, and joint arthrosis. During the last decade, treatment of an anterior cruciate ligament (ACL) injury and the results thereof were reported in 52 articles in the *Journal of Bone and Joint Surgery* (American volume) or the *American Journal of Sports Medicine*. The results were determined according to 38 different rating scales. The variability of the patient populations and of the knee rating scales makes it difficult to compare the relative effectiveness of the many treatment programs that were reported.

Knee evaluation systems have been evolving over the past 40 years. O'Donoghue[1] used clinical findings and a subjective rating scale to evaluate the results of knee ligament repairs. In his experience there was not a consistent correlation between the subjective assessment and the objective evaluation.[2,3] Slocum recognized the value of comparing preoperative and postoperative evaluations;[4,5]

Hughston advocated quantification of joint laxity in millimeters;[6] and Larson added functional tests to the evaluation.[7]

The Hospital for Special Surgery Knee Score (HSSKS), the first comprehensive method designed specifically for evaluating knee ligament injuries, was used most frequently during the past decade.[8] This scale included subjective evaluation of symptoms and function, objective tests of function, and clinical examination. Objective stability evaluation was accorded 40% of the total score. The Lysholm scale,[9] which was the second most commonly used, was based on symptoms of instability. Feagin and Blake[10] emphasized that a single number evaluation (total score) lacks discrimination and recommended using individual scores for subjective symptoms, subjective function, and objective stability testing. Windsor and associates[11] revised the HSSKS to include current concepts in documenting ligament laxity and functional testing. Function of the ACL was the predominant component of this scale. The Noyes rating system is the most comprehensive.[12] This rating system was developed for assessing return to sports, recognizing the importance of identifying the functional level, intensity level, and frequency of participation. The Noyes system uses a point scale to evaluate patients who are operated on for chronic ligament deficiency and categories of excellent, good, fair, and poor for patients who are operated on for acute ligament tears. The Zarins scale was equally divided into symptoms and impairments and objective examination.[13]

Anderson performed a prospective study to compare and determine the differences in the six rating scales that were most commonly used during the last decade. These scales were used to evaluate 70 patients a minimum of five years after ACL reconstructive surgery. The surgical procedure consisted of an intra-articular semitendinosus and gracilis ACL reconstruction and a Losee extra-articular reconstruction.

Comparison of the six rating scales is difficult. The scales have different categories, and the components of these categories vary as does the relative weight accorded the components (Table 1). Another factor that complicates comparison is that the definition of a component in one scale may be distinctly different from that in another scale. For example, swelling was considered a subjective symptom in five scales, but an objective measurement in the HSSKS. Still another type of discrepancy in the scales relates to differences in the numerical values. For purposes of comparison, the total number of points for the HSSKS (50), Feagin/Blake (15), and Noyes (450) were adjusted to yield comparable totals of 100. The results of evaluating the 70 patients and the length of time taken to administer the evaluations are presented in Table 2. The correlation coefficients between the different scales are given in Table 3. The total scores may not be important in the context of a rating scale that uses a classification system to categorize results. Four of the scales describe a classification system that depends on fulfillment of

Table 1 Components of rating scales with weighting points for each

Component of Scale	Scale					
	HSSKS (MR)	Revised HSSKS (WI)	Feagin/ Blake (FB)	Noyes Profile (NY)	Lysholm (LY)	Zarins (ZR)
Subjective						
Symptom						
1. Pain	1		1	40	30	10
2. Swelling	1	2	1	20	10	8
3. Clicking	1					
4. Giving way-Instability	4	20	2	40	30	10
5. Locking		3				
6. Stiffness			1			4
7. Limp					5	
8. Support (needs crutch)					5	
Function						
9. Stair difficulty	1			*	10	
10. Walking				*		
11. Running				**		
13. Return to work	3	4		0		
14. Sports-Athletics		4	5	100		10
15. Ability to decelerate		4		**		
16. Cut/cutting		4				
18. Jump		4		**		
19. Ability to pivot				**		8
20. Squatting/Kneeling	2			*	5	
22. Composite activities of daily living*				50		
23. Composite problems with sports**				100		
Objective						
Indicator						
24. Tender	1					
25. Effusion	1	4		14.3		
26. Swelling	1					
27. Crepitation	1					
28. Power-Muscle strength	3			14.3		
29. Thigh size-Atrophy	2	2			5	
30. Range of motion (ROM)	3	3				5
31. Patellofemoral				14.3		
32. Medial tibial				14.3		
33. Lateral tibial				14.3		
34. Alignment				14.3		
Function						
35. Duck walk		2				
36. Run in place		1				
37. Jump on 1 leg		2				
38. Forward jump (hop) % diff		10				
Stability						
39. Lachman (ACL+PCL)	5	4	#	#		15
40. Anterior drawer (ACL)		2	#			
41. Posterior drawer (PCL+)	5	5		#		
42. Pivot shift (PS) (ACL+)		10	#	#		20
43. Reverse PS (PCL+)		5		#		
44. Valgus (MCL)	5	5		#		5
45. Varus (LCL)	5	5		#		5
46. Composite Stability#		5	14.3			
Total	50	100	15	450	100	100

Table 2 Statistics of rating scales for evaluation of 70 patients with reconstructed ACL

| | Score | | | | | |
	Mean	Median	Standard Deviation	Minimum Value	Maximum Value	Time to Administer
Lysholm	93.04	95	8.87	58	100	4
Zarins	90.31	91.5	8.04	60	99	9
Feagin-Blake	89.44	93	10.64	53	100	8
Noyes	85.86	87.5	10.61	50	98	17*
HSSKS	82.49	84	10.10	42	96	14
Revised HSSKS	81.67	84	10.36	33	95	15

*No CYBEX

certain outcome criteria. The mean total score for the 70 patients was classified as "good" according to the criteria of the HSSKS, revised HSSKS, Noyes profile, and Lysholm scales, although significant differences exist in the patient rankings (Table 4).

If the scales were equally sensitive and specific, each lowest decile would include the same 10% with the poorest knee function; however, this is not the case. Fourteen of the 70 patients fall into the lowest decile on at least one scale. Of these 14, only three fall into the lowest decile on all scales, while five were classified in the lowest decile by only one scale.

Evaluation of patient scores, rankings, scattergrams, and the lowest decile of patients demonstrated that the differences in the scales are sufficiently great to preclude predicting individual results from one scale based on another.

International Knee Documentation Committee

In an effort to develop a standardized examination system, the International Knee Documentation Committee (IKDC) was formed in 1987 under the auspices of the European Society for Knee Surgery and Arthroscopy (ESKA) and the American Orthopaedic Society for Sports Medicine (AOSSM). The committee reviewed basic terminology[14] and identified a core of observations and measurements that describe the patient population and document the patients' symptoms, impairments, and joint instability. The list is intentionally short so it may be used as part of a routine office evaluation program. Research protocols are expected to add items to the list. The evaluation form is presented in Figure 1. Each component of the evaluation system will be discussed below. To date, a point system has not been developed for the IKDC form.

Patient Population

A cohort is a designated group of patients[15] who are selected from a specific population. Criteria are established to define who will be admitted into a study. Admission criteria consist of eligibility criteria, which give the conditions required for participation in the study,

Future Directions

Develop methods to document knee instability, joint kinematics, joint function, and patient impairment related to knee dysfunction.

The outcome of the ligament-injured knee with or without treatment is incompletely documented. There is a need to develop measures of knee stability and function as well as patient impairment that can be used in clinical studies. In particular, there is a need for instruments and techniques to measure compartment motion during passive testing and for techniques to measure joint subluxation during physiologic activities. There is also a need to develop a universally acceptable outcome evaluation system.

Perform prospective controlled outcome studies with follow-ups of five, ten, or more years to document the history of a knee ligament injury with and without surgical treatment.

Few controlled studies have been reported that document the results of surgical and nonsurgical treatment of a knee ligament injury. Studies should be prospective, include control groups, and be randomized if possible. Issues to be studied for nonsurgical treatment include activity modification, braces, and rehabilitation techniques. Issues to be studied for surgical treatment include timing of surgery; graft source (autograft, allograft, prosthetic); graft placement, tensioning, and fixation; and postoperative rehabilitation programs.

Define the relationship between instability, patient impairment, and joint deterioration.

Research should be done to identify what level of instability is compatible with good limb function and avoidance of joint arthrosis in surgically and nonsurgically treated patients.

Determine the biology of graft remodeling in the human knee.

The patient's postoperative rehabilitation program and scheduled return to work and sports after ligament surgery is based on our perception of the structural and mechanical properties of the implanted graft over time. The biology and biomechanics of implanted grafts (autograft, allograft, and prosthetic grafts) should be determined by imaging methods, percutaneous biopsies, and harvest of graft material in total knee replacement surgery or in deceased subjects.

Measure in vivo ligament forces during physiologic activity.

The inability to protect the graft from destructive loads during the rehabilitation period may be a cause of graft failure. Knowledge of the in-vivo ligament forces and strains during activity is needed for the development of rehabilitation programs that optimize patient function and are not deleterious to the healing/remodeling ligament.

585

Evaluate allograft procurement, sterilization, and use in ligament surgery.

Allograft surgery avoids the morbidity of graft harvest. Documentation of the risks, benefits, and cost effectiveness of allograft ligament surgery compared to those of other options needs to be established. The effect of sterilization techniques on disease transmission and on the mechanical and biologic properties of the graft should be evaluated.

Index